**Please Note:** Since the publication of this text, the Joint Commission on Accreditation of Healthcare Organizations (JCAHO) has changed its name to The Joint Commission (TJC).

## The Joint Commission (TJC) Prohibited Abbreviations and Notations

| Abbreviation | Write |
|---|---|
| U, u | unit |
| IU | International Unit |
| Q.D. | daily |
| Q.O.D. | every other day |
| Trailing zero (X.0 mg)* | Delete the trailing zero (X) |
| Lack of leading zero (.X mg) | Insert a leading zero (0.X) |
| MS $MSO_4$ | morphine sulfate |
| $MgSO_4$ | magnesium sulfate |

## Institute for Safe Medication Practices (ISMP) Dangerous Abbreviations and Notations

| Abbreviation | Write | Abbreviation | Write |
|---|---|---|---|
| A.D., A.S., A.U. | right ear, left ear, both ears | $\times$ 3d | for 3 days |
| O.D., O.S., O.U. | right eye, left eye, both eyes | S.C., S.Q., sub q | subcut or subcutaneously |
| B.T. | bedtime | ss | one half' |
| Cc | mL for milliliters | SSI | sliding scale (insulin) |
| H.S. | bedtime | $\mu$g | mcg |
| q.h.s. | nightly | > | greater than |
| q6 PM, etc | 6 PM every night (or daily) | < | less than |
| q.i.d. | 4 times a day | + | plus, or and |
| q.n. | nightly | @ | at |

Please note: This is a partial list. For a more complete list, refer to www.ISMP.org.

# JOYCE M. MULHOLLAND, APRN, B.C.

Adult Nurse Practitioner, Tucson, Arizona
Nursing Education Consultant, Tucson, Arizona
M.S. California State University, Long Beach, California
M.A. Arizona State University, Tempe, Arizona
B.S. Fairleigh Dickinson College, Rutherford, New Jersey

# The Nurse, The Math, The Meds

## DRUG CALCULATIONS USING DIMENSIONAL ANALYSIS

5 mcg/kg/min

120 mL/hr

Ordered

MOSBY
ELSEVIER

11830 Westline Industrial Drive
St. Louis, Missouri 63146

THE NURSE, THE MATH, THE MEDS: DRUG CALCULATIONS USING DIMENSIONAL ANALYSIS

ISBN-13: 978-0-323-03031-1
ISBN-10: 0-323-03031-9

**Copyright © 2007 by Mosby, Inc., an affiliate of Elsevier Inc.**

ISBN-13: 978-0-323-03031-1
ISBN-10: 0-323-03031-9

*Senior Editor:* Yvonne Alexopoulos
*Senior Developmental Editor:* Danielle Frazier
*Publishing Services Manager:* Peggy Fagen
*Design Direction:* Amy Buxton

Printed in Canada

Last digit is the print number: 9 8 7 6 5 4 3

# CONTENT AND MATH REVIEWERS

**Jeanette M. Anderson,** RN, BSN, MSN
Owner
JMA Nursing Consultant
Associate Professor of Nursing,
    Emeritus
Tarrant County College
Fort Worth, Texas

**Lou Ann Boose,** RN, BSN, MSN
Associate Professor
Department of Nursing
Harrisburg Area Community College
Harrisburg, Pennsylvania

**Linda Fluharty,** BSN, MSN
Associate Professor
Ivy Tech Community College
Staff Nurse
Clarian Hospitals
Indianapolis, Indiana

**Deborah L. Freyman,** RN, MA, MSN
Faculty
Department of Nursing
National Park Community College
Hot Springs, Arkansas

**Janis E. Grimland,** RN, BSN
Program Director
Clifton Vocational Nursing Program
Hill College
Clifton, Texas

**Paula D. Hopper,** MSN, RN
Professor
Department of Nursing
Jackson Community College
Jackson, Mississippi

**Cordia A. Starling,** RN, BSN, MS, EdD
Professor and Division Chair
Division of Nursing
Dalton State College
Dalton, Georgia

**Ann B. Tritak,** RN, EdD, MA, BS
Associate Professor
Farleigh Dickinson University
Henry P. Becton School of Nursing
    and Allied Health
Teaneck, New Jersey

**Jo A. Voss,** RN, PhD, CNS
Assistant Professor
South Dakota State University
College of Nursing
Rapid City, South Dakota

# TO THE INSTRUCTOR

This first edition is designed for classroom and independent use by students at all levels in full-time, part-time, and accelerated nursing courses, as well as a refresher for nurses and physician assistant students.

Because the course is brief, only one method of calculation—dimensional analysis—is presented, in order to permit adequate time for mastery. There are entire texts devoted to other methods. Dimensional analysis was selected because the method is known by many students who have taken science courses. It is simple and offers superior insight into the proper setup of problems, a most challenging area for many students.

Chapter 1 is a general math review. Chapter 2 is a separate introductory chapter on dimensional analysis based on practical everyday problems. These two chapters form a base that is repeated and reinforced throughout the rest of the text. When a student has only 3 to 8 weeks to master medication calculations, repetition becomes very important.

It is strongly recommended that students complete and demonstrate mastery of Chapters 1 and 2 by the beginning of the second class session. A random-question 20-point test covering these two chapters combined is offered for convenience in the Instructor Manual following separate quizzes on math and dimensional analysis.

Use of a calculator is discouraged until the student has completed several chapters. Some familiarity with the calculator is useful, and calculators are frequently employed in the clinical setting. But dependence on the calculator should be avoided until the student has a firm grasp of the logic of medication calculations. Also, the student must not be helpless at those times when a calculator is not available.

Emphasis is placed on reading the problem for identification of the desired answer, estimation of a reasonable answer, and evaluation of the solution in terms of the equation setup and the estimate. This critical thinking approach will serve the user well as a habit for all courses. Brief quizzes are included consisting of five questions, which can be completed in approximately 5 to 30 minutes. Worked-out answers are provided.

A word about multiple-choice questions: Approximately 98 out of 100 questions in the current NCLEX examination are in multiple-choice format. The instructor has the option of requiring that students show all calculations. Guessing an answer is not recommended. The multiple-choice format itself is also beneficial as an adjunctive learning tool because it teaches the student to analyze potential answers and to eliminate those that are wrong. This reinforces understanding.

Medication calculation does not occur in a vacuum. Administering medications safely requires integration of a great deal of theory derived from many courses as well as clinical experience. Anecdotes, based on my own experience as well as that of colleagues, pharmacists, reviewers, and current journals, are included to expand the concept of the role of the medication administrator. Students without clinical experience particularly appreciate these anecdotes.

## Instructional Design Features

- Selected **essential vocabulary** relevant to chapter contents is provided for convenient reference at the beginning of each chapter.
- Selected **mnemonics** are supplied to facilitate memorization. These memory shortcuts conserve learning time.
- A **red arrow alert** included throughout calls attention to critical math and patient safety theory as well as to issues related to practice.
- **FAQ and Answers** included in each chapter are derived from years of medication and math-related classroom questions compiled by the author. These break up text, add to comprehension, and provide needed additional knowledge. FAQs enjoy high readership and are of particular benefit to students who are studying outside a classroom environment.
- **Ask Yourself questions** within each chapter are based on content previously covered in the chapter to help students synthesize and reinforce comprehension of content.
- **Communication boxes** display sample nurse-patient or nurse-prescriber dialogues that help reduce medication errors. This increases motivation and interest in learning by relating the math to the medications and to clinical application.
- **Cultural boxes** describe selected math notation and medication-related cultural practices.
- **Clinical Relevance boxes** in each chapter offer additional information for integration of medication-related clinical practice concepts such as nursing practice, legal aspects, high-risk drugs, and common errors.

## Ancillaries

*Instructor's Resource Manual for The Nurse, The Math, The Meds: Drug Calculations Using Dimensional Analysis, First Edition* is available to enhance student instruction. This printed resource corresponds with the main book and includes:

- Suggested Teaching Strategies
- Test Bank with over 175 questions

This resource is also available online on the Evolve site at: ***http://evolve. elsevier.com/Mulholland/themath/***

**Romans & Daugherty Dosages and Solutions CTB, Version II** is a generic computerized test bank that has been completely updated and is provided as a gratis item to instructors upon adoption of this book. It contains over 700 questions on general math, converting within systems of measurement, oral dosages, parenteral dosages, flow rates, pediatric dosages, intravenous calculations, and more. This CTB is available online on the Evolve site at: http://evolve.elsevier.com/Mulholland/themath/

*Dimensional Analysis Companion CD for The Nurse, The Math, The Meds* is an interactive student tutorial that includes an extensive menu of various topic areas within drug calculations such as oral, parenteral, pediatric, and intravenous calculations, to name a few. It includes interactive exercises where students can fill in syringes to answer problems. Covering the dimensional analysis method, this CD contains over 500 practice problems, including a comprehensive post-test.

# TO THE STUDENT

*The Nurse, The Math, The Meds: Drug Calculations Using Dimensional Analysis, First Edition* has been designed not only to teach you what you need to know but also to save you valuable time. Here are a few time-tested tips:

- It will be to your great advantage to take an hour or two to review and master Chapters 1 and 2. They contain all the math and concepts of dimensional analysis you will need.
- Set aside at least three study periods for each chapter; the first shortly after the initial presentation and the last shortly before the next class session or quiz. Working with a focused study buddy may be very helpful. Working a practice problem or two each day will improve your retention.
- Take the time to review Essential Vocabulary provided at the beginning of each chapter.
- Try to complete a topic and quiz in one sitting. Most of the quizzes within the chapters contain only five questions and can usually be completed within 30 minutes.
- If you have the opportunity, visit a laboratory setting on campus to view and handle the equipment that is mentioned in the chapters, such as syringes, calibrated medicine cups, and intravenous devices. The label on a bottle of aspirin would be very useful to have on hand for the topic of metric measurements and labels when it arises. Fifteen minutes spent studying medication labels in the over-the-counter drug section of a pharmacy will greatly help to clarify information needed about medication labels and drug measurements.
- Don't use your calculator until you get to the final chapters. The methods of solving the problems need to be fully understood before you try to use a calculator. You also need an independent method of calculation to verify answers. The discipline of writing out equations and solutions will make you competent quickly and help you avoid errors. This is a critical safety issue. Indeed, there will be times when no calculator is available.
- As you proceed through the text, some useful math operation shortcuts will occur to you. They have their place, but only after you are sure you understand what you are doing.
- Write numbers as neatly as you can, using the metric notation guidelines. Sloppy writing of numbers, decimals, and commas contributes to major errors.
- Be sure to review and refresh your memory after holidays and long breaks as well as before entering new clinical areas. And remember, think metric!

This text also offers key features to enhance your learning experience. Take a look at the following features so that you may familiarize yourself with this text and maximize its value:

**ix**

**FAQ and Answers** included in each chapter are derived from years of medication and math-related classroom questions compiled by the author. They break up text, add to comprehension, and provide needed additional knowledge.

---

**FAQ** | *What is the quickest way to learn selection of syringe and needle sizes?*

**ANSWER:** There is no substitute for supervised and, later, independent experience, but learning can be greatly expedited. Assuming that you have learned to identify syringe capacities and calibration amounts (covered in Chapter 6), focus on a commonly used syringe size for each route and an approximate needle size and amount for an *average-sized adult*. Try to learn syringe and needle size selection in sequential order from the intradermal to intramuscular or vice versa (Table 8-1). Then, in the clinical setting, modifications and the selection of needles and the appropriate angle of injection for specific-sized patients can be added to the body of knowledge.

---

1   What does U 100 on the label of the insulin vial mean?

_____

2   What is the most common adverse effect of insulin therapy?

_____

Q: *Ask Yourself*

A: *My Answer*

**Ask Yourself questions** within each chapter are based on content previously covered in the chapter to help you synthesize and reinforce comprehension of content.

---

▲ **Cultural Note**

In some countries, such as the United States, a comma is used to separate groups of three numbers within large numbers, as in 20,000. In other countries, a *space is* used. Thus, 25,000 or 25 000 might be seen. In the past, the British used a comma to designate a *decimal point* between a whole number and a fraction: 5,5 would be read as 5.5. ("5 point 5" or "5 and 5 tenths"). This type of notation can still be seen in scientific math.

**Cultural boxes** describe selected math notation and medication-related cultural practices.

---

**Clinical Relevance**

There is an automatic expiration date on narcotics and medications that have the potential for dependence or abuse or that are ineffective if given beyond a specified period. Check agency policy. It is usually 48-72 hours for controlled substances. In order to continue the medications, the order must be renewed in a timely manner so that the medication schedule proceeds without interruption.

**Clinical Relevance boxes** in each chapter offer additional information for integration of medication-related clinical practice concepts such as nursing practice, legal aspects, high-risk drugs, and common errors.

*Dimensional Analysis Companion CD for The Nurse, The Math, The Meds* is an interactive student tutorial that includes an extensive menu of various topic areas within drug calculations such as oral, parenteral, pediatric, and intravenous calculations, to name a few. It includes interactive exercises where students can fill in syringes to answer problems. Covering the dimensional analysis method, this CD contains over 500 practice problems including a comprehensive post-test. See sample screen shots below:

Here is an outline of the table of contents for the *Dimensional Analysis Companion CD for The Nurse, The Math, The Meds*

Look for this icon at the end of the chapters. It will refer you to the *Dimensional Analysis Companion CD for The Nurse, The Math, The Meds* for additional practice problems and content information.

Best wishes. You've chosen a great profession!
**Joyce M. Mulholland**

# ACKNOWLEDGMENTS

A first edition is a challenge for reviewers and editors as well as for the author. I am very grateful to all those who gave suggestions for inclusions and revisions. Each suggestion was given serious consideration.

A special thanks to Martha Mulholland, Penny Lutsi, and Janet Corey for many hours of assistance and support with formatting, editing, and/or proofing. Also thank you to Arlene Copley, RN, Diabetic Educator; Shirley Lesure, RN, Nurse Educator; Shari Robinson, RN, MS, Nurse Faculty; Barbara Robinson, CCRN; Pharm D's Brad Peters, Ching Lum Clum, and Amy Kopfer, who answered questions about medication practices at their respective agencies; and Sandra Dinwiddie, nursing student, who assisted with answer keys. Yvonne Alexopoulos, Danielle Frazier, and Peggy Fagen, nursing editors at Elsevier, have been incredibly patient and supportive through several draft revisions.

# CONTENTS IN BRIEF

# DETAILED TABLE OF CONTENTS

## Part II  Modern Metric System and Medication Calculations 77

## Part III  Reconstituted Medications *195*

## Part IV  Parenteral Medication Calculations *253*

# PART I
## ESSENTIAL MATH REVIEW
## FOR MEDICATION CALCULATIONS

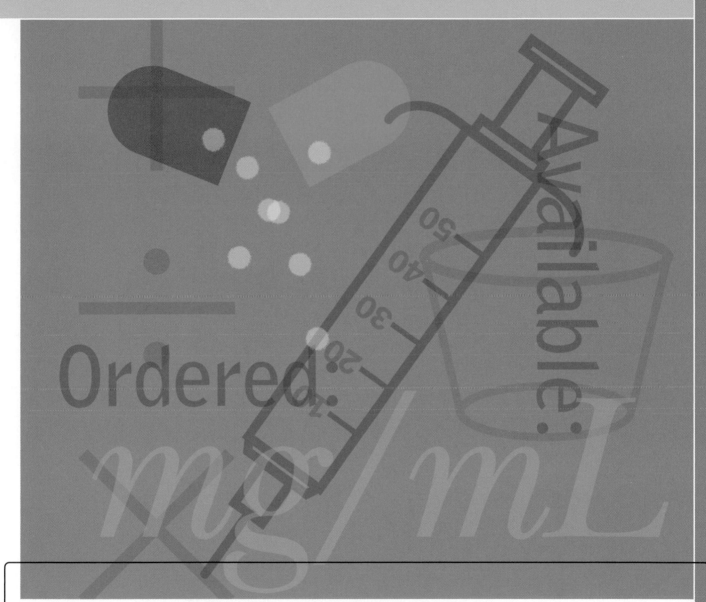

# ESSENTIAL MATH SELF-ASSESSMENT

**Estimated Completion Time: 20 to 30 Minutes**

## Introduction

Time spent mastering any unfamiliar material in this basic review will be time very well spent. To increase your speed, this material is organized in a specific sequence, building on prior questions.

The basic mathematics in this review chapter is critical to subsequent medication calculations. Chapter 1 provides an essential math review for further study. Be able to define all the terms and do all of the operations in Chapter 1 with ease before proceeding to Chapter 2 or other chapters.

**Directions:** Answer all of the questions using paper and pencil when necessary. Circle the problems that may need review. After you are finished, check your answers on p. 499. Review Chapter 1 for the areas needing further study.

A calculator is not necessary for most medicine calculations. However, mental calculations and occasional quick use of pencil and paper are necessary for most medicine calculations. A calculator will be helpful later with more complex medication problems. Remember, you have to understand the math well enough to know how to enter it into the calculator and to be able to function when the batteries cease to function.

## Symbols (explanation on p. 6)

*Write out the meaning of the following symbols:*

1 $>$ _____

2 $<$ _____

3 $\geq$ _____

4 $\leq$ _____

5 Fill in the appropriate symbol: Take two aspirin if your fever is _____ (greater than or equal to) 100 degrees F.

## Whole Numbers (explanation on p. 7)

6 Write the whole number as a fraction without changing the value: 300 _____

7 Write the whole number *425* with a decimal point in the implied decimal place for whole numbers. _____

8 Edit the whole number to avoid misinterpretation: 434.000 _____

9 Use the whole number 256 to write a fraction that equals the number one (1). _____

## Roman Numerals (explanation on p. 9)

10 Write the Arabic numeral 5 as a Roman numeral: _____

11 Write the Roman numeral X as an Arabic numeral: _____

# Products, Factors, Multiples, Multipliers, Common Factors (explanation on pp. 10-13)

**12** Write the *product* of 10 and 9. _____

**13** Write 5 *factors* of the number 16. _____

**14** Write the *common factors* of the numbers 10 and 20. _____

**15** Write the first 3 *multiples* of the number 15: _____

# Squares, Square Roots, Powers (explanation on pp. 14-16)

**16** Write $10^3$ out in the sequence, illustrating the process you would use to calculate it. _____

**17** Write the *square* of 5. _____

**18** Write the *square root* of 36. _____

**19** Which number is the *base?* $10^8$ _____

**20** Which number is the *exponent?* $10^8$ _____

# Fractions (explanation on pp. 24-34)

**21** Write 2 divided by 5 as a fraction. _____

**22** Label the numerator and denominator: $\frac{2}{3}$ _____

**23** Which is greater: $\frac{1}{10}$ or $\frac{1}{100}$? _____ $\frac{1}{9}$ or $\frac{1}{6}$? _____

**24** Change the improper fraction $\frac{31}{6}$ to a whole number and a fraction. _____

**25** Change the mixed fraction $7\frac{1}{5}$ to an improper fraction. _____

**26** Find the lowest common denominator (LCD) in the pairs of fractions:

$\frac{1}{2}$ and $\frac{5}{8}$ _____ $\qquad\qquad$ $\frac{2}{3}$ and $\frac{9}{10}$ _____

**27** Find a common factor (if available) other than 1 for the numerator and denominator: $\frac{10}{15}$ _____

**28** Reduce the fractions to lowest terms: $\frac{8}{10}$ _____ $\frac{4}{100}$ _____

**29** Add the fractions: $\frac{3}{4} + \frac{2}{3}$ _____ $\frac{1}{2} + \frac{1}{9}$ _____

**30** Subtract the fractions: $\frac{7}{8} - \frac{1}{6}$ _____ $\frac{5}{8} - \frac{1}{4}$ _____

**31** Multiply the fractions and use cancellation to simplify:

$\frac{2}{3} \times \frac{6}{8}$ _____ $\qquad\qquad$ $\frac{4}{5} \times 4\frac{3}{4}$ _____

**32** Divide the fractions and use cancellation to simplify:

$\frac{1}{2} \div \frac{1}{9}$ _____ $\qquad\qquad$ $2\frac{2}{3} \div \frac{1}{6}$ _____

**33** Write each of the following expressions in fraction form:

10 diapers *per* package _____ $2.00 *each* gallon _____ $30 *an* hour _____

## Decimals (explanation on pp. 17-24)

**34** Change the following fractions to a decimal and round to the nearest hundredth:

$\frac{1}{4}$ _____          $\frac{5}{6}$ _____

**35** Write the following decimals in fraction form: 0.461 _____     5.09 _____

**36** Round the following decimals to the nearest tenth: 0.541 _____     0.084 _____

**37** Round the decimals to the nearest hundredth: 1.34481 _____

**38** Round the decimals to the nearest thousandth: 0.23456 _____

**39** Which is greater? 0.23 or 0.023 _____

**40** Which is smaller? 0.15 or 0.1 _____

**41** Change the following decimals to a fraction and reduce to lowest terms:

0.3 _____     0.16 _____     0.125 _____

**42** Multiply 0.4 by 1.04 _____

**43** Divide 0.5 by 0.125 _____

## Percent (explanation on pp. 34-37)

**44** Change the following decimals to a percent:

0.1 _____     0.32 _____     0.032 _____

**45** A 5% annual raise for a salary of $32,000 a year = _____ dollars increase.

**46** What is 25% of 300? _____

**47** What is the numerical value of the *constant* used to convert hours to minutes? _____

**48** How is a period inserted midway between numbers as illustrated below *interpreted mathematically?* $5 \cdot 6 \cdot 3$ _____

**49** What is the required written spatial placement for a decimal point?

_____

**50** Write and solve an equation to illustrate the product of $\frac{1}{2}$ and $\frac{1}{6}$.

_____

*"Review and repetition are the mother of retention."*

—AUTHOR UNKNOWN

# ESSENTIAL MATH REVIEW

## Objectives

- Define and interpret the symbols and vocabulary of basic mathematics.
- Create fractions from whole numbers.
- Insert leading zeros and eliminate trailing zeros.
- Convert Arabic and Roman numerals.
- Calculate sums, products, and multiples of numbers.
- Identify factors and multipliers.
- Calculate squares and square roots.
- Interpret and calculate values of bases and exponents.
- Use mental arithmetic to calculate powers of base 10.
- Multiply and divide whole numbers and decimal numbers with powers of 10 by moving decimal places.
- Distinguish decimal fractions from other fractions.
- Read and write decimal numbers.
- Round whole numbers and decimal numbers.
- Add, subtract, multiply, cancel, divide, and reduce simple, mixed, and improper fractions.
- Find lowest common denominators for fractions.
- Compare fraction size by creating equivalent fractions.
- Convert fractions, decimal numbers, and percents.
- Solve basic equations with fractions, decimal fractions, and whole numbers.
- Estimate and evaluate answers.
- Calculate unit values.

## Essential Prior Knowledge

1 Basic addition, subtraction, division, and multiplication operations
2 Multiplication tables

## Equipment

- No special equipment is needed for this chapter. It is recommended that this chapter be mastered using mental arithmetic and pencil and paper. You may wish to have a calculator on hand only for verification of paper and pencil calculations. There are two reasons for this suggestion: the underlying processes must be known in order to enter the data correctly in a calculator, and calculators may not always be available or function.

## Estimated Time to Complete Chapter

- 1-2 hours (assuming some arithmetic background)

➤ Please do not skip this chapter if you missed questions on the Essential Math Self-Assessment.

5

# Introduction

This chapter contains all of the mathematics needed for calculating medicine dosages. The math is basic. Being confident in one's own ability to understand and interpret basic arithmetic and do the basic math reduces chances of error.

Time is precious for students, staff nurses, and patients. Being skilled with the medication arithmetic speeds up the delivery of medicines and frees up sorely needed time for other aspects of nursing care. No one wants to wait a half-hour for a medication while the nurse laboriously attempts to calculate the dosage.

For those students who are interested in accelerated learning, this is the key chapter in the text. Arithmetic comprehension provides a strong foundation for all of the material covered in this text.

The short answers requested in writing are useful. Writing activity, even a very brief notation, will reinforce memory.

It is assumed that the reader has completed mathematics prerequisite courses and may only need occasional extra practice exercises. For that reason, Rapid Practice quizzes related to each of the concepts are placed at the end of Chapter 1.

# Directions

Set aside the time to complete this chapter in one sitting if you have a recent arithmetic background or in two or three sittings if you need a refresher.

Skim the chapter objectives. Skim each concept in the chapter and answer the Ask Yourself questions. When more review of a topic is needed, take the designated Rapid Practice quiz for that topic. The depth of your review depends on your assessment of your comprehension. A review *before* taking a test boosts scores. Be sure you can answer all of the questions provided. Answer the text questions in brief *written* phrases to check understanding and reinforce memory. Revisit any content areas where questions are missed.

When your review is completed, take the Multiple-Choice Review and the Chapter 1 Final Practice.

Refer to a basic mathematics text if further explanation is needed.

**Remember:** An investment of an hour or two in the basics will greatly accelerate your mastery of the rest of the text.

# Essential Math Vocabulary and Concepts

Basic mathematical symbols are graphic representations of a mathematical expression. Symbols speed comprehension and reduce writing time. For instance, writing and reading numbers in symbolic numeric form is faster than writing out the word for a number (e.g., 174 versus one hundred seventy-four). Here are several other examples:

| Symbol | Meaning | Example |
|---|---|---|
| $<$ | Less than arrow points to the Left | The baby weighs $<$ 5 pounds. |
| $>$ | Greater than arrow points to the Right | His weight was 2 pounds $>$ last week. |
| $\geq$ | Greater than or equal to | Give the medications if the blood pressure $\geq$ 160/100. |
| $\leq$ | Less than or equal to | Hold the medication if his temperature is $\leq$ 100. |
| $\sqrt{\phantom{x}}$ | Square root | $\sqrt{16}$ means the square root of 16. |

**✳ Mnemonic**

Note the "L" in *less than* and *left*.

The smaller end of the arrow *always* points to the *smaller* number:

5 is $>$ 3 but 5 is $<$ 10

The larger open end of the arrow always faces the *larger* number.

➤ These symbols have been misinterpreted in medical records.
➤ They should be written out to prevent confusion. Write out "is greater than" rather than use the $>$ symbol. This will probably be a requirement for

handwritten medical records in the future. These symbols are included in the text to increase understanding and avoid medicine errors when reading printed drug labels, current pharmacology references, and laboratory reports.

> **Clinical Relevance**
>
> Keep in mind the potential effect on a patient receiving a medication that was supposed to be withheld for a pulse $<50$ because the nurse misinterpreted that symbol as "greater than." If this results in a patient medication error, remember that ignorance is not a defense.

**Q:** *Ask Yourself*

**A:** *My Answer*

1   How will I remember the difference between *less than* and *greater than* when I read the symbols?

   _____

2   Write a brief sentence using your age and the symbols for *less than* and *greater than* to illustrate that the arrow always points to the lower number.

   _____

> **FAQ** | *Are these symbols really used much in medicine and nursing?*
>
> **ANSWER:** Yes. These symbols are frequently seen in nursing journals, laboratory reports, drug package inserts, and pharmacology references. They are used to delineate age limits and weight limits for medications. They are used in laboratory reports to differentiate normal and abnormal values. Research findings include symbols.

For additional practice on symbols, refer to Rapid Practice 1-1 on p. 38 and Rapid Practice 1-2 on p. 39.

# Whole Numbers

A whole number is a number that is evenly divisible by the number 1.

## Multiplying and Dividing Whole Numbers by the Number 1

Working with whole numbers is easier than working with fractions and decimals.

➤ Remember that a number divided by or multiplied by 1 will not change in value.

To write a whole number as a fraction, write the whole number as a numerator with the number 1 as the denominator.

The *numerator (N)*, the number above the dividing line, indicates the number of parts out of a total number of equal parts, the *denominator (D)*, designated below the dividing line.

**EXAMPLES**

Division by 1:

$$\frac{500 \text{ Numerator}}{1 \text{ Denominator}} = 500 \qquad 30 = \frac{30 \text{ N}}{1 \text{ D}} = 30 \qquad \frac{10}{1} = 10$$

# Implied Decimal Points and Trailing Zeros

A *whole* number has an *implied* decimal point immediately *following* the whole number (e.g., 1. and 20.).

➤ Do write 1 and 20; do not write 1. and 20.

Implied decimal points, if written, can be misread as commas, zeros, or the number one.

Zeros that follow the last number after a decimal point are called *trailing zeros*. Do write 1.3; do *not* write 1.30. Trailing zeros are only appropriate for printed laboratory reports and statistical reports.

➤ Avoid writing implied decimal points and trailing zeros.

| EXAMPLES | Decimals can be mistaken for commas. Trailing zeros contribute to a reading error. |
|---|---|
| | 20.~~0~~     403.~~00~~     8.~~000~~     50.9~~0~~     400.~~000~~     2.4~~00~~ |

➤ Do *not* remove zeros that occur *within* a number. The number 3.08 would be read as 3.8 if this error was made, resulting in a tenfold error.
➤ Do not remove zeros that occur before a decimal point. They *alert* the reader to a decimal that follows the zero immediately:

$$0.04 \qquad 0.4 \qquad 0.8$$

➤ Always place a zero in front of a decimal point that is not preceded by a whole number.
➤ Always eliminate implied decimal points and trailing zeros that follow a whole number. Implied decimal points and trailing zeros do not change the value, but they do lead to reading errors and medication dosage errors.

**1**  How might the whole number 200 written improperly with a decimal and/or trailing zeros (e.g., 200.00) be misinterpreted if the decimal point was read as a comma or as a number 1?

 *Ask Yourself*

*My Answer* _____

## Dividing a Number or Fraction by Itself

A number or fraction divided by itself equals 1.
A number or fraction divided by 1 equals itself.

| EXAMPLES | | | | |
|---|---|---|---|---|
| Equals the number 1: | $\frac{500}{500} = 1$ | | $\frac{3}{3} = 1$ | $\frac{10}{10} = 1$ |
| Equals itself: | $\frac{500}{1} = 500$ | | $\frac{3}{1} = 3$ | $\frac{10}{1} = 10$ |

*Ask Yourself*

**1.** Can you write your age as a whole number in fraction form that will equal itself? Now create a fraction using your age that will equal 1.

*My Answer*

| My Age Whole Number | Fraction Equals Itself | Fraction Equals 1 |
|---|---|---|
| _____ | _____ | _____ |

For practice editing whole numbers, converting whole numbers to fractions, and dealing with implied decimal points, refer to Rapid Practice 1-3 on p. 39 and Rapid Practice 1-4 on p. 40.

# Arabic Numerals and Roman Numerals

There are many numbering systems. We are accustomed to the Arabic numeral system: 1, 2, 3, 4, and so on.

- The Roman numeral system uses letters to designate numbers. Occasionally you may see Roman numerals, such as I, II, III, IV, and V, denoting the year of construction on public buildings, time on the face of a clock, and numbering of book chapters. Rarely, but occasionally, uppercase and lowercase Roman numerals will be seen in a medication order, such as *Aspirin gr* $\overline{xv}$.
- Roman numerals are usually written in capital letters, such as I, X, L, C, and D.
- Some prescribers write Roman numerals in lowercase, such as ī, īi, īii, v̄, and x̄. Lowercase numerals have a line placed over them.

The Roman numbering system does not repeat more than three *consecutive* symbols of the *same* value (e.g., III, XXX, CCC, and MMM). After three consecutive repetitions of same-value symbols, *smaller*-value symbols are used to add or subtract from the larger value.

Examine the example that follows. Pay special attention to numbers that end in the Roman numerals for 4, 6, and 9. They illustrate the simple system of addition and subtraction.

- A number (e.g., I) that *precedes* a larger-value symbol, as in IV, shoud be subtracted (subtract 1 from 5).
- A number (e.g., I) that *follows* a symbol signals *addition*, as in VI and XXI.

| ARABIC | ROMAN | ARABIC | ROMAN |
|--------|-------|--------|-------|
| 1, 2, 3 | I, II, III | 11, 12, 13 | XI, XII, XIII |
| 4 | IV | 14, 15*, 16 | XIV, XV, XVI |
| 5* | V | 20, 24 | XX, XXIV |
| 6 | VI | 40, 50, 60 | XL, L, LX |
| 7, 8 | VII, VIII | 100 | C |
| 9 | IX | 500 | D |
| 10* | X | 1000 | M |

*More commonly seen if written with a medication order. Focus on the 5, 10, and 15.

**EXAMPLES**

**FAQ** | *If Roman numerals are so seldom used in current medication orders, why should I learn to read them?*

**ANSWER:** ➤Infrequent and/or unfamiliar events require extra careful scrutiny to avoid error. A "V" for "5" can be misread as a "U" for "Unit." At one time, Roman numerals were used exclusively for medications. Some providers in the United States and from a few other countries may still occasionally write them. In order to avoid a medication dosage interpretation error, the nurse must recognize and verify the rare order that may occur with a Roman numeral dosage. Fortunately, the metric system and Arabic numbers now prevail for most orders.

**EXAMPLES**

| CORRECT | INCORRECT* |
|---|---|
| IV (4) 1 less than 5 | IIII |
| VIII (8) 5 plus 3 | IIIIIIII |
| IX (9) 1 less than 10 | VIIII |
| XLV (45) 10 less than 50 plus 5 | XXXXV |
| CXI (111) 100 plus 10 plus 1 | CIIIIIIIIIII |
| MCMLXXX (1980) 1000, plus 1000 minus 100, plus 50 plus 10, 10, 10 | MDCCCCLXXX |

**✳ Mnemonic**

C = 100
There are 100 cents in a dollar.
Centennials take place every 100 years.
A century spans 100 years.

*Cannot have more than 3 consecutive symbols of same value.

Note: *Addition* is employed when the *larger* value is to the *left* in the sequence. (VI, XV, XXI).

*Subtraction* is employed when the *larger* value is to *the right* in the sequence. (IV, IX, XL, CM).

**✳ Mnemonic**

LCD: from smallest to largest, the Roman numeral letter order for 50, 100, and 500 is the same as the first letters in the phrase *liquid crystal display*.

**Q** *Ask Yourself*

**A** *My Answer*

1   Can you write the number 14 in Roman numerals to illustrate the subtraction process?

   _____

2   How would you write your age in Roman numerals?

   _____

3   How would you write this year in Roman numerals?

   _____

For further practice with the conversion of Roman and Arabic numerals, refer to Rapid Practice 1-5 on p. 40 and Rapid Practice 1-6 on p. 41.

## Sum

A sum is the result of addition.

**EXAMPLES**

The sum of 3 and 6 is 9.

The sum of 2 and 2 is 4.

The sum of 1 and 9 is 10.

## Product

A product is the result of multiplication of numbers, decimals, fractions, and other numerical values.

**EXAMPLES**

The product of 3 and 6 is 18.

The product of $\frac{1}{3}$ and $\frac{1}{8}$ is $\frac{1}{24}$.

The product of 1.2 and 4 is 4.8.

**1**   What is the product of 10 and 10?

Q: *Ask Yourself*

_____

**2**   What is the sum of 10 and 10?

A: *My Answer*

_____

# Factor

A factor is any whole number that can *divide another number evenly without* a *remainder*. For example, in addition to 1 and 18, the numbers 2, 3, 6, and 9 are factors of 18. Seventeen only has factors of 1 and 17. No other whole numbers divide 17.

> 25 has factors of 1, 5, and 25.
>
> 60 has factors of 1, 2, 3, 4, 5, 6, 10, 12, 15, 20, 30, and 60.
>
> 3 has factors of 1 and 3.

**EXAMPLES**

➤ A factor can only be less than or equal to a given whole number. One and the number itself are always factors. "Factoring" the number 25 gives you 1, 5, and 25.

*Factor* also has other meanings. It also can be used as a general term to describe relevant data. For example, "He examined all the factors in the case" or "A dimensional analysis equation permits all the factors to be entered in one equation."

**1**   Can you quickly jot down all six factors of 12?

Q: *Ask Yourself*

_____

**2**   Can a fraction be a factor? (Review the definition.)

A: *My Answer*

_____

# Common Factors

A common factor is a whole number that divides every number in a pair or group of numbers evenly. The number 1 is always a common factor of whole numbers.

## Common Factors Other Than 1

> 5 and 10 have the common factor: 5. (It helps to see first whether the smaller or smallest number divides the other number or numbers evenly.)
>
> 4 and 16 have common factors of 4 and 2. (8 is not a common factor because the fraction $\frac{1}{2}$ will be the result of dividing into 4 and the factor must be a whole number.)
>
> 12 and 8 have common factors of 2 and 4. (If the smaller number does not divide the larger number evenly, it helps to try dividing by 2.)

**EXAMPLES**

➤ A common factor can never be greater than the smallest number in the group. First, try to divide the numbers in the group by the smallest number. If that does not work, try to divide them by 2, 3, and so on.

**Q:** *Ask Yourself*

**A:** *My Answer*

**1** Is the characteristic of dividing a number evenly a key feature of factors? (Review the definition.)

_____

**2** Can you quickly jot down some common factors of 100 and 50, other than 1?

_____

**3** Can any of the factors referred to in the previous question be larger than 50?

_____

**4** Can a common factor be greater than the smallest whole number in the group?

_____

**✳ Mnemonic**

Multiply *factors* to arrive at a multiple (MM).

A multiple must be greater than or equal to the given numbers.

A multiple is a product, but it is a specific kind of product.

## Multiple

A multiple is the product of a *whole* number multiplied by two or more factors (*whole* numbers).

**EXAMPLES**

Five *multiples* of the number 5 are 5 (5 × 1), 10 (5 × 2), 15 (5 × 3), 20 (5 × 4), and 25 (5 × 5).

6 is a multiple of factors 2 and 3, and 6 and 1.

50 is a multiple of factors 10 and 5, 25 and 2, and 50 and 1.

**Q:** *Ask Yourself*

**A:** *My Answer*

**1** Can you jot down three multiples of the number 4?

_____

**2** Ten is a multiple of which factors other than the number 1?

_____

## Factors Versus Multiples

**EXAMPLES**

5 has factors of 1 and 5. 5 has multiples of 5, 10, 15, . . .

8 has factors of 1, 2, 4, and 8. 8 has multiples of 8, 16, 24, . . .

20 has factors of 1, 2, 4, 5, 10, and 20. 20 has multiples of 20, 40, 60, . . .

## Multiplier

A multiplier is the number used to multiply; it immediately follows the times sign.

**EXAMPLES**

Right: The *multiplier* of 9 × 4 is 4.

Right: The *multiplier* of 2 × 5 is 5.

Right: The *multiplier* of 10 × $\frac{1}{2}$ is $\frac{1}{2}$.

A multiplier does *not* need to be a whole number.

1   How will I distinguish the following terms: factors, multipliers, multiples, and products?

   _____

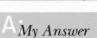

2   Find some factors of your age.

   _____

3   Find three multiples of your age.

   _____

4   Name the product of 2 and 6.

   _____

For further practice with multiplication terms and concepts, refer to Rapid Practice 1-7 on p. 41.

## Divisor

A divisor is the opposite of a multiplier. It is the number used to *divide* another number into smaller parts.

## Dividend

A dividend is the number being divided up, or the number the divisor is dividing.

## Quotient

A quotient is the result of division, or the answer.

## Remainder

The remainder is the amount left over in the answer when a divisor does not divide a dividend *evenly*.

| | **EXAMPLES** |
|---|---|

$$\text{Dividend} \quad \text{Divisor} \qquad \frac{\text{Dividend}}{\text{Divisor}} \qquad 20\frac{2}{5} \text{ (Quotient and Remainder)}$$

$$100 \;\div\; 5 \qquad \frac{100}{5} \qquad 5 \text{ (Divisor)}\overline{)102} \text{ (Dividend)}$$

1   What is the name for the number being divided?

   _____

2   What is the name for the answer to a division operation?

   _____

3   What is the name for the number used to divide?

   _____

For practice with division terms, refer to Rapid Practice 1-8 on p. 41.

## Square

The square is the product of a number multiplied by itself one time.

<table>
<tr><td>EXAMPLES</td><td>

$4 \times 4 = 4^2 = 16$

$10 \times 10 = 10^2 = 100$

$2 \times 2 = 2^2 = 4$

</td></tr>
</table>

Squares can also can be written and spoken as follows:

2 squared ($2^2$) = 4; 4 is the square of 2.

4 squared ($4^2$) = 16; 16 is the square of 4.

10 squared ($10^2$) = 100; 100 is the square of 10.

Think of the dimensions of a square box. To be a square, the sides must all be of equal size.

**FAQ** | *When are squares used in medication administration?*

**ANSWER:** Squares are used to denote square meters of body surface area. The most appropriate dosage for powerful drugs for pediatric and patients with cancer may be determined by milligrams per square meter ($m^2$) of body surface area rather than by weight. Nurses encounter the symbol when investigating the safe dosage ranges in a pharmacology reference. The symbol may also be on a record sent from the agency pharmacy on the patient's medical chart.

*Ask Yourself*

*My Answer*

1   What are two additional terms used for a product?

_____

## Square Root

The square root is the (root) number used to arrive at a square when multiplied *by itself*. It is the inverse of a square.

<table>
<tr><td>EXAMPLES</td><td>

2 is the square *root* of 4.

3 is the square *root* of 9.

10 is the square *root* of 100.

</td></tr>
</table>

The square root symbol is used to reduce writing and increase speed and comprehension:

$$\sqrt{4} = 2, \sqrt{9} = 3, \sqrt{100} = 10$$

To obtain a square root on a calculator, enter the number followed by the square root symbol.

1   How will I remember the difference between a square root and a square? Does the word *root* help?

_____

2   What is the square root of 36?

_____

3   What is the square of 6?

_____

4   How will I distinguish among the terms *factor, multiple, square,* and *product?*

_____

For additional practice with multiplication terms and concepts such as factors, multiples, squares, and products, refer to Rapid Practice 1-9 on p. 41 and Rapid Practice 1-10 on p. 42.

## Bases and Exponents

Bases and exponents are numbers written with two parts: $2^{3 \rightarrow \text{exponent}}$

$\uparrow$
base

The *base* is the number that must be multiplied by *itself*. The *exponent*, also known as *power*, is the small superscript number that indicates *how many times* the base must be multiplied *by itself*. Some examples were given in the section on squares. The expression $2^3$ is a type of shorthand for $2 \times 2 \times 2$. Writing powers saves a lot of math time.

Examine the difference in the values for $4^5$ and $5^4$ and for $3^2$ and $2^3$.

base | base | base | base |
exponent exponent   exponent exponent

$$5^4 = 5 \times 5 \times 5 \times 5 = 625$$

$$4^5 = 4 \times 4 \times 4 \times 4 \times 4 = 1024$$

$$3^2 = 3 \times 3 = 9$$

$$2^3 = 2 \times 2 \times 2 = 8$$

Multiply the *base* the specified *number of times* by *itself*.

You would *say* or *read* $2^3$ as, "2 to the third power" *or*, alternatively, "the third power of 2." The exponent is read as "power."

1   Which is the base and which is the exponent in $5^2$?

_____

2   Does $5^2 = 2^5$?

_____

3   What are the differences in the results for these two calculations?

_____

## Powers of 10 Calculations

When working with powers of 10, such as $10^2$, $10^3$, $10^4$, and so on, note the number of zeros in the answers.

| EXAMPLES | |
|---|---|
| | $10^2 = 10 \times 10 = 100$ |
| | $10^3 = 10 \times 10 \times 10 = 1000$ |
| | $10^4 = 10 \times 10 \times 10 \times 10 = 10,000$ |

The number of zeros in the result is equal to the number in the exponent.

**FAQ** | *How are powers and exponents used in medication administration?*

**ANSWER:** Using powers of 10 and exponents makes it much easier to understand decimals and metric system conversions. The metric system is a decimal system based on powers of 10. Most medications are delivered in milligrams and grams, which are converted using powers of 10. The nurse who understands these conversions will learn the metric system much more quickly and will be less likely to make errors when converting the units within the metric system. It only takes a few minutes to comprehend powers and exponents of 10, and doing so will save time in the clinical arena.

**Q:** *Ask Yourself*

**A:** *My Answer*

1 How would you write the following in short form: 10 to the tenth power?

_____

2 How would you write the following in short form: 8 to the second power?

_____

3 What are two ways you can read or say $10^2$?

_____

For additional practice with powers of 10, refer to Rapid Practice 1-11 on p. 42.

## Multiplying and Dividing by 10, 100, and 1000 the Fast Way

Dividing and multiplying by a multiple of 10—such as 10, 100, and 1000—involves moving the decimal place to the left or right by a number of places that is *equal to the number of zeros* in the *divisor* or *multiplier:* 10, 100 or 1000, and so on. These three numbers are the most frequently used numbers in metric medication calculations. They are powers of 10: $10^1$, $10^2$, and $10^3$.

To divide, examine the *divisor*—10, 100, or 1000—for the number of zeros. In the dividend, move the decimal point (real or implied) to the left by a number of places that is equal to the number of zeros:

$$1000 \div 10 = 100$$

To multiply, examine the *multiplier*—10, 100, or 1000—for the number of zeros. In the number being multiplied, move the decimal point to the right by a number of places that is equal to the number of zeros:

$$10 \times \underset{1\,2\,3}{1000} = 10,000$$

| Whole Number × Multiplier = Answer | Whole Number ÷ Divisor = Answer |
|---|---|
| 50 × 10   = 500 | 500 ÷ 10   = 50.0 = 50 |
| 400 × 100   = 40,000 | 40 ÷ 100   = .40 = 0.4 |
| 10 × 1000 = 10,000 | 4 ÷ 1000 = .004 = 0.004 |

**EXAMPLES**

➤ Whenever there are more than four numbers in a group, insert a comma in front of every three digits from right to left to ease the reading: e.g, 1000000 becomes 1,000,000 (1 million), and 20000 becomes 20,000 (20 thousand).

Insert zeros in front of decimals, and avoid trailing zeros after whole numbers.

For additional practice with multiplication and division with powers of 10, refer to Rapid Practice 1-12 and Rapid Practice 1-13 on p. 43.

# Decimal Fractions

A decimal fraction is any fraction with a denominator that is a *power of 10*. It is easier to read and write decimal *fractions* in *abbreviated* form with a decimal point to replace the denominator, for example, 0.1 for $\frac{1}{10}$ and 0.06 for $\frac{6}{100}$. In this abbreviated form, these decimal fractions are called *decimals*. Our money system is based on decimals.

| Decimal = Fraction | Decimal = Fraction |
|---|---|
| $0.1 = \frac{1}{10}$ | $0.4 = \frac{4}{10}$ |
| $0.05 = \frac{5}{100}$ | $0.35 = \frac{35}{100}$ |
| $0.005 = \frac{5}{1000}$ | $0.025 = \frac{25}{1000}$ |
| $0.0009 = \frac{9}{10,000}$ | $0.0005 = \frac{5}{10,000}$ |

**EXAMPLES**

➤ Decimals replace the division bar and the denominator of a fraction with a decimal point in the specified place that identifies power of 10 in the denominator. Zeros are used to hold the place values. When you read a decimal fraction, you read it and say it in the fraction form: four tenths, five one-hundredths.

**FAQ** | *How does the denominator of a decimal fraction differ from the denominators of other fractions?*

**ANSWER:** The decimal fraction has a denominator that is a power of 10. Other fractions, such as $\frac{2}{3}$, $\frac{5}{6}$, and $\frac{1}{5}$, do not have a power of 10 in the denominator.

Fractions with denominators other than powers of 10 are covered in more detail on p. 24.

Like other fractions, decimal fractions—or decimals—are numbers that indicate less than a whole unit.

Observe the number line below, which represents numbers as points on a line. The numbers to the *left* of the decimal point are whole numbers. The numbers to the *right* of the decimal point are decimal fractions.

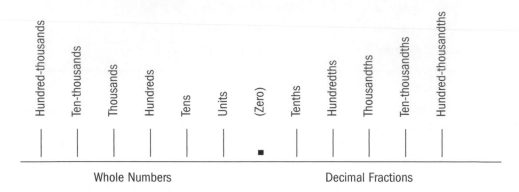

Read the number to the right of the decimal point as the numerator.

The number of places to the right of the decimal point determines the power of 10 in the denominator. One place denotes tenths, two places denote hundredths, three places denote thousandths, and so on.

| EXAMPLES | 1 Decimal Place | 2 Decimal Places | 3 Decimal Places | 4 Decimal Places |
|---|---|---|---|---|
| | 0.5, | 0.12, | 0.375, | 0.0005, |
| | 5 tenths | 12 hundredths | 375 thousandths | 5 ten-thousandths |

## Reading Numbers and Decimals

Decimals are read as fractions. Decimal points separate whole numbers from fractional parts of a number. The fractional part follows to the immediate *right* of the decimal point.

Read the number or numbers that appear to the left of the decimal point out loud.

Read the decimal *point* as "and" or "point."

Read the decimal in *fraction* form.

| EXAMPLES | Written | Read and Spoken as |
|---|---|---|
| | 0.5 | "five tenths" |
| | 1.5 | "one and 5 tenths" "or one point 5" |
| | 1.06 | "one and 6 hundredths" or "one point zero 6" |
| | 42.005 | "42 and 5 thousandths" |
| | 2.0008 | "2 and 8 ten-thousandths" or "2 point zero, zero, zero, 8" |

For additional practice reading decimals, refer to Rapid Practice 1-14 on p. 44.

➤ Note that the decimal point is placed at the *baseline* between the numbers. If it is elevated, it may be read as a symbol to multiply. This symbol appears in mathematics texts.

| | |
|---|---|
| 1.4 is 1 and four *tenths.*<br><br>1 · 4 is 1 times 4. | **EXAMPLES** |

# Writing Decimals in Fraction Form

Write the number or numbers that appear to the right of the decimal point as the *numerator.*

Write the power of 10 (e.g., 10, 100, or 1000) according the decimal places in the *denominator.*

The number of zeros in the denominator is equal to the number of decimal places.

Eliminate the decimal point.

## Say and Read

| Decimal | | Fraction Form | | | |
|---|---|---|---|---|---|
| 0.5 | 5 "tenths" | $\frac{5}{10}$ | One zero in the denominator because there is one place after the decimal point | | **EXAMPLES** |
| 0.25 | 25 "hundredths" | $\frac{25}{100}$ | Two zeros in the denominator because there are two places after the decimal point | | |
| 0.025 | 25 "thousandths" | $\frac{25}{1000}$ | Three zeros in the denominator because there are three places after the decimal point | | |

Be sure to include a zero for *each* decimal place, the *place value* of the decimal number (tenths, hundredths, thousandths, etc.), in the *denominator.*

To avoid 10-, 100-, and 1000-fold errors, the decimal point must be clearly identified and in the correct place:

0.5, *not* .5
0.025, *not* .025
625, *not* 625.00

➤ Insert leading zeros before decimal points and remove trailing zeros. Commas, decimal points, and the number 1 must be clearly distinguished to avoid errors.

| Decimal | Fraction | Decimal | Fraction | Decimal | Fraction | |
|---|---|---|---|---|---|---|
| 0.5 | $\frac{5}{10}$ | 0.01 | $\frac{1}{100}$ | 0.025 | $\frac{25}{1000}$ | **EXAMPLES** |

| EXAMPLES | Decimal | Fraction | |
|---|---|---|---|
| | 0.5 | $\frac{5}{10}$ | The decimal point *replaces* the division bar and the denominator of the decimal fraction |
| | 0.01 | $\frac{1}{100}$ | |
| | 0.025 | $\frac{25}{1000}$ | |

➤ Tenths are the *largest* decimal fraction denominator. A tenth is 10 times larger than a hundredth.

The decimal point *replaces* the division bar and the denominator of the decimal fraction.

**Q:** *Ask Yourself*

**1** How would you write the decimal 0.25 as a fraction?

_____

**A:** *My Answer*

**2** How would you write 0.14 as a fraction?

_____

**3** How would you write 0.1 as a fraction?

_____

For additional practice reading decimal fractions, refer to Rapid Practice 1-15 on p. 44.

## Comparing Decimals to see Which is Larger

Evaluate the *whole* number first. The higher number has the higher value (e.g., 1.21 < 2.21; 1.04 > 0.083).

If there are no whole numbers, examine the *tenths* column for the higher number (e.g., 0.82 > 0.593; 0.632 < 0.71).

If the tenths columns are equal, examine the *hundredths* column (e.g., 0.883 > 0.87).

For practice reading and comparing decimal fractions, refer to Rapid Practice 1-15 and Rapid Practice 1-16 on p. 44.

**Q:** *Ask Yourself*

**1** Which is greater: 0.002 or 0.012? (Examine the hundredths column.)

_____

**A:** *My Answer*

**2** How do you write 0.015 and 0.06 using fraction notation (i.e., a denominator with a power of 10)?

For additional practice writing decimals using fraction notation, refer to Rapid Practice 1-17 on p. 44.

## Rounding Decimals and Whole Numbers

To round a number to an approximate number, examine the *specified place value* (e.g., round to the nearest *tenth, hundredth, thousandth*, etc.).

If the number immediately following the specified place is ≤5, leave the specified place value unchanged and eliminate all the subsequent numbers.

If the number after the specified place is ≥5, round the specified place value up to the next number.

*Do not* round *down. Do not* decrease the last digit.

Examine the Specified Column and the Number that Follows

| Number | Result | |
|--------|--------|---|
| Round to the nearest *tenth:* | | |
| 4.54 | 4.5 | 5 is in the tenths (specified) column and the number immediately following it in the hundredths is 4. The 5 remains unchanged because 4 is less than 5. The last 4 is dropped. |
| 0.92 | 0.9 | 2 is less than 5. No change. |
| 0.375 | 0.4 | 7 is greater than 5; increase the 3 to 4. |
| Round to the nearest *hundredth:* | | |
| 3.0256 | 3.03 | 2 is in the hundredths (specified) column. The number immediately following it in the thousandths column is 5. Round 2 up to 3. |
| 0.125 | 0.13 | The 2 is rounded up to 3. Any number greater than or equal to 5 is rounded up 1 digit. The last number is dropped. |
| 0.550 | 0.56 | 0 is less than 5. The 5 is unchanged. Drop the 0. |
| Round to the nearest *whole number:* | | |
| 400.9 | 401 | 0 is in the last whole number column. The 9 is the number immediately following the decimal point. The 0 is rounded to 1 and the decimal point and decimals are eliminated. |
| 25.4 | 25 | 4 is less than 5; 25 remains unchanged. |
| 99.8 | 100 | 8 is greater than 5. Round 99 to 100. |

**FAQ** | *Why do nurses need to learn how to round numbers?*

**ANSWER:** Most syringe medications are rounded to the nearest tenth. Very small amounts may be rounded to the nearest hundredth. Drops need to be rounded to the nearest whole number. Medicines may be administered by dropper, and some intravenous solutions are delivered in drops per minute. Drops cannot be split.

1   Can you round 0.007 to the nearest hundredth?

_____

2   Can you round 2.19 to the nearest whole number?

_____

3   Can you round 0.75 to the nearest tenth?

_____

*Q: Ask Yourself*

*A: My Answer*

For additional practice rounding, refer to Rapid Practice 1-18 on p. 45.

## Adding and Subtracting Decimal Numbers

To add and subtract decimal numbers, line them up in a column with the decimal points directly under each other. Add or subtract the columns, proceeding from right to left, as with whole numbers. Insert the decimal point in the answer directly under the decimal points in the problem.

| EXAMPLES | Addition | | Subtraction | |
|---|---|---|---|---|
| | 0.26 | 1.36 | 4.38 | 12.4 |
| | +1.44 | +2.19 | −1.99 | −0.6 |
| | 1.70 | 3.55 | 2.39 | 11.8 |

It is important to keep the decimal points aligned in addition, subtraction, and division.

## Multiplying Decimals

To multiply decimals, multiply the numbers as for any multiplication of whole numbers.

Counting from right to left, insert the decimal point in the answer in the place equal to the *total number of decimal places* in the two numbers that are multiplied.

| EXAMPLES | 1.2 →1 Decimal Place | 3.4 →1 Decimal Place | 0.08 →2 Decimal Places |
|---|---|---|---|
| | ×0.4 →1 Decimal Place | ×0.0001 →4 Decimal Places | ×0.0123 →4 Decimal Places |
| | 0.48 →2 Total Decimal Places | 0.00034 →5 Total Decimal Places* | 0.000984 →6 Total Decimal Places* |

Insert a zero in front of the decimal point in the answer if the answer does not contain a value to the left of the decimal point. The decimal points in multiplication are *not* aligned with other decimal points in the problem, as in addition, subtraction, and division.

Insert zeros in the answer to hold the place for the decimal point if there are insufficient digits in the answer.

**Q: Ask Yourself**

**A: My Answer**

1 If you multiply 10.45 × 1.246, how many decimal places must there be in the product?

_____

2 Do you count decimal places from left to right or right to left?

_____

For additional decimal multiplication practice, refer to Rapid Practice 1-19 on p. 45.

## Dividing Decimals

Division of decimals is the same as division of whole numbers, with one exception: decimal point placement is emphasized. Examine the divisor.

## Division of Decimals When the Divisor Is a Whole Number

Examine the divisor. If it is a *whole* number, place the decimal point in the answer *directly above* the decimal point in the dividend, as shown in the examples that follow.

Proceed as with division for whole numbers.

| A | B | C |
|---|---|---|
| 2.6 Quotient | 0.43 Answer | 0.05 Answer |
| 4 Divisor)10.4 Dividend | 5)2.15 | 8)0.40 |

**EXAMPLES**

The alignment of decimal points must be exactly as shown in examples A, B, and C.

Insert a zero in front of a decimal that does not have an accompanying whole number, as shown in example B in red.

Add zeros if necessary to the dividend in order to arrive at a numerical answer, as shown in example C in red.

## Division of Decimals When Divisor Contains Decimals

If the divisor contains decimals, first change the divisor to a *whole* number by *moving* the real or implied decimal place in the dividend to the right by the number of decimal places *equal* to the decimal places in the *divisor*.

*Place the decimal point in the answer directly* above the new decimal place in the dividend. Proceed with the division as for whole numbers.

| A | B | C |
|---|---|---|
| 45 | 401 | 0.5 |
| 0.4)18.0 | 0.51)204.51 | 5)2.5 |

**EXAMPLES**

Add zeros if necessary as placeholders, as shown in example C.

Moving the decimal place an equal number of places in both the divisor and the dividend to make a whole number in the divisor is the equivalent of multiplying both figures by 10, 100, or 1000. The value of the answer will be *unchanged*, as seen in the following example.

| Dividend/Divisor = Quotient | Multiplying Divisor and Dividend × 10 | Multiplying Divisor and Dividend × 100 |
|---|---|---|
| $\frac{18}{0.4} = 45$ | $\frac{180}{4} = 45$ | $\frac{1800}{40} = 45$ |

**EXAMPLES**

**FAQ** | *Why not just let a calculator do the division?*

**ANSWER:** Before using a calculator, the "operator" must understand the underlying process sufficiently to enter the data correctly in the absence of a calculator.

**Q** *Ask Yourself*

**A** *My Answer*

**1** If the dividend 3.85 is divided by 2.9, where will the decimal be moved in the dividend before the division takes place?

_____

**2** If the dividend 253 is divided by 62.1, what change will be made to the dividend before the division takes place?

_____

For additional practice with division of decimals, refer to Rapid Practice 1-20 on p. 45 and Rapid Practice 1-21 on p. 46.

## Fractions

A fraction is a number that describes the *parts* of a whole number. It is a form of division. A fraction has a numerator and a denominator. The numerator is the top number in the fraction and tells the number of parts in the fraction. The denominator is the bottom number in the fraction and tells the number of equal parts in which the whole number is divided. For math calculations or data entry on a calculator, the numerator is to be *divided by the denominator.*

✳ **Mnemonic**

DDD: Denominator, divisor, down under or down below the *divide by* line

➤ A denominator is the same as a divisor.

_____

**EXAMPLES**

$$\frac{2}{3 \text{ (denominator, divisor)}} = 2 \div 3$$

This fraction denotes two parts of a whole that is divided into three equal parts. The division line that divides the numerator and denominator, reading *top to bottom*, indicates "2 divided by 3."

The whole pizza below is divided into six equal pieces (the denominator).

If you eat one piece of pizza, you have consumed $\frac{1}{6}$ of the pizza.

**EXAMPLES**

$$\frac{1 \text{ Numerator}}{2 \text{ Denominator}} \text{ Division Bar, Dividing Line} \quad \frac{1 \text{ part}}{2 = \text{total number of equal parts}}$$

The denominator is a *divisor.*

**Q** *Ask Yourself*

**A** *My Answer*

**1** How would you write "the number 5 divided by the number 8" as a fraction?

_____

**2** Which part of the answer identifies the number of *parts of the whole?*

_____

**3**  Which part of the answer identifies the *total number* of parts in the whole?

_____

## Alternative Fraction Forms

The fraction $\frac{1}{2}$ can be expressed in the following forms:

decimal with a decimal point: 0.5 (numerator ÷ denominator, or 1 divided by 2)

percent with a percent sign: 50% (fraction × 100 with a percent sign added)

The forms above express one part of two equal parts.

**1**  Can you express the fraction $\frac{1}{4}$ in decimal form and as a percent?

_____

**2**  How will you remember the difference between the numerator and the denominator?

_____

**3**  Can you write $\frac{1}{8}$ out using the traditional long division symbol?

_____

**Q** *Ask Yourself*

**A** *My Answer*

## Mixed Fractions

A fraction that consists of a *mixture* of a whole number and a fraction is called a *mixed fraction*.

| |
|---|
| $1\frac{2}{3}, 41\frac{5}{6}, 8\frac{1}{8}$ |

**EXAMPLES**

Be sure to leave a space between the whole number and the fraction to avoid misinterpretation as a larger number.

✻ **Mnemonic**

A mixed fraction represents a *mixture* of whole and part of a whole. An improper fraction is improper because it is top heavy.

## Improper Fractions

A fraction that consists of a numerator that is *equal to* or *larger than* the denominator is called an improper fraction.

| |
|---|
| $\frac{10}{8}, \frac{12}{7}, \frac{4}{4}$ |

**EXAMPLES**

**1**  Can you write an example of an improper fraction using your age for the numerator?

_____

**2**  Can you write an example of a mixed fraction using your age for the whole number?

_____

**Q** *Ask Yourself*

**A** *My Answer*

# Converting Mixed and Improper Fractions

To convert a mixed fraction to an improper fraction, *multiply* the denominator by the whole number and *add* it to the numerator.

Place the new numerator over the original denominator of the fraction.

**EXAMPLES**

$$3\frac{1}{2} = \frac{7}{2} \ (2 \times 3 + 1), \ 4\frac{1}{3} = \frac{13}{3} \ (3 \times 4 + 1), \ 1\frac{1}{5} = \frac{6}{5} \ (5 \times 1 + 1)$$

**Q: Ask Yourself**

1   Can you quickly write an example of conversion of a small mixed fraction to an improper fraction?

**A: My Answer**

# Converting an Improper Fraction to a Mixed Fraction

To convert an improper fraction to a mixed fraction, *divide* the numerator by the denominator to obtain a whole number and a remainder.

Write the remainder as a fraction.

**EXAMPLES**

$$\frac{20}{6} = 3\frac{2}{6} \text{ or } 3\frac{1}{3} \qquad \frac{10}{8} = 1\frac{2}{8} \text{ or } 1\frac{1}{4} \qquad \frac{27}{23} = 1\frac{4}{23}$$

➤   Be careful when writing mixed fractions. Leave space between the whole number and the fraction. The mixed number $3\frac{1}{2}$ without adequate space could be misread as $\frac{31}{2}$ (thirty-one over two, or $15\frac{1}{2}$).

**Q: Ask Yourself**

1   Can you quickly write an example of a small improper fraction and convert it to a mixed fraction?

**A: My Answer**

For more practice with basic mixed and improper fractions, refer to Rapid Practice 1-22 on p. 46.

# Reducing Fractions

**✳ Mnemonic**

The definition of the word *reduce* gives a clue to the operation.

Reducing fractions to the lowest (simplest) terms simplifies the math. Reducing a fraction is usually requested for the final answer to a fraction problem, but this step can be performed at any point in a calculation to make it easier.

To reduce a fraction, divide the numerator and the denominator by the same (common) factor until it *cannot be divided* further into whole numbers.

Try using the numerator as the common factor. Divide it directly into the denominator, as shown in the first example that follows.

If that does not work, try dividing the numerator and denominator by 2.

If the numerator and denominator are not divisible by 2, find all factors of the numerator and denominator. The common factors will divide both the numerator and the denominator evenly.

A fraction *cannot* be further reduced if the numerator is 1.

CHAPTER 1

The numerator is the largest common factor.

Dividing the numerator and denominator by 100 reduces the fraction to its simplest terms.

$$\frac{\overset{1}{\cancel{100}}}{\underset{2}{\cancel{200}}} = \frac{1}{2}$$

Dividing by the common factor, 2, reduces the fraction to its lowest terms.

$$\frac{\overset{3}{\cancel{6}}}{\underset{4}{\cancel{8}}} = \frac{3}{4}$$

$\frac{1}{8}$, $\frac{1}{200}$, and $\frac{1}{9}$ cannot be reduced because a numerator less than 1 is not a whole number. $\frac{3}{7}$ cannot be reduced because there are no common factors.

**1**  Does the value of a fraction change when it is reduced?

_____

**2**  Is it important to focus on whole numbers when reducing a fraction?

_____

**3**  Can you reduce $\frac{15}{75}$ to its lowest terms? $\frac{10}{12}$?

_____

For more practice reducing fractions, refer to Rapid Practice 1-23 on pp. 46-47.

Q: *Ask Yourself*

A: *My Answer*

## Common (Same) Denominator and Lowest Common Denominator

Fractions are easier to compare and interpret if they have the *same* denominator.

Comparing the size of $\frac{8}{24}$ and $\frac{9}{24}$ is easier than comparing the size of $\frac{1}{3}$ and $\frac{3}{8}$ because you only have to compare the numerators when the denominators are equal.

**1**  If the denominators are the same, as in $\frac{1}{4}$, $\frac{2}{4}$, and $\frac{3}{4}$, which fraction is largest?

_____

Q: *Ask Yourself*

A: *My Answer*

## Lowest Common Denominator (LCD)

Fractions can be added and subtracted if they share a common denominator. Finding the lowest common denominator simplifies the calculation.

### Finding the Lowest Common Denominator (LCD)

To find the lowest common denominator (LCD), reduce fractions first where applicable.

If the larger denominator can be divided by the other denominator or denominators with a whole-number result, the larger denominator will be the LCD.

*Or,* if the denominators are low numbers, multiply the denominators by each other.

*Or* test each multiple of the largest denominator, starting with × 1, × 2, and so on, until a common multiple is located.

Reduce the answer to lowest terms.

---

**EXAMPLES**

$\frac{1}{4}$ and $\frac{1}{8}$: 8 is the larger denominator. 4 will divide evenly into 8. $\frac{1}{4} = \frac{2}{8}$. 8 is the LCD.

$\frac{1}{2}$ and $\frac{1}{3}$: 3 is the larger denominator. 2 will not divide evenly into 3. Multiply the denominators by each other. 3 × 2 = 6. 6 is the LCD.

$\frac{1}{4}$ and $\frac{5}{6}$: 6 is the larger denominator. 4 will not divide evenly into 6. Try using multiples of 6. 6 × 1 = 6; 6 × 2 = 12. 12 is a multiple for both 4 and 6. 12 is the LCD.

---

**Q: Ask Yourself**

**1** Can you determine the LCD for $\frac{1}{10}$ and $\frac{1}{20}$?

_____

**A: My Answer**

For more practice finding the LCD, refer to Rapid Practice 1-24 on p. 47.

## Equivalent Fractions

Equivalent fractions are fractions that have the same value.

To create an equivalent fraction, multiply the denominator (D) and then the numerator (N) in that fraction by the *same factor*. The value will be *unchanged* because you are really multiplying by a fraction that equals 1 (e.g., $\frac{2}{2} = 1$)

You can also divide the numerator and denominator by the same factor to arrive at smaller equivalent fractions.

---

**EXAMPLES**

| Original Fraction | Factor 2 | Equivalent Fraction | Original Fraction | Factor 3 | Equivalent Fraction | Original Fraction | Factor 4 | Equivalent Fraction |
|---|---|---|---|---|---|---|---|---|
| $\frac{5}{6}$ | × $\frac{2}{2}$ | = $\frac{10}{12}$ | $\frac{5}{6}$ | × $\frac{3}{3}$ | = $\frac{15}{18}$ | $\frac{5}{6}$ | × $\frac{4}{4}$ | = $\frac{20}{24}$ |
| $\frac{24}{36}$ | ÷ $\frac{2}{2}$ | = $\frac{12}{18}$ | $\frac{24}{36}$ | ÷ $\frac{3}{3}$ | = $\frac{8}{12}$ | $\frac{24}{36}$ | ÷ $\frac{4}{4}$ | = $\frac{6}{9}$ |

---

For practice creating equivalent fractions, refer to Rapid Practice 1-25 on p. 47.

**Q: Ask Yourself**

**1** Which would you rather have: $\frac{1}{100}$ or $\frac{1}{10}$ of a million-dollar lottery? A lottery that is divided 10 ways or 100 ways?

**A: My Answer**

_____

# Comparing Fractions

To compare fractions with the *same denominator*, compare the numerators.

Comparing $\frac{1}{8}$, $\frac{3}{8}$, and $\frac{7}{8}$, the largest is $\frac{7}{8}$ and the smallest is $\frac{1}{8}$.

There are two ways to compare fractions when the denominators are *different*.

The first way is to find the lowest common denominator and create equivalent fractions.

The faster way to compare sizes of fractions is to multiply diagonally from the denominator of one fraction to the numerator of the next fraction. This is called *cross-multiplication*.

The *numerator* of the fraction with the higher product indicates which is the larger fraction. Examine the example of cross-multiplication that follows.

---

Cross-multiply the *numerator* of each fraction by the *denominator* of the other.
If the products are equal, the fractions are equivalent.

| Equivalent | Larger | Larger |
|---|---|---|
| 40    40 | 12    15 | 200    100 |
| $\frac{5}{10} \times \frac{4}{8}$ | $\frac{2}{3} \times \frac{5}{6}$ | $\frac{1}{100} \times \frac{1}{200}$ |
| $40 = 40$ | 15 is the *larger* product. | 200 is the larger product. |
| $\frac{5}{10} = \frac{4}{8}$ | $\frac{5}{6}$ is the larger fraction. | $\frac{1}{100}$ is the larger fraction. |

**EXAMPLES**

---

**1**  Which is smaller: $\frac{3}{8}$ or $\frac{2}{6}$?

For practice comparing fraction sizes, refer to Rapid Practice 1-26 on p. 48.

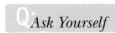

**Q** *Ask Yourself*

**A** *My Answer*

# Adding and Subtracting Fractions

To add or subtract fractions that have the *same denominator*, just add or subtract the numerators.

Place the result over the denominator. Reduce the answer to simplest terms.

If the denominators are *not* the same, identify the LCD, create an equivalent fraction, and then use the numerators to add and subtract while retaining the new common denominator.

## Denominators the Same

---

$$\frac{2}{4} - \frac{1}{4} = \frac{1}{4}$$
$$\frac{1}{8} + \frac{3}{8} + \frac{5}{8} = \frac{9}{8} = 1\frac{1}{8}$$
$$\frac{1}{6} + \frac{5}{6} = \frac{6}{6} = 1$$

**EXAMPLES**

---

## Denominators Not the Same

| EXAMPLES | Fractions (LCD) | Equivalent Fractions with LCD | Solution |
|---|---|---|---|
| | $\dfrac{2}{3}$ | $\dfrac{8}{12}$ | $\dfrac{8}{12}$ |
| | $+\dfrac{1}{4}$ (12) | $+\dfrac{3}{12}$ | $+\dfrac{3}{12}$ |
| | | | $\dfrac{11}{12}$ |
| | $1\dfrac{1}{4}$ | $1\dfrac{2}{8}$ | $1\dfrac{2}{8}$ |
| | $-\dfrac{1}{8}$ (8) | $-\dfrac{1}{8}$ | $-\dfrac{1}{8}$ |
| | | | $1\dfrac{1}{8}$ |
| | $3\dfrac{1}{6}$ | $3\dfrac{4}{24}$ | $3\dfrac{4}{24}$ |
| | $-2\dfrac{1}{8}$ (24) | $-2\dfrac{3}{24}$ | $-2\dfrac{3}{24}$ |
| | | | $1\dfrac{1}{24}$ |

**Q: Ask Yourself**

**1** What is the LCD for $2\frac{1}{9}$ and $4\frac{1}{6}$?

_____

**A: My Answer**

**2** How would you subtract $\frac{1}{3}$ from $\frac{5}{8}$?

_____

For practice adding and subtracting fractions using an LCD, refer to Rapid Practice 1-27 on p. 48.

## Mixed Fraction Subtraction and Borrowing

A mixed fraction consists of a whole number and a fraction (e.g., $1\frac{2}{3}$).

If the fractions have common denominators, subtract the numerator of the lower fraction from the numerator of the upper fraction and then subtract the whole numbers, if applicable (see Example A on following page).

If the lower fraction is larger than the upper one, _borrow_ one whole number from the whole number accompanying the _upper_ fraction and _add_ it in _fraction form_ to the upper fraction (see Example B on following page).

Subtract the numerators of the fractions. Reduce the answer (see Example B on following page).

Be sure the fractions have common denominators and that the upper fraction is larger than the lower fraction (see Examples A, B, and C on following page).

**EXAMPLES**

A.  $2\frac{3}{4}$      The fractions have common denominators.

$-1\frac{1}{4}$      The upper fraction, $\frac{3}{4}$, is larger than the lower fraction, $\frac{1}{4}$.

$1\frac{2}{4} = 1\frac{1}{2}$      Subtract the fraction numerators first. Then subtract the whole numbers.

$\overset{1}{}$

B.  $\overset{\,}{2}\frac{1}{4}$   $1\frac{5}{4}$      The fractions have a common denominator: 4.

$-1\frac{3}{4}$   $-1\frac{3}{4}$      $\frac{3}{4}$ cannot be subtracted from $\frac{1}{4}$.

$\frac{2}{4} = \frac{1}{2}$      Borrow (subtract) 1 from 2, and convert it to a fraction: $\frac{4}{4}$.

Add it to $\frac{1}{4}$ to arrive at $\frac{5}{4}$. $\frac{5}{4}$ is equal to $1\frac{1}{4}$.

Subtract the fraction numerators: $\frac{5}{4} - \frac{3}{4}$.

Reduce the answer to its simplest terms.

$\overset{7}{}$

C.  $\overset{\,}{8}\frac{1}{6}$   $7\frac{7}{6}$      Make $\frac{1}{6}$ and $\frac{2}{3}$ equivalent fractions with a common denominator: 6.

$-3\frac{2}{3}$   $-3\frac{4}{6}$      Borrow 1 from 8, and convert it to a fraction: $\frac{6}{6}$.

$4\frac{3}{6}$      Add it to the upper fraction to make $\frac{7}{6}$.

$= 4\frac{1}{2}$      Subtract the fraction numerators first: $\frac{7}{6} - \frac{4}{6}$.

Subtract the whole numbers: $7 - 3$.

Reduce the answer to its simplest terms.

1   Can a fraction with a numerator of 1, such as $\frac{1}{4}$, $\frac{1}{70}$, or $\frac{1}{200}$ be reduced?

_____

**Q:** *Ask Yourself*

2   Which digit do you borrow from in the following subtraction problem: $25\frac{1}{4} - \frac{3}{4}$?

_____

**A:** *My Answer*

For practice subtracting fractions, refer to Rapid Practice 1-28 on p. 48.

## Multiplying Fractions

To multiply fractions, multiply the numerators straight across. Then multiply the denominators straight across.

Reduce the answer to its simplest terms.

**EXAMPLES**

$$\frac{1}{2} \times \frac{1}{4} = \frac{1}{8} \qquad\qquad \frac{1}{4} \times \frac{1}{2} = \frac{1}{8}$$

$$\frac{1}{4} \times \frac{2}{3} = \frac{2}{12} = \frac{1}{6} \qquad\qquad \frac{2}{3} \times \frac{1}{4} = \frac{2}{12} = \frac{1}{6}$$

$$\frac{1}{4} \times \frac{4}{5} = \frac{4}{20} = \frac{1}{5} \qquad\qquad \frac{1}{100} \times \frac{1}{100} = \frac{1}{10{,}000}$$

▲ **Cultural Note**

In some countries, the word *of* is used instead of *times* for multiplication of fractions. It might be simpler to understand multiplication of fractions by substituting the word *of* for *times*. For example, $\frac{1}{2}$ of 4 is 2, $\frac{1}{2}$ of $\frac{1}{4}$ is $\frac{1}{8}$, and $\frac{1}{4}$ of $\frac{1}{2}$ is $\frac{1}{8}$.

➤ The answer will be the same regardless of the order of the fractions.

**Q:** *Ask Yourself*

**A:** *My Answer*

**1** If you divided $\frac{1}{4}$ in half, what would you have? If you divided $\frac{1}{2}$ in quarters, what would you have?

_____

**2** Could you also say that $\frac{1}{3}$ divided into quarters $= \frac{1}{12}$, or $\frac{1}{4}$ of $\frac{1}{3}$ is the same as $\frac{1}{3}$ of $\frac{1}{4}$?

_____

**3** Could you say that, when you multiply fractions, the answer becomes smaller than either of the fractions? If so, would this be a useful check when you review your answer for accuracy?

_____

For practice multiplying fractions, refer to Rapid Practice 1-29 on p. 49.

# Fraction Multiplication and Canceling Fractions

Simplification of fractions is very helpful in reducing math errors. Canceling fractions is a method of simplifying fraction *multiplication* by reducing numerators and denominators diagonally in *front* of the equals sign (the left side of the equation) by a common factor.

*Diagonal reduction* can be done only *before* the equals sign, *not* after it.

Cancellation must be on a one-for-one basis: one numerator for one denominator.

## Canceling When the Numerators and Denominators Are the Same

**EXAMPLES**

$$\frac{\overset{1}{\cancel{2}}}{3} \times \frac{1}{\underset{1}{\cancel{2}}} \times \frac{5}{7} = \frac{5}{21}$$

A numerator and denominator of 2 are the same. They cancel each other out.

## Canceling When the Numerators and Denominators Are *Not* the Same but Have Common Factors

**EXAMPLES**

$$\frac{1}{\underset{5}{\cancel{15}}} \times \frac{\overset{1}{\cancel{3}}}{6} = \frac{1}{30}$$

A common factor of 3 and 15 is 3.

Select only *one* numerator for *each* denominator.

In multiplication of fractions, cancel diagonally on the left side of the equation. Then reduce the answer.

Examine the differences between reduction and cancellation of fractions in the examples that follow:

| Reduction | Cancellation |
|-----------|--------------|

$$\frac{\overset{3}{\cancel{6}}}{\underset{4}{8}} = \frac{3}{4} \qquad \frac{\overset{1}{\cancel{6}}}{\underset{2}{8}} \times \frac{\overset{1}{\cancel{4}}}{\underset{2}{\cancel{12}}} = \frac{1}{4}$$

Cancellation is used to simplify math only during *multiplication* of fraction forms. *Cancellation occurs diagonally* with two or more fractions on the *left* side of the equation.

*Reduction* is *vertical.* Reduction is used in addition, subtraction, and simplification of answers.

Cancellation is used in all dimensional analysis equations to cancel units.

**1**   How would you cancel $\frac{5}{6} \times \frac{2}{15}$?

For practice with cancellation and multiplication of fractions, refer to Rapid Practice 1-30 on p. 49.

## Multiplication With Mixed Fractions

Before multiplying fractions that contain a mixed fraction, the mixed fraction must be changed to an *improper* fraction.

$$1\frac{1}{3} \times \frac{2}{5} = \frac{4}{3} \times \frac{2}{5} = \frac{8}{15}$$

$$2\frac{5}{8} \times 2\frac{1}{7} = \frac{\overset{3}{\cancel{21}}}{8} \times \frac{15}{\underset{1}{\cancel{7}}} = \frac{45}{8} = 5\frac{5}{8}$$

$$5\frac{1}{8} \times \frac{1}{8} = \frac{41}{8} \times \frac{1}{8} = \frac{41}{64}$$

Use cancellation to simplify the improper form of the fraction.

**1**   Can you multiply $1\frac{2}{5} \times \frac{2}{6}$?

For practice multiplying mixed fractions, refer to Rapid Practice 1-31 on p. 49.

## Dividing Fractions

To divide fractions, invert the dividing fraction, as shown in red in the examples on p. 34.

Proceed as for multiplication of fractions, using cancellation to simplify before multiplying.

Reduce the answer.

Dividend Divisor

$$\frac{1}{3} \div \frac{1}{7} = \frac{1}{3} \times \frac{7}{1} = \frac{7}{3} = 2\frac{1}{3}$$

How many sevenths are there in $\frac{1}{3}$?

Answer: There are $2\frac{1}{3}$ sevenths in $\frac{1}{3}$.

$$\frac{4}{5} \div \frac{5}{9} = \frac{4}{5} \times \frac{9}{5} = \frac{36}{25} = 1\frac{11}{25}$$

How many times will $\frac{5}{9}$ go into $\frac{4}{5}$?

Answer: $1\frac{11}{25}$.

$$\frac{1}{4} \div \frac{1}{8} = \frac{1}{4} \times \frac{8}{1} = \frac{2}{1} = 2$$

How many eighths are there in $\frac{1}{4}$?

Answer: There are 2 eighths in $\frac{1}{4}$.

➤ The most common error is to invert the dividend instead of the *dividing fraction*, the *divisor* (e.g., $\frac{1}{4} \div \frac{1}{8} = \frac{4}{1} \times \frac{1}{8} = \frac{1}{32}$).

Cancellation can be used to simplify during the multiplication process.

**Q: Ask Yourself**

**1** Which fraction is inverted in division of fractions: the dividend or the divisor?

_____

**A: My Answer**

**2** Which is the simplest fraction operation: addition, subtraction, multiplication, or division? Why?

_____

**3** Can I divide $\frac{8}{9}$ by $\frac{3}{16}$?

_____

For practice in division of fractions, refer to Rapid Practice 1-32 on p. 49.

# Percentages

**✳ Mnemonic**

To remember the 100 divisor, it might be helpful to view a % as a "jumbled" 100.

Percent means parts per 100. Percentages reflect the numerator of a fraction that has a denominator of 100. A percentage is the ratio of a number to 100. For example, $50\% = \frac{50}{100}$ $\left(\frac{1}{2}\right)$ or 50:100 or 0.5, and $2\% = \frac{2}{100}$ or 2:100 $\left(\frac{1}{50}\right)$ or 0.02.

**FAQ** | *Why do nurses need to learn percentages?*

**ANSWER:** Percentages may appear in orders for dilution of nutritional formulas for babies and adults as well as solutions such as those used for wound irrigations.

## Changing a Fraction to a Percentage

To change a *fraction* to a *percentage, multiply* the fraction by 100 and add a percent sign to the answer, as shown in the examples that follow.

It is helpful to remember one easy example, such as 50% and its fraction and decimal equivalents ($\frac{1}{2}$ and 0.5) when you work with other percentage conversions.

$$\frac{1}{2} \times 100 = \frac{100}{2} = 50\%$$

$$\frac{2}{3} \times 100 = \frac{200}{3} = 66\frac{2}{3}\%$$

$$\frac{1}{8} \times 100 = \frac{100}{8} = 12\frac{1}{2}\%$$

1   Can you write the fraction $\frac{1}{5}$ as a percentage?

CHAPTER 1

Q: *Ask Yourself*

A: *My Answer*

_____

## Changing a Percentage to a Fraction

To change a percentage to a fraction, *divide* the percentage by a denominator of 100. Reduce the fraction. Eliminate the percent sign.

> $$50\% = 50 \div 100 = \frac{1}{2}$$
> $$66\frac{2}{3}\% = 66\frac{2}{3} \div 100 = \frac{2}{3}$$
> $$75\% = 75 \div 100 = \frac{3}{4}$$

**EXAMPLES**

A percentage is just another form of a fraction. It has a denominator of 100.

1   What root word gives you the clue that, when working with percentages and conversions of percentages, you always use the number 100?

Q: *Ask Yourself*

A: *My Answer*

_____

For practice converting percentages and fractions, refer to Rapid Practice 1-33 on p. 50.

## Changing a Decimal to a Percentage

To change a decimal to a percentage, multiply the decimal by 100 by moving the decimal point two places to the right and adding a percent sign. Remember: whenever percentages are involved, the number 100 is involved.

Retain the decimal point if there are numbers remaining after the decimal point (e.g., $0.003 = 0.3\%$).

Eliminate the decimal point and subsequent zeros if there are no numbers higher than zero remaining after the decimal point (e.g., $0.590 = 59\%$).

Examine the following examples. Note that the decimal point placement is the starting point when changing a decimal to a percentage.

| | | | | |
|---|---|---|---|---|
| $0.45 = 45\%$ | $0.459 = 45.9\%$ | $0.20 = 20\%$ | $1.23 = 123\%$ | **EXAMPLES** |
| $0.3 = 30\%$ | $0.03 = 3\%$ | $0.003 = 0.3\%$ | $0.019 = 1.9\%$ | |

You are moving the decimal point two places to the right.

Again, do not forget to insert the *leading zero* in front of any decimal that does not have a whole number accompanying it, so that the reader will know there is a decimal to follow.

# Changing a Percentage to a Decimal

To change a percentage to a decimal, *divide* the percentage by 100 by moving the decimal point or implied decimal point two places to the left.

Insert zeros as placeholders and leading zeros where needed.

Remove the percent sign, and eliminate trailing zeros.

| EXAMPLES | 25% = 0.25 | 38% = 0.38 | 96% = 0.96 | 1.25% = 0.0125 | 5.9% = 0.059 |

0.059 has a leading zero in front of the decimal point and a zero placeholder after the decimal point.

**Q: Ask Yourself**

**A: My Answer**

1   Can a percentage contain a decimal?

_____

2   Write an example of a decimal that has more than two places so that it still has a decimal point after it has been converted to a percentage. (See the examples above.)

_____

3   Can you convert 3.8% to a decimal by moving the decimal place?

_____

4   Can you convert 0.15 to a percentage by moving the decimal place?

_____

For practice converting percentages and decimals, refer to Rapid Practice 1-34 on p. 50.

1   Can you convert the fraction $\frac{1}{6}$ to a decimal and to a percentage?

**Q: Ask Yourself**

**A: My Answer**

_____

For practice converting fractions, decimals, and percentages, refer to Rapid Practice 1-35 on p. 50.

# Calculating the Percentage of a Whole Number

Change the percentage to a decimal (by dividing by 100) by moving the decimal point two places to the left. Then multiply the result by the number.

| EXAMPLES | 200% of 35 |
|---|---|
| | 2.00 × 35 = 70 (no decimals in answer) |

➤ Trailing zeros are eliminated after decimals.

| EXAMPLES | % | % to Decimal | Number | Result | |
|---|---|---|---|---|---|
| | 5% of 25 | 0.05 | × 25 = | 1.25 | (2 decimal places in answer) |
| | 20% of 80 | 0.20 | × 80 = | 16.00 | (2 zeros because 20 and 80 each have 1 zero to carry to answer) |
| | 1.25% of 50 | 0.0125 | × 50 = | 0.0625 | (4 decimal places in answer) |

# Constants

A constant is a number or quantity that does *not* change. It can be used to simplify such calculations as intravenous flow rates.

> To change dimes to dollars, divide by the constant 10.
>
> To change pounds to kilograms, divide by the constant 2.2.
>
> Calculating percentages involves using the numerical constant 100.

**EXAMPLES**

**1**   What is the constant used to change inches to feet?

_____

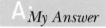

# Finding Unit Values and Totals

When performing calculations, comprehension is increased and the margin of error decreased if numbers can be simplified. If we buy more than one of something, we want to know the cost of each unit. Stores now assist us in comparing the value of similar products more quickly by posting the unit price on many items. If we pay $40 to fill our car's tank with gas, we usually are interested in the price *per* gallon: the unit price.

One of the common needs in medication math calculation is to find the value of *one part* of the whole of something. The math is very simple.

To find the unit value, divide the total by the number of units.

> What is the cost of *each pencil?*
>
> 4 *pencils* for $1 or 25 cents *per* (1) unit ($1.00 ÷ 4)
>
> How many dollars are earned *per hour?*
>
> $200 *every 8 hours* = $25.00 *each* hour ($200 ÷ 8)

**EXAMPLES**

**Test Tip:** The unit and number in the question following "each" or "per" one unit become the divisor. The unit quantity in relation to another quantity expresses a *ratio* (e.g., $200 dollars/8 hr; give 3 ounces/hr).

Drug concentrations are also expressed as ratios, for example, 100 milligrams/ tablet, 10 grams/ vial, or 15 milligrams/ milliliter.

**1**   An intravenous solution contains 500 mg/ 1000 mL. How many *milligrams per milliliter* are in the solution?

_____

**Q:** *Ask Yourself*

**A:** *My Answer*

# Finding the Total Value

Determine the unit value.

Multiply the unit value by the total quantity.

Problem: 4 cups cost $1. How much will 16 cups cost?
Solution: Each unit costs $0.25. 0.25 × 16 = $4.00 total cost.

Problem: You earn $30 an hour. If you work 90 hr in two weeks, how much will you earn?
Solution: $30 × 90 = $2700.

Problem: You walk 30 miles per week. How many miles will you walk in a month?
Solution: 30 × 4 = 120 miles.

**Q** Ask Yourself

**1** If a patient averages a urine output of 60 mL/ hr, what will the output for 8 hours be?

**A** My Answer

_____

For practice calculating unit and total values, refer to Rapid Practice 1-36 on p. 51.

## Equations

*Equations* describe an *equal* relationship between two mathematical expressions. The expressions on both sides of the equals sign are equivalent when solved. The equation is said to be balanced.

**EXAMPLES**

$1 + 1 = 2$ $\qquad$ $3 - 2 = 1$ $\qquad$ $\frac{3}{1} = 3$ $\qquad$ $4 \times 5 = 20$ $\qquad$ $\frac{1}{2} \times \frac{1}{4} = \frac{1}{8}$

$$\frac{1}{2} \div \frac{1}{4} = \frac{1}{2} \times \frac{4}{1} = 2$$

**Q** Ask Yourself

**1** Can you write and solve an equation to express the sum of 10 and 8?

_____

**A** My Answer

**2** Can you write and solve an equation to express the product of $\frac{1}{2}$ and $\frac{1}{4}$?

_____

**3** Can you write and solve an equation to express the square of 4?

_____

## RAPID PRACTICE 1-1 Interpreting Symbols

**Estimated completion time: 5 minutes** **Answers on page 500.**

**Directions:** *Circle the correct definition for the symbols.*

**Test Tips:** *Keep the initial statement (stem) of the multiple-choice test questions in mind, and as you read each choice, say to yourself, "True or false."*

*Put a mark to the right of the incorrect responses as you go through them. Marks on the right are suggested because if the answers are entered on a computer response sheet, any stray marks on the left or within the choices may cause the scanner to read them as a desired response. Eliminating wrong answer choices speeds a second review of the material if time is available.*

**1** A blood pressure goal for healthy adults is ≤120/80.

    **1.** less than                    **3.** less than or equal to
    **2.** greater than               **4.** greater than or equal to

**2** If the pulse is <50, notify the physician.

**1.** less than            **3.** less than or equal to
**2.** greater than         **4.** greater than or equal to

**3** When a blood pressure is ≥120/ 80 in an otherwise healthy adult, lifestyle changes need to be instituted.

**1.** less than            **3.** less than or equal to
**2.** greater than         **4.** greater than or equal to

**4** According to the Centers for Disease Control and Prevention (CDC), one of the characteristics of SARS disease is a temperature >100.4°F (38°C).

**1.** less than            **3.** less than or equal to
**2.** greater than         **4.** greater than or equal to

**5** Identify the symbol used for square root.

**1.** £                  **3.** $\sqrt{\phantom{x}}$
**2.** ®                **4.** ≥

*The square root symbol does not appear in handwritten medical records. It appears in dosage formulas for body surface area.*

## RAPID PRACTICE 1-2  Writing Math Symbols

**Estimated completion time: 5 minutes**   Answers on page **500.**

**Directions:** *Write in the appropriate symbol in the space provided.*

**Test Tip:** *Writing a response is another way to reinforce memory and learning for visual and kinesthetic learners. It is emphasized that the nurse will write out the definition for the symbols in the nursing notations on the medical record to avoid misinterpretation.*

**1** Inject the medicine in the baby's thigh if he has walked _____ a year. (less than)

**2** Give the patient 1 teaspoon of medicine if his age is _____ 5 years. (less than or equal to)

**3** The risk of cancer from smoking is greatly accelerated when the patient has a history of smoking _____ 20 years. (greater than or equal to)

**4** If the blood pressure is _____ 180/90, notify the physician. (greater than)

**5** The _____ symbol is used in medication math to determine body surface area for safe dosages for very powerful medicines. (square root)

## RAPID PRACTICE 1-3  Whole Numbers

**Estimated completion time: 5 minutes**   Answers on page **500.**

**Directions:** *Circle the correct equivalent for the whole number supplied.*

**1** Identify the correct location of an implied decimal point for the *whole number* 10. _____

**1.** 0.10            **3.** 1.0
**2.** 100.           **4.** 10.

**2** Identify the correct editing of decimals and trailing zeros for the number 350.000. _____

**1.** 350,000        **3.** 350
**2.** 3500           **4.** 35

**3** When a whole number such as 30 is divided by itself, the numerical result is _____

   **1.** 1                       **3.** 30

   **2.** 3                       **4.** 900

**4** Which fraction retains the value of the whole number 30? _____

   **1.** $\frac{30}{1}$                   **3.** $\frac{30}{30}$

   **2.** $\frac{30}{10}$                  **4.** $\frac{30}{1000}$

**5** What is the numerical value of 50 multiplied or divided by 1? _____

   **1.** 1                       **3.** 10

   **2.** 5                       **4.** 50

---

## RAPID PRACTICE 1-4   Whole Numbers

**Estimated completion time: 5 minutes**   **Answers on page 500.**

**Directions:** *Fill in the answers pertaining to whole numbers in the space provided.*

**1** Write the whole number 100 as a fraction without changing the value of the whole number. _____

**2** Write the whole number 100 with a decimal point in the implied decimal place. _____

**3** Edit the number 192.0200 to eliminate any trailing zeros. _____

**4** Why is it necessary to remove decimals after whole numbers and trailing zeros? _____

**5** Write a fraction that equals 1 with 100 in the numerator. _____

---

## RAPID PRACTICE 1-5   Interpreting Roman Numerals

**Estimated completion time: 3 minutes**   **Answers on page 500.**

**Directions:** *Fill in the Arabic numeral equivalent for the Roman numeral supplied.*

| Roman Numeral | Arabic Numeral |
|---|---|
| 1  XV | _____ |
| 2  XIV | _____ |
| 3  XXII | _____ |
| 4  VIII | _____ |
| 5  IV | _____ |
| 6  XLI | _____ |
| 7  LIX | _____ |
| 8  CCC | _____ |
| 9  CD | _____ |
| 10  MMM | _____ |

## RAPID PRACTICE 1-6  Writing Roman Numerals

**Estimated completion time: 5 minutes**    Answers on page **501**.

**Directions:** *Fill in the equivalent Roman numeral for the Arabic numeral supplied.*

| Arabic Numeral | Roman Numeral | Arabic Numeral | Roman Numeral |
|---|---|---|---|
| 1  10 | _____ | 6  64 | _____ |
| 2  15 | _____ | 7  14 | _____ |
| 3  30 | _____ | 8  1903 | _____ |
| 4  49 | _____ | 9  2000 | _____ |
| 5  60 | _____ | 10  44 | _____ |

## RAPID PRACTICE 1-7    Multiplication Terms

**Estimated completion time: 10 minutes**    Answers on page **501**.

**Directions:** *Multiply or factor the numbers as requested.*

1  Write the product of 10 and 4. _____

2  Write four factors of the number 12 (excluding 1 and 12). _____

3  Write the two common factors of 8 and 12 (excluding 1). _____

4  Write the product of 3 and 4. _____

5  Write the first three multiples of the number 5. _____

## RAPID PRACTICE 1-8    Division Terms

**Estimated completion time: 5 minutes**    Answers on page **501**.

**Directions:** *Identify the division terms requested:*

1  Circle the *divisor*: $20 \div 5 = 4$.

2  Circle the *quotient*: $\frac{100}{40} \div 5 = 0.5$.

3  Circle the *dividend*: $50\overline{)2000}$.

4  Circle the *divisor*: $\frac{500}{50} = 10$.

5  Circle the *remainder*: $\frac{45}{6} = 7\frac{1}{2}$.

## RAPID PRACTICE 1-9    More Multiplication Terms

**Estimated completion time: 5 minutes**    Answers on page **501**.

**Directions:** *Select the correct answer. Narrow your choices by eliminating the obviously wrong answers with a lightly penciled mark on the right of the paper.*

**Test Tip:** *Create a different type of penciled reminder if you wish a reminder to revisit a question or response.*

1  Which is a common factor of the numbers 8 and 10? _____

   **1.** $\frac{4}{5}$                       **3.** 5

   **2.** 2                           **4.** 80

**2** Which is a multiple of 36? _____

   **1.** 6                        **3.** 18

   **2.** 12                      **4.** 72

**3** What is the square of 4? _____

   **1.** 2                        **3.** 8

   **2.** 4                        **4.** 16

**4** Which is the multiplier of $8 \times \frac{1}{4}$? _____

   **1.** $\frac{1}{4}$                     **3.** 8

   **2.** 2                        **4.** 32

**5** What is the square root of 16? _____

   **1.** 2                        **3.** 6

   **2.** 4                        **4.** 256

---

## RAPID PRACTICE 1-10  Multiplication, Squares, and Division

**Estimated completion time: 5 minutes**  Answers on page **501.**

**Directions:** *Fill in the answers to the multiplication and division problems in the space provided.*

**1** Write the *product* of $3 \times 4$.            _____

**2** Write the *square* of 7 ($7^2$).            _____

**3** Write the *divisor* of $10 \div \frac{1}{2}$.        _____

**4** Identify the *dividend* in 100 divided by 10. _____

**5** Write the product of 3 and 5.          _____

## RAPID PRACTICE 1-11  Powers

**Estimated completion time: 5-10 minutes**  Answers on page **501.**

**Directions:** *Use your understanding of powers and exponents to answer the following questions:*

**1** Write $10^2$ out in the sequence to illustrate the process you would use to arrive at the answer. _____

**2** Write $2^5$ out in the sequence to illustrate the process you would use to arrive at the answer. _____

**3** Write in numerical shorthand: 10 to the eighth power. _____

**4** Which number is the base in $10^4$? _____

**5** Which number is the exponent in $10^4$? _____

## RAPID PRACTICE 1-12  Multiplying and Dividing by 10, 100, and 100

**Estimated completion time: 5-10 minutes**   Answers on page **502.**

**Directions:** *Select the correct notation for multiplication and division using mental arithmetic and moving decimal places. Narrow the field of choices by quickly eliminating the obviously wrong answers.*

**Test Tip:** *Since only the multiplier or divisor determines the number of places to move the decimal point,* first *identify the multiplier or divisor and the number of zeros in it. Then move the decimal point to the left or the right.*

1  30 multiplied by 100 = _____.
  **1.** 300
  **2.** 3,000
  **3.** 30,000
  **4.** 300,000

2  0.4 multiplied by 1000 = _____.
  **1.** 0.004
  **2.** 4
  **3.** 400
  **4.** 4,000

3  5000 divided by 100 = _____.
  **1.** 5
  **2.** 50
  **3.** 100
  **4.** 500

4  250 divided by 1000 = _____.
  **1.** 0.0025
  **2.** 0.025
  **3.** 0.25
  **4.** 2.55

5  1500 divided by 100 = _____.
  **1.** 0.15
  **2.** 1.5
  **3.** 15
  **4.** 150

## RAPID PRACTICE 1-13  Multiplying and Dividing by 10, 100, and 1000

**Estimated completion time: 10 minutes**   Answers on page **502.**

**Directions:** *Fill in the answer in the table by moving decimal points to the left for division and to the right for multiplication.*

| Number | ÷ 10 | ÷ 100 | ÷ 1000 | Number | × 10 | × 100 | × 1000 |
|--------|------|-------|--------|--------|------|-------|--------|
| 1  50 | _____ | _____ | _____ | 6  0.125 | _____ | _____ | _____ |
| 2  125 | _____ | _____ | _____ | 7  0.5 | _____ | _____ | _____ |
| 3  10 | _____ | _____ | _____ | 8  0.25 | _____ | _____ | _____ |
| 4  250 | _____ | _____ | _____ | 9  0.005 | _____ | _____ | _____ |
| 5  1000 | _____ | _____ | _____ | 10  0.1 | _____ | _____ | _____ |

**RAPID PRACTICE 1-14**  Reading Decimal Numbers

**Estimated completion time: 5 minutes**   Answers on page **502.**

**Directions:** *Write the following decimals in fraction notation.*

1  0.5   $\frac{5}{10}$

2  0.003 _____

3  0.25 _____

4  1.56 _____

5  2.0345 _____

**RAPID PRACTICE 1-15**  Reading Decimal Fractions

**Estimated completion time: 5-10 minutes**   Answers on page **502.**

**Directions:** *Write the decimal fractions in decimal form.*

1  $\frac{25}{100}$ _____

2  $\frac{2}{10}$ _____

3  $\frac{25}{1000}$ _____

4  $\frac{4}{10}$ _____

5  $\frac{5}{100}$ _____

6  $\frac{15}{100}$ _____

7  $\frac{6}{10}$ _____

8  $\frac{10}{100}$ _____

9  $\frac{4}{100}$ _____

10  $\frac{5}{1000}$ _____

**RAPID PRACTICE 1-16**  Comparing Decimal Values

**Estimated completion time: 5-10 minutes**   Answers on page **502.**

**Directions:** *Circle the* larger-value *decimal in each pair:*

**Test Tip:** *Examine the place value of the denominators (e.g., tenths, hundredths, and thousandths), and read them as decimal fractions. Do not reduce to lowest terms.*

1  0.3 and 0.03

2  1.24 and 1.32

3  0.01 and 0.005

4  0.6 and 0.16

5  0.5 and 0.25

6  0.0006 and 0.006

7  0.01 and 0.05

8  0.05 and 0.5

9  1.06 and 1.009

10  0.1 and 0.5

**RAPID PRACTICE 1-17**  Reading and Writing Decimal Numbers in Fraction Form

**Estimated completion time: 5 minutes**   Answers on page **503.**

**Directions:** *Write the decimal in fraction notation. Do not reduce to lowest terms.*

1  0.8 _____

2  0.35 _____

3  0.005 _____

4  1.25 _____

5  3.5 _____

6  0.25 _____

7  0.015 _____

8  0.9 _____

9  2.08 _____

10  0.0004 _____

## RAPID PRACTICE 1-18   Rounding Decimal Numbers

**Estimated completion time: 5 minutes**   Answers on page **503.**

**Directions:** *Round to the desired approximate value in the space provided:*

**1** Round to the nearest *tenth.*

   **1.** 0.34 _____

   **2.** 1.27 _____

   **3.** 0.788 _____

   **4.** 1.92 _____

   **5.** 0.06 _____

**3** Round to the nearest *whole* number.

   **1.** 2.38 _____

   **2.** 10.643 _____

   **3.** 0.9 _____

   **4.** 1.52 _____

   **5.** 3.47 _____

**2** Round to the nearest *hundredth.*

   **1.** 0.6892 _____

   **2.** 3.752 _____

   **3.** 0.888 _____

   **4.** 2.376 _____

   **5.** 0.051 _____

## RAPID PRACTICE 1-19   Multiplying Decimals

**Estimated completion time: 10 minutes**   Answers on page **503.**

**Directions:** *Multiply the numbers. Count the total decimal places and insert the decimal point in the answer.*

**1**     2
    $\times$ 0.4

**3**     0.5
    $\times$ 0.3

**5**     0.14
    $\times$ 0.0001

**2**     3.21
    $\times$ 0.02

**4**    1.5
    $\times$ 6

## RAPID PRACTICE 1-20   Division of Decimals: Placing the Decimal Point

**Estimated completion time: 10-15 minutes**   Answers on page **503.**

**Directions:** *Move the decimal points in the divisor and dividend as necessary, in contrasting ink, to illustrate the correct placement of decimal points for division, as shown in the examples on p. 23. Place the decimal point prominently in the* answer *line in the correct place. Do* not *perform the math. Add zeros as necessary as placeholders in the dividend.*

**1** $4\overline{)10}$

**5** $0.025\overline{)0.1}$

**8** $2.6\overline{)4.003}$

**2** $3.05\overline{)20.32}$

**6** $0.1\overline{)0.5}$

**9** $0.04\overline{)2.1}$

**3** $0.25\overline{)100}$

**7** $9\overline{)12.035}$

**10** $0.125\overline{)2.5}$

**4** $1.2\overline{)5.06}$

## RAPID PRACTICE 1-21 Dividing Decimals

**Estimated completion time: 10-15 minutes**   Answers on page **504.**

**Directions:** *Perform the division. Do not use a calculator.*

**Test Tip.** *Move the decimal points and place the decimal point prominently in the answer* before *proceeding with the division.*

1  $5\overline{)20.5}$

3  $0.02\overline{)0.03}$

5  $250\overline{)200}$

2  $0.5\overline{)20.5}$

4  $4\overline{)1}$

## RAPID PRACTICE 1-22 Basic Fraction Vocabulary

**Estimated completion time: 5 minutes**   Answers on page **504.**

**Directions:** *Identify the appropriate terms and forms for the fractions.*

1  Identify the numerator of $\frac{5}{8}$. _____

   **1.** 1

   **2.** 5

   **3.** 8

   **4.** 40

2  Identify the denominator of $\frac{2}{6}$. _____

   **1.** 1

   **2.** 2

   **3.** 3

   **4.** 6

3  Identify the improper fraction. _____

   **1.** $\frac{1}{2}$

   **2.** $1\frac{1}{3}$

   **3.** $10\frac{1}{2}$

   **4.** $\frac{11}{2}$

4  Identify the correct conversion of an improper fraction to a mixed fraction. _____

   **1.** $\frac{1}{4} = \frac{4}{16}$

   **2.** $\frac{4}{3} = 1\frac{1}{3}$

   **3.** $\frac{21}{2} = 10\frac{1}{21}$

   **4.** $\frac{11}{3} = 33\frac{1}{3}\%$

5  Identify the correct conversion of a mixed fraction to an improper fraction. _____

   **1.** $\frac{1}{2} = \frac{4}{8}$

   **2.** $5\frac{1}{2} = \frac{11}{2}$

   **3.** $2\frac{1}{4} = 2\frac{2}{8}$

   **4.** $\frac{1}{3} = 1:3$

## RAPID PRACTICE 1-23 Reducing Fractions

**Estimated completion time: 5 minutes**   Answers on page **504.**

**Directions:** *Identify the correctly reduced fraction.*

**Test Tip:** *Put a light "X" to the right to the obviously incorrect answers.*

1  $\frac{4}{8}$ can be reduced to _____.

   **1.** $\frac{8}{4}$

   **2.** $\frac{2}{3}$

   **3.** $\frac{1}{2}$

   **4.** $\frac{8}{16}$

2  $\frac{100}{500}$ can be reduced to _____.

   **1.** $\frac{100}{250}$

   **2.** $\frac{10}{25}$

   **3.** $\frac{2}{5}$

   **4.** $\frac{1}{5}$

**3** $\frac{25}{75}$ can be reduced to which lowest terms? _____

   **1.** $\frac{1}{4}$                  **3.** $\frac{2}{3}$

   **2.** $\frac{1}{3}$                  **4.** $\frac{5}{25}$

**4** The lowest terms for the fraction $\frac{15}{26}$ are _____.

   **1.** $\frac{3}{13}$                  **3.** $\frac{15}{26}$

   **2.** $\frac{5}{26}$                  **4.** $\frac{30}{52}$

**5** The lowest terms for the fraction $\frac{1}{12}$ are _____.

   **1.** $\frac{1}{12}$                  **3.** $\frac{2}{24}$

   **2.** $\frac{2}{6}$                  **4.** $\frac{3}{36}$

---

## RAPID PRACTICE 1-24 Finding the LCD

**Estimated completion time: 15 minutes**   Answers on page **504.**

**Directions:** *Calculate the LCD for the fractions supplied.*

**Test Tip:** *Since the LCD cannot be smaller than the largest denominator, start by examining the largest denominator to see if the smaller denominator or denominators divide the largest denominator evenly.*

**1** $\frac{1}{3}$, $\frac{1}{9}$, and $\frac{1}{18}$ _____     **4** $\frac{1}{10}$ and $\frac{1}{25}$ _____

**2** $\frac{1}{5}$ and $\frac{2}{6}$ _____     **5** $\frac{1}{100}$, $\frac{1}{50}$, and $\frac{1}{200}$ _____

**3** $\frac{1}{2}$, $\frac{1}{3}$, and $\frac{1}{4}$ _____

---

## RAPID PRACTICE 1-25 Creating Equivalent Fractions

**Estimated completion time: 5-10 minutes**   Answers on page **504.**

**Directions:** *Using the common factor supplied, create an equivalent fraction.*

| Fraction | Common Factor | Equivalent Fraction |
|---|---|---|
| **1** $\frac{1}{3}$ | 2 | _____ |
| **2** $\frac{4}{5}$ | 3 | _____ |
| **3** $\frac{1}{2}$ | 4 | _____ |
| **4** $\frac{3}{4}$ | 2 | _____ |
| **5** $\frac{3}{8}$ | 3 | _____ |

## RAPID PRACTICE 1-26 Comparing Fraction Sizes

**Estimated completion time: 5-10 minutes**   Answers on page **505.**

**Directions:** *Circle the greater fraction in the pairs by calculating the LCD and creating equivalent fractions with common denominators.*

| Fractions | LCD | Equivalent Fractions | Result |
|---|---|---|---|
| 1  $\frac{3}{7}$ and $\frac{1}{2}$ | 14 | $\frac{6}{14}$ and $\frac{7}{14}$ | $\frac{1}{2}$ is larger |
| 2  $\frac{1}{8}$ and $\frac{2}{24}$ | _____ | _____ | _____ |
| 3  $\frac{1}{100}$ and $\frac{1}{200}$ | _____ | _____ | _____ |
| 4  $\frac{4}{5}$ and $\frac{5}{6}$ | _____ | _____ | _____ |
| 5  $\frac{1}{250}$ and $\frac{4}{50}$ | _____ | _____ | _____ |

## RAPID PRACTICE 1-27 Adding Fractions

**Estimated completion time: 10 minutes**   Answers on page **505.**

**Directions:** *Find the LCD, and create equivalent fractions if necessary. Add the fractions, as indicated. Reduce the answer to its lowest terms.*

1   $\begin{array}{r} \frac{1}{2} \\ +\ \frac{1}{2} \\ \hline \end{array}$
3   $\begin{array}{r} \frac{4}{8} \\ +\ \frac{1}{3} \\ \hline \end{array}$
5   $\begin{array}{r} \frac{2}{3} \\ +\ \frac{1}{4} \\ \hline \end{array}$

2   $\begin{array}{r} \frac{1}{2} \\ +\ \frac{1}{4} \\ \hline \end{array}$
4   $\begin{array}{r} \frac{6}{8} \\ +\ \frac{3}{5} \\ \hline \end{array}$

## RAPID PRACTICE 1-28 Subtracting Fractions

**Estimated completion time: 15 minutes**   Answers on page **505.**

**Directions:** *Identify the LCD. Create an equivalent fraction. Reduce the answer to its lowest terms.*

| Fraction | LCD | Answer | Fraction | LCD | Answer |
|---|---|---|---|---|---|
| 1  $\begin{array}{r} 1\frac{1}{2} \\ -\ \frac{1}{2} \\ \hline \end{array}$ | | | 4  $\begin{array}{r} 10\frac{1}{4} \\ -\ 4\frac{5}{8} \\ \hline \end{array}$ | | |
| 2  $\begin{array}{r} \frac{3}{5} \\ -\ \frac{1}{2} \\ \hline \end{array}$ | | | 5  $\begin{array}{r} 4\frac{1}{20} \\ -\ 3\frac{7}{20} \\ \hline \end{array}$ | | |
| 3  $\begin{array}{r} 1\frac{1}{6} \\ -\ \frac{3}{4} \\ \hline \end{array}$ | | | | | |

## RAPID PRACTICE 1-29 Multiplying Fractions

**Estimated completion time 10-15 minutes**   Answers on page **505.**

**Directions:** *Multiply the following fractions. Reduce the answer to its lowest terms.*

1  $\frac{1}{3} \times \frac{1}{9} =$ _____

2  $\frac{1}{2} \times \frac{3}{4} =$ _____

3  $\frac{2}{5} \times \frac{1}{6} =$ _____

4  $\frac{1}{100} \times \frac{1}{250} =$ _____

5  $\frac{9}{10} \times \frac{3}{5} =$ _____

## RAPID PRACTICE 1-30 Cancellation and Multiplication of Fractions

**Estimated completion time: 10-15 minutes**   Answers on page **506.**

**Directions:** *Multiply the following fractions using cancellation to simplify the process.*

1  $\frac{1}{2} \times \frac{6}{8} =$ _____

2  $\frac{2}{3} \times \frac{3}{2} =$ _____

3  $\frac{3}{5} \times \frac{5}{6} =$ _____

4  $\frac{4}{5} \times \frac{10}{12} =$ _____

5  $\frac{100}{200} \times \frac{200}{250} =$ _____

## RAPID PRACTICE 1-31 Multiplication of Mixed Fractions

**Estimated completion time: 20 minutes**   Answers on page **506.**

**Directions:** *Multiply the fractions* after *changing mixed fractions in the equation to improper fraction. Cancel if appropriate. Reduce the answer to its lowest terms:*

1  $\frac{1}{4} \times 1\frac{1}{4} =$ _____

2  $3\frac{1}{6} \times 1\frac{1}{3} =$ _____

3  $2\frac{1}{2} \times \frac{1}{2} =$ _____

4  $\frac{1}{5} \times 4\frac{1}{3} =$ _____

5  $\frac{1}{6} \times 2\frac{1}{8} =$ _____

## RAPID PRACTICE 1-32 Division of Fractions

**Estimated completion time: 10 minutes**   Answers on page **506.**

**Directions:** *Divide the following fractions* after *converting any mixed fractions to improper fraction. Reduce the answer to its lowest terms.*

1  $\frac{1}{2} \div \frac{1}{6}$

2  $\frac{1}{3} \div \frac{1}{8}$

3  $\frac{2}{5} \div \frac{1}{4}$

4  $1\frac{1}{4} \div \frac{1}{4}$

5  $2\frac{1}{2} \div \frac{1}{2}$

## RAPID PRACTICE 1-33 Converting Fractions and Percentages

**Estimated completion time: 15-20 minutes**   Answers on page **506.**

**Directions:** *Change the fractions to percentages. Round the answer to the nearest tenth. Change the percentages to a fraction. Reduce the answer to its lowest terms.*

| Fraction | Percentage | Percentage | Fraction |
|---|---|---|---|
| 1 $\frac{1}{4}$ | _____ | 6  10% | _____ |
| 2 $\frac{3}{4}$ | _____ | 7  15% | _____ |
| 3 $\frac{1}{6}$ | _____ | 8  50% | _____ |
| 4 $\frac{1}{3}$ | _____ | 9  $12\frac{1}{2}$% | _____ |
| 5 $\frac{5}{6}$ | _____ | 10  25% | _____ |

## RAPID PRACTICE 1-34 Converting Decimals and Percentages by Moving Decimal Points

**Estimated completion time: 10 minutes**   Answers on page **507.**

**Directions:** *Calculate the decimal or percentage by moving the decimal points two places to the left or right as needed.*

| Percentage | Decimal | Decimal | Percentage |
|---|---|---|---|
| 1  1% | 0.01____ | 6  0.1 | 10%____ |
| 2  35% | _____ | 7  0.05 | _____ |
| 3  75% | _____ | 8  0.125 | _____ |
| 4  5.5% | _____ | 9  0.0525 | _____ |
| 5  200% | _____ | 10  0.5 | _____ |

## RAPID PRACTICE 1-35 Converting Fractions, Decimals, and Percentages

**Estimated completion time: 15 minutes**   Answers on page **507.**

**Directions:** *Examine the example in the first row. Fill in the table with the requested numbers.*

**Test Tip:** *Make equivalent fraction have a denominator with a power of ten.*

| Fraction | Decimal | Percent |
|---|---|---|
| $\frac{1}{4} = \frac{25}{100}$ | 0.25____ | 25%____ |
| 1 $\frac{2}{10}$____ | _____ | _____ |
| 2 _____ | 1.5____ | _____ |
| 3 _____ | _____ | 75%____ |
| 4 $\frac{1}{5}$____ | _____ | _____ |
| 5 _____ | 0.6____ | _____ |

## RAPID PRACTICE 1-36 Finding Unit and Total Values

**Estimated completion time: 15 minutes**   Answers on page **507.**

**Directions:** *Examine the worked-out first problem and calculate the unit values requested.*

1  You worked 20 hours this week. This week's gross paycheck is $600. How many *dollars per hour* did you earn?

Answer: $\frac{\$600}{20 \text{ hr}}$ = $30 per hour (the question asks for dollars *per hour*, which indicates that the divisor will be *20 hours*)

2  The patient has a water pitcher that contains 960 mL or 4 cups of water. How many mL (milliliters) of water per cup does the pitcher contain?

_____

3  Your car runs 300 miles on a tank of gas. The tank holds 12 gallons. How many miles per gallon does your car drive?

_____

4  Your computer has 6000 megabytes of memory storage. This equals 6 gigabytes. How many megabytes are there in 1 gigabyte?

_____

5  You are on a diet that is limited to 80 g of carbohydrate daily. This amounts to 320 calories of carbohydrates. How many *calories* are there in each gram of carbohydrate?

_____

## CHAPER 1 MULTIPLE-CHOICE REVIEW

Answers on page **507.**

**Directions:** *Circle the correct answer.*

1  Interpret the symbol on a label of medicine in the following sentence: For children ≥ age 3 years, give 2 teaspoons of the medicine.

**1.** less than                    **3.** less than or equal to
**2.** greater than                 **4.** greater than or equal to

2  Identify the statement that describes a whole number that does not change in value.

**1.** a whole number divided by itself
**2.** a whole number divided or multiplied by 1
**3.** a whole number multiplied by itself
**4.** a whole number from which 1 is added or subtracted

3  Multiples of 50 are:

**1.** 5, 10, 15                    **3.** 5, 10, 20, 50
**2.** 10, 20, 30, 40               **4.** 100, 150, 200

4  Factors of 30 include:

**1.** 60, 90, 120                  **3.** 3 and 0
**2.** 3, 5, 8                      **4.** 1, 10, 15

5  Common factors of 15 and 30 include:

**1.** 1, 3, 5, 15                  **3.** 3, 6, 10
**2.** 10, 15, 30                   **4.** 1, 2, 30

6 Five hundredths is written in decimal form as:

  **1.** 0.5                                      **3.** 0.005
  **2.** 0.05                                    **4.** 5.00

7 Identify 5% as a decimal.

  **1.** 0.0005                             **3.** 0.05
  **2.** 0.005                              **4.** 0.5

8 Identify 2.5% as a fraction.

**Test Tip:** *Change the percentage to a decimal first.*

  **1.** $\frac{25}{100}$                             **3.** $\frac{2.5}{100}$
  **2.** $\frac{25}{1000}$                           **4.** $\frac{0.025}{1000}$

9 If you were going to give one tenth of 0.01 milliliters of a certain amount of medication, how much would you give?

  **1.** 0.0001                            **3.** 0.1
  **2.** 0.001                             **4.** 1

10 A fraction equivalent to $\frac{4}{5}$ is

  **1.** $\frac{2}{3}$                               **3.** $\frac{8}{10}$
  **2.** $1\frac{1}{5}$                             **4.** $1\frac{1}{4}$

11 Identify the improper fraction.

  **1.** $\frac{1}{8}$                               **3.** $2\frac{1}{3}$
  **2.** $\frac{6}{5}$                               **4.** $\frac{100}{200}$

12 The fraction $\frac{10}{15}$ can be reduced to which lowest terms?

  **1.** $\frac{2}{3}$                               **3.** $\frac{24}{30}$
  **2.** $\frac{3}{5}$                               **4.** $\frac{100}{150}$

13 Find the sum of $1\frac{1}{3}$ and $\frac{1}{5}$.

  **1.** $1\frac{1}{15}$                             **3.** $1\frac{8}{15}$
  **2.** $2\frac{1}{8}$                             **4.** $2\frac{2}{5}$

14 Identify the multiplier in the problem $5 \times 100$:

  **1.** 5                                     **3.** 100
  **2.** 20                                    **4.** 500

15 The product of $\frac{1}{2}$ and 3 is:

  **1.** $3\frac{1}{2}$                             **3.** $1\frac{1}{2}$
  **2.** $\frac{1}{2}$                               **4.** 10

16 $\frac{1}{8} \div \frac{1}{2} =$

  **1.** $\frac{1}{16}$                             **3.** $\frac{2}{16}$
  **2.** $\frac{1}{4}$                               **4.** $\frac{2}{8}$

17 Which is a definition of cancellation of fractions?

  **1.** Changing mixed whole numbers and fractions to improper fractions
  **2.** Reducing fraction answers to the lowest terms
  **3.** Diagonal reduction of fractions in fraction multiplication
  **4.** Converting fractions to percentages

18 The square of 4 is:

**Test Tip:** *Distinguish* square root *from* square.

**1.** 1                                   **3.** 4
**2.** 2                                   **4.** 16

19 The sequence for writing out $10^3$ would be:

**1.** $10 \times 3$                       **3.** $3 \times 3 \times 3$
**2.** $3 \times 10$                       **4.** $10 \times 10 \times 10$

20 If a package of medicine cups costing $20 contains 40 cups, what is the unit value per cup?

**1.** $0.50                              **3.** $20
**2.** $2.00                              **4.** $80

## CHAPTER 1 FINAL PRACTICE

**Answers on page 508.**

**Directions:** *Supply the answer in the space provided.*

**Test Tip:** *Answer the easiest questions first. The easier questions will boost your confidence and, it is hoped, increase relaxation and jog memory for more complex processes.*

1  The nurse looks up an unfamiliar medication in a current pharmacology reference. It says that, for children <2 years, the physician should be consulted for dosage. Write out the meaning of the symbol. _____

2  Formulas for medications based on body surface area require that a square root be obtained. Write out the symbol that illustrates the square root of 9.
_____

3  Fill in the symbol found in many laboratory reports indicating that a total cholesterol level ≥200 is abnormal. _____

4  Write the whole number 85 as a fraction *without* changing the value. _____

5  Write the whole number 85 with a decimal point in the *implied* decimal place for whole numbers. _____

6  Edit the trailing zeros in the following whole number to avoid misinterpretation: 500.00. _____

7  Use the whole number 500 to write a fraction that equals the number 1.
_____

8  Write the Arabic numeral for XV. _____

9  Write the Roman numeral for 16. _____

10 Write the *sum* of 8 and 7. _____

11 Write the *product* of 8 and 7. _____

12 Write all the *factors* of the number 12. _____

13 Write the *common factors* of the numbers 10 and 20. (Do not include 1.) _____

14 Write a multiple of both 4 and 3. _____

**15** Write 3 *multiples* of the number 5. _____

**16** Which number is the *multiplier* in $8 \times \frac{1}{2}$? _____

**17** Write $10^4$ out to illustrate the sequence you would use to calculate the result. _____

**18** Write the *square* of 12. _____

**19** Write the *square root* of 100. _____

**20** Which number is the *base* in $10^8$. _____

**21** Which number is the exponent in $10^8$? _____

**22** Write *3 divided by 4* as a fraction. _____

**23** Label the numerator and denominator in $\frac{7}{8}$ _____

**24** Which is a decimal fraction: $\frac{1}{100}$ or $\frac{2}{3}$? _____

**25** Write out 0.114 as if it were being read or spoken. _____

**26** Which is larger: 0.089 or 0.42? _____

**27** Divide 125.9 by 100 by moving the decimal place. _____

**28** Multiply 8.03 by 1000 by moving the decimal place. _____

**29** Round 0.893 to the *nearest* tenth. _____

**30** Round 0.012 to the *nearest* hundredth. _____

**31** Round 50.389 to the *nearest* whole number. _____

**32** Write the decimal 0.5 as a fraction in simplest terms. _____

**33** Change 0.025 to a fraction. _____

**34** Change $\frac{5}{100}$ to a decimal. _____

**35** Multiply $0.1 \times 2.32$. _____

**36** Divide 20 by 5.9. _____

**37** Which is greater: $\frac{1}{8}$ or $\frac{1}{10}$? _____

**38** Which is smaller: $\frac{1}{12}$ or $\frac{1}{15}$? _____

**39** Write the fraction $\frac{1}{100}$ as a percentage. _____

**40** Change the improper fraction $\frac{25}{4}$ to a mixed fraction. _____

**41** Change the mixed fraction $1\frac{1}{6}$ to an improper fraction. _____

**42** Find the lowest common denominator (LCD) in the following group of fractions: $\frac{10}{12} + \frac{1}{3} + \frac{1}{4} =$ _____

**43** Write two equivalent fractions for $\frac{2}{3}$. _____

**44** The current pharmacology literature says, "Withhold the drug for a systolic blood pressure >180. Write out the meaning of the symbol. _____

**45** Which is greater: $\frac{4}{5}$ or $\frac{5}{6}$? _____

**46** Find the greatest common factor for the numerator and denominator: $\frac{12}{20}$. _____

**47** Reduce the fraction to its lowest terms: $\frac{15}{60}$. _____

**48** Add: $\frac{1}{2} + \frac{1}{6} + \frac{1}{8}$ _____

**49** Subtract: $\frac{1}{5} - \frac{1}{8}$ _____

**50** Multiply: $1\frac{1}{4} \times 2\frac{3}{7}$ _____

**51** Divide: $\frac{2}{3} \div \frac{1}{6}$ _____

**52** Change $\frac{3}{5}$ to a decimal and a percentage. _____

**53** Change 0.01 to a percentage and a fraction. _____

**54** There are 50 syringes in a package that costs $75. What is the unit value of a syringe? _____

**55** Write and solve an equation that reflects the product of 10 and 8. _____

## Suggestions for Further Reading

www.aaamath.com/gwpg.html
www.jcaho.org
www.math.com
www.mathworld.com
www.usp.org

  Additional information can be found on the CD

Chapter 2 teaches the basic dimensional analysis style of solving equations. This method is used throughout the text to solve and verify medication dosage calculations.

**2**

*"It isn't that they can't see the solution. It is that they can't see the problem."*

—G. K. CHESTERTON

# DIMENSIONAL ANALYSIS CALCULATIONS

## Objectives

- Examine a problem to identify the desired units for the answer.
- Examine a problem to identify the units on hand that need to be converted.
- Select and orient appropriate conversion formulas.
- Analyze the dimensional analysis (DA) setup to determine whether it will yield the desired answer units.
- Estimate answers.
- Solve basic arithmetic and simple metric medication equations using DA and units and number cancellation.
- Evaluate answers.

## Essential Prior Knowledge

Contents of Chapter 1

## Equipment

- No special equipment is needed for this chapter. Find a pencil and a quiet place.

## Estimated Time to Complete Chapter

- 1 hour

## Introduction

Derived from the sciences, DA is a simple mathematical process. It begins with the identification of the desired answer. Equations are set up and solved in fraction multiplication format according to the *units* of measurement. The learner can see at a glance if the setup is incorrect. The math is as straightforward as simple multiplication of fractions. Other names for this method are *factor analysis, factor* or *label method,* and *unit method,* reflecting the emphasis on factors, labels, and units of measurement, respectively.

It is important to have a solid foundation in basic arithmetic and equation solving so that the focus in the clinical setting can be on the patient, the written order, the medication available, and safe administration in a timely manner. The nurse needs to know how to calculate rapidly and independently and must have a thorough command of a method such as DA for verifying results and for more complex calculations.

Medication errors based on the wrong dosage can and do occur. Technical competence, including medication mathematics, is as important as communication skills when it comes to medications and treatments. The nurse cannot rely on colleagues and calculators for accuracy. The patient and employer cannot afford to wait a half-hour while the nurse refreshes math skills.

**56**

There are several advantages to learning the DA method of solving equations:

1   It is a fast, simple, organized system for setting up problems.
2   It allows the nurse to easily identify incorrect setup before calculations are carried out; a key factor in accuracy and efficiency.
3   It can be used for all medication problems, which cannot be said for all medication calculation methods.
4   An incorrect answer resulting from incorrect setup can be immediately identified.

Once the method is mastered with simpler problems, it can easily be applied to more complex dosage problems. For students who have used DA in science courses, this chapter will require only a brief review.

## ESSENTIAL Vocabulary

| | |
|---|---|
| **Conversion Formula** | An expression of *equivalent* amounts for two entities, such as 12 inches = 1 foot, 3 feet = 1 yard, 5280 feet = 1 mile, 1000 mg = 1 g, 250 mg/ 1 tablet, $20/ 1 hr, and 5 mg/ 10 mL |
| **Dimensional Analysis** | A practical scientific method used to solve mathematical equations with an emphasis on units of measurement to set up the equation. The method requires three elements: desired answer, original factors, and conversion formula or formulas. |
| **Dimension** | Unit of mass (or weight), volume, length, time, and so on, such as milligram (mass or weight), teaspoon (volume), liter (volume), meter (length), and minute (time) |
| **Equation** | Expression of an equal relationship between mathematical expressions on both sides of an equals sign, such as $2x = 4$, $3 \times 2 = 6$, and $\frac{10}{2} = 5$. When an equation is solved, the values on both sides of the equals sign have equivalent value. |
| **Factors** | In DA, the data (numbers and units) that are entered in an equation in fraction form. In general, the word *factor* denotes anything that contributes to a result. The term has different meanings in different contexts. |
| **Label** | Descriptor of type, not necessarily a unit of dimension, such as 4 eggs, 4 dozen eggs, 1 tsp Benadryl, 100 mg tablets, 2 liters of 5% dextrose in water |
| **Numerical Orientation of a Fraction Form** | Contents of the numerator (N) and denominator (D), such as $\frac{12 \text{ inches (N)}}{1 \text{ foot (D)}}$ and $\frac{1 \text{ foot (N)}}{12 \text{ inches (D)}}$ |
| **Ratio** | Relationship between two different entities, such as 10 mg/ tablet, 1 g/ capsule, and 2 boys/ 2 girls |
| **Unit\*** | Descriptor of *dimension,* such as length, weight, and volume, for example, 2 inches ointment, 3 m height, 1 qt water, 250 mg antibiotic, 2 tbs Milk of Magnesia, and 6 kg body weight. In the first example, 2 is a quantity and inches is the unit of dimension. In the last example, 6 is a quantity and kilograms is the unit of dimension. |

\*The word unit has different meanings in different contexts. Other definitions will be provided later in the text when relevant to the topic.

## RAPID PRACTICE 2-1   Essential Vocabulary Review

**Estimated completion time: 10 minutes**   Answers on page **510.**

**Directions:** *Study the vocabulary to supply the requested information.*

1   What are the three required elements of a DA-style equation? _____

2   What is the difference between a quantity and a unit? _____

3 What is a conversion formula? _____

4 In the fraction $\frac{3}{4}$, what is the numerical orientation of 3? (Is it in the numerator or the denominator?) _____

5 In the fraction $\frac{1}{8}$, what is the numerical orientation of 8? (Is it in the numerator or the denominator?) _____

**Q** *Ask Yourself*

1 How will you remember the difference between a unit and a label when both appear?

**A** *My Answer*

_____

# Required Elements of a Dimensional Analysis Equation

**Memorize:**

1 Desired answer units
2 Conversion formula or formulas (which contain the desired answer units and the units that need to be converted)
3 Original factors to convert (quantity and units)

Analyze the following simple problem and the illustrated setup: Question: How many inches are in 2 feet? Conversion formula: 12 inches = 1 foot.

1 Desired answer units are inches only.
2 Conversion formula needs to contain inches and feet: 12 inches = 1 foot. Feet need to be converted to inches. Feet will not appear in the answer.
3 Original factors to convert (quantity and units): 2 feet

With all questions in any course of study, it is a good idea to read the question initially to find out exactly what is being asked.

# The Setup of a Dimensional Analysis–Style Equation

**Memorize:** The goal of a DA equation is to take a known quantity and multiply it by one or more conversion factors to solve an equation.

Study the setup and explanations in each of the following examples and then take the next quiz.

**EXAMPLES**

Question: How many inches are there in 2 feet? Conversion formula: 12 inches = 1 foot.
➤ Identify the required elements of the DA equation:
　1 Desired answer units: inches
　2 Conversion formula: 12 inches = 1 foot (a conversion ratio that contains the desired answer unit and the unit to be converted: feet)
　3 Original factors to convert: 2 feet

These elements are multiplied in fraction form to solve the problem. Identify all the required elements of the equation. Use the following systematic approach to place the elements in an equation:

1 Enter the desired answer units after identifying the required elements.
2 Enter the selected conversion formula or formulas with the desired answer units in the numerator.

3 Enter the original factors that need to be converted.
   **a.** Cancel all unwanted units that appear in steps 2 and 3.
   **b.** Pause and check that only desired answer units remain.
4 Estimate a reasonable answer. Multiply the remaining factors to obtain the desired answer. Evaluate the answer.

Answer: Conversion Formula × Original Known Factors = Desired Answer

| Step 1 | Step 2 | Step 3 | Step 4 |
|---|---|---|---|
| Identify Desired Answer Units | Enter Conversion Formula | Enter Original Factors to Convert (Quantity plus Units) | Estimate, Multiply, Evaluate |
| | ➤ Enter the conversion formula that will change feet to inches with the desired answer units (inches) in the numerator. | ➤ Enter the factors that need to be converted (2 feet) in the numerator. | ➤ Estimate: Answer will be double the inches in 1 foot. |
| | ➤ Place the rest of the formula in the denominator (1 foot), the unit that will be converted. | ➤ Cancel the unwanted units diagonally. | ➤ Solve the equation by multiplying the factors. |
| | ➤ (Plan to cancel feet next step.) | ➤ Stop! Evaluate the equation. Are all unwanted units cancelled? Are the desired answer units the only units remaining? | ➤ Evaluate the answer. |
| ? inches = | $\dfrac{12 \text{ inches}}{1 \text{ foot}}$ | × 2 ~~feet~~ | = 24 inches |

Take the time now to analyze and evaluate the process. It will speed up comprehension and reduce errors later.

**Analysis:** Inches appear first and last in the equation (steps 1 and 4).
The numerical orientation of the conversion formula, $\frac{12 \text{ inches}}{1 \text{ foot}}$, places the desired answer units in the numerator.
The factors that contain the unwanted units, feet, appear *twice:* once in a denominator and again in a subsequent *numerator* in order to be canceled diagonally.
Check: Were the unwanted units canceled *before* the math was carried out? Yes
Check: After all remaining undesired units were canceled, were the *only* units remaining for the answer the same as those identified initially from the question (inches)? If the answer is yes, then the equation setup is complete.

**Evaluation:** The answer gives the desired *answer units*: inches.
The estimate supports the answer.
Both sides of the equation are equal (math check: 12 × 2 = 24). Therefore the equation is balanced.

**FAQ** | *Why are the units canceled before multiplying?*

**ANSWER:** This ensures a correct setup of the equation. Incorrect math setups pose problems for some students. DA permits a fast check of setup to ensure that only the desired answer units will remain in the answer. Analyzing the setup *before* multiplying is a timesaver.

**Q** *Ask Yourself*

**A** *My Answer*

1   What are the three main elements of a DA equation that must be identified before setting up an equation? (Use brief phrases, as stated in the text.)

_____

➤   In DA, the placement of units, not of numbers, guides the setup. The orientation of the conversion formula fraction is the first element to check if the answer does not make sense. Are the desired answer units in the numerator? The math is elementary fraction-style cancellation and multiplication.

Examine the following example. It includes different terms than those used in the previous example, but the process is the same.

| **EXAMPLES** | Question: How many milligrams are in 6 grams (g)? Conversion formula: 1000 mg = 1 g. |
|---|---|

Identify the required elements of the DA equation:
  **1**  Desired answer units: milligrams
  **2**  Conversion formula: $\frac{1000 \text{ mg}}{1 \text{ g}}$
  **3**  Original factors to convert: 6 g

| Step 1 | Step 2 | Step 3 | Step 4 |
|---|---|---|---|
| Identify Desired Answer Units | Enter Conversion Formula | Enter Original Factors to Convert (Include Quantity) | Estimate, Multiply, Evaluate |
| | ➤ Enter the conversion formula for grams to mg with the desired answer units (mg) in the numerator. | ➤ Enter the original factors (quantity and units) to convert (6 grams) in the numerator. | ➤ Estimate: Answer will be about 6 times the available mg. |
| | ➤ Place the rest of the formula (1 gram) in the denominator. | ➤ Cancel the unwanted units diagonally. | ➤ Solve the equation by multiplying the factors. |
| | ➤ (Plan to cancel grams next step.) | ➤ Stop! Evaluate the equation. Are all unwanted units cancelled? Are the desired answer units the only units remaining? | ➤ Evaluate the answer. |
| ? milligrams = | $\frac{1000 \text{ milligrams}}{1 \text{ gram}}$ | × 6 ~~grams~~ | = 6000 milligrams |
| | | | Answer: There are 6000 milligrams in 6 grams. This is a reasonable answer. The equation is balanced. |

Take a second look at the setup. In order to cancel undesired units, each set of undesired units (grams) must appear *twice* in the final equation. They must be in a denominator and a numerator in order to be canceled.

**FAQ** | *Does it matter in which order the data are entered in the equation?*

**ANSWER:** The order of data does not matter from a mathematical perspective. The data can be entered in any order as long as the desired answer units match up in numerical orientation and the undesired units cancel diagonally. However, the method shown is designed to reduce errors by providing a systematic approach, and many students find it easier to learn.

See the Example on p. 62 for an illustration of an incorrect setup. Eventually, after sufficient practice, a slightly shorter process will be introduced.

**FAQ** | *Which are the commonest types of errors?*

**ANSWER:** Math errors and incorrect setup of the units will result in the wrong answer.

➤ Even if the setup is correct and even if both sides of the equation are equal, the answer may be wrong. Wrong data entry and incorrect multiplication will yield a wrong answer. DA is one of the best methods of preventing a setup error, and the final math equality on both sides of the equation is very easy to prove. However, DA cannot prevent operator numerical entry errors and careless handwriting that can be misread.

# Conversion Formula Review

Conversion formulas

1   Must contain a *quantity* and a *unit of measurement* and/or a *label* (e.g., 12 inches = 1 foot, 250 mg/ 1 tablet, 10 employees/ 1 supervisor).
2   Are equivalent.
3   Are inserted in an equation in fraction form.
4   Do not change the value of the other units in the equation because they equal the number 1. (Multiplying numbers by 1 does not alter the value.)
5   Must be positioned (oriented) to match the desired answer units and permit cancellation of the unwanted units.

Note that there are *three* methods of writing a conversion formula: an equation, fraction orientation 1, and fraction orientation 2. The three ways are equivalent. For DA equations, the fraction form of conversion formulas must be used.

**EXAMPLES**

| Equation | Fraction Form 1 | Fraction Form 2 |
|---|---|---|
| 3 feet = 1 yard | $\dfrac{3\text{ feet}}{1\text{ yard}}$ | $\dfrac{1\text{ yard}}{3\text{ feet}}$ |
| 1000 mg = 1 g | $\dfrac{1000\text{ mg}}{1\text{ g}}$ | $\dfrac{1\text{ g}}{1000\text{ mg}}$ |
| 2 g/ tablet (per tablet) | $\dfrac{2\text{ g}}{1\text{ tablet}}$ | $\dfrac{1\text{ tablet}}{2\text{ g}}$ |
| $5/ box (per box) | $\dfrac{\$5}{1\text{ box}}$ | $\dfrac{1\text{ box}}{\$5}$ |
| 20 mg/ capsule (per capsule) | $\dfrac{20\text{ mg}}{1\text{ capsule}}$ | $\dfrac{1\text{ capsule}}{20\text{ mg}}$ |

> **FAQ** | *How will I know when the setup is incorrectly positioned?*
>
> **ANSWER:** The answer *does not* make sense. It does not match the *desired answer units*. Undesired units cannot be canceled.

Study the following example for incorrectly positioned units.

| EXAMPLES |
|---|

**Incorrect Setup**

Question: How many yards are in 6 feet? Conversion formula: 3 feet = 1 yard

| Step 1 | Step 2 | Step 3 | Step 4 |
|---|---|---|---|
| Identify Desired Answer Units | Enter Conversion Formula | Enter Original Factors to Convert (Include Quantity) | Estimate, Multiply, Evaluate |
| ? yards | $\dfrac{3 \text{ feet}}{1 \text{ yard}}$ | × 6 feet = | $\dfrac{18 \text{ feet squared}}{1 \text{ yard}}$ |
| | ➤ Observe that this is an incorrect set up. The desired answer units (yards) should be in the numerator. | ➤ Observe that the undesired units (feet) cannot be canceled. | ➤ The answer and the units for the answer do not make sense. The setup was not correctly positioned. |

➤ Pay attention to the desired answer units when setting up step 2. Then position the undesired units diagonally.

Rapid Practice 2-2 provides quick insight into the correct conversion formula entry.

## RAPID PRACTICE 2-2 Selecting the Correct Conversion Formula Orientation

**Estimated completion time: 5 minutes**   Answers on page **510.**

**Directions:** *Read the problem. Identify the required elements. Place a* circle *around the correctly oriented conversion formula fraction (ensuring that numerator and denominator placement* matches *the desired answer units in the numerator and permits* cancellation *of the undesired units). Evaluate your setup. Review the previous examples if necessary.* **Do not** *carry out the math to solve the equation.*

**1** How many eggs are in 10 dozen? Conversion formula: 12 eggs = 1 dozen.

| Step 1: Desired Answer Units | Step 2: Conversion Formula | Step 3: Original Factors to Convert (Quantity and Units) |
|---|---|---|
| ? eggs | $\dfrac{1 \text{ dozen}}{12 \text{ eggs}}$ *or* $\dfrac{12 \text{ eggs}}{1 \text{ dozen}}$ | 10 dozen |
| | ➤ Circle the correct conversion formula placement. | |

**2** How many kilometers are in 5 miles? Conversion formula: 1 km = 0.6 mile.

| Step 1: Desired Answer Units | Step 2: Conversion Formula | Step 3: Original Factors to Convert (Quantity and Units) |
|---|---|---|
| ? km | $\dfrac{0.6 \text{ mile}}{1 \text{ km}}$ *or* $\dfrac{1 \text{ km}}{0.6 \text{ mile}}$ | 5 miles |
| | ➤ Circle the correct conversion formula placement. | |

**3** How many quarts are in 10 gal? Conversion formula: 4 qt = 1 gal.

| Step 1:<br>Desired Answer Units | Step 2:<br>Conversion Formula | Step 3:<br>Original Factors to Convert<br>(Quantity and Units) |
| --- | --- | --- |
| ? quarts | $\dfrac{4 \text{ qt}}{1 \text{ gal}}$ or $\dfrac{1 \text{ gal}}{4 \text{ qt}}$<br><br>➤ Circle the correct con-<br>version formula placement. | 10 gal |

**4** How many seconds are in 30 minutes? Conversion formula: 60 seconds = 1 minute.

| Step 1:<br>Desired Answer Units | Step 2:<br>Conversion Formula | Step 3:<br>Original Factors to Convert<br>(Quantity and Units) |
| --- | --- | --- |
| ? seconds | $\dfrac{1 \text{ min}}{60 \text{ sec}}$ or $\dfrac{60 \text{ sec}}{1 \text{ min}}$<br><br>➤ Circle the correct con-<br>version formula placement. | 30 minutes |

**5** How many milligrams are in 2 grams? Conversion formula: 1000 mg = 1 g.

| Step 1:<br>Desired Answer Units | Step 2:<br>Conversion Formula | Step 3:<br>Original Factors to Convert<br>(Quantity and Units) |
| --- | --- | --- |
| ? mg | $\dfrac{1 \text{ g}}{1000 \text{ mg}}$ or $\dfrac{1000 \text{ mg}}{1 \text{ g}}$<br><br>➤ Circle the correct con-<br>version formula placement. | 2 grams |

The conversion formula permits the undesired units to be changed to the units for the desired answer without changing the value of the answer.

**RAPID PRACTICE 2-3** Identifying Desired Answer Units, Conversion Formulas, and Original Factors to Convert

**Estimated completion time: 10 minutes**    Answers on page **511.**

**Directions:** *Read the question, identify the required elements, and fill in the quantities and units in the space provided, as illustrated in problem 1. Select the correct conversion formula and place it with the desired answer in the numerator.* **Do not** *solve the equation. Conversion formulas: 3 feet = 1 yard, 4 cups = 1 quart, 1 yard = approximately 1 meter, 12 dozen = 1 gross, 1 eurodollar = approximately $1.20 U.S. dollars.*

**1** How many feet are in 8 yards?

| Step 1:<br>Desired Answer Units | Step 2: Conversion<br>Formula (With Desired<br>Answer in Numerator) | Step 3:<br>Original Factors to Convert<br>(Quantity and Units) |
| --- | --- | --- |
| ? feet | $\dfrac{3 \text{ feet}}{1 \text{ yard}}$ | 8 yards |

Since the step 2 denominator unit (yard) is repeated in the numerator in step 3 (yards), it can be canceled.

2 How many quarts are in 8 cups?

| Step 1: Desired Answer Units | Step 2: Conversion Formula | Step 3: Original Factors to Convert (Quantity and Units) |
| --- | --- | --- |
| | | |

**Q** *Ask Yourself*

How many times must an undesired unit be entered in order to cancel out?

**A** *My Answer*

3 Approximately how many yards are in 50 meters?

| Step 1: Desired Answer Units | Step 2: Conversion Formula | Step 3: Original Factors to Convert (Quantity and Units) |
| --- | --- | --- |
| | | |

4 How many dozen are in 2 gross?

| Step 1: Desired Answer Units | Step 2: Conversion Formula | Step 3: Original Factors to Convert (Quantity and Units) |
| --- | --- | --- |
| | | |

5 If you have $500, how many eurodollars can you buy?

| Step 1: Desired Answer Units | Step 2: Conversion Formula | Step 3: Original Factors to Convert (Quantity and Units) |
| --- | --- | --- |
| | | |

# Two Kinds of Conversions That Must be Identified

Two kinds of conversions are commonly used for calculations:

1   Conversion formulas within the same dimension, such as 12 eggs = 1 dozen (quantity), 4 qt = 1 gal (volume), or 1000 mg = 1 g (weight or mass)
2   Conversions formulas within different dimensions (ratios), such as 10 pills/day (10 pills per 1 day), 250 mg/tablet (250 mg in 1 tablet), 1 g/capsule (1 g in 1 capsule), 10 workers/ 1 supervisor, $12 per hr, or 10 tickets/ 2 free passes.

➤   These formulas are entered as conversion units in the same way, with the desired answer unit placed in the numerator of the first conversion formula.

**RAPID PRACTICE 2-4** Identifying Correct Equation Setup

**Estimated completion time: 5-10 minutes**   **Answers on page 511.**

**Directions:** *Identify the required elements. Focus on the setup. Correct the incorrect setup. Do not solve the equation.*

1  If there are approximately 2.5 cm in 1 inch, how many centimeters are there in 50 inches?

| Step 1:<br>Desired Answer Units | Step 2:<br>Conversion Formula | Step 3:<br>Original Factors to Convert |
| --- | --- | --- |
| ? cm | $\dfrac{2.5\ cm}{1\ inch}$ | 50 inches |

**a.** Is the DA setup correct? _____
**b.** If it is incorrect, correct it._____

_____

**c.** Estimate: Will the numerical answer be larger or smaller than the units to be converted? _____

2  The average baby weighs 7 lb at birth. There are 2.2 lb in 1 kg. How many kilograms does the average baby weigh? _____

| Step 1:<br>Desired Answer Units | Step 2:<br>Conversion Formula | Step 3:<br>Original Factors to Convert |
| --- | --- | --- |
| ? kg | $\dfrac{2.2\ lb}{1\ kg}$ | 2.2 lb |

**a.** Is the DA setup correct? _____
**b.** If it is incorrect, correct it.   _____

_____

**c.** Estimate: Will the numerical answer be larger or smaller than the units to be converted? _____

3  A bottle contains 2500 milliliters of fluid. There are 1000 mL in 1 liter. How many liters are in the bottle? _____

| Step 1:<br>Desired Answer Units | Step 2:<br>Conversion Formula | Step 3:<br>Original Factors to Convert |
| --- | --- | --- |
| ? mL | $\dfrac{1000\ mL}{1\ Liter}$ | 2500 mL |

**a.** Is the DA setup correct? _____
**b.** If it is incorrect, correct it.   _____

_____

**c.** Will the numerical answer be larger or smaller than the units to be converted? _____

4 There are 1000 mg in 1 g. If you have 5.5 grams, how many milligrams do you have? _____

| Step 1: Desired Answer Units | Step 2: Conversion Formula | Step 3: Original Factors to Convert |
|---|---|---|
| ? mg | $\dfrac{1000\ mg}{1\ g}$ | 5.5 g |

   **a.** Is the DA setup correct? _____
   **b.** If it is incorrect, correct it. _____

   **c.** Will the numerical answer be larger or smaller than the units to be converted? _____

5 The patient takes 10 pills per day. How many pills will the patient need for 7 days? _____

| Step 1: Desired Answer Units | Step 2: Conversion Formula (Ratio) | Step 3: Original Factors to Convert |
|---|---|---|
| ? pills | $\dfrac{10\ pills}{1\ day}$ | 7 days |

   **a.** Is the DA setup correct? _____
   **b.** If it is incorrect, correct it. _____

   **c.** Will the answer be larger or smaller than the units to be converted? _____

**FAQ** | *Why practice the DA method with problems that can easily be calculated mentally?*

**ANSWER:** This is a learning technique. The goal is to practice the method to perfection with simple problems and to plant it in long-term memory so that the setup can be recalled when the solutions to more complex calculations are needed. Some problems call for more entries. If you can set up simple problems, you will be able to apply the technique to more complex problems.

**Clinical Relevance**

Many medications ordered do not require calculations for administration, but some do. The nurse needs to know a calculation method very well. A calculation method is frequently needed with liquid oral doses or to determine whether an intravenous flow rate is delivering the correct amount of drug at the correct rate per hour.

➤ Even when a calculator is used, the nurse must understand the math process well enough to enter the data correctly. Frail and at-risk populations may require fractional doses, which involve calculations of a small dose from a large amount on hand. Almost all intravenous solutions require some calculations.

## RAPID PRACTICE 2-5  Solving DA Equations

**Estimated completion time: 10-20 minutes**  Answers on page **511.**

**Directions:** *Set up and solve the equation as shown in Problem 1. Select the conversion formula from the list supplied. Even though you can do these problems mentally, the goal is to practice the method so that you can apply it easily to more complex, unfamiliar problems. For credit, label each answer.*

*Conversion formulas: 32 oz = 1 qt, 1000 megabytes = 1 gigabyte, 1000 mg = 1 g, 1000 mL = 1 liter, and 4 liters = approximately 1 gal, 5 RNs per 2 LPNs, $20 = 1 hr pay.*

**1** You have 3 qt of milk. How many ounces is that?

| Step 1: Desired Answer Units | Step 2: Conversion Formula | Step 3: Original Factors to Convert | Step 4: Answer |
|---|---|---|---|

DA Equation:

$$\text{oz} = \frac{32 \text{ oz}}{1 \text{ qt}} \times 3 \text{ qt} = 96 \text{ oz}$$

**2** Your salary is $20/hr. You earned $500. How many hours did you work?

| Step 1: Desired Answer Units | Step 2: Conversion Formula | Step 3: Original Factors to Convert | Step 4: Answer |
|---|---|---|---|

DA Equation:

**3** Your computer has 4 gigabytes. How many megabytes is this?

| Step 1: Desired Answer Units | Step 2: Conversion Formula | Step 3: Original Factors to Convert | Step 4: Answer |
|---|---|---|---|

DA Equation:

**4** You buy 40 liters of gas for your car in Mexico. About how many gallons did you buy?

| Step 1: Desired Answer Units | Step 2: Conversion Formula | Step 3: Original Factors to Convert | Step 4: Answer |
|---|---|---|---|

DA Equation:

**5** The hospital has 40 CNAs. How many LPN slots are there?

| Step 1: Desired Answer Units | Step 2: Conversion Formula | Step 3: Original Factors to Convert | Step 4: Answer |
|---|---|---|---|

DA Equation:

# Problems That Call for More Than One Conversion Formula

Once the basic DA setup is mastered, entering more conversion formulas becomes very simple. Analyze the following simple example:

Question: How many seconds in 5 hours? Desired answer units: seconds. Units to be canceled: hours.

There is no formula for directly converting seconds to hours. There are formulas for converting seconds to minutes and minutes to hours. Therefore, two conversion formulas are needed to solve this problem: 60 seconds = 1 minute, and 60 minutes = 1 hour.

To solve the problem:

1 Set up the basic DA grid as in previous examples, allowing room for additional conversion formulas.

When there is more than one conversion formula to be entered, the *numerator* of the next conversion formula must *match the denominator* of the previous conversion formula (minutes in the example shown).

2 Solve the equation and evaluate.

| Step 1: Desired Answer Units | Step 2: Conversion Formula | Step 2A: Second Conversion Formula (60 min = 1 hr) | Step 3: Convert Original Factors (5 hr) | | Step 4: Desired Answer |
|---|---|---|---|---|---|
| ? sec = | $\dfrac{60 \text{ sec}}{1 \text{ min}}$ | × $\dfrac{60 \text{ min}}{1 \text{ hr}}$ | × 5 hr | = | 18,000 sec |
| | Plan to cancel minutes next. | Plan to cancel hours next. | | | There are 18,000 sec in 5 hr. |

➤ Remember that a whole number is considered a *numerator* with an implied denominator of 1.

When you set up your equation on paper, it should look like this:

$$? \text{ seconds} = \frac{60 \text{ sec}}{1 \text{ min}} \times \frac{60 \text{ min}}{1 \text{ hr}} \times 5 \text{ hr} = 18{,}000 \text{ sec}$$

➤ Note the *flow* of the canceled units from denominator to numerator: minutes to minutes and hours to hours.

The only difference between this and earlier simpler examples is that there are two conversion formulas because there are two units to be canceled. You do not have a conversion formula that goes directly from seconds to hours. Start with seconds and work your way through with the available formulas to get to hours.

If the first entry is correct, the rest flows easily if all undesired units are entered and canceled. Continue with the systematic approach you have learned. Each denominator leads to the next numerator.

Note how a DA-style equation can be set up using *three* and *four* conversion formulas.

Question: How many inches are in a mile? Conversion formulas: 12 inches = 1 foot, 3 feet = 1 yard, and 1760 yards = 1 mile.

$$? \text{ inches} = \frac{12 \text{ inches}}{1 \text{ foot}} \times \frac{3 \text{ feet}}{1 \text{ yard}} \times \frac{1760 \text{ yards}}{1 \text{ mile}} = 63{,}360 \text{ inches in 1 mile}$$

• Inches are entered first with the appropriate conversion equivalent (foot).
• Examine the natural flow as each denominator identifies the next numerator.

Do not forget that the original question called for converting 1 mile to inches. The equation setup is *complete* when the original unit to be converted (mile) is entered and canceled.

The following example illustrates how to set up a DA equation using four conversion formulas.

Question: How many seconds are in the month of June?

Conversion formulas: 60 seconds = 1 minute, 60 minutes = 1 hour, 24 hours = 1 day, and 30 days = month (June).

$$? \text{ sec} = \frac{60 \text{ sec}}{1 \text{ min}} \times \frac{60 \text{ min}}{1 \text{ hr}} \times \frac{24 \text{ hr}}{1 \text{ day}} \times \frac{30 \text{ day}}{1 \text{ month}} \times 1 \text{ month} = 86,430 \text{ sec}$$

The following exercise will make the process of adding one more conversion fraction easily understood.

## RAPID PRACTICE 2-6  DA Equations Using Two Conversion Formulas

**Estimated completion time: 25 minutes**   Answers on page **511.**

**Directions:** *Circle A or B to indicate the correct setup of the equations for the following problems; then solve the equation using the correct setup as shown in Example 1. Label the answer.*

➤ Test principle: If *any part* of a solution is incorrect, the entire solution is incorrect.

Before beginning, remember the four parts for solving a DA equation:
1. Desired answer units
2. Conversion formula(s)
3. Known quantity
4. Answer

1  How many cups in 5 qt? Conversion formulas: 2 cups = 1 pt, and 2 pt = 1 qt.

| Step 1 | Step 2 × Step 2A | × | Step 3 | = | Step 4 |
|---|---|---|---|---|---|
| A. ? cups | $\frac{2 \text{ cups}}{1 \text{pt}} \times \frac{2 \text{ pt}}{1 \text{ qt}}$ | × | 5 quarts | = | 20 cups |
| B. ? cups | $\frac{1 \text{ pt}}{2 \text{ cups}} \times \frac{2 \text{ pt}}{1 \text{ qt}}$ | × | 5 quarts | = | |

DA Equation:

$$\text{cups} = \frac{2 \text{ cups}}{1 \text{ pint}} \times \frac{2 \text{ pints}}{1 \text{ quart}} \times 5 \text{ quarts} = 20 \text{ cups}$$

Evaluate your choice. Is the desired answer unit the only remaining unit?

2  How many inches are in 20 yards? Conversion formulas: 12 inches = 1 foot, and 3 feet = 1 yard.

| Step 1 | Step 2 × Step 2A | × | Step 3 | = | Step 4 |
|---|---|---|---|---|---|
| A. ? inches | $\frac{1 \text{ yard}}{3 \text{ feet}} \times \frac{1 \text{ foot}}{12 \text{ inches}}$ | × | 20 yards | = | Answer |
| B. ? inches | $\frac{12 \text{ inches}}{1 \text{ foot}} \times \frac{3 \text{ feet}}{1 \text{ yard}}$ | × | 20 yards | = | Answer |

DA Equation:

Evaluate your choice. Is the desired answer unit the only remaining unit?

**3** How many millimeters (mm) are in 10 inches? Conversion formulas: 2.5 cm = 1 inch, and 10 mm = 1 cm.

| Step 1 | Step 2 × Step 2A | | × | Step 3 | = | Step 4 |
|---|---|---|---|---|---|---|
| A. ? millimeters | $\dfrac{1\text{ cm}}{10\text{ mm}}$ × | $\dfrac{1\text{ inch}}{2.5\text{ cm}}$ | × | 10 inches | = | Answer |
| B. ? millimeters | $\dfrac{10\text{ mm}}{1\text{ cm}}$ × | $\dfrac{2.5\text{ cm}}{1\text{ inch}}$ | × | 10 inches | = | Answer |

DA Equation:

Evaluate your choice. Is the desired answer unit the only remaining unit?

**4** Approximately how many weeks are in 4 years? Conversion formulas: 12 months = 1 year, and 4 weeks = 1 month.

| Step 1 | Step 2 × Step 2A | | × | Step 3 | = | Step 4 |
|---|---|---|---|---|---|---|
| A. ? weeks | $\dfrac{4\text{ weeks}}{1\text{ month}}$ × | $\dfrac{1\text{ year}}{12\text{ months}}$ | × | 4 years | = | Answer |
| B. ? weeks | $\dfrac{4\text{ weeks}}{1\text{ month}}$ × | $\dfrac{12\text{ months}}{1\text{ year}}$ | × | 4 years | = | Answer |

DA Equation:

Evaluate your choice. Is the desired answer unit the only remaining unit?

**5** How many grams are in 4000 micrograms (mcg)? Conversion formulas: 1000 mg = 1 g, and 1000 mcg = 1 mg.

| Step 1 | Step 2 × Step 2A | | × | Step 3 | = | Step 4 |
|---|---|---|---|---|---|---|
| A. ? grams | $\dfrac{1\text{ g}}{1000\text{ mg}}$ × | $\dfrac{1000\text{ mcg}}{1\text{ mg}}$ | × | 4000 mcg | = | Answer |
| B. ? grams | $\dfrac{1\text{ g}}{1000\text{ mg}}$ × | $\dfrac{1\text{ mg}}{1000\text{ mcg}}$ | × | 4000 mcg | = | Answer |

DA Equation:

Evaluate your choice. Is the desired answer unit the only remaining unit?

**FAQ** | *Which are the commonest errors when using two or more conversion formulas?*

**ANSWER:** Assuming that the desired answer unit is entered correctly, the second conversion formula may be positioned incorrectly. The second conversion formula numerator must cancel the denominator of the previous conversion formula. Also, the numbers may be transposed if the writer is not focused. Finally, each *undesired unit* must be entered *two* times, once in a denominator and once in a numerator.

## RAPID PRACTICE 2-7 Solving DA Equations Using 1 or 2 Conversion Formulas

**Estimated completion time: 20 minutes**   Answers on page **512.**

**Directions:** *Identify the required elements. Solve the equations using the 4-column systematic approach presented in this chapter. Allow space for an extra conversion formula if needed. Evaluate your equation. Even if you can solve the equations mentally, the benefit of this practice is to reinforce a solid method of verification for more complex problems using DA.*

**1** How many pounds are in 80 kilograms? Conversion formula: 2.2 lb = 1 kg. _____

**2** How many pints are in 5 gal? Conversion formulas: 2 pt = 1 qt, and 4 qt = 1 gal. _____

**3** How many inches are in 25 millimeters (mm)? Conversion formulas: 10 mm = 1 cm, and 2.5 cm = 1 inch. _____

**4** How many hours are in 7200 seconds? Conversion formulas: 60 seconds = 1 minute, 60 minutes = 1 hour. _____

**5** How many grams are in 25,000 micrograms (mcg)? Conversion formulas: 1 g = 1000 mg, and 1 mg = 1000 mcg. _____

## CHAPTER 2 MULTIPLE-CHOICE REVIEW

**Estimated completion time: 20 minutes**   Answers on page **512.**

**1** What is the *first* step in analyzing a problem and solving a DA equation? _____
   **1.** Identify the on-hand units and quantities.
   **2.** Estimate the answer.
   **3.** Identify the desired answer units.
   **4.** Set up the equation.

**2** Which of the following is a key process *that guides* the setup of DA equations? _____
   **1.** Placement of units          **3.** Multiplication of units
   **2.** Placement of numbers          **4.** Multiplication of numbers

**3** Which of the following statements about DA setup is *incorrect?* _____
   **1.** The quantities must always be accompanied by the unit of measure.
   **2.** The units of measure are canceled after the numbers are multiplied.
   **3.** More than one conversion formula may be needed to solve the equation.
   **4.** Units of measure are addressed before quantities in solving DA equations.

**4** Which conversion formula setup is correct for the following question?
   Question: How many yards are in 72 inches?
   Conversion formulas: 12 inches = 1 foot, and 3 feet = 1 yard.
   Circle the correct choice.

**Test Tip:** *If the first or any entry is incorrect, the rest of that selection is incorrect.*

| Step 1<br>Desired Answer Units | Step 2<br>Conversion Formula | × | Step 2 A<br>Conversion Formula |
|---|---|---|---|
| **1.** ? yards | $\dfrac{72 \text{ inches}}{1 \text{ foot}}$ | × | $\dfrac{3 \text{ feet}}{1 \text{ yard}}$ |
| **2.** ? yards | $\dfrac{1 \text{ yard}}{3 \text{ feet}}$ | × | $\dfrac{1 \text{ foot}}{12 \text{ inches}}$ |
| **3.** ? yards | $\dfrac{12 \text{ inches}}{1 \text{ foot}}$ | × | $\dfrac{3 \text{ feet}}{1 \text{ yard}}$ |
| **4.** ? yards | $\dfrac{1 \text{ yard}}{72 \text{ inches}}$ | × | $\dfrac{3 \text{ feet}}{12 \text{ inches}}$ |

**5** Which DA equation is correct for solving the following question?

Question: How many kilobytes (KB) are in 2 gigabytes (GB)?
Conversion formulas: 1000 (KB) = 1 megabyte (MB), and 1000 MB = 1 GB.
Circle the correct conversion formula.

| Step 1<br>Desired Answer<br>Units | Step 2<br>Conversion<br>Formula | Step 2A<br>Conversion<br>Formula | × | Step 3<br>Original Factors<br>to Convert |
|---|---|---|---|---|
| **1.** ? kilobytes | $\dfrac{1000 \text{ GB}}{1 \text{ MB}}$ | $\dfrac{1 \text{ GB}}{1000 \text{ MB}}$ | × | 2 GB |
| **2.** ? kilobytes | $\dfrac{1 \text{ MB}}{1000 \text{ KB}}$ | $\dfrac{1 \text{ GB}}{1000 \text{ MB}}$ | × | 2 GB |
| **3.** ? kilobytes | $\dfrac{1000 \text{ KB}}{1 \text{ MB}}$ | $\dfrac{1000 \text{ MB}}{1 \text{ GB}}$ | × | 2 GB |
| **4.** ? kilobytes | $\dfrac{1000 \text{ MB}}{1 \text{ GB}}$ | $\dfrac{25000 \text{ KB}}{1 \text{ MB}}$ | × | 2 GB |

**6** Solving an equation using DA requires which of the following processes? _____

    **1.** Cancellation of units followed by multiplication
    **2.** Multiplication of units followed by cancellation
    **3.** Cancellation of desired answer units
    **4.** Division of desired and undesired units

**7** The analysis of the DA equation setup to ensure that all unwanted units are canceled should take place at which step of the process? _____

    **1.** After entering the first conversion fraction
    **2.** When entering the original factors
    **3.** After all the data are entered but before multiplication of quantities
    **4.** After all the data are entered and after the multiplication of quantities

**8** The two types of conversion formulas are as follows: _____

    **1.** Data and factors
    **2.** Units and fractions
    **3.** Those that contain the same dimensions and those that contain different dimensions
    **4.** Fraction equivalents and decimal equivalents

**9** The *final* evaluation of a DA equation should include which of the following critical steps? _____

**1.** Ensuring the desired answer units are the only remaining units
**2.** Checking the conversion fraction for correct placement in the numerator and denominator
**3.** Estimating the answer
**4.** Identifying the known quantity

**10** Which of the following choices reflects the *correct* setup for a DA equation? Circle the number of the correct choice.

Question: How many micrograms are in 0.5 g? Conversion formulas: 1000 mcg = 1 mg, and 1000 mg = 1 g.

| Step 1: Desired Answer Units | Step 2: Conversion Formula × Step 2A: Conversion Formula | × | Step 3: Original Factors to Convert | = | Answer |
|---|---|---|---|---|---|
| **1.** ? grams = | $\dfrac{1000 \text{ mcg}}{1 \text{ mg}} \times \dfrac{0.5 \text{ g}}{1000 \text{ mg}}$ | × | 1000 mcg | | |
| **2.** ? micrograms = | $\dfrac{1 \text{ mg}}{1000 \text{ mcg}} \times \dfrac{1000 \text{ mg}}{0.5 \text{ g}}$ | × | 0.5 g | | |
| **3.** ? milligrams = | $\dfrac{0.5 \text{ g}}{1000 \text{ mg}} \times \dfrac{1 \text{ mg}}{1000 \text{ mcg}}$ | × | 0.5 g | | |
| **4.** ? micrograms = | $\dfrac{1000 \text{ mcg}}{1 \text{ mg}} \times \dfrac{1000 \text{ mg}}{1 \text{ g}}$ | × | 0.5 g | | |

## CHAPTER 2 FINAL PRACTICE

**Estimated completion time: 1-2 hours**   Answers on page **512.**

**Directions:** *Set up and solve the following problems using the four-step DA method even if you can obtain the answer with mental arithmetic. Label all data. Evaluate your equations.*

**1** Write the three required *elements* of dimensional style equations.

   a. _____
   b. _____
   c. _____

**2** How many eggs are in 10 dozen? Conversion formula: 12 eggs = 1 dozen. _____

DA Equation:

**3** How many kilometers are in 50 miles to the nearest tenth? Conversion formula: 1 km = 0.6 mile. _____

DA Equation:

4  How many pounds are in 60 kg? Conversion formula: 2.2 lb = 1 kg.
_____

DA Equation:

5  How many inches are in 50 yards? Conversion formulas: 12 inches = 1 foot, and 3 feet = 1 yard. _____

DA Equation:

6  How many millimeters are in 1 inch? Conversion formulas: 10 mm = 1 cm, and 2.5 cm = 1 inch. _____

DA Equation:

7  How many meters are in 30 yards? Conversion formula: 1 m = 1.09 yards.
_____

DA Equation:

8  How many DVDs can you buy for a gift certificate worth $100? How much money will you have left over? Ratio: $8/DVD. _____

DA Equation:

9  How many prescriptions (Rx) can be bought with an insurance policy that has a $2000 limit? Conversion formula: $50 average cost per prescription.
_____

DA Equation:

10  How many nurses will be needed for a new 480-bed hospital? Ratio: 1 nurse for 12 beds. Round answer to nearest whole number. _____

DA Equation:

➤ Use two conversion formulas in a DA-style equation for the next 10 questions.

**11** How many liters are in 8 gal? Conversion formulas: 1 L = 1 qt, and 4 qt = 1 gal. _____

DA Equation:

**12** How many inches are in 10 yards? Conversion formulas: 12 inches = 1 foot, and 3 feet = 1 yard. _____

DA Equation:

**13** How many tablespoons are in a cup of fluid? Conversion formulas: 3 tbs = 1 oz, and 8 oz = 1 cup. _____

DA Equation:

**14** How many cups are in 2 qt? Conversion formulas: 2 cups = 1 pt, and 2 pt = 1 qt. _____

DA Equation:

**15** How many seconds are in 2 hours? Conversion formulas: 60 seconds = 1 minute, and 60 minutes = 1 hour. _____

DA Equation:

**16** How many milliliters are in 3 tbs of milk? Conversion formulas: 5 mL = 1 tsp, and 3 tsp = 1 tbs. _____

DA Equation:

**17** How many nurse assistants are needed for a 300-bed hospital? Conversion formulas: 1 nurse for 10 beds, and 2 nurse assistants for each nurse. _____

DA Equation:

**18** How many inches are in a meter? Conversion formulas: 2.5 inches = 1 cm; 100 cm = 1 m. _____

DA Equation:

**19** How many centimeters are in a foot? Conversion formulas: 2.5 cm = 1 inch, and 12 inches = 1 foot. _____

DA Equation:

**20** How many micrograms are in 2 grams (g) of sugar? Conversion formulas: 1000 mcg = 1 mg, and 1000 mg = 1 g. _____

DA Equation:

## Suggestions for Further Reading

www.cogsci.princeton.edu
www.mathforum.org
www.worldscinet.com

 Additional information can be found on the CD.

Chapter 3 focuses on the measurement units currently used for medications. Medications are primarily ordered and supplied in terms of metric system measurements, a system used in most parts of the world. DA-style equations are useful for verifying conversions and solving metric-equivalent medication dose problems.

# PART II
# MODERN METRIC SYSTEM AND MEDICATION CALCULATIONS

*"Metric is easy for anyone who can count up to ten."*
—**CONTRIBUTOR M** (source: www.woodweb.com)

# MEASUREMENT UNITS AND CONVERSIONS FOR MEDICATIONS

## Objectives

- Memorize the units of metric measurement used in medication orders.
- State equivalent values of weight (mass) and volume used in metric dose calculations: micrograms, milligrams, grams, kilograms, milliliters, and liters.
- Distinguish milligram, milliliter, and milliequivalent.
- Define the uses of the term *Unit* related to measurements and medications.
- Calculate basic metric oral medication problems using mental arithmetic and decimal placement.
- Verify metric conversions using dimensional analysis.
- Use approved abbreviations for metric units.
- Distinguish metric, household, and apothecary measurements.

## Essential Prior Knowledge

Mastery of Chapters 1 and 2

## Equipment

- Yardstick measured in centimeters and meters or ruler measured in millimeters and centimeters
- Food package labels measured in grams
- Measuring cup illustrating ounces and milliliters
- 30-ml plastic medicine cup showing 1 and 2 tbs
- Several medication labels, prescription or over-the-counter

## Estimated Time To Complete Chapter

- 2 hours

## Introduction

Three systems of measurement are used for medication doses: metric, household, and apothecary. The metric system is the main system now used for medication doses. Household measures are used for some medications taken at home, primarily liquids. The apothecary system has been almost completely phased out of use. Nurses need to know the metric-household equivalents for home care practice and family teaching. They also need to distinguish the metric and apothecary systems in case a prescriber writes an order in the apothecary system.

The U.S. Metric Association, Inc. was founded in 1916 to advocate U.S. conversion to the French International System of Units (SI), now known as the Modern Metric System. Resistance to change shared by many since Napoleonic times has slowed the U.S. "metrication" progress. In fact, there are anti-metric system associations.

Membership in the European Union requires the use of the metric system. Medicines are now almost entirely ordered and supplied in the metric system. If you would rather count by tens, hundreds, and thousands, then this is the system for you. The metric system is precise and easy to work with because it is a standardized decimal measurement system using multiples (powers) of 10. Memorization of a selected number of conversions is necessary. With a little practice and repetition, nurses will be more comfortable with metric system vocabulary than with ounces, cups, gallons, pounds, inches, and yards.

The United States still uses the imprecise, old English system of measurement for popular purchases, such as food, fuel, lumber, fabric, and many other items.

In the metric system, the meter (m) is the *only* descriptor of *length*. It is a precise measurement that is modified by prefixes to change it by multiples of 10. In contrast, the English system uses various descriptors of length, including inches, feet, square feet, yards, square yards, miles, square miles, acres, and nautical miles. To convert one length descriptor to another in the English system, one must use a different equivalent for each, for example, 12 inches = 1 foot, 3 feet = 1 yard, 9 square feet = 1 square yard, and 5280 feet = 1 mile.

This chapter describes metric measurements used in the nursing field and includes examples of and exercises in converting to other measurement systems.

## ESSENTIAL Vocabulary

| | |
|---|---|
| **Apothecary System** | Imprecise old English system of weights and measures. *Feet, yards, gallons, teaspoons,* and *cups* are apothecary terms. The system was formerly used for medication doses but has now been mostly replaced with precise metric system measurements for medications. |
| | The grain is the basic unit of weight in the apothecary system. |
| | *Apothecary* means "pharmacist." |
| **Base Units of Metric Measurement** | Three base units are commonly used for metric measurement of medications to indicate weight (or mass), volume, and length: **gram** (g), **liter** (L), and **meter** (m). |
| | ➤ Memorize these base units of measurement. |
| | The abbreviation for *liter* is capitalized, *L,* to avoid confusion with the number 1. |
| **Household System of Measurement** | Utensils used in the home, such as cups, teaspoons, tablespoons, droppers, etc. Their use can create a safety risk for measuring medication doses because of inconsistent capacities. |
| **Modern Metric System** | Standardized international system of units and measurements based on powers of 10, established in France in the late 1800s and adopted for uniform measurement in most countries. Now used for most medication doses in the United States. |
| **TJC** | The Joint Commission, the accrediting body for health care organizations. TJC issues a variety of directives, including some related to abbreviations and medication practices designed to improve patients' safety. |
| **Units** | Units in the metric system refer to a dimension, such as weight (or mass), volume, and length. Examples of metric units of measurement include kilogram (kg), microgram (mcg), milligram (mg), gram (g), liter (L), and meter (m). |
| | ➤ Write out the words *Unit* and *Units;* do not use abbreviations such as U. |

## RAPID PRACTICE 3-1  Vocabulary Review

**Estimated completion time: 10-15 minutes**   **Answers on page 513.**

**Directions:** *Study the vocabulary and write the answers in the space provided.*

1  What is the name of the basic unit of weight in the apothecary system?

_____

2  What are the three base units of the metric system? _____

3  Why is the abbreviation for liter capitalized? _____

4  What is one problem with using household utensils for medication doses?

_____

5  What system of measurement is currently used for most medication doses in the United States? _____

## Metric Measurements: Base Units

Three base units are commonly used in the medical field. Two are used mainly for medication doses (gram and liter) and one (meter) is used occasionally for topical medications.

➤  Memorize these three base units.

| Base Units | | |
| --- | --- | --- |
| Dimension | Metric Base Unit | Approximate English System Equivalent |
| Weight (or mass) | gram (g) | About $\frac{1}{3}$ ounce dry weight |
| Volume | liter (L) | About 4 measuring cups, a little more than a quart |
| Length | meter (m) | About 39 inches, a little more than a yard |

The abbreviation for the base unit liter is capitalized (L) to avoid misreading as the number 1. The base unit abbreviations for gram (g) and meter (m) are written in lowercase letters. No other abbreviations are authorized.

*Ask Yourself*

*My Answer*

1  What are the three base units of metric measurement used for medications and their abbreviations?

_____

## Metric Units Number Line

The following Metric Units Number Line illustrates the relationship of the values for selected metric prefixes.

| Prefix | Abbreviation | | Value |
| --- | --- | --- | --- |
| kilo- | k | | 1,000 |
| hecto- | h | | 100 |
| deka- | da | | 10 |
| | | | 0 (zero) |
| deci- | d | | 0.1 |
| centi- | c | | 0.01 |
| milli- | m | | 0.001 |
| micro- | mc | | 0.000001 |

## Metric Prefixes and Values

Four prefixes are commonly used for medication dose calculations:

• centi- (meaning hundredth)
• milli- (meaning thousandth)
• micro- (meaning millionth)
• kilo- (meaning a thousand times)

| TABLE 3-1 | **Metric Measurements, Prefixes, Values, and Meaning** | | | | |
|---|---|---|---|---|---|
| **Prefix** | **Multiplier** | **Exponential Power of 10** | **Meaning** | **Examples** | **Meaning** |
| deci- (d) | .1 | $10^{-1}$ | tenth part of | deciliter (dL) | one tenth of a liter |
| centi- (c) | .01 | $10^{-2}$ | hundredth part of | centimeter (cm) | one hundredth of a meter |
| milli- (m) | .001 | $10^{-3}$ | thousandth part of | milliliter (mL) milligram (mg) | one thousandth of a liter one thousandth of a gram |
| micro- (mc) | .000001 | $10^{-6}$ | millionth part of | microgram (mcg) | one millionth of a gram |
| kilo- (k) | 1000 | $10^{3}$ | 1000 times | kilogram (kg) | one thousand grams |

**Note:** The prefix value never changes when combined with a base unit (e.g., the prefix *milli* [m] = .001).
1 mm = 0.001 (one thousandth of a meter).
1 mL = 0.001 (one thousandth of a liter).
1 mg = 0.001 (one thousandth of a gram).

A fifth prefix, deci-, is used in laboratory reports.

➤ Memorize the prefixes and definitions.

Study Table 3-1, and note the numerical values and relationships. Metric prefixes are combined with bases to create new quantities, as shown in the examples in the table.

**1**  What are the numerical values of the prefixes *m, c, d,* and *k?*

_____

• For review, write out the four prefixes and three base units used for medication administration. Memorize them in preparation for analyzing medication orders.

**Q** *Ask Yourself*

**A** *My Answer*

**Prefixes and Abbreviations**              **Base Units and Abbreviations**

1. _____              1. _____

2. _____              2. _____

3. _____              3. _____

4. _____

➤ The abbreviation for the prefix micro- (mc) is preferred over the Greek letter mu ($\mu$) in handwritten patient medical records. A handwritten $\mu$g (microgram) can be mistaken for mg (milligram).

It is very important to recognize the $\mu$ and distinguish it from zero and from mg. Either misinterpretation could lead to serious errors in medication dosage. The nurse should clarify the meaning of the symbol with the prescriber.

**Clinical Relevance**

## RAPID PRACTICE 3-2  Writing Metric Units and Abbreviations

**Estimated completion time: 10 minutes**    Answers on page **514.**

**Directions:** *Study the metric units and abbreviations. Write the metric name and abbreviation in the space provided.*

**1**  Write the name and abbreviation for the prefix that means $\frac{1}{1000}$. _____

**2**  Write the name and abbreviation for the prefix that means $\frac{1}{100}$. _____

**3**  Write the name and abbreviation for the prefix that means $\frac{1}{1,000,000}$. _____

**4**  Write the name and abbreviation for the prefix that means $\frac{1}{10}$. _____

5 Write the name and abbreviation for the prefix that means 1000 times. _____

6 Write the name and abbreviation for the base unit of volume. _____

7 Write the name and abbreviation for the base unit of length. _____

8 Write the name and abbreviation for the base unit of weight, or mass. _____

9 Write the name for the base unit *m*. _____

10 Write the name for the prefix *m*. _____

# Metric Notation

## Writing Metric Unit Combinations and Equivalents

Study the example and note the correct order of writing as follows:
1 Numeral or numerals
2 Space
3 Prefix
4 Base unit

| EXAMPLES | The following are examples of correctly written metric quantities: 100 mg, 1000 mL, 250 cm, 2500 mcg, and 1,000,000 kg. |
| --- | --- |

Do not write an *m* to look like a *w* or a *u*.
Do capitalize *L* for *liter*.
Do not close up a *c* so that *cm* looks like *am*.
Do use commas to group numbers with more than three consecutive zeros in groups of three from right to left.

| Guide to Metric Notation | Examples |
| --- | --- |
| Abbreviations are always used when accompanied by a number. The number, followed by a space, precedes the abbreviation. | 10 mg, 2 g, 5 L |
| | Metric terms are written out when unaccompanied by a number, as illustrated in the following sentence: "Write out grams and milligrams." |
| When the number of units following the slash meaning *per* is 1, the number 1 may be omitted from the abbreviation. It is implied. | 40 mg/ g (40 mg per 1 g) |
| Metric *abbreviations* are always singular. They are *not* pluralized. | *Milligrams* is abbreviated *mg*. |
| | *Liters* is abbreviated *L*. |
| | Write *mg*, not *mgs; g*, not *gs;* and *L*, not *Ls*. |
| There is no period after metric abbreviations except when they fall at the end of a sentence. | Give 2 mg, not 3 mg. |
| | He drank 2 L of water, followed by 1 L. |

## RAPID PRACTICE 3-3 Writing Metric Measurements

**Estimated completion time: 5-10 minutes**   **Answers on page 514.**

**Directions:** *Write the metric measurement in the space provided.*

1 Write out the base unit that is capitalized so that it will not be confused with the number 1. _____

2 Which prefix shown in Table 3-1 equals 1000 times the base unit? _____

**3** If a laboratory report indicated that a blood sugar level was 80 mg/dL, how would that quantity be written out and read aloud? _____

**4** Which abbreviation is preferred over the Greek $\mu$ for micro? _____

**5** Write the names and abbreviations for the three base units in the metric system. _____

## RAPID PRACTICE 3-4 Metric Abbreviations

**Estimated completion time: 3 minutes**   Answers on page **514.**

**Directions:** *Circle the* recommended *abbreviation for the metric units of measurement:*

**1** grams

   **1.** gr                          **3.** G

   **2.** gms                      **4.** g

**2** milligrams

   **1.** mgm                    **3.** Mgs

   **2.** mg                      **4.** mcg

**3** liters

   **1.** L                          **3.** ls

   **2.** l                          **4.** Ls

**4** milliliters

   **1.** m                         **3.** mg

   **2.** mL                     **4.** mLs

**5** microgram

   **1.** $\mu$g                      **3.** mcg

   **2.** mg                      **4.** mc

## RAPID PRACTICE 3-5 Combining Metric Measurements

**Estimated completion time: 5 minutes**   Answers on page **514.**

**Directions:** *Write the recommended abbreviation for the metric unit combinations in the space provided:*

**1** milligram _____

**2** microgram _____

**3** millimeter _____

**4** milliliter _____

**5** kilogram _____

**1** Are there 100 or 1000 cm in a meter?

_____

**2** Are there 100 or 1000 mg in a gram?

_____

**3** Are there 10 or 100 dL in a liter?

_____

**Q** *Ask Yourself*

**A** *My Answer*

## RAPID PRACTICE 3-6 Metric Base Units

**Estimated completion time: 5 minutes**   Answers on page **514.**

**Directions:** *Write the requested metric base units in the correct form in the space provided.*

1 Which metric base unit abbreviation presented in this chapter must be capitalized? _____

2 Which metric base unit abbreviation would be added to the prefix *c* in a measurement of the length of a scar? _____

3 Which metric base unit abbreviation would be added to the prefix *m* in a measurement of fluids consumed? _____

4 Which metric base unit abbreviation would be added to the prefix *k* in a measurement of current weight? _____

5 Which metric base unit abbreviation would be added to the prefix *m* in a measurement of drug weight? _____

➤ To accelerate mastery of the metric system, begin to THINK METRIC.

Read the labels on food, beverages, medicines, and vitamins to speed learning of the uses of *g* and *mg*.

**Q:** *Ask Yourself*

**A:** *My Answer*

1 The average American consumes 5-6 g of table salt per day. The recommended amount is 1-2 g/day. Approximately how many grams of salt do you consume on an average day?

_____

## Equivalent Metric Measurements of Weight or Mass

**Memorize:**

1000 mcg = 1 mg,   1000 mg = 1 g,   1000 g = 1 kg

**Clinical Relevance**

In clinical agencies, the kilogram is used for weight reporting and dose calculations. At birth the average baby weighs 3200 g, or 3.2 kg (approximately 7 lb). Low-birth-weight infants are those who weigh ≤2500 g (2.5 kg, or 5.5 lb) at birth. Many drug doses are ordered and adjusted on the basis of kilogram weight. Oral medications contain large ranges of doses in milligrams, such as 0.5 mg, 50 mg, 100 mg, 250 mg, or 500 mg. Doses of some oral medications are very small, such as those found in Synthroid (0.175 mg, or 175 mcg). Examine the doses on the following labels:

N 3 0087-6060-10 9

Each tablet contains 500 mg of metformin hydrochloride.
See enclosed package insert for dosage information.
Caution: Federal law prohibits
dispensing without prescription.
Store between 15°–30° C (59°–86° F).
Dispense in light resistant container.
Glucophage is a registered trademark of LIPHA s.a.
Licensed to Bristol-Myers Squibb Company.
Distributed by
Bristol-Myers Squibb Company
Princeton, NJ 08543 USA
606010DRL-2
34-007102-01

**500 Tablets**   NDC 0087-**6060-10**

**GLUCOPHAGE®**
(metformin hydrochloride tablets)

**500**
mg

Bristol-Myers Squibb Company

Some medications, particularly antibiotics, are supplied in grams.

## Metric Equivalent Measurements of Volume

**Memorize:**

$$1000 \text{ mL} = 1 \text{ L}$$

A liter is slightly greater than a quart (1 L = 1.06 qt, 1 qt = 0.9 L). Most intravenous solutions are delivered in 1 L containers. Examine a water or soda bottle.

Does it contain 750 ml or 1 L? Write *240 mL* on an 8-oz measuring cup at home. Drink 240 mL of water several times a day instead of 8 ounces or 1 cup.

In many parts of the world, gasoline is purchased and paid for by the liter. If you normally buy 10 gal, you would buy about 40 L. While this conversion is not exact, using it when buying gas abroad will assist you in deciding how much to buy and give you an idea of what you will owe. Making a quick conversion is safer than saying, "Fill the tank."

➤ The abbreviation for cubic centimeter (cc) is often written to indicate milliliters (mL). The recommended and preferred abbreviation for milliliter is mL because cc has been misread as two zeros (00), resulting in medication errors.

| **Clinical Relevance** | In clinical agencies, liquids are usually ordered and supplied in milliliters and liters. When calculating liquid dose problems, the answer should be in milliliters. A special calibrated medicine teaspoon holds 5 mL of fluid. Plastic liquid medicine cups, referred to as *ounce cups,* hold 30 mL, which is approximately 1 oz. Think *30 mL* for an ounce. Intravenous medications are also supplied in milliliters and liters. |
|---|---|

## Metric Measurements of Length

**Memorize:**

$$10 \text{ mm} = 1 \text{ cm}$$

$$100 \text{ cm} = 1 \text{ meter}$$

$$1000 \text{ mm} = 1 \text{ meter}$$

| **Clinical Relevance** | When you are assisting with cardiopulmonary resuscitation (CPR), it is helpful to know that fully dilated pupils (10 mm, or 1 cm) can indicate that the patient has been without oxygen for more than 4 minutes. Assessment of the pupils of the eye provides a clue as to a patient's response to CPR. The pinpoint pupil (1-2 mm) may be a reaction to strong light or to certain narcotics or other medications (Figure 3-1). Familiarity with millimeters and centimeters is also helpful in gauging the length of specified areas, such as wounds or scars, or in documenting the application of ointments in the clinical setting. |
|---|---|

**Q:** *Ask Yourself*

**1** What is the width of a friend's, family member's, or friendly pet's eye pupil in millimeters? (Caution: Do not place the ruler on the eye or face.)

**A:** *My Answer*

**2** Do you have any arm scars, freckles, or skin lesions you can measure in millimeters and/or centimeters? If so, what is the length?

Figure **3-1.** Pupil gauge (mm).

**3**   What is your height in centimeters? Multiply your height in inches by 2.5 (2.5 cm = approximately 1 inch).

_____

**4**   If you had to put 10 mm of ointment on a wound, how many centimeters would you need?

_____

> Once you have established some personal landmarks in millimeters and centimeters, you can estimate the size of skin lesions at the bedside by comparing them with your own lesions without searching for a ruler. Topical prescription ointments usually supply paper tape rulers when exact measurements are needed. Note that ointments may be prescribed in inches.

**Clinical Relevance**

## RAPID PRACTICE 3-7 Metric Abbreviations Review

**Estimated completion time: 5 minutes**   Answers on page **514.**

**Directions:** *Identify the correct units of measurement.*

**1**   The three *base* units of measurement, noted correctly, in the metric system are: ____

  **1.** c, k, m

  **2.** g, l, m

  **3.** cm, mL, g

  **4.** g, L, m

**2**   Which of the following metric units is 0.001 of a liter? _____

  **1.** mL (cc)

  **2.** kL

  **3.** mg

  **4.** 1L

**3**   Which of the following metric units is a measure of liquid volume? _____

  **1.** mg

  **2.** cm

  **3.** mL

  **4.** mcg

**4**   Which of the following metric units is a measure of mass or weight? _____

  **1.** g

  **2.** m

  **3.** L

  **4.** cc or mL

**5**   Which of the following metric units is 0.001 of a meter? _____

  **1.** millimeter

  **2.** centimeter

  **3.** milligram

  **4.** kilometer

**1**   What are two abbreviations for the unit *microgram,* and which one is preferred?

**Q** *Ask Yourself*

_____

➤   Metric measurements do *not* require *conversions* within the system. The prefixes *c, m,* and *k* denote the *equivalent* amount in powers of 10.

**A** *My Answer*

## Metric Equivalents

Study the following major metric equivalents. The *values* are evident from the prefix and suffix combinations.

| Weight, or Mass | Volume | Length |
|---|---|---|
| 1000 mcg = 1 mg | 1000 mL = 1 L | 1000 mm = 1 m |
| 1000 mg = 1 g | | 100 cm = 1 m |
| 1000 g = 1 kg | | 10 mm = 1 cm |

After you learn the major equivalent values, you can infer such values for quarters, halves, and one and a half. You find metric equivalents by moving the decimal place.

## Sample Equivalent Metric Values

| Row | Length | Volume | Volume | Weight | Weight | Weight | Weight | Weight | Weight |
|-----|--------|--------|--------|--------|--------|--------|--------|--------|--------|
| A | 10 mm | 500 mL | 1000 mL | 1000 mcg | 250 mg | 500 mg | 1000 mg | 1500 mg | 1000 g |
| B | 1 cm | 0.5 L | 1 L | 1 mg | 0.25 g | 0.5 g | 1 g | 1.5 g | 1 kg |

➤ Do not confuse micrograms with milligrams. Note the difference in value between 1 mcg and 1 mg. The metric system uses only decimals for numbers less than 1. Note the leading zeros in front of decimals and the elimination of trailing zeros after numbers.

Use the examples in the table above to answer the following questions:

**Q: Ask Yourself**

1 Can you identify the base unit in each abbreviation?

_____

**A: My Answer**

2 Can you identify the numerical value (e.g., $\frac{1}{10}$ or $\frac{1}{1000}$) of the prefix (e.g., *milli-*, *centi-*, *micro-*, or *kilo-*) when you read them in an abbreviation?

_____

3 Can you distinguish when to read *m* as *meter* and when to read *m* as *milli-*? One is a prefix, and the other is a base. Which would be placed on the left and which would be placed on the right?

_____

4 Which dimension (weight or volume) does milliliter measure, as opposed to milligram?

_____

# Finding Equivalents: Changing Milligrams to Grams and Grams to Milligrams

Grams and milligrams are the units most frequently encountered in the administration of tablets and capsules.

Equivalent amounts within units of the metric system are found by moving decimal places. Moving a decimal point three places to the right or left is needed to convert grams and milligrams.

Conversion formula: 1000 mg = 1 g.

## Finding Metric Equivalents by Moving Decimals

➤ To change milligrams to grams, divide milligrams by 1000.

Divide milligrams by 1000 by moving the decimal place (implied or existing) three places to the left: 2500 mg = 2.5 g

➤ To change grams to milligrams, multiply grams by 1000.

Multiply grams by 1000 by moving the decimal place (implied or existing) three places to the right: 2.5 g = 2500 mg

**Clinical Relevance**

Moving decimals carefully is a timesaver when calculating drug doses.

**Question:** How many milligrams are in 1.5 g? Conversion formula: 1000 mg = 1 g (mg = g × 1000).

    A.  Move the decimal place: 1.5 g = 1.500 mg

    B.  Verify with a dimensional analysis (DA) equation. Identify required elements of the DA equation as shown below.

| 1. Desired Answer | 2. Conversion Formula | 3. Original Factors to Be Converted | 4. Answer |
|---|---|---|---|
| ? mg | $\dfrac{1000 \text{ mg}}{1 \text{ g}}$ | × 1.5 g | 1500 mg |
| | Place desired answer units in numerator of conversion formula. | Cancel units. Stop and check. Multiply. | Evaluate answer. |

This is how the completed equation will be written:

$$mg = \frac{1000 \text{ mg}}{1 \text{ g}} \times 1.5 \text{ g} = 1500 \text{ mg}$$

See Chapter 2 for a more extensive review of DA equations.

> **FAQ** | *How can I decide whether to divide or multiply in order to move the decimal point to the left or the right of a number for metric equivalents?*
>
> **ANSWER:** You know that *m* stands for *milli-*, or 0.001. The (memorized) conversion formula (e.g., 1000 mg = 1 g) reveals the direction in which to move the decimal point. Converting milligrams to grams requires division. Converting grams to milligrams requires multiplication. Write out the relevant conversion formulas when taking a test so that they are in front of you for reference until the conversions become automatic.

**1**   How many places would I move decimals to change mg to g? to the left or to the right?

   Q: *Ask Yourself*

   A: *My Answer*

## RAPID PRACTICE 3-8   Milligram and Gram Equivalents

**Estimated completion time: 10-20 minutes**   Answers on page **515**.

**Directions:** *Determine the direction in which the decimal place is to be moved, note the prefix, and move the decimal point accordingly to convert milligrams to grams and grams to milligrams. Insert leading zeros and eliminate trailing zeros when necessary. Label the answer using correct notation. It would be helpful to write out the relevant conversion formula.*

| Milligrams | Grams | | Grams | Milligrams |
|---|---|---|---|---|
| 150 | _____ | | 3.5 | _____ |
| 500 | _____ | | 0.25 | _____ |
| 2000 | _____ | | 0.6 | _____ |
| 250 | _____ | | 0.125 | _____ |
| 100 | _____ | | 0.04 | _____ |
| 1500 | _____ | | 2 | _____ |
| 375 | _____ | | 0.3 | _____ |
| 60 | _____ | | 0.75 | _____ |
| 175 | _____ | | 5 | _____ |
| 400 | _____ | | 0.006 | _____ |

RAPID PRACTICE 3-9 Basic Milligram-to-Gram Medication Conversions

**Estimated completion time: 5-10 minutes**   Answers on page **515.**

**Directions:** *Analyze the questions for the desired metric equivalent dose and move the decimal places accordingly to arrive at the correct equivalents. Insert leading zeros and remove trailing zeros from the answer. (Refer to p. 8 for a review of leading and trailing zeros.) Confirm your answer with a DA equation.*

**1** The physician ordered 1.5 g of a medication. What is the equivalent dose in milligrams? _____

DA Equation:


**2** The physician ordered 0.15 g of a medication. What is the equivalent dose in milligrams? _____

DA Equation:


**3** The physician ordered 4 g of a medication. What is the equivalent dose in milligrams? _____

DA Equation:


**4** The physician ordered 500 mg of a medication. What is the equivalent dose in grams? _____

DA Equation:


**5** The physician ordered 60 mg of a medication. What is the equivalent dose in grams? _____

DA Equation:


**FAQ** | *Why verify these decimal movements with a DA-style equation?*

**ANSWER:** Both methods require practice. Mastery of a verification method for backup proof of any calculation is essential. If a nurse practices and masters DA with some simple equations, the more complex conversions requiring DA will be simple also.

## RAPID PRACTICE 3-10 Identifying Metric Equivalents

**Estimated completion time: 5 minutes**   Answers on page **515**.

**Directions:** *Circle the correct metric* equivalent *for the amount presented:*

1 Ordered: 0.2 g

  **1.** 0.002 mg   **3.** 200 mg
  **2.** 0.02 mg    **4.** 2000 mg

2 Ordered: 400 mg

  **1.** 0.04 g   **3.** 40 g
  **2.** 0.4 g    **4.** 4000 g

3 Ordered: 1.6 g

  **1.** 1600 mg   **3.** 1.6 mg
  **2.** 160 mg    **4.** 0.016 mg

4 Ordered: 5 mg

  **1.** 0.005 g   **3.** 500 g
  **2.** 50 g     **4.** 5000 g

5 Ordered: 0.04 g

  **1.** 0.004 mg   **3.** 4 mg
  **2.** 0.04 mg    **4.** 40 mg

# Examining Micrograms

The metric equivalents of micrograms are as follows:

1000 mcg = 1 mg

1,000,000 mcg = 1 g

Milligrams and grams are among the commonest measurements in medications. Of the two, milligrams are used more frequently. In order to avoid errors, it is advisable to avoid using decimals and to select an equivalent that can be stated in whole numbers.

Micrograms are very small units. Microgram and milligram conversions are needed for intravenous calculations and occasionally for very small doses of powerful medications. Just as with milligrams and grams, it is helpful to examine the prefix to determine the equivalent units.

➤ To change micrograms to milligrams, divide micrograms by 1000.
➤ To change milligrams to micrograms, multiply milligrams by 1000.

## RAPID PRACTICE 3-11 Mental Math: Micrograms to Milligrams, Milligrams to Micrograms, and Micrograms and Grams

**Estimated completion time: 10 minutes**   Answers on page **515**.

**Directions:** *Fill in the equivalent metric measure in the spaces provided by moving decimal points.*

| MICROGRAMS TO MILLIGRAMS | | MILLIGRAMS TO MICROGRAMS | | MICROGRAMS AND GRAMS | |
| --- | --- | --- | --- | --- | --- |
| mcg | mg | mg | mcg | mcg | g |
| 5000 | _____ | 2 | _____ | _____ | 0.001 |
| 300 | _____ | 0.5 | _____ | 500,000 | _____ |
| 1500 | _____ | 1.8 | _____ | _____ | 0.0002 |
| 20,000 | _____ | 0.15 | _____ | 10,000 | _____ |
| 2500 | _____ | 0.6 | _____ | _____ | 0.03 |

▲ **Cultural Note**

In some countries, such as the United States, a comma is used to separate groups of three numbers within large numbers, as in 20,000. In other countries, a *space is* used. Thus, 25,000 or 25 000 might be seen. In the past, the British used a comma to designate a *decimal point* between a whole number and a fraction: 5,5 would be read as 5.5. ("5 point 5" or "5 and 5 tenths"). This type of notation can still be seen in scientific math.

➤ Write numbers, commas, and decimals neatly and use the custom of the country where you work.

<table>
<tr><td>**Clinical Relevance**</td><td>As with mastering arithmetic, mastery of the metric system frees precious time for other priorities, such as</td></tr>
</table>

- patient and medical record assessments
- patient and family communications
- medication preparation and administration
- clinical theory
- patient treatments
- documentation in the patient record

## RAPID PRACTICE 3-12  Review: Defining and Abbreviating Metric Units

**Estimated completion time: 10 minutes**   Answers on page **516.**

**Directions:** *Fill in the full word or approved abbreviation for the metric units in the space provided:*

| Full Word | Approved Abbreviation |
|---|---|
| 1  cm _____ | 6  liter _____ |
| 2  mL _____ | 7  meter _____ |
| 3  mg _____ | 8  kilogram _____ |
| 4  mm _____ | 9  kilometer _____ |
| 5  mcg _____ | 10  centiliter _____ |

## RAPID PRACTICE 3-13  Metric Equivalents Review

**Estimated completion time: 10 minutes**   Answers on page **516.**

**Directions:** *Convert to equivalent metric units by moving decimal places.*

| | | | | | |
|---|---|---|---|---|---|
| 1  1 g = | _____mg | | 6  1 L = | _____mL |
| 2  1 kg = | _____g | | 7  2.5 g = | _____mg |
| 3  1 cm = | _____mm | | 8  500 mg = | _____g |
| 4  1 mg = | _____mcg | | 9  2500 mg = | _____g |
| 5  1 g = | _____mcg | | 10  50 mcg = | _____mg |

# Milliequivalents (mEq)

**FAQ** | *What is a milliequivalent (mEq), and what is the difference between a milliequivalent and a milligram (mg)?*

**ANSWER:** The milliequivalent is another way of expressing the contents of a medication in solution. A milliequivalent is the number of grams of solute in 1 mL of solution. It reflects the *chemical combining power* of the ingredients. Milligrams are a measure of *weight*.

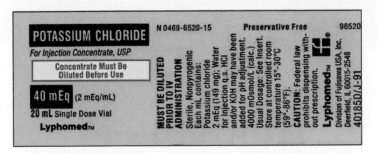

Figure 3-2. Potassium chloride label.

Solutions of electrolytes, such as potassium, sodium, and magnesium, are usually ordered and supplied in numbers of mEq/ mL or mEq/ L. The medication label may also state the amount of milligrams of drug contained in the product.

➤ Milligrams and milliequivalents are not equivalent.

| | |
|---|---|
| Many intravenous solutions administered by nurses contain electrolytes. The sample medication label in Figure 3-2 includes both milliequivalents and milligrams. In small print, the label lists 2 mEq (149 mg). | **Clinical Relevance** |

➤ When interpreting the label shown in Figure 3-2, it is important for the nurse to recognize that 2 mEq *cannot be substituted for* 149 mg in dose calculations.

## Other Medication Measurement Systems

### Household Measurements

Most people are familiar with household (kitchen) measurement terms. It is important to realize that household utensils are usually not calibrated precisely. There are small and large teaspoons and tablespoons, cups, and glasses. Medicines taken at home should be taken with specially calibrated droppers, measuring teaspoons, and cups. Patients and their families need instruction about the use of precisely calibrated household measuring devices before being discharged from the hospital.

### Apothecary System

The apothecary system of weights and measures was transported from Greece to England in 1602 and from there to the U.S. Most of the terms used for medications have now been replaced by the metric system. Some of the Apothecary terms are being used occasionally and can lead to error if they are misinterpreted.

Compare the systems in Table 3-2.

| | |
|---|---|
| Apothecary minims measurements used to be seen on syringes. If they appear, there will be a second scale in milliliters on the other side of the syringe (Figure 3-3).<br>➤ Read the milliliter calibrations and ignore the minims. Note the large difference between minims and milliliters: 16.2 minims = 1 mL. | **Clinical Relevance** |

➤ Errors have been caused by nurses who assumed a minim was the same as a milliliter.

| TABLE 3-2 | Comparison of Metric, Household, and Apothecary Liquid Measurements Used for Medications | |
| --- | --- | --- |
| **Metric** | **Household** | **Apothecary** |
| 1 mL | 1 drop | 15-16 minims* |
| 5 mL | 1 teaspoon (tsp) | 1 dram* (1 tsp) |
| 15 mL | 1 tablespoon (tbs) (½ oz) | 4 drams (oz s̄s̄) |
| 30 mL | 2 tablespoons (1 oz) | 8 drams (oz i) |
| 240 mL | 1 measuring cup (8 oz) | 8 oz (oz viii) |
| 500 mL | 1 pint (16 oz) | 1 pint (16 oz) |
| 1000 mL (1 L ) | 1 quart (32 oz) | 1 quart (32 oz) |
| 4 L | 1 gallon (gal) (4 quarts) | 1 gallon (4 quarts) |

**Note:** All equivalents with Household and Apothecary are approximate. Equivalents within the metric system are precise. Apothecary numbers used for medications are usually written in lowercase Roman numerals followed by numbers or fractions. The fraction $\frac{1}{2}$ is written as s̄s̄ (with the overbar).

*Minims and drams are no longer seen in medication orders.

Figure 3-3. 1-mL tuberculin syringe with minim and milliliter measurements. (From Clayton BD, Stock YN: Basic pharmacology for nurses, ed. 13, St. Louis, 2004, Mosby.)

## Household and Metric Liquid Measuring Containers

➤ Syringes, calibrated medicine cups, and calibrated droppers are used in clinical practice to prepare small amounts of liquid doses (Figure 3-4).

Figure **3-4**. Household and metric measuring liquid containers. (From Brown M, Mulholland J: Drug calculations: process and problems for clinical practice, ed 7, 2004, St. Louis, Mosby.)

1  If an order calls for 1 tsp of cough medicine, how many milliliters will the nurse prepare?

_____

2  If an order calls for 1 tbs of a laxative, how many milliliters will the nurse prepare?

_____

3  If an order calls for $\frac{1}{2}$ oz of an antacid, how many milliliters will the nurse prepare?

_____

The terms ounces and pounds are familiar, but the term grain (gr) as a unit of measurement is not. The grain is a basic unit of mass, or weight, in the apothecary system and is based on the weight of a grain of wheat. The numbers that accompany grains are written in Roman numerals and fractions following the unit name grain (Table 3-3).

➤ Do not make up abbreviations. For example, writing gr for gram (g) might be misread as grain. A gram is 15 times larger than a grain. Writing gm for gram (g) can also lead to errors.

➤ A line is placed over lowercase Roman numerals in the apothecary system, as noted with $\overline{xv}$ and $\overline{ss}$. Lowercase numerals are used for numbers less than 20.

The apothecary symbol for $\frac{1}{2}$ is two lowercase s's with a line over them: gr $\overline{ss}$ (as shown in Table 3-3).

➤ Refer to the inside back cover for the metric apothecary conversion clock.

**Q** *Ask Yourself*

**A** *My Answer*

### TABLE 3-3

### Comparison of Metric And Apothecary Weights

| Metric | Apothecary |
|---|---|
| 1000 g = 1 kg | 2.2 lb |
| 1000 mg = 1 g | 15 grains (gr $\overline{xv}$)* |
| 60 mg | gr $\dagger$ |
| 30 mg | gr $\frac{1}{2}$ or $\overline{ss}$ |
| 0.6 mg | gr $\frac{1}{100}$* |
| 0.4 mg | gr $\frac{1}{150}$* |
| 0.3 mg | gr $\frac{1}{200}$* |

*Metric measurements have replaced the use of these apothecary measurements.

### Converting Pounds to Kilograms

➤ Review the required elements of a DA equation

- Desired answer units
- Conversion formula or formulas
- Original factors to be converted

To change pounds to kilograms, create a DA equation using the conversion formula 2.2 lb = 1 kg. Kilograms are metric units of measurement. Pounds are units used in the apothecary and household systems of measurement. Medications are often ordered on basis of kilograms of a patient's body weight.

| **EXAMPLES** | Change 120 lb to kg. Conversion formula: 2.2 lb = 1 kg. Identify the required elements for the equation. |
|---|---|

| Step 1:<br>Desired<br>Answer Units | | Step 2:<br>Conversion<br>Formula (ratio) | | Step 3:<br>Original Factors<br>to Be Converted | | Step 4:<br>Answer |
|---|---|---|---|---|---|---|
| kg | = | $\dfrac{1 \text{ kg}}{2.2 \text{ lb}}$ | × | 120 lb | = | 54.5 kg |

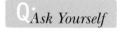

**Q:** *Ask Yourself*

**A:** *My Answer*

1  A 150-lb adult weighs 68.2 kg (150 lb ÷ 2.2 rounded to the nearest tenth). What is your weight in kilograms to the nearest tenth? (Divide your weight in pounds by 2.2.)

_____

**RAPID PRACTICE 3-14** Metric, Household, and Apothecary Equivalents

**Estimated completion time: 5 minutes   Answers on page 516.**

**Directions:** *Examine Tables 3-2 and 3-3 and supply the correct approximate metric, household, or apothecary equivalent.*

1  How many grains are in a gram? _____

2  How many milliliters are in 2 tsp? _____

3  How many milliliters are in a tablespoon? _____

4  How many milliliters are in half an ounce? _____

5  How many mL are in 2 tbs? _____

The figure below is an example of a medication label on which both the metric and the apothecary equivalents appeared in the past:

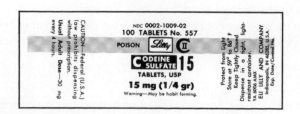

Medicines now are labeled in the metric system even if an apothecary equivalent may remain on a few of the labels. Drug orders that may occasionally be written in grains include the following:

- Aspirin or acetaminophen (Tylenol): gr $\overline{x}$

- Codeine: gr $\frac{1}{4}$ or $\frac{1}{2}$

- Morphine: gr $\frac{1}{8}$, $\frac{1}{4}$, or $\frac{1}{2}$

➤ Use metric. Recognize apothecary. Clarify any orders with the prescriber and/or the pharmacist that are not written in metric terms.

➤ Document the clarification in the medical record.

## Key Points About the Three Measurement Systems

**1** The metric system uses Arabic numerals and decimals. The apothecary system employs Roman numerals and fractions. Double-check any order written in Roman numerals.

**2** The metric system basic unit for mass, or weight, is the gram. The apothecary system uses grains.

**3** A gram is 15 times the size of a grain. If *gram* is abbreviated incorrectly as *gm*, it can be *misread* as *gr*

**4** The metric system measures *liquids* in milliliters and liters. The apothecary system measures liquids in minims, drams, teaspoons, tablespoons, ounces, pints, and quarts.

**5** Household measurements have many implications for patient discharge teaching.

**6** A teaspoon order for medication doses must be calibrated for 5 mL capacity.

**7** A tablespoon order is for 15 mL (3 calibrated tsp) or $\frac{1}{2}$ of a calibrated medication 30-mL cup.

**8** An ounce is 30 mL (2 measuring tbs). Teach patients to use calibrated ounce measurement cups at home. Do not substitute liquor "shot" glasses for ounce cups at home.

**9** The milliliter is the preferred metric unit for liquid measurements. The abbreviation *mL* may be used interchangeably with *cc* (the abbreviation for cubic centimeters) by some prescribers.

**10** A liter is a little more than a quart. Liters are used in clinical agencies. Quarts are not.

**11** If the l in lb is written next to the number without a space (i.e., 2.2lb), it may be misread as the number 1.

**12** Think metric but be prepared to see occasional apothecary orders. Verify the equivalent measurement with pharmacy. Never guess.

➤ The nurse who confuses mg with mcg, mL and mg with g or mEq, or gr and g is at extreme risk for making medication dose errors.

Nurses must learn the metric system in order to read and interpret physicians' orders and medication labels. For the sake of patients' safety, nurses must master and become comfortable using all the metric units employed in medications.

A nurse who has committed the relevant metric system terminology and values to memory will never have to say, "I thought *mg* and *mcg* were the same thing," after administering a dosage that was in error by a thousand-fold.

| **Clinical Relevance** | Examples of errors in the clinical setting include the following:<br>• Giving 10 mL of a liquid drug instead of 10 mg<br>• Converting 1 g to 100 mg instead of 1000 mg, a ten-fold error.<br>• Giving 20 mg instead of 200 mg for a 0.2 g order, a ten-fold error<br>• Reading 100U as 1000 because *Units* was not spelled out or a space was not left between the number and the *U*, or the *U* was closed and looked like a zero, resulting in a ten-fold overdose<br>• Reading 7.5 mg as 75 mg because the decimal was not seen<br>• Reading 100 mEq as 100 mg, two different measurements |
| --- | --- |

➤ Knowing the value of the difference between a microgram, a milligram, and a gram is critical. Knowing that a milliequivalent is not a milligram is critical.

➤ Note that hospital policy may require that the prescriber be contacted for use of nonmetric terms and unapproved abbreviations.

➤ Table 3-4 lists some recommendations on how to avoid metric abbreviation errors.

➤ For the "Do Not Use" list, refer to the inside front cover.

➤ Keep an eye out for TJC's "Do Not Use" abbreviations in the clinical setting and in written references. They are likely to cause errors.

| TABLE 3-4 | **Metric Abbreviations That May Generate Errors** | | |
| --- | --- | --- | --- |
| **Unit** | **Abbreviation to Use** | **Abbreviations to Avoid** | **Potential Errors** |
| milliliter(s) | mL | cc (cubic centimeter), ccs, mls | Misread when written poorly; *L* for *liter* capitalized to prevent misreading as the number 1; metric abbreviations not pluralized |
| gram(s) | g | gm, gms, gs, G, Gs | Misread as *gr* (grain) when poorly written; should not be capitalized or pluralized |
| microgram(s) | mcg | $\mu$g, $\mu$gs, $\mu$ | Misread as *mg* (milligram) or zero (0) |
| milligram(s) | mg | mgm, mgms | Misread as microgram |
| Units | Write out Units (do not abbreviate) | U,* u* | Misread as zero (0) |
| International Units | Write out International Units (do not abbreviate) | IU* | Misread as the number 10 |

*Metric units included in TJC's "Do Not Use" list as of 1/1/2004. Their use has been banned in clinical agency handwritten medical records. Refer to inside front cover for complete TJC's "Do Not Use" list.

## CHAPTER 3 MULTIPLE-CHOICE REVIEW

**Estimated completion time: 10-20 minutes**   Answers on page **516.**

**Directions:** *Circle the correct answer.*

1  The correct abbreviations for metric prefixes are

   **1.** L, m, g
   **2.** m, c, k, mc
   **3.** mg, ml, cc
   **4.** mm, cm, mg, kg

2  Select the correct equivalent for 0.003 g.

   **1.** 3 mcg
   **2.** 3 mg
   **3.** 30 mg
   **4.** 300 mg

3  Select the correct equivalent for 50 mg.

   **1.** 5 g
   **2.** 0.5 g
   **3.** 0.05 g
   **4.** 0.005 g

4  Select the correct equivalent for 3 kg.

   **1.** 1 g
   **2.** 3 g
   **3.** 3000 g
   **4.** 30,000 g

5  Which is the appropriate way to write *Units* in the medical record?

   **1.** Units
   **2.** U
   **3.** u
   **4.** U's

6  Select the correct equivalent for 0.5 L.

   **1.** 50 mL
   **2.** 500 mL
   **3.** 0.5 mL
   **4.** 5000 mL

7  Select the correct equivalent for 0.2 g:

   **1.** 2000 mg
   **2.** 20 mg
   **3.** 2 mg
   **4.** 200 mg

8  Select the correct equivalent for 3500 g.

   **1.** 3.5 kg
   **2.** 350 kg
   **3.** 3500 kg
   **4.** 35 kg

9  Select the correct equivalent for 0.25 g.

   **1.** 2500 mg
   **2.** 250 mg
   **3.** 25 mg
   **4.** 2.5 mg

10  Select the correct equivalent for 100 mg.

   **1.** 1 g
   **2.** 10 g
   **3.** 0.1 g
   **4.** 0.05 g

## CHAPTER 3 FINAL PRACTICE

**Estimated completion time: 15-20 minutes**   Answers on page **516.**

1  Write out the three approved base SI units and the four prefixes and their abbreviations covered in this chapter.

| Base Units Abbreviation | | Prefixes Abbreviation | |
|---|---|---|---|
| a. _____ | _____ | d. _____ | _____ |
| b. _____ | _____ | e. _____ | _____ |
| c. _____ | _____ | f. _____ | _____ |
| | | g. _____ | _____ |

2 The physician ordered 0.15 g of a medication. How many milligrams would be the equivalent? _____ Use the DA method to back up your answer. Label all work.

DA Equation:

3 The physician ordered 400 mg of a medication. How many grams would be the equivalent? _____ Use the DA method to back up your answer. Label all work.

DA Equation:

4 If you drank 0.25 L, how many milliliters would you have consumed? _____

DA Equation:

5 How many milligrams are in a medication that contains 150 mcg? _____

DA Equation:

6 A baby weighs 1.5 kg. How many grams would be the equivalent? _____

DA Equation:

7 The physician ordered 0.1 g of a medication. How many milligrams would be the equivalent? _____

DA Equation:

8 If a scar measured 15 mm, how many centimeters would be the equivalent? _____ Use the appropriate conversion formula and DA style method to solve.

DA Equation:

**9** The physician ordered 0.2 mg of a medication. How many micrograms would be the equivalent? _____

DA Equation:

**10** How many grams are in 256,000 mcg? _____

DA Equation:

**11** If you were giving medications in home care, how many milliliters would you prepare for 3 tsp? _____

DA Equation:

**12** If 2 tbs were ordered for a home-care patient, how many milliliters would be prepared? _____

DA Equation:

**13** How many milliliters are in 1.5 oz of medication? _____

DA Equation:

**14** How many teaspoons are in a medication tablespoon? _____

DA Equation:

**15** How many medication tablespoons are in 2 ounces? _____

DA Equation:

**16** How many grams are in a kilogram? _____

DA Equation:

**17** How many pounds are in a kilogram? _____

DA Equation:

**18** How many milliliters are in a half-liter (0.5 L)? _____

DA Equation:

**19**

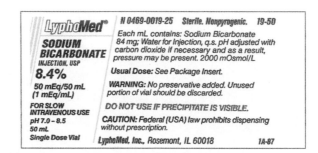

**a.** How many milligrams per milliliter of sodium bicarbonate are contained in the medication with the label shown above? _____

**b.** How many milliequivalents of sodium bicarbonate are contained in 1 milliliter? _____

**20**

**a.** How many milligrams per milliliter of potassium chloride are noted on the label shown above? _____

**b.** How many milliequivalents per milliliter of potassium chloride are noted on the label? _____

## Suggestions for Further Reading

www.guideline.gov/summary
www.ismp.org
www.jointcommission.org
www.lamar.colostate.edu
www.mathforum.org/library
www.wordiq.com/definition/SI

 Additional information can be found in the Introducing Drug Measures section on the enclosed companion CD.

Chapter 4 incorporates the material that has been learned in Chapters 1-3—arithmetic, metric units, mental math, and dimensional analysis—and applies that knowledge to interpretation of medication orders, drug labels, and medication records.

*"Perplexity is the beginning of knowledge."*
**KHALIL GIBRAN**

# PATIENT RECORDS, MEDICATION ORDERS, AND LABELS

## Objectives

- Interpret medication orders and labels.
- Identify abbreviations that cannot be used for handwritten medical records.
- Identify abbreviations that can lead to medication errors.
- Identify forms of medications.
- Read and write time using the 24-hour clock.
- Describe the data from the order and label that must be entered in all medication calculations.
- Interpret Medication Administration Records (MAR).
- Describe medication-related nurse actions that may lead to medication errors.
- Identify patients' rights.

## Essential Prior Knowledge

Mastery of Chapters 1-3

## Equipment

While not essential, the following items will be useful:

- Several medication labels (over-the-counter and/or prescription)
- 30-mL plastic medicine cup
- Glass measuring cup marked in ounces and milliliters

## Estimated Time To Complete Chapter

- 1-2 hours

## Introduction

Physicians and other prescribers write medication and treatment orders on the patient's medical record on a page usually designated "Physician's Order Sheet" or "Doctor's Order Sheet." Several timesaving abbreviations are used to write medication orders, labels, and records.

The medication orders are sent to the pharmacy. The trend has been for the pharmacy to transfer the orders to computerized forms. In most hospitals, medications are charged to the patient and delivered to the patient's area by the pharmacy in unit-dose (single-serving) packages labeled in metric system measurements. The medications may be stocked in a locked cabinet or in drawers of a locked medication cart until needed and restocked periodically by the pharmacy, usually every 24 hours.

The nurse must check the complete written order against the label on the medication supplied. If there is any discrepancy, the physician or pharmacist, whoever is more appropriate for the situation, must be contacted. If the amount of the dose is ordered based on the patient's weight or the amount of drug on hand is not identical to the amount ordered, a calculation may be needed. Usually, such calculations can be performed mentally, but sometimes written mathematics or a calculator is needed.

**103**

There is potential for error in each step of the written process, including the order, the medication administration record, the supplied medication and its label, and the preparation and administration. The nurse who administers the medication is legally responsible for the medications given even if the order was wrong or the medication and/or dose supplied by the pharmacy was in error. The nurse provides the final protection for patients in the medication chain.

This chapter focuses on reading and interpreting medication dose orders, labels, and abbreviations within the context of patients' safety. Abbreviations and measurements learned in earlier chapters are incorporated.

## ESSENTIAL Vocabulary

| | |
|---|---|
| Drug Form | The composition of a drug: liquid or solid; tablet, capsule, or suppository, etc. |
| Drug Route | The body location where the drug will be administered, e.g., mouth, nasogastric (nose to stomach), vein, muscle, subcutaneous tissue, rectum, or vagina. |
| FDA | Food and Drug Administration, the federal agency responsible for approving tested drugs for consumer use in the United States. |
| Generic Drug | *Official* name used for a drug by all companies that produce it. For example, there are many brands and trade names for *acetaminophen,* the *generic* name for Tylenol. *Acetaminophen* is the official name. Tylenol is a brand name. |
| | Generic drugs are identical or bioequivalent to brand-name drugs in dosage form, safety, strength, route of administration, quality, performance, and intended use. |
| MAR | Medication administration record, the official record of all medications ordered for and received by each patient during an inpatient visit. It is maintained by nurses. Each page may reflect one or more hospital days. |
| NF | National Formulary, the official resource for the contents of generic drugs. *NF* is occasionally seen on medication labels. |
| NKA | No known allergies |
| NKDA | No known drug allergies |
| OTC Drug | Drug sold and purchased "over the counter" in drugstores, grocery stores, and health food stores without a prescription. Some were formerly required to be dispensed only by prescription and have been released from that requirement by the FDA. |
| Patent | Official permission from the U.S. Patent Trade Office to market a drug exclusively for 20 years from the time of application. The patent period compensates the first company to market a drug for the costs of drug research and development. |
| | After the patent period expires, other manufacturers may apply to sell the generic form of the drug and must meet the same standards as the original company. |
| TJC | The Joint Commission |
| Trade Name | Name assigned to a product by its manufacturer. The symbol ® written as a superscript after a trade name indicates that the manufacturer has officially registered that name for the product with the U.S. Patent Trade Office. |
| 24-Hour Clock | System for telling time that begins with 0001 (1 minute after midnight) and ends with 2400 (midnight). Also known as the international clock or military time. |
| | The system is used internationally and has been adopted in the United States by many agencies to avoid potential confusion caused by duplication of AM and PM hours. |

| Unit Dose | The usual dose serving of a solid or liquid medication for the target population, child and/or adult. |
|---|---|
| Unit-Dose Packaging | Unit-dose packaging has the advantage of serving as a safety net, because it helps limit the amount of overdose that might occur. |
| USP | United States Pharmacopoeia, the official drug reference that lists all FDA-approved 60 generic drugs. *USP* can be seen next to the generic name on some drug labels. |
| Usual Dose | Manufacturer's recommendation for the average dose strength (concentration) that usually achieves the desired therapeutic effect for the target population (e.g., "for adults with fever, 1-2 tablets every 4-6 hours, not to exceed 6 tablets in 24 hours"). |
| | Based on clinical trials, the usual dose is often specified by the patient's weight and occasionally by body surface area or age. |

1  What is the difference between a trade-name product and a generic product and why must the nurse know the difference?

$Q$ *Ask Yourself*

_____

$A$ *My Answer*

2  What are some examples of drug forms?

_____

3  How may unit-dose packaging help prevent a medication error?

_____

4  What is the abbreviation for the daily medication record maintained by the nurses?

_____

## RAPID PRACTICE 4-1  Essential Vocabulary

**Estimated completion time: 5 minutes**  Answers on page **518**

**Directions:** *Circle the correct answer.*

1  The term that describes the difference between a medication capsule, suppository, tablet, or liquid solution is

**1.** form            **3.** trade
**2.** generic         **4.** OTC

2  Medications, vitamins, and minerals that can be purchased without a prescription are designated

**1.** generic         **3.** OTC
**2.** trade           **4.** Rx

3  The official organization that approves the sales of new drugs for consumers based on laboratory and clinical testing is

**1.** USP             **3.** NF
**2.** FDA             **4.** PTO

4  The name for a single-serving package of a tablet, capsule, or liquid is

**1.** dose concentration   **3.** total dose
**2.** unit dose            **4.** form

5 The name for a drug that can be sold under a variety of trade names by a variety of manufacturers after the original patent has expired is

1. proprietary
2. generic/official

3. over-the-counter
4. USP

# Medication Storage and Security

Medications for institutional use are stored in locked cabinets, carts, and drawers (Figure 4-1).

Bar codes are increasingly used to reduce medication errors. The pharmacy enters the patients' drug information, records, and medication orders into a com-

**A**

Figure 4-1. **A,** One-cell Omni supplier module. **B,** The Lighted Matrix Drawer. **C,** Safety stock scanning bin bar code. **D,** Safety stock scanning item code. (From Omnicell, Inc., Palo Alto, CA.)

**B**

**C**

**D**

**Figure 4-2.** Bar code reader. (From Kee JL, Marshall SM: Clinical calculations: with applications to general and specialty areas, ed. 5, St. Louis, 2004, Saunders.)

puter. Each dose is bar-coded in the pharmacy. The nurse uses a hand-held scanner to scan the drug and the patient's wrist bracelet (Figure 4-2). The computer checks that it is the right medication for the right patient. Unit-dose medications supplied by the pharmacy also reduce medication errors.

## Medication Forms and Packaging

Medications are supplied in a variety of solid and liquid forms, including tablets, capsules, suppositories, and various liquid preparations. The physician's order must specify the form of the medication. A single medication may be prepared in several forms and marketed and packaged in several single and/or multidose sizes. Multidose sizes are convenient for pharmacy and home use (Figure 4-3). At most clinical facilities, the pharmacy packages smaller single-serving-size amounts from the multidose containers to reduce medication errors (Figure 4-4).

**Figure 4-3.** Dilantin label.

**Figure 4-4.** Unit dose packages. (From Clayton BD, Stock YN: Basic pharmacology for nurses, ed. 13, St. Louis, 2004, Mosby.)

Since medications are supplied in a variety of forms to meet patients' needs, it is important to select the form that matches the physician's order. This is done by matching the order to the medication label. The orders for medication forms are abbreviated.

# Solid Drug Forms

Table 4-1 lists solid medication abbreviations, terms, and forms. Since the nurse must be able to interpret the abbreviations and terms, the contents of Table 4-1 should be memorized.

➤ A single medicine may be available as a tablet, a capsule, a gel cap, and an enteric-coated tablet. When there is a choice, the prescriber offers the one that is best for the patient.

| **TABLE 4-1** Solid Medication Forms | |
| --- | --- |
| **Abbreviation or Term** | **Description** |
| cap: capsule | Medication covered in hard or soft gelatin. They are supplied in various sizes. The entire contents may be sprinkled in food such as applesauce or a liquid if the physician so specifies. Capsules should never be cut or divided into partial amounts. |
| caplet | Smooth, lightly coated, small oval tablet. The name is derived from capsule and tablet. It may or may not be scored. |
| compound | Medication consisting of a combination of two or more drugs. Each ingredient may be available in one or more strengths. The order will specify the number of tablets. If there is more than one strength, the order will specify the strength. |
| ent: enteric-coated tablet (Do not use this abbreviation. Always write out.) | Tablet containing potentially irritating substances and covered with a coating that delays absorption until it reaches the intestine. This protects the oral, esophageal, and gastric mucosa. Should not be crushed, cut, or chewed. *Enteric* should be written out to avoid misunderstanding. |
| gelcap, soft-gel | Capsule cover made of a soft gelatin for ease of swallowing |
| powders and granules | Pulverized fragments of solid medication, to be measured and sprinkled in a liquid or a food such as applesauce or cereal |
| scored tablet | Tablets scored with a dividing line that may be cut in half |
| supp: suppository | Medication distributed in a glycerin-based vehicle for insertion into the rectum, vagina, or urethra and absorbed systemically |
| tab: tablet | Medication combined with a powder compressed into small round and other shapes |
| ung: ointment | Medication contained within a semisolid petroleum or cream base |
| CD: controlled-dose (sustained action) | Terms reflecting the use of various processing methods to extend or delay the release and absorption of the medication. They need to be differentiated from a regular form of the same medicine. |
| DS: double-strength* LA: long-acting | A regular medication may be ordered, for example, every 4 hours. An XR version may be given only every 12 or 24 hours. Some medications, such as Celexa, are marketed in both SR and XL forms. |
| SR: slow-release | |
| XL: extra-long-acting | |
| XR: extended-release | |

*Does not mean long-acting or extended-release. However, a DS pill probably will be given less frequently than a "regular" counterpart.

*Ask Yourself*

*My Answer*

**1** How is DS different from medications marked XL, XR, CD, and LA?

## RAPID PRACTICE 4-2 Abbreviations and Terms for Solid Medication Forms

**Estimated completion time: 5-10 minutes**   Answers on page **518**

**Directions:** *Study the abbreviations in Table 4-1. Supply the abbreviation that may be seen in the prescriber's orders for the following types of medication:*

1  capsule _____

2  double-strength _____

3  extended-release _____

4  suppository _____

5  tablet _____

6  long-acting _____

7  extra-long-acting _____

8  enteric _____

9  controlled dose (sustained action) _____

10  ointment _____

## RAPID PRACTICE 4-3 Solid Medication Forms

**Estimated completion time 5-10 minutes**   Answers on page **518**

**Directions:** *Study the abbreviations in Table 4-1. Give the requested information pertaining to oral medication forms. Use brief phrases.*

1  Name the only oral medication form that may be *cut* in order to give a half-serving. _____

2  What is the abbreviation for the kind of oral medication that is packaged in a soft or hard gelatin covering? _____

3  Name two solid medication forms that should never be crushed or cut.

   _____

4  What is the name for a medication that contains more than one drug, will be ordered by the *quantity* to be given, and may include the strength of each medication within the form supplied? _____

5  Give five abbreviations for *longer-acting* oral medications that would be given less often than a regular medication. _____

# Liquid Drug Forms

Liquid drug forms are packaged in small prefilled unit-dose-serving containers and larger stock bottles, such as the containers seen for multidose home prescriptions. The liquids are supplied and administered through a variety of routes to the patient in an amount of milliliters.

Liquid drug forms are administered using specially calibrated equipment: cups; teaspoons; needles attached to tubing; syringes with needles; needle-less syringes; droppers for the mouth, eye, or ear; or tubes for the stomach and intestine. See Figures 4-5 and 4-6 for examples.

Doses of oral liquid medications such as milk of magnesia (MOM) can be supplied in small unit-dose packages or larger multidose bottles. As stated in Chapter 3, 5 mL and 15 mL are the equivalents of 1 calibrated teaspoon and 1 calibrated tablespoon, respectively. The manufacturer attempts to provide the usual drug dose for the target population within those two measurements because they are reasonable volumes to swallow.

Abbreviations appear in most patients' orders and medication records. They may be handwritten or printed. Memorize the abbreviations in Table 4-2.

**Figure 4-5. A,** Liquid medication in single-dose package. **B,** Liquid measured in medicine cup. **C,** Oral liquid medicine in syringe. (From Potter PA, Perry AG: Fundamentals of nursing, ed. 6, St. Louis, 2005, Mosby.)

**Figure 4-6. A,** Medicine dropper. **B,** Measuring teaspoon. (From Clayton BD, Stock YN: Basic pharmacology for nurses, ed. 13, St. Louis, 2004, Mosby.)

| TABLE 4-2 | Liquid Medication Forms |
|---|---|
| **Abbreviation** | **Form** |
| aq: aqueous | Medication supplied in a water-based solution |
| elix: elixir | Liquid medication sweetened with alcohol, e.g., elixir terpin hydrate (ETH), a cough medicine |
| emul: emulsion | A mixture of two liquids, such as oil and water, that normally do not mix |
| fld: fluid | Of liquid composition |
| gtt (do not use) | Drop(s) (always write out) |
| HS: half-strength (Do not use this abbreviation. Always write out: mistaken for "bedtime.") | Half-strength solution that has been diluted 50% |
| mixt: mixture | Compound medicine consisting of more than one liquid medication |
| sol: solution | Water-based liquid medication |
| susp: suspension | Solid particles mixed in liquid that must be gently but thoroughly mixed immediately before administration; should not be shaken vigorously |

➤ Liquid forms such as suspensions and elixirs cannot be distinguished without reading the label.

---

**RAPID PRACTICE 4-4** Liquid Medication Abbreviations

**Estimated completion time: 5-10 minutes**   Answers on page **518**

**Directions:** *Study Table 4-2 and supply the abbreviations requested if approved. If recommended, write out the term.*

| Liquid Type | Abbreviation |
| --- | --- |
| 1 Suspension | _____ |
| 2 Mixture | _____ |
| 3 Solution | _____ |
| 4 Elixir | _____ |
| 5 Aqueous | _____ |

1   Which of the oral liquid drug forms contains alcohol?

_____

2   Which of the liquid drug forms must be gently and thoroughly mixed before administration?

_____

3   Which of the liquid drug forms is the most concentrated?   _____

_____

Q: *Ask Yourself*

A: *My Answer*

# Medication Routes

Medication routes can be divided into two types:

- Nonparenteral (noninjectable)
- Parenteral (injectable)

➤ The nurse may *not* substitute a different route for the one ordered. Only the prescriber can write and change the medication order.

Nonparenteral routes through which medications are delivered include the following:

- Oral
  - Mouth
  - Buccal and sublingual
- Nasogastric
- Enteric (intestinal)
- Eye and ear
- Gastric
- Rectal
- Skin (topical)
- Vaginal

Several abbreviations are used in medication orders to describe specific nonparenteral routes of administration (Table 4-3). Some of these abbreviations are derived from Latin and Greek. The abbreviations must be learned even though the trend is to write more of them out in English to avoid misinterpretation.

➤ Refer to the inside cover for TJC's "Do Not Use" list. These abbreviations were banned for all handwritten medical records as of 2004.

---

**✳ Mnemonic**

Associate *O* with *oral* and *N* with *nothing* or *no.* (*NPO* is the abbreviation for the Latin phrase *non per os,* meaning *"nothing by mouth."*)

---

| TABLE 4-3 | Nonparenteral Medication Routes |
| --- | --- |
| **Abbreviation or Term** | **Route** |
| AD (Do not use this abbreviation. Always write out.) | Right ear |
| AS (Do not use this abbreviation. Always write out.) | Left ear |
| AU (Do not use this abbreviation. Always write out.) | Both ears |
| buccal (bucc) | To be dissolved in the cheek, not swallowed |
| enteral (ent) | Administered through a tube or port to the small intestine |
| GT | Gastrostomy tube; given through a tube or port directly to the stomach |
| inh | Per inhaler |
| MDI | Metered dose inhaler |
| NG | Nasogastric; given through a tube inserted in the nose to the stomach |
| NPO | Nothing by mouth |
| OD (Do not use this abbreviation. Always write out.) | Right eye |
| OS (Do not use this abbreviation. Always write out.) | Left eye |
| OU (Do not use this abbreviation. Always write out.) | Both eyes |
| PO | Given by mouth |
| PR (Do not use this abbreviation. Always write out.) | Given by rectum |
| SL, subl | Sublingual, meaning "under the tongue"; to be dissolved, not swallowed |
| Top | Topical, meaning "applied to the skin" (e.g., ointments and lotions) |
| Vag | Given per vagina |

➤ The routes accompanied by "write out" on Table 4-3 have abbreviations that have led to medication errors and are best avoided. They had not been prohibited at the time of publication.
There are several routes that must be spelled out.

1 What is the difference between NPO and PO?

_____

2 What is the difference between the buccal and sublingual routes?

_____

**Q:** *Ask Yourself*

**A:** *My Answer*

---

**FAQ** | *What is an example of the kind of error that can occur from administering medication via the wrong route?*

**ANSWER:** A student nurse did not interpret the route GT for a medication. The patient was acutely ill and had a gastric tube as well as a tracheotomy tube. The student administered the medication without supervision into the tracheotomy tube. The tracheotomy tube is an airway tube, and the liquid medication went into the patient's lungs.

---

**RAPID PRACTICE 4-5** Nonparenteral Routes

**Estimated completion time: 5-10 minutes**    Answers on page **518**

**Directions:** *Memorize the nonparenteral routes. Supply the abbreviation for the route in the space provided. If an abbreviation is listed as not recommended, write out the term.*

1  cheek _____

2  sublingual _____

3  nasogastric _____

4  left ear _____

5  gastric tube _____

6  topical _____

7  by mouth _____

8  metered dose inhaler _____

9  vaginal _____

10  nothing by mouth _____

1  Some Latin-derived abbreviations for routes of medication administration include *OS* for left eye, *OD* for right eye, *OU* for both eyes, *AS* for left ear, *AD* for right ear, and *AU* for both ears. Why do you think these abbreviations have been discontinued in favor of spelling the words out?

_____

2  What cue will help you remember that *PO* means "by mouth"?

_____

3  How will you distinguish *subl* and *subcut*?

_____

4  How will you distinguish *GT* and *NGT*?

_____

**Q:** *Ask Yourself*

**A:** *My Answer*

The routes listed in Table 4-4 are for parenteral, or injectable, medications. Parenteral medications are administered under the skin into soft tissue, muscle, vein, or spinal cord. Memorize the abbreviations and terms in the table.

| TABLE 4-4 | Parenteral Medication Routes |
|---|---|
| **Abbreviation or Term** | **Route** |
| epidural | Injected into the epidural space, usually in the lumbar region |
| hypo | Hypodermic; injected under the skin; refers to subcutaneous and intramuscular routes |
| ID | Intradermal; given under the skin in the layer just below epidermis (e.g., skin test)* |
| IM | Intramuscular, intramuscularly; given into the muscle layer, usually the gluteal muscles, the thigh, or the deltoid |
| intrathecal | Given into the spinal canal |
| IV | Intravenous, intravenously; given into vein |
| IVP | Intravenous push; given directly into vein with syringe or syringe pump |
| IVPB | Intravenous piggyback; given into vein via a small container attached to an established intravenous line. |
| subcut† | Subcutaneous, subcutaneously; given beneath the skin, usually into the fat layer of abdomen, upper arm, or thigh |
| TPN | Total parenteral nutrition; nutritional feedings per intravenous line into a large vein |

*Do not confuse ID route with the word "identify."
†Do not write SC or Subc for subcutaneous.

**Q:** *Ask Yourself*

**A:** *My Answer*

5  Why should the route for rectal medications be spelled out rather than abbreviated with the letter *R*?

_____

6  How will you distinguish *IV, IVP,* and *IVPB*?

_____

7  What is the abbreviation for the intramuscular route?

_____

8  What is the abbreviation for the intradermal route?

_____

9  What is the abbreviation for *inhaler*?

_____

10  What kind of solution is TPN?

_____

# Frequency and Times of Medication

**✳ Mnemonic**

tid (three times daily)— "tricycle"
bid (two times daily)—"bicycle"

Table 4-5 lists abbreviations for terms that denote the frequency and times of medication administration. Memorize the abbreviations in the table.

➤  "Give with food" and "Give after meals" are usually orders for medications that irritate the gastric mucosa.

| TABLE 4-5 | Medication Frequency and Time |
| --- | --- |
| **Abbreviation or Term** | **Meaning** |
| $\overline{a}$ or a | Before |
| $\overline{p}$ | After |
| $\overline{c}$ | With (e.g., with meals) |
| $\overline{s}$ | Without |
| $\overline{ac}$ | Before meals |
| $\overline{pc}$ | After meals |
| ad lib | Give as desired; pertains to fluids and activity, *not* to medication |
| bid | Two times a day |
| tid | Three times a day |
| qid (Do not use this abbreviation. Always write out.) | Four times a day |
| qod (Do not use this abbreviation. Always write out.) | Every other day |
| D/C, DC, d/c (Do not use this abbreviation. Always write out.) | Discontinue; discharge |
| hs (Do not use this abbreviation. Always write out.) | Bedtime |
| min | Minute |
| on call | Give the medication when the x-ray department or the operating room (OR) calls for the patient |
| prn | As needed |
| q (Do not use this abbreviation by itself. Always write out.) * | Each, every |
| qh | Every hour |
| q2h | Every 2 hours |
| q4h | Every 4 hours |
| q6h | Every 6 hours |
| q8h | Every 8 hours |
| q12h | Every 12 hours |
| stat | Immediately and only one dose |

* The abbreviation "q" may be used in combination with other letters as listed in Table 4-5.

➤ "Give 1 hour before meals" and "Give 2 hours after meals" are orders for medications that have reduced absorption if given with food.

1  How will you remember to distinguish the abbreviations for *before* and *after* meals?

_____

Q: *Ask Yourself*

A: *My Answer*

| TABLE 4-6 | Selected Abbreviations and Symbols That May Lead to Misinterpretation and Medication Errors | |
|---|---|---|
| **Abbreviation** | **Term to Write Out** | **Error** |
| BT | Bedtime | Mistaken for "twice a day" |
| HS, hs | Bedtime, half-strength | Confused with each other |
| qhs | At bedtime | Mistaken for "every hour" |
| SQ, SC, subq | Subcutaneous, subcut | S mistaken for the number 5, Q for "every" or zero, and C for zero |
| AD, AS, AU | Right ear, left ear, both ears | Confused with the abbreviations for eyes |
| OD, OS, OU | Right eye, left eye, both eyes | Confused with the abbreviation for ears |
| QD, QID, QOD | Everyday, four times a day, every other day | Confused with each other |
| OD | Once a day | Mistaken for "right eye" |
| D/C, DC | Discontinue | Mistaken for "discharge" |
| ss | Half | Mistaken for "sliding scale" |
| + | Plus | Mistaken for the number 4 |
| 0 | Hour | Mistaken for a zero |

➤ Always write out the terms listed in Table 4-6 to avoid medication errors. These abbreviations will probably be banned in the future.

For examples of prohibited abbreviations, refer to TJC's "Do Not Use" list on the inside front cover. Refer also to Table 3-4 and to www.ISMP.org for a more extensive list of abbreviations that have not been banned but that may result in errors and should not be used.

➤ If a medication order contains an abbreviation that has been banned or may be misinterpreted, clarify it with the prescriber.

## RAPID PRACTICE 4-6   Abbreviations for Time and Frequency

**Estimated completion time: 10-15 minutes**   Answers on page **519**

**Directions:** *Study the terms and abbreviations for time and frequency on p. 115. Write in the term or abbreviation requested in the space provided. If an abbreviation is listed as not recommended, write out the term.*

1  pc _____

2  bid _____

3  prn _____

4  s̄ _____

5  stat _____

6  q4h _____

7  NPO _____

8  ac _____

9  c̄ _____

10  ad lib _____

11  with _____

12  as needed _____

13  discontinue _____

14  enteric _____

15  before meals _____

16  each, every _____

17  three times a day _____

18  every 2 hours _____

19  without _____

20  every 12 hours _____

## RAPID PRACTICE 4-7 Terms and Abbreviations for Time and Frequency

**Estimated completion time: 5 minutes**    Answers on page **519**

**Directions:** *Answer the following questions pertaining to abbreviations for times of medication administration in brief phrases.*

1 What commonly used words that begin with *t* and *b* will you use to distinguish the abbreviations for three times a day (tid) and two times a day (bid)? _____

2 What abbreviation would be used if the physician's order indicated to take acetaminophen only *when needed?* _____

3 What would be the *total times* a day a patient would receive a medication q4h? _____

4 How would you interpret the following orders?

  **a.** Give Tears No More gtt $\overline{ii}$ each eye prn itching or burning.

  _____

  **b.** Give antacid Mylanta 1 oz. tid ac. _____

  _____

  **c.** Whom would you consult if you were unfamiliar with these abbreviations?

  _____

5 If you were going to administer two medications, one four times a day (within 12 hours) and the other q4h (within 24 hours), how many doses would you give of each? four times a day: _____ q4h: _____

---

1 Why would it be very important for the nurse to differentiate the meaning of *ad lib* and *prn* in medication orders?

_____

2 What are two abbreviations that may be seen for "hour"?

_____

**Q:** *Ask Yourself*

**A:** *My Answer*

**FAQ** | *Why are orders written for four times a day versus q6h?*

**ANSWER:** Many medications, such as a cough medicine, may be given totally within waking hours, such as 0900, 1300, 1700, and 2100. The patient will not have to be disturbed during sleep. Other medications, such as some antibiotics, need to have a more stable blood level concentration to be effective and/or safe and are ordered at equal intervals around the clock, such as q6h, q4h, or q8h.

▲ **Cultural Note**

Note that there are significant differences in the way abbreviations are used in different countries. In the United Kingdom, *QD* means "four times day." In the United States, *qid* or *QID* means "four times a day," and *qd* or *QD* means *daily*. (These abbreviations are now on TJC's "Do Not Use" list.)

## RAPID PRACTICE 4-8 Abbreviations for Form, Route, and Times

**Estimated completion time: 10 minutes**    Answers on page **520**

**Directions:** *Write the medical abbreviation in the space provided.*

1 suspension _____

2 elixir _____

3 solution _____

4 fluid _____

5 fluid extract _____

6 as needed _____

7 nothing by mouth _____

8 intramuscular _____

9 immediately _____

10 apply to the skin _____

**Directions:** *Write the meaning in the space provided.*

**11** bucc _____    **16** prn _____

**12** ad lib _____    **17** NPO _____

**13** MDI _____    **18** IVP _____

**14** bid _____    **19** on call x-ray _____

**15** ID _____    **20** q6h _____

 **Ask Yourself**

**My Answer**

**1** What are two meanings for the abbreviation *HS*, which, if misinterpreted, may result in an error?

_____

➤ Look up unfamiliar abbreviations. Contact the prescriber when a banned or unclear abbreviation is used. Do not guess. Document the clarification.

## RAPID PRACTICE 4-9 Abbreviations Review

**Estimated completion time: 5-10 minutes**   Answers on page **520**

**Directions:** *Define the abbreviations and terms in the space provided.*

**1** SL _____    **11** PO _____

**2** sol _____    **12** G tube _____

**3** IM _____    **13** ac _____

**4** DS _____    **14** buccal _____

**5** qh _____    **15** pc _____

**6** elix _____    **16** prn _____

**7** q6h _____    **17** bid _____

**8** NGT _____    **18** q8h _____

**9** q4h _____    **19** tid _____

**10** NPO _____    **20** stat _____

➤ Memorize these two important abbreviations seen on medication records:
NKDA, no known *drug* allergies
NKA, no known allergies
➤ These are not interchangeable.

## Medication Orders

The following terms and abbreviations may be seen in medication orders and prescriptions:

| Abbreviation | Meaning | Example |
| --- | --- | --- |
| Rx | Prescription | Rx Sig aspirin 325 mg q4h prn |
| Sig | Take | Sig aspirin 325 mg q4h prn |
| TO | Telephone order | TO Dr. Smith |
| VO | Verbal order | VO Dr Smith |

## Complete Medication Orders

In order to be *complete*, a medication order *must be legible* and contain the following elements:

- Patient's name
- Date and time ordered
- Medication name
- Form
- Total amount in strength to be given
- Route
- Frequency schedules
- Additional instructions if needed
- Signature

## Sample Physician's Order Sheet

**Directions:** *Cover the interpretations below the red line in the sample physician's order sheet below. See if you can read and translate the orders. Check your interpretation.*

---

John Q. Smith          Hospital # _____          Allergies: NKDA

*Male 45*

1/05/06 0900 Ampicillin cap 250 mg PO q6h × 5d

1/05/06 0900 ASA tab 325 mg ent tab PO q4h prn headache $\bar{c}$ food

1/05/06 0900 Compazine SR cap 10 mg PO q12h prn nausea

1/05/06 0900 MOM $\frac{1}{2}$ oz po bid

      1/05/06 William Smith, MD

1/07/06 1000 DC ampicillin

1/07/06 1000 Bactrim DS 1 cap PO stat and daily × 3d

      1/7/06 William Smith, MD

1/09/06 1800 NPO $\bar{p}$ midnight TO Dr. Smith, Jan Brown, RN

1/10/06 0700 Atropine 0.4 mg IM on call OR TO Dr. Smith, Cal Pearce, RN

---

Interpretation                                        No known drug allergies.

Ampicillin 250-milligram capsule by mouth every 6 hours for 5 days.

Aspirin 325-milligram enteric-coated tablet by mouth every 4 hours as needed for headache. Give with food.

Compazine sustained-release capsule 10 milligrams by mouth every 12 hours as needed for nausea.

Milk of magnesia $\frac{1}{2}$ ounce by mouth at bedtime when needed.

Discontinue ampicillin.

Bactrim double-strength capsule by mouth immediately and daily for 3 days.

Nothing by mouth after midnight 1/09/06

1800 telephone order Dr Smith, Jan Brown, RN

1/10/06 7 AM Atropine 0.4 milligram intramuscular route when receive call from operating room, telephone order Dr Smith, Cal Pearce, RN

---

➤ Consult a current drug reference text, glossary, or the pharmacy for interpretation of unfamiliar abbreviations such as ASA (aspirin) or MOM (milk of magnesia).

➤ The nurse cannot give medications more often or earlier than ordered. The prescriber must always be contacted if there is a need to revise the order, such as a need for a prn pain or nausea medication before the prescribed interval.

➤ When orders are handwritten, capitalization, periods, and decimal guidelines are often obscured or ignored. Be very careful with interpretation of handwritten orders.

# Interpreting Labels and Orders

Medication labels must be read carefully and compared with the prescriber's order before preparing a medication. Many drug names look and sound alike, for example, Flonase and FluMist; dopamine and dobutamine, prednisone and prednisolone; digoxin and digitoxin; phentermine and phentolamine; and Norcet and Nordette, to name a few. Analyze the contents, abbreviations, and *differences* among the labels for solid and liquid medications shown in this section.

Most of the information on a medication label is self-explanatory if one understands metric measurements and abbreviations. The unit dose concentration is usually specified in milligrams per tablet or capsule for *solid* forms and micrograms or milligrams per milliliter for *liquid* forms.

➤ Keep in mind as you read medication labels that two key pieces of information are used in all medication calculations:
  1 Ordered dose
  2 Unit dose concentration (on the label)
➤ Misreading a label usually results in a medication error. Accurate medication administration is the responsibility of the nurse.

The nurse focuses on the order in the medical record and on the label. For example,

**Order: Principen 250 mg cap PO tid**

Trade name: Principen®

Generic name: ampicillin, United States Pharmacopeia (USP)

Form: capsules

Total contents of multidose container: 500 capsules

Unit dose strength (concentration): 250 mg/ capsule

Total daily dose ordered: 250 mg × 4, or 1000 mg/ day

Individual dose ordered: 250 mg

Note that the drug is contained in capsules. Oral solid drugs are usually placed in some type of *capsule* or *tablet*. Read the cautions; the expiration date; the usual dose, if mentioned; and storage directions, if any. The nurse seldom has access to the multidose container in large institutions. The pharmacy dispenses the unit doses from the multidose containers. The *label* must match the medication *order*, either the trade name or the generic name.

**FAQ** | *What should the nurse do if the name of the drug on the order is not the same as the name on the label?*

**ANSWER:** Check carefully to see whether the ordered name is the generic equivalent of the name on the label. The order may be written with either the trade or the generic name. Look in a drug reference. Then call the pharmacy if you are uncertain.

**Order: Tegretol susp 100 mg bid c̄ food for a patient with seizures**

Trade name: Tegretol®

Generic name: carbamazepine USP

Form: liquid suspension

Total contents of multidose container: 450 mL

Unit dose strength (concentration): 100 mg/ 5 mL

Total daily dose ordered: 200 mg

Individual dose ordered: 100 mg

Route: oral

**1**  How large an error would a nurse make who did not read the entire label, assumed that it was a unit-dose container instead of a multidose container, and administered the entire contents to the patient?

Q: *Ask Yourself*

A: *My Answer*

2    Examine the Tegretol label above. How could an examination of the label have prevented this kind of error?

_____

**Order: ferrous sulfate 648 mg PO bid pc**

Trade name: none

Generic name: ferrous sulfate (USP)

Form: tablets

Total contents of multidose container: 100 tablets

Total daily dose ordered: 1296 mg

Individual dose ordered: 648 mg

Unit dose strength (concentration): 324 mg/ tablet (5 gr). Note the apothecary measurement. Focus on the metric measurement (mg).

_____

**Order: Septra DS 1 tablet daily**

Trade name: Septra®

Generic name: trimethoprim and sulfamethoxazole

Total contents of multidose container: 100 tablets

Form: scored tablet compound drug

Unit dose strength (concentration): double-strength (DS) compound containing two drugs; 800 mg trimethoprim and 160 mg sulfamethoxazole (If a medication has *DS* on the label, it is available in at least one other strength: regular. It is important to read the order and label carefully to find a match for dosage in a regular-strength or a DS order.)

Route: oral*

_____

* When the route is not mentioned on the label of an unfamiliar medication, check the route with a current reference or pharmacy.

Compound medications can be ordered by the quantity (i.e., the number of tablets or capsules, e.g., Septra DS 1 capsule daily). Compound medications are combined in one capsule.

➤ Tablets can be administered through various routes.

---

**Order: Nitrostat 0.6 mg SL q 5 min × 3 prn angina (chest pain). Call MD if relief is not obtained.**

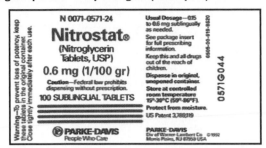

Trade name: Nitrostat®

Generic name: nitroglycerine

Total contents of multidose container: 100 tablets

Form: tablet

Unit dose strength (concentration): 0.6 mg/ tablet (written in two systems, using milligrams and grains)

Route: sublingual (subl)

---

➤ Sublingual tablets must be held under the tongue until they are absorbed. They are not to be swallowed.

1   What are the key differences among the following terms: total contents, total daily dose, dose ordered, unit dose, and usual dose? (Give brief answers.)

**Q:** *Ask Yourself*

**A:** *My Answer*

---

**RAPID PRACTICE 4-10** Interpreting Labels

**Estimated completion time: 10-20 minutes**   Answers on page **520**

**Directions:** *Examine the labels provided, and write the requested information.*

1

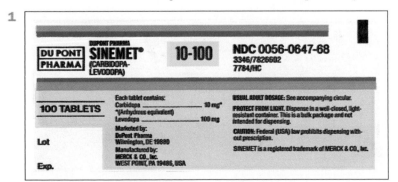

  **a.** Trade name: _____

  **b.** Number of drugs contained in the tablet: _____

  **c.** Generic names and doses within the compound: _____

**a.** Generic name: _____

**b.** Total number of tablets in container: _____

**c.** Unit dose concentration per tablet: _____

**a.** Single- or multiple-dose vial? _____

**b.** Unit dose concentration in micrograms: _____

**c.** Unit dose concentration equivalent in milligrams: _____

**a.** Generic name:_____

**b.** Unit dose concentration:_____

**c.** Total amount in container:_____ mL

**a.** Trade name:_____

**b.** Generic name: _____

**c.** Unit dose in gram equivalent: _____

**6**

a. Trade name: _____

b. Generic name: _____

c. Unit dose concentration: _____

**7**

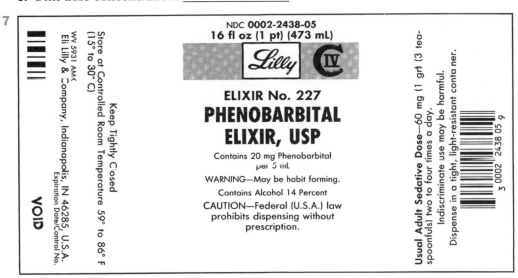

a. Form of medication: _____

b. Unit dose concentration: _____

c. What percent alcohol is contained in this medicine? _____

**8**

| Each tablet contains 600 mg gemfibrozil. | N 0071-0737-20 |
| --- | --- |

Each tablet contains 600 mg gemfibrozil.

Usual Adult Dosage– See package insert for full prescribing information.

Keep this and all drugs out of the reach of children.

Dispense in tight container as defined in the USP.

Store at controlled room temperature 20°- 25°C (68° - 77°F) [see USP]. Protect from light and humidity.

Manufactured by:
Parke Davis
Pharmaceuticals, Ltd.
Vega Baja, PR 00694

Distributed by:
PARKE-DAVIS
Div of Warner-Lambert Co
Morris Plains, NJ 07950 USA
© 1987-'99, PDPL

N 0071-0737-20

**Lopid**®
(Gemfibrozil
Tablets, USP)

**600 mg**

℞ only

60 TABLETS

℗ PARKE-DAVIS

6505-01-290-1762

0737G116

0071-0737-20

Exp date and lot

a. Generic name: _____

b. Unit dose concentration in gram equivalent: _____

c. Unit dose or multidose container? _____

9

NDC 0006-0021-68

**100 TABLETS**
**COGENTIN® 0.5 mg**
(BENZTROPINE MESYLATE)

Dist. by:
**MERCK & CO., INC.**
West Point, PA 19486, USA

USUAL ADULT DOSAGE:
See accompanying circular.

Dispense in a well-closed container.

CAUTION: Federal (USA) law prohibits dispensing without prescription.

100 / No. 3397   7603912

This is a bulk package and not intended for dispensing.

Lot        Exp.

**a.** Generic name: _____
**b.** Unit dose concentration in microgram equivalent: _____
**c.** Total number of tablets in container: _____

10

LOT                    EXP

**200 mg**                    2B0832
                              NDC 0338-1005-02
**Dopamine**                  **50**
(800 mcg/mL)
**Dopamine Hydrochloride**
**and 5% Dextrose Injection USP**   **100**

**250 mL**
EACH 100 mL CONTAINS 80 mg DOPAMINE   **150**
HYDROCHLORIDE USP   5 g DEXTROSE HYDROUS USP
5 mEq/L SODIUM BISULFITE ADDED AS A STABILIZER   pH
ADJUSTED WITH HYDROCHLORIC ACID   pH 3.5 (2.5 TO
4.5)   OSMOLARITY 261 mOsmol/L (CALC)   STERILE
NONPYROGENIC   SINGLE DOSE CONTAINER   DRUG
ADDITIVES SHOULD NOT BE MADE TO THIS SOLUTION
DOSAGE   INTRAVENOUSLY AS DIRECTED BY A PHYSICIAN
SEE DIRECTIONS   CAUTIONS   MUST NOT BE USED IN   **200**
SERIES CONNECTIONS   DO NOT ADMINISTER
SIMULTANEOUSLY WITH BLOOD   DO NOT USE UNLESS
SOLUTION IS CLEAR AND IS NOT DARKER THAN SLIGHTLY
YELLOW   FEDERAL (USA) LAW PROHIBITS DISPENSING
WITHOUT PRESCRIPTION

**Baxter**
BAXTER HEALTHCARE CORPORATION Viaflex® Plus CONTAINER
DEERFIELD IL 60015 USA        PL 2207 PLASTIC
MADE IN USA                   FOR PRODUCT INFORMATION
                             CALL 1-800-933-0303

**a.** Unit dose concentration in mcg/ mL: _____
**b.** Unit dose concentration in mg/ mL: _____
**c.** Specified route of administration: _____

**Q** *Ask Yourself*

**A** *My Answer*

1   What is the *amount* of difference between a microgram and a milligram?

_____

# Calculating Dose Based on Label and Order Information

Interpreting orders and labels provides the information for dose calculation, mental arithmetic, and/or DA equations.

**Memorize:**

The prescribed dose ordered and the unit dose concentration on the label are two factors that must be entered in *every medication dose* calculation. The only other entries in the calculation are conversion formulas as needed.

1   The desired answer unit will almost always be tablets, capsules, or milliliters.
2   The unit dose concentration, such as 10 mg/ tablet, will be placed in the first conversion formula, step 2, in fraction form, just as 5 RN/ 1 LPN and $120/ package were entered in fraction form in earlier DA-style equations.

3   The original factors to be converted will be the prescriber's original ordered drug and quantity.

4   An additional metric conversion formula may need to be entered if the units ordered do not match the units supplied (e.g., milligrams and grams; see step 2A in the example that follows).

➤   If the units ordered are the same as those supplied (e.g., ordered, 650 mg; unit dose supplied, 325 mg), omit step 2A in the equation setup. Mental arithmetic may suffice.

---

**EXAMPLES**

Ordered: aspirin (ASA) 0.65 g. Label unit dose concentration: 325 mg/ tablet.
Conversion formula: 1000 mg = 1 g.

| Step 1: Desired Answer Units | Step 2: Conversion Formula | Step 2A: Conversion Formulas (as Needed) | Step 3: Original Factors to Be Converted (Quantity and Units) | Step 4: Answer |
|---|---|---|---|---|
| | Enter unit dose concentration. | | Enter dose ordered. Cancel units first. ➤ Stop: Will all unwanted units cancel? | Estimate: Ordered dose is about twice the unit dose (mental conversion of g to mg). Multiply: |
| **tablets** = | $\dfrac{1\ \text{tab}}{325\ \cancel{\text{mg}}}$ × | $\dfrac{1000\ \cancel{\text{mg}}}{1\ \text{g}}$ | × 0.65 $\cancel{\text{g}}$ | = $\dfrac{650}{325}$ = 2 tabs  Answer: 2 tabs  Evaluate: The answer matches the estimate. The equation is balanced. |

The final equation will be written like this:

$$\text{tablets} = \frac{1\ \text{tab}}{325\ \cancel{\text{mg}}} \times \frac{1000\ \cancel{\text{mg}}}{1\ \text{g}} \times 0.65\ \cancel{\text{g}} = \frac{650}{325} = 2\ \text{tabs}$$

---

➤   Remember that the label will contain the desired answer units. It will be the first conversion formula, the unit dose concentration conversion formula, or ratio (e.g., 10 mg/ capsule, 1 g/ 5 mL, or 250 mcg/ tablet) to be entered in the equation in fraction form.

➤   The ordered dose and quantity will be entered as the original factors.

➤   One or more conversion factors may need to be entered in the middle (in step 2A) if the units of measurement do not match.

Reminder: The goal of DA is to multiply a known quantity (the ordered dose) by one or more conversion formulas to solve an equation.

1   What are the two critical pieces of information for a DA equation that will be obtained from the order and the label?

_____

2   What are the additional factors that may need to be added if the units ordered and supplied do not match?

_____

**Q:** *Ask Yourself*

**A:** *My Answer*

Some unofficial abbreviations for medications will be learned with clinical experience, for example:

Aspirin (ASA for its chemical name: acetylsalicylic acid)
Penicillin (PCN)
Codeine (Cod)
Hydrochlorothiazide (HCTZ)

These are given so often that they are abbreviated. There have been recommendations to ban the use of abbreviations for names of medicines.

**FAQ** | *Why is the medication not administered in milligrams?*

**ANSWER:** Milligrams are the unit of measurement for the amount of drug contained *within the prepared medication form,* as shown in the following examples:

| **Drug/ Form** | **Drug/ Form** | **Drug/ Form** | **Drug/ Form** |
| 1 mg/ 1 tablet | 1 mg/ 2 capsules | 1 mg/ 1 suppository | 1 mg/ 1000 mL |

If you were going to dissolve 2 tbs of cocoa in 8 oz of hot milk to give to a child, you would administer it in the *form* of 8 oz of the *prepared beverage,* not 2 tbs of cocoa.

**Memorize:**

When all the calculations are completed, the correct amount of medication is given in the form of solids or liquids (e.g., $\frac{1}{2}$, 1, or 2 tablets; 1 or 2 capsules; or a number of milliliters).

## RAPID PRACTICE 4-11 Order and Label Interpretation for DA Equations

**Estimated completion time: 20-30 minutes**   Answers on page **521**

**Directions:** *Examine the example shown in problem 1. Read the order and the label to obtain the answers. Be sure you can read the abbreviations in the order.*

1   Ordered: aspirin tab 0.65 g tid and at bedtime.

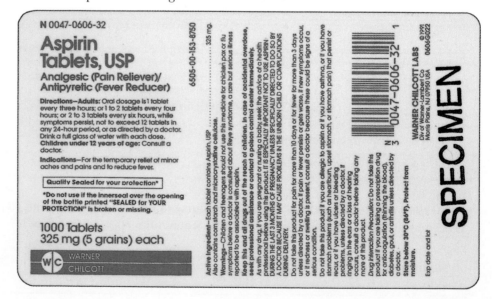

a. Identify desired answer units: <u>tablet</u>
b. Identify the unit dose concentration (first conversion): <u>325 mg/tablet</u>.
   Note the apothecary equivalent: 5 gr per tablet.
c. Identify the original factors to be converted: <u>0.65 g</u>
d. State the second conversion formula if needed: <u>1000 mg = 1 g</u>
e. How often should the medication be administered? <u>3 times a day and</u>
   <u>at bedtime</u>
f. What is the ordered dose equivalent in mg? (Use mental arithmetic.) <u>650 mg</u>

**2** Ordered: cephalexin cap 0.5 g PO q8h × 5 days for a patient with an infection.

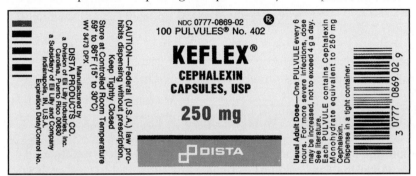

a. Identify desired answer units._____
b. Identify the unit-dose concentration to be entered in a DA
   equation._____
c. Identify the original factors to be converted. _____
d. State the second conversion formula needed. _____  ____
e. What is the total daily dose ordered? _____
f. What is the ordered dose equivalent in milligrams? (Use mental arithmetic.)
   _____

**3** Ordered: cephalexin susp 0.25 g PO q6h × 10 days for a child discharged with
an infection

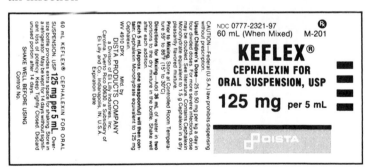

a. Identify the desired answer units. _____
b. Identify the unit dose concentration to be entered in a DA
   equation._____
c. Identify the original factors to be converted. _____
d. State the second conversion formula needed. _____
e. What is the total daily dose ordered? _____
f. What is the ordered dose equivalent in milligrams? (Use mental arithmetic.)_____

**4** Ordered: morphine sulfate 15 mg IM stat for pain.

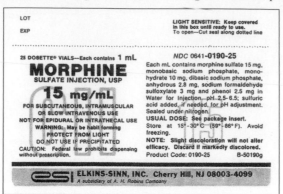

a. Identify desired answer units. _____

b. Identify the unit dose concentration to be entered in a DA equation._____

c. What is the route ordered? _____

d. When is the drug to be administered? _____

e. Three routes by which the label states the drug can be administered:

_____

**5** Ordered: loracarbef susp 0.2 g PO bid.

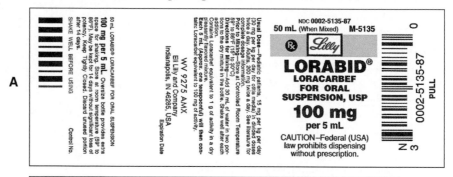

a. What is the generic name? _____

b. What is the form? _____

c. What is the unit dose strength of the medication you would select?

_____

d. What are the original factors to be converted? _____

e. What conversion formula would convert the original factor to the dose supplied?_____

➤ Morphine has a capital C II (Class 2) printed on the label. This means that it is regulated under the Controlled Substances Act, which is enforced by the Drug Enforcement Agency (DEA). There are five classifications or schedules for these drugs. C II drugs have a high potential for abuse but are permitted by prescription for medical use. C II drugs include barbiturates, Percodan, and methylphenidate (Ritalin) as well as other medications.

**1** Morphine is a powerful opioid narcotic. What would probably happen to a patient if the nurse gave the total contents instead of the unit dose strength?

Q: *Ask Yourself*

A: *My Answer*

➤ Do not abbreviate morphine sulfate as MS. It has been mistaken for magnesium sulfate.

Remember that liquid medications are delivered in milliliters. Solid drugs are supplied in many forms, including tablets, capsules, powders, and suppositories.

For reinforcement, the next time you are in a pharmacy section of a store, spend 5 or 10 minutes browsing the cold, cough, and headache medication section and examine the labels. Note the variety of forms and strengths on the labels. Look for the registered sign ®, the generic name, the total dose, and the unit dose on the container. Stores sell drugs in multidose containers so that the customer does not have to return hourly or daily for refills.

**1** What are the *sources* of the two key pieces of information that must be entered in all DA equations for medications?

Q: *Ask Yourself*

A: *My Answer*

## Orders for Two or More Medications To Be Combined

Examine this sample order:

| 9/9/06 1800 | { meperidine 50 mg <br> Vistaril 25 mg } | IM stat and q4h prn pain TO Dr. John Smith, <br> Jane Nurse, RN |
|---|---|---|

Translation:
9/9/06, 6 PM. Give meperidine 50 mg and Vistaril 25 mg together, intramuscular route, immediately and every 4 hours as needed for pain, telephone order, Dr. John Smith per Jane Nurse, RN.

## Telephone and Verbal Orders

➤ Telephone and verbal orders are reserved for urgent situations and must be countersigned at the next visit or within 24 hours by the person who gave the order. Check TJC and agency policies. They are strict. Some agencies forbid verbal medication orders.

TJC recommends that telephone orders be written or entered in a computer and then *read back* for confirmation from the person who gave the order. Be sure to write the name of the person giving the order. Check TJC and agency policies regarding telephone orders.

✳ **Communication**

➤ It is safer to read back and restate numbers individually, such as "three five zero milligrams" as opposed to "350 mg."

## ➤ Examples of Orders That Must Be Clarified

**Order: Tylenol (acetaminophen) 650 mg PO 2 tablets q4h fever over 38 C.**

The prescriber wrote "2 tablets." The medication is supplied as 325 mg/ tablet. Does the order mean 2 tablets of 650 mg, 2 tablets of 325 mg, or 4 tablets of 325 mg? Guidelines require the total dose to be written. This order is confusing and could result in a toxic overdose. Most medicines are supplied in more than one strength. The prescriber cannot second guess which strength the pharmacy will supply. The nurse cannot guess what dose the prescriber meant.

➤ Clarify unclear dose orders, such as total dose desired, with the *prescriber*.

The order should read: Tylenol (acetaminophen) tab 650 mg PO q4h fever over 38 C. The nurse will calculate the number of tablets to give depending on the strength supplied.

---

**Order: Children's Tylenol 1 tsp q4h.**

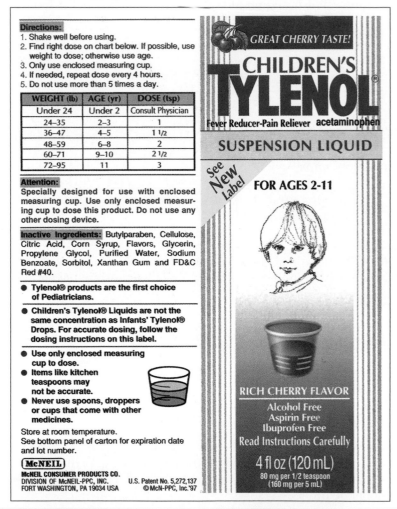

---

➤ The dose strength and form need to be specified.

The order should read: Children's Tylenol susp 160 mg q4h.

## RAPID PRACTICE 4-12  Review of Abbreviations Used for Medication Orders

**Estimated completion time: 15 minutes**   Answers on page 521

**Directions:** *Use brief phrases to describe the hazards of the following types of abbreviations.*

1 How will you distinguish the Latin-derived abbreviation for the word *with* from the abbreviation for *without*?

**2** With whom will you consult if the order contains unapproved or questionable unclear abbreviations?

_____

**3** What do you think may be some of the safety hazards of TO and VO?

_____

**4** If a medication order appeared as follows, would the medications be given separately or together?

[Morphine sulfate 10 mg]
[Atropine 0.4 mg] } IM stat

_____

**5** How can handwritten abbreviations, numbers, decimals, and slashes result in medication errors?

_____

➤ Do not attempt to interpret incorrectly written or confusing orders. Contact the prescriber promptly.

**FAQ** | _How do I go about questioning orders?_

**ANSWER:**

➤ Keep in mind that only the prescriber or designated physician can change the order.

There are a few ground rules:

➤ Illegible or incomplete order: be prepared to contact the prescriber.
➤ Questionable dose or total dose unspecified: contact the prescriber.
➤ Form or dose supplied is a mismatch with the order: contact the pharmacy.

An experienced nurse may not find the order illegible or incomplete. Verify all questions with your instructor after investigation. Students need to review the prescriber's recent progress notes, check a current drug reference, and then clarify with the instructor.

➤ Just because someone else has been giving this medication on earlier shifts does not mean that it is right. Decide whether the pharmacy or the prescriber is the appropriate first contact.

➤ Document all clarifications in the patient's record.

✴ **Communication**

"This is Rose Quartz, RN at General Hospital, Unit 4 A. I'm calling Dr. Doe to clarify a medication order written by Dr. John Doe for patient Mark Smith, aged 60, admitted with appendicitis in room 222." (Read the whole order.) "Please confirm the order for _____(dose, medication, route, times, etc.). The telephone number here is _____." One more sentence may be added regarding the reason for clarification, for example, "The patient is allergic to_____," "The patient is having difficulty swallowing solids," or "The patient had only been receiving half that dose in the past," and so on.

# The 24-Hour Clock

Medications and many other medical records are documented using the 24-hour clock (Figure 4-7). Most institutions use the international 24-hour clock for pharmacy and medication administration records to avoid mistaking AM hours with PM hours. The clock starts at midnight, 0000, and ends at 2400, the following midnight. It is _reset_ to 0000 at midnight for the AM hours. Instead of repeating 1 through 12 twice, the 24-hour clock has one number for each hour, minute, and second. Seconds are not usually written in medication administration records.

- The 24-hour clock is written in hundreds from 0000-2400: midnight to midnight.
- The time designations include a minimum of four digits, two for hours and two for minutes. They do not contain colons.

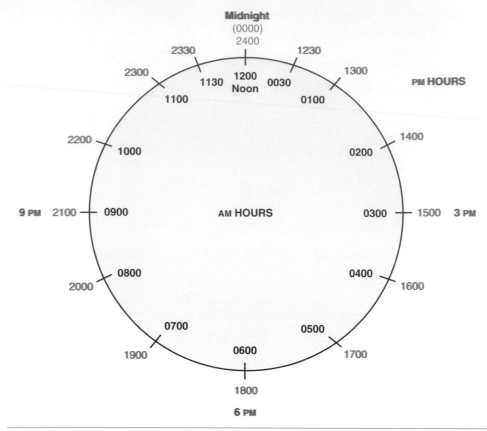

Figure 4-7. The 24-hour clock. (From Brown M, Mulholland J: Drug calculations: process and problems for clinical practice, ed. 7, St. Louis, 2004, Mosby.)

- The AM hours *begin* at midnight, or 12 AM, when the 2400 is *reset* to 0000.
- The AM hours *end* at 11:59 AM, or 1159 hours.
- The clock changes to PM hours at noon. 12 PM (noon) =1200 hours.
- The PM hours end at midnight, which is 12 AM, or 2400 hours, when the clock resets to 0000.
- The AM hours are unchanged except for being written in a four-digit format without a colon. 11:30 AM becomes 1130.

➤ The *major change is at 1 PM,* when the time becomes 1300, to avoid the duplication of writing a second set of 1-12.

**Q:** *Ask Yourself*

**A:** *My Answer*

1  Can you describe an acute problem that might arise if there was confusion about carrying out an urgent order at "2" as opposed to the clarity of 1400 hours or 0200 hours?

_____

2  If you were going to set your timer for a television show at 12 noon, would you set it for 12 AM or 12 PM? Would 1200 or 2400 hours be more helpful? If you set it for 2 minutes after noon, what would the time be on the 24-hour clock?

_____

**Remember:**

| PM Hours | AM Hours |
|---|---|
| 12 PM = noon = 1200 hours | 12 AM = *midnight* = 2400 hours and resets to 0000 hours |
| 1 PM = 1300 hours | 1 AM = 0100 hours |

Medicines given 1 minute after noon are written 1201 hours because the PM hours start at noon. Medicines given 1 minute after midnight are written 0001 hours because the AM hours start at midnight.

## Converting Standard Time to the 24-Hour Clock

**PM Hours**

➤ Add 12 to the PM time: 1 PM + 12 = 13 hours.
➤ Add the minutes or zeros for the last two digits: 10 PM + 12 = 2200 hours.

**AM Hours**

➤ Write the standard time.
➤ For 1 AM to 9 AM, add a leading zero: 1 AM = 0100, 4 AM = 0400.
➤ Add minutes or zeros for the last two digits: 1:30 AM = 0130, 4:00 AM = 0400.
➤ Remove the colon.

## Converting 24-Hour Clock PM Hours to Standard Time

➤ Subtract 1200 from the PM hours 1300 to 2400.
➤ Insert a colon between the minutes and hours. Add PM: 2358 − 1200 = 11:58 PM.

### RAPID PRACTICE 4-13  The 24-Hour Clock

**Estimated completion time: 10-20 minutes**  Answers on page **522**

**Directions:** *Analyze the question to determine whether AM or PM hours are to be identified. Calculate the time using mental arithmetic. Circle the correct answer.*

1  Which is the correct 24-hour clock designation for 1:10 AM?

**1.** 0100                    **3.** 0110
**2.** 1000                    **4.** 2410

2  The maximum hour for the 24-hour clock is

**1.** 1200                    **3.** 2400
**2.** 0001                    **4.** 2459

3  A medication given at 1:30 AM would be written in the medication administration record (MAR) as

**1.** 1300                    **3.** 1030
**2.** 0130                    **4.** 01:30

4  A medication given at 1 PM would be charted in international time as

**1.** 1300                    **3.** 0001
**2.** 1000                    **4.** 0100

5  A change of shift at 4 PM would be noted on the MAR as

**1.** 0400                    **3.** 1400
**2.** 4000                    **4.** 1600

1  At what time, in 24-hour terms, do you usually wake up, eat dinner, and go to bed?

Q: *Ask Yourself*

A: *My Answer*

Write all your appointments from now on in 24-hour clock terms, and in a couple of days the time will be automatic for you.

# Medication Administration Records

The MAR is the official record of all the medications given to the patient. It is maintained by the nurses. The forms are usually computerized in large agencies, but some smaller agencies may use handwritten records (Figures 4-8 and 4-9). The MAR must match the original medication orders.

The nurse enters data as *soon as possible* after administering medications so that no other personnel will mistakenly think a medication was not given and give it again. A medication that is ordered but not given for any reason, including refusal by patient, must also be noted on the MAR. The codes for abbreviations on the MAR differ among departments and agencies, but they are similar enough that they are self-explanatory or can be understood after only a few minutes of consultation with the staff.

**Figure 4-8.** Example of a handwritten medical administration record for 24 hours day of admission.

Mary Laura Rowen
ID 13254444
Age: 49 Rm 250-B

Adm. 06/01/06

GENERAL HOSPITAL

<u>Allergies</u>
*Penicillin (PCN); Aspirin (ASA)*

Today's Date: 6/03/06

| Date Ordered | Medication Dose Rte, Freq | Start Date | Stop Date | 1st shift 2400–0659 | 2nd shift 0700–1459 | 3rd shift 1500–2359 |
|---|---|---|---|---|---|---|
| 6/01/06 | Lasix 20mg po daily AM | 6/01 | | | (0930) Xray JP | |
| 6/01/06 | Humalog 75/25 mix 20 units subcut daily 15 min before bkst | 6/01 | | 0630 MS RA | | |
| 6/01/06 | Digoxin 0.25mg PO daily | 6/01 | | | (P76) 09/30 JP | |
| 6/01/06 | Minocin 100mg PO q12h | 6/01 | 6/05 | 0600 MS | | 1800 LG |

Handwritten MARs may be seen in smaller clinical agencies. They also may be seen on admission until pharmacy computerizes the admission orders. The information contained in MARs is fairly similar. Check agency protocols for data entry requirements. Medications that are withheld typically have the time due encircled with a brief reason for the omission such as NPO, Xray, Lab, or See notes. Some medications such as antibiotics and control drugs have an automatic stop date. Agency policies must to be consulted for those automatic expirations. Take special care with interpretation of handwritten medications and numbers, decimal points and zeros. Also be aware that these records have been hand-copied from prescriber order sheets. Any copying increases risk for error.

PRN and ONE TIME ONLY MEDICATIONS

| 6/01/06 | Meperidine HCL 50mg IM q4h prn pain | 14/00 LJ JP | | |
|---|---|---|---|---|
| | | | | |
| | | | | |

| Signature | Init. | Signature | Init. |
|---|---|---|---|
| Mary Smith | MS | | |
| John Pauli | JP | | |
| Louise Gray | LG | | |

| Patient ID stamp<br>John Douglas Gray<br>523469<br>Room 569-A | MEDICATION<br>ADMINISTRATION<br>RECORD<br><br>GENERAL HOSPITAL | ALLERGIES:<br><br>**NKDA** | |
|---|---|---|---|

| DATE<br>START<br>STOP | MEDICATION DOSAGE, ROUTE<br>ADMINISTRATION TIME | First Shift<br>07:00 to 14:59 | Second Shift<br>15:00 to 22:59 | Third Shift<br>23:00 to 06:59 |
|---|---|---|---|---|
| | Ord. 08-01-06<br>5% Lactated Ringer's<br>Sol. 1000 mL IV<br>TKO at 20 mL/hour<br>continuous | | | |
| | Ord. 08-01-06<br>losartan (Cozaar) tablet<br>50 mg once daily AM and HS<br>Hold for systolic BP less than 130.<br>Call MD. | | | |
| | Ord. 08-01-06<br>Insulin glargine (Lantus)<br>20 units subcut. daily at 8 AM<br>Give on time.<br>Record on insulin MAR.<br>Do not mix with other insulins or medications. | | | |
| | Ord. 08-02-06<br>norfloxacin (Noroxin)<br>400 mg q12h × 3 days<br>STOP 8-05-06 aftor 6 doses<br>Take with glass water 1 hr before or 2 hr after meals | | | |
| | | | | |
| | | | | |

This type of a 24-hour printed MAR for routine scheduled medications can be computer or pharmacy generated. It mentions some administration priorities and includes both the generic and the trade name to reduce chance of error. Separate MARs may be used for one-time-only and prn orders (refer to p.138) and certain drugs such as heparin and insulin, which require coagulation or blood glucose assessment prior to administration.

| SIGNATURES<br>(FIRST & LAST NAME) | INITIALS | SIGNATURES<br>(FIRST & LAST NAME) | INITIALS |
|---|---|---|---|
| | | | |
| | | | |
| | | | |
| | | | |
| | | | |
| | | | |
| | | | |
| | | | |
| | | | |

| SITE CODES | | MEDICATIONS NOT GIVEN | |
|---|---|---|---|
| LU | - L Gluteus | NPO | - NPO |
| RU | - R Gluteus | RF | - Refused |
| LT | - L Thigh | WH | - Withheld |
| RT | - R Thigh | | |
| LA | - L Abdomen | | |
| RA | - R Abdomen | | |
| LV | - L Ventrogluteal | | |
| RV | - R Ventrogluteal | | |
| LM | - L Arm | | |
| RM | - R Arm | | |
| LD | - L Deltoid | | |
| RD | - R Deltoid | | |

**Figure 4-9. A,** Example of a computerized medical administration record.              *Continued*

```
        **** PRN ****
        ACETAMINOPHEN 650MG SUPP
     650 MG PR    Q4H PRN PAIN DOC
    DO NOT GIVE > 4000 MG APAP/24H
          * AS NEEDED FOR TEMP
  Start: 9/23      Stop:
```

```
            50% INJ 50ML
            MP  IV   PRN
            PRN BS <70

  Start: 9/23      Stop:
```

```
  PURALUBE NP OPTH OINT (LACRI-LUBE) UD
     1.00  OU     BID PRN
         FOR THE EYE

  Start: 9/23      Stop:
```

```
  POTASSIUM CL 10MEQ ER TAB (KLOR-CON) UD
     20 MEQ PO      PRN
        MAY GIVE Q8H X 3 FOR K=3-3.4
        OR Q12H X 2 FOR K=3.5-3.8
  Start: 9/23      Stop:
```

RN/LPN SIGNATURE & INIT:

**Figure 4-9, cont'd.  B,** Example of computer-generated medication administration record for PRN medications.

Spaces in rows are avoided as each medication order is entered to prevent overlooked medication order errors.

## RAPID PRACTICE 4-14 Interpreting MARs

**Estimated completion time: 10-15 minutes    Answers on page 522**

**Directions:**  *Add handwritten MAR in Figure 4-8 to answer these questions.*

1 What are the patient's medication allergies? _____

2 When is the next dose of meperidine for pain available for the patient if needed? _____

3  Which medication must be given before breakfast? _____

4  Which drug was withheld because the patient was in x-ray? _____

5  At what time will a new MAR be used? _____

**Directions:** *Read the computerized MARs in Figure 4-9, A and B, and answer the following questions.*

6  Does the patient have medication allergies? (MAR 4-9, *A*) _____

7  Which medication order for a tablet is based on a bedside physical assessment? (MAR 4-9, *A*) _____

8  Which prn medication is given per rectum? (MAR 4-9, *B*) _____

9  The prn ophthalmic ointment route uses a "Do Not Use" abbreviation: OU.
   **a.** What does that mean? _____
   **b.** If you did not know, how would you find out and what action would you take about a prohibited abbreviation? _____

10  How often may the patient have acetaminophen if needed? _____

---

You must witness patients taking their medications in order to document on the MAR that they were administered. Often, when administration is unsupervised, medications have been found in the bedding or have gone back to the kitchen on a food tray. Check your agency's policies for any exceptions to this rule.

**Clinical Relevance**

## Patients' Rights

Meeting the patient's basic rights makes sense to everyone and is an accreditation requirement of TJC. The process of guaranteeing them involves several steps that must be followed consistently to be permanently embedded in practice. The means to ensure each of these rights is addressed throughout the text. Think of *yourself* as a patient as you read the patient's rights regarding medications.

### Seven Basic Rights

| | |
|---|---|
| Right patient | Right route |
| Right drug | Right documentation |
| Right dose | Right to refuse treatment |
| Right time | |

**Right Patient**  TJC requires that two methods be used to identify the patient for medications and treatments. Identify the patient by asking for the patient's full name and checking the wristband identification number or birth date. A patient who is hard of hearing may respond to a wrong name. A room number or bed number does not constitute a valid identification. Medication errors have occurred from relying on room and bed numbers as means of identifying patients.

**Right Drug**  Name the drug and dose you are administering. Ask the patient and family about allergies or problems with medications. The stress on admission may cause patients to forget some of these details. Mention the class and purpose of the drug. Many patients do not know their medications by name.

★ **Communication**

"What is your name?" is best. Asking, "Are you Mr. Smith?" may yield a "Yes" answer from a confused or hard-of-hearing patient. You need to check the full first and last names.

**Q** *Ask Yourself*

**A** *My Answer*

1   Do you think that giving a "look-alike" generic drug to a patient instead of the ordered drug because the spelling was very similar would constitute a valid legal defense (e.g., AndroGel, which is testosterone, for Amphojel, an antacid)?

---

**Right Dose** The dose prepared must be the same as the *ordered* dose. The ordered dose may involve giving 1 to 2 tablets or 1 to 2 unit-dose servings of an injectable or oral liquid. When the dose to be administered exceeds 1 to 2 portions of the unit-dose serving, withhold the medication and promptly recheck the order. Clarify the order with the prescriber. Remember that the unit dose is the usual average dose ordered.

➤ Beware of decimal-reading errors, and look up unfamiliar drugs and doses in current drug references.

**Right Time** Medications generally should be given within 30 minutes of the designated time. The need to give medications on time can present delivery difficulties if the institution schedules all daytime medications at the same time for all patients, for example, at 9, 1, 5, and 9 o'clock or 8, 12, 4, and 8 o'clock.

➤ Some priority medications must be given very promptly:

  • Stat and emergency medications
  • Medications for acute pain or nausea and powerful intravenous medications
  • Medications to be taken with meals or before or after meals, such as insulin and other antidiabetic agents

If the nurse is delivering many medications to a group of patients, the delivery schedule must be prioritized. Safe prioritization can be achieved through experience and study. Students need to consult with an instructor and/or clinical mentors.

➤ Ask for help when the medication work load is too heavy to deliver medications in a timely manner.

**Right Route** Many medications are packaged in several forms: solids and liquid, oral and injectable, or for intravenous or intramuscular injection. The name will be the same, but the routes may differ.

Compare the ordered route with the fine print on the label. Students in particular need to ask for help from the appropriate source when they meet the unfamiliar.

The *route* was not specified in the order. Occasionally, the physician may omit writing the PO route when the medication is a tablet or capsule. That is an error. The front of labels specifies tablets or capsules, but the oral route is not always mentioned on the label. All other routes are specified on the label. Suppository labels contain the words *suppository* and *the route*. It is understandable that some very large pills and capsules might seem too large to swallow, but giving them rectally would not be effective or wise. The form (suppository) of a drug and the route (rectal) must be specified in the order and on the label.

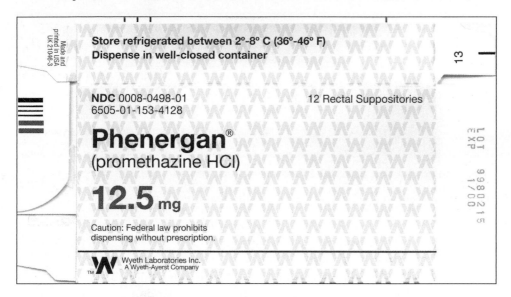

**Right Documentation** Prompt documentation on the correct MAR prevents duplication errors. Such errors can occur when another nurse gives the medication again because the first nurse did not record it in the right record or in a timely manner.

➤ Document soon *after* medication is given, never *before* it is given. Include drugs that had to be held or omitted.
➤ Remember the cliché, "If it wasn't documented, it wasn't done."

**Right to Refuse Treatment** Promptly report and document the refusal and the reason given for it.

## RAPID PRACTICE 4-15 Identifying Patients' Basic Rights

**Estimated completion time: 5-10 minutes**   Answers on page **522**

**Directions:** *Match the nurse action to the letter that corresponds to the appropriate basic patient right:*

### Patient's Basic Rights

**a.** Right patient
**b.** Right drug
**c.** Right dose
**d.** Right route
**e.** Right time
**f.** Right documentation
**g.** Right to refuse

**1** Instruct the patient to hold a sublingual tablet under the tongue until dissolved. _____

**2** Check wrist identification band with full written name. _____

3 Give the stat medication 10 minutes after order is received. _____

4 Compare the order and name of the drug on the label three times before administering it. _____

5 Calculate and question an order that exceeds 2 times the unit dose supplied by the manufacturer and pharmacy. _____

6 Record medication administration promptly on the MAR.

➤ Write out the seven basic patient's rights in abbreviated form.

_____

_____

## CHAPTER 4 MULTIPLE-CHOICE REVIEW

**Estimated completion time: 10-15 minutes**  Answers on page **522**

**Direction:** Circle the correct answer. Consult Chapter 2 if necessary.

1 Which is the correct interpretation for the following physician's order: Amphojel antacid 15 mL tid pc and hs?
   **1.** Amphojel 15 mL 3 times a day after meals and at bedtime
   **2.** Amphojel 15 mg twice a day before meals and at bedtime
   **3.** Amphojel 15 mL twice a day before meals and at bedtime
   **4.** Amphojel 15 mL 4 times a day after meals and at bedtime

2 Which is the correct interpretation for the following physician's order: ampicillin 500 mg IM stat and q8h?
   **1.** Ampicillin 500 mg intramuscular whenever necessary and three times a day
   **2.** Ampicillin 0.5 g intramuscular immediately and every 8 hours
   **3.** Ampicillin 500 mg intravenously and every 8 hours
   **4.** Ampicillin 500 mg intramuscularly at discharge and every 8 hours

3 What is the correct interpretation for the following abbreviations: *tid ac?*
   **1.** Twice a day after meals and periodically
   **2.** Twice a day before meals and periodically
   **3.** Three times a day before meals
   **4.** Three times a day after meals

4 What would be the appropriate interpretation for the following order: morphine sulfate 10 mg IM stat?
   **1.** Give morphine sulfate 10 mg IM when needed
   **2.** Give morphine sulfate 10 mg IM as desired
   **3.** Give morphine sulfate 10 mg on call to X ray
   **4.** Give morphine sulfate 10 mg immediately

5 How would you interpret the following order: NPO p midnight?
   **1.** May not eat after 1200
   **2.** Nothing by mouth after 2400 hours
   **3.** No physical activity after midnight
   **4.** Do not wake after midnight

6  What would be an appropriate schedule for the following order: 8 oz $H_2O$ q6h?

**1.** 0800, 1400, 2000, and 0200
**2.** 0900, 1300, 1700, and 2100
**3.** 0900, 1300, 1700, 2100, 0100, and 0500
**4.** 0800, 1200, 1800, and 2400

7  How would you interpret the following military hours in standard time: 0001 and 1425?

**1.** 1 AM and 4:25 PM
**2.** 1 PM and 2:25 AM
**3.** 12:01 AM and 2:25 PM
**4.** 12:01 PM and 2:25 AM

8  How many times a day is a q4h medicine given?

**1.** 4
**2.** 6
**3.** 8
**4.** 12

9  How should a susp be prepared for administration?

**1.** Shake well until completely dissolved.
**2.** Shake vigorously until completely dissolved.
**3.** Administer as supplied without shaking.
**4.** Shake gently until completely dissolved.

10  If a medicine was ordered PO and the patient had a GT, what action would the nurse take?

**1.** Mix the PO medicine with liquid and place in the gastric tube.
**2.** Clarify the route with the physician who wrote the order.
**3.** Give the medicine PO as ordered.
**4.** Clarify the route with another, more experienced nurse on duty.

**Directions:** *For problems 11-20, read the labels supplied to obtain the answer. Use mental arithmetic to calculate a dose if requested. Circle the correct answer.*

11  Ordered: Synthroid 0.05 mg.

The unit dose concentration is

**1.** 100 tablets
**2.** 50 mcg/ tab
**2.** 0.5 mg/ tab
**4.** 50 mg/ tab

**12** Ordered: Lanoxin (digoxin) 62.5 mcg for a child.

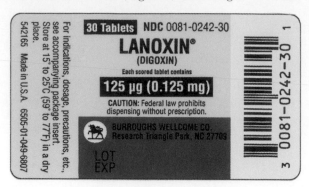

**1.** You would give 1 tablet

**2.** You would give $\frac{1}{2}$ tablet

**3.** You would hold this tablet and clarify with the physician

**4.** You would give two tablets

**13** Ordered: Ery-tab 250 mg q8h PO for a patient with an infection.

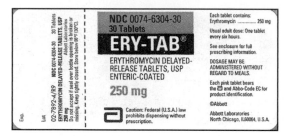

What is the form of this drug?

**1.** Milligrams

**2.** Enteric-coated tablets

**3.** Capsules

**4.** Double-strength tablets

**14** Ordered: Decadron tablets 0.5 mg PO daily in AM.

The nurse would administer (use mental arithmetic)

**1.** 1 tablet

**2.** 2 tablets

**3.** 3 tablets

**4.** 5 tablets

**15** Ordered: Percodan 1 tab q4h PO prn severe pain.

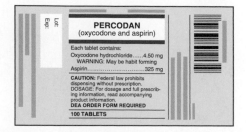

What form of medication is this?

1. Compound
2. Elixir
3. Mixture
4. Suspension

16 Ordered: Indocin SR 150 mg AM pc daily for an adult with a chronically painful shoulder.

What would be the appropriate complete nurse interpretation?

1. Prepare 2 capsules of double-strength Indocin and give every day in the morning.
2. Prepare 2 capsules of sustained-release-type Indocin, a medication that probably is irritating to gastric mucosa, and give after breakfast.
3. Prepare 2 capsules of Indocin and give on an empty stomach for better absorption.
4. Prepare 2 capsules of sustained-release Indocin and give before breakfast.

17 Ordered: epinephrine 1:10,000 0.3 mg IV stat for a patient who is having a severe allergic reaction.

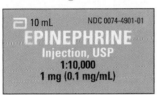

How much *total drug* is in the vial?

1. 1:10,000
2. 1 mg
3. 0.1 mg/ mL
4. 10 mL

18 Ordered: Glucophage 1 g bid with meals.

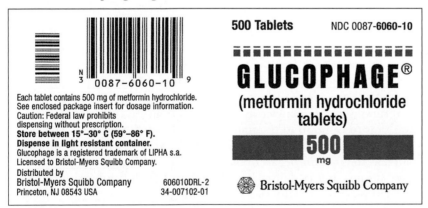

What is the information from the label that would need to be entered in a complete DA equation to calculate the dose?

1. The total amount supplied in the container, the unit dose supplied, and a conversion formula
2. The generic name of the drug
3. The unit dose concentration supplied
4. The ordered dose

19　Ordered: Lopid 0.6 g PO daily

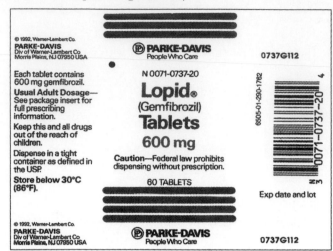

How many tablets would the nurse administer to the patient? Move decimals to obtain the metric equivalent.

**1.** 1 tablet　　　　　　　　　　**3.** $\frac{1}{2}$ tablet

**2.** 2 tablets　　　　　　　　　　**4.** 0.3 g

20　Who should the nurse consult if a handwritten medication order is incomplete or unclear?

**1.** the prescriber
**2.** a nurse who gave the medication during the preceding shift
**3.** a drug reference
**4.** the pharmacy

## CHAPTER 4 FINAL PRACTICE

**Estimated completion time: 10-20 minutes**　　Answers on page **523**

**Directions:** *As you read the following paragraph, write out the definition of each italicized abbreviation in the space provided. Reread the paragraph as often as necessary to become comfortable with the abbreviations.*

A patient was admitted to the hospital in a diabetic coma. X-rays and laboratory tests were ordered **1** _____ (*stat*). The vital signs were assessed **2** _____ (*qh*) and **3** _____ (*prn*). All of the medications were given **4** _____ (*IV*) because the patient was **5** _____ (*NPO*). Patients who are in a coma cannot swallow **6** _____ (*PO*) medications. Oral medications and feedings may go into their airways. The patient's mental status was slow to respond to treatment. Feedings were administered via **7** _____ (*TPN*) with a tube inserted into the subclavian vein. Later, as the patient began to be more alert, an **8** _____ (*NG*) tube was inserted to deliver liquid food and medications with the patient in an upright position. Insulin was discontinued **9** _____ (*IV*) and given **10** _____ (*subcut*). The patient still had difficulty swallowing for a while but eventually graduated to sips and chips: sips of water and chips of ice. Because that was tolerated well, the **11** _____ (*NG*). tube was removed and small **12** _____ (*PO*) soft feedings were introduced **13** _____ (*q2h*) during the daytime hours and **14** _____ (*qHS*). The nurse always assessed the patient's mental status and ability to swallow before giving a feeding. Medications for pain were given **15** _____ (*IM q4h prn*). Rectal **16** _____ (*supp*) were given for complaints of nausea. Medications for coexisting problems were now given **17** _____ (*po*), such as **18** _____ *(elix* and *susp bid)* because they were easy to swallow **19** _____ (s̄) choking incidents. The patient had a history of angina and chest pain attacks and now was able to take nitroglycerine pills **20** _____ *(subl)*. The nurse checked at each visit to find out how many the patient had taken because the physician needed to be called if more than a maximum of 3 tablets, 5 minutes apart, did not provide relief. The nurse knew that all chest pain signals a heart attack unless proven otherwise. The patient was discharged to home to family.

**Directions:** *For questions 21-27, state the seven patient's basic rights.*

**21** _____

**22** _____

**23** _____

**24** _____

**25** _____

**26** _____

**27** _____

**28** Ordered: 0.1 g of a medication. It is supplied in 50-mg capsules.

How many capsules will you give? _____ Show the decimal movement to obtain the metric equivalent.

**29 a.** Write the two required pieces of information from the medication order and the label which must be entered in all medication dose calculations.

_____

_____

**b.** Write the variable piece or pieces of information that may need to be entered in medication dose calculations. _____

_____

_____

**30** Ordered: erythromycin 0.5 g ent coated, delayed-release c̄ food bid.

NDC 0074-6304-30
30 Tablets
**ERY-TAB®**
ERYTHROMYCIN DELAYED-
RELEASE TABLETS, USP
ENTERIC-COATED
**250 mg**

Caution: Federal (U.S.A.) law
prohibits dispensing without
prescription.

Each tablet contains:
Erythromycin .............. 250 mg

Usual adult dose: One tablet
every six hours.

See enclosure for full
prescribing information.

DOSAGE MAY BE
ADMINISTERED WITHOUT
REGARD TO MEALS.

Each pink tablet bears
the Ⓔ and Abbo-Code EC for
product identification.

©Abbott

Abbott Laboratories
North Chicago, IL60064, U.S.A.

**a.** What is the trade name of this medication? _____

**b.** What is the total daily dose in grams and milligrams? _____

**c.** What is the unit dose concentration? _____

**d.** How many tablets will you give per dose? _____

## Suggestions for Further Reading

Lilley LL, Harrington S, Snyder JS: Pharmacology and the nursing process, ed 4, St. Louis, 2005, Mosby.

www.dea.gov/pub/abuse/1-CSA.htm
www.fda.gov/cder
www.health.rutgers.edu/quality
www.ismp.org
www.jointcommission.org

 Additional information can be found in the Safety in Medication Administration section on the enclosed companion CD.

Chapter 5 introduces a large variety of metric medication problems using dimensional analysis to calculate and verify results.

# SOLID AND LIQUID ORAL DOSE CALCULATIONS

**5**

## Objectives

- Estimate, calculate, and evaluate a variety of solid and liquid medication doses.
- Calculate dosages for liquid medications to the nearest tenth of a milliliter.
- Measure oral liquids in a calibrated measuring cup.
- Measure syringe volumes in 3- and 5-mL syringes.
- Calculate and evaluate safe dose ranges (SDR) for medication doses.

## Essential Prior Knowledge

Mastery of Chapters 1-4

## Equipment

- Calculator for converting pounds to kilograms and calculating SDR

## Estimated Time to Complete Chapter

- 2 hours

---

*"The scientists had another idea which was totally at odds with the benefits to be derived from the standardization of weights and measures; they adapted to them the decimal system, on the basis of the metre as a unit; they suppressed all complicated numbers. Nothing is more contrary to the organization of the mind, of the memory, and of the imagination. . . . The new system of weights and measures will be a stumbling block and the source of difficulties for several generations. . . . It's just tormenting the people with trivia!"*

**NAPOLEON BONAPARTE** (Comments on the French adoption of the metric system)

## Introduction

This chapter builds on prior knowledge to solve many basic and complex medication dose problems using DA, with an emphasis on estimation and evaluation of the answer. Calculations based on weight are included.

Medication doses are not calculated in a vacuum. Assessments and safety checks are critical before, during, and after medication administration.

It is always helpful to have a simple example in mind to build on for more complex equations. This chapter covers situations involving a variety of orders, medications, and metric units of measurement. Analysis, repetition, and practice are the keys to ease of problem solving.

**149**

## ESSENTIAL Vocabulary

| | |
|---|---|
| **Calibration** | Set of graduations that indicate capacity or size in standard units of measure. Measuring devices for precise doses of medications have calibrations, such as the lines on a measuring cup or a syringe. |
| **Concentration, Liquid** | Ratio of a specific amount of drug in a specified amount of solution, for example, 10 mg/ mL or 5 mg/ 5 mL. |
| **Concentration, Solid** | Ratio of a specific amount of drug contained in the solid drug form supplied, for example, 50 mg/ cap. The concentration of a medication, solid or liquid, is always found on the label. |
| **Divided Doses** | Total dose for the day divided by a frequency schedule |
| **Precise** | Having sharply defined, accurate, limits based on a standard. For example, syringes, special medication droppers, and teaspoons have precise capacities. Household equipment does not. |
| **Ratio** | The relationship between two quantities. |
| **Safe Dose Range (SDR)** | Manufacturer's dosage guidelines for minimum and maximum safe medication doses based on laboratory and clinical trials of therapeutic effectiveness. For example, the SDR for aspirin for adults is 325 to 650 mg q4h. |

## RAPID PRACTICE 5-1 Vocabulary Review

**Estimated completion time: 5-10 minutes**   Answers on page **524**

**Directions:** *Indicate whether the statement is true or false.*

1 When a reference states that a drug must be given in divided doses, the total dose must be administered in parts at specified intervals during the 24-hour period. _____

2 50 mg/ mL refers to the concentration of a drug in solution. _____

3 An SDR specifies the safe minimum and maximum dose for patients. _____

4 The concentration of a liquid is the amount of solution in the liquid. _____

5 The concentration of a medication is always found on the label. _____

## RAPID PRACTICE 5-2 Metric Solid Oral Dose Calculations and Review

**Estimated completion time 10-20 minutes**   Answers on page **524**

**Directions:** *Convert the dose ordered to the desired dose using mental arithmetic and decimal movement.*

| Ordered | Dose Concentration Supplied | Amount to Give |
|---|---|---|
| 1  0.25 mg | 0.125 mg/ tab scored | _____ |
| 2  150 mg | 0.1 g/ tab scored | _____ |
| 3  0.5 mg | 0.25 mg/ cap | _____ |
| 4  125 mg | 250 mg/ tab scored | _____ |
| 5  350 mcg | 0.175 mg/ tab scored | _____ |

| | | |
|---|---|---|
| **6** 0.5 mg | 0.25 mg/ tab scored | _____ |
| **7** 0.1 mg | 0.2 mg/ tab scored | _____ |
| **8** 1 g | 500 mg/ cap | _____ |
| **9** 2.5 g | 1000 mg/ tab scored | _____ |
| **10** 250 mg | 0.5 g/ tab scored | _____ |

➤  Make it a habit to estimate the dose before calculations.

Ordered: 250 mg.

Available: dose concentration 125 mg/ cap.

The nurse can see at a glance that the order is about *twice* the amount on hand. If the numbers do not divide evenly, an *approximate* amount of the unit dose is estimated.

## RAPID PRACTICE 5-3   Metric Oral Solid Dose Calculations Using Estimation and DA Equations

**Estimated completion time: 30-60 minutes**   Answers on page **524**

**Directions:** *Review the metric equivalents in Chapter 4. Study worked-out problem 1, and solve problems 2-5. Estimate answers by moving decimals for needed conversions, and verify with a DA equation. Evaluate answers: Is the equation balanced? Does the estimate support the answer? It would be helpful to write out the four steps of the DA equation before proceeding to problem 2.*

➤  Remember that the unit concentration supplied and the dose ordered must be part of every medication dose calculation.

**1**  Ordered: 0.5 g tab PO daily. Label: dose concentration 250 mg/ tab.

  **a.** Metric conversion formula needed: 1000 mg = 1g

  **b.** Estimated dose: 0.5 g = 500 mg; 500 mg = 2 × 250 mg, or 2 tab

  **c.** Amount of tablets to administer:
     DA equation

$$\text{Tab} = \frac{1 \text{ tab}}{\underset{1}{250 \text{ mg}}} \times \frac{\overset{4}{1000 \text{ mg}}}{1 \text{ g}} \times 0.5 \text{ g} = 2 \text{ tab}$$

  **d.** Evaluation: The equation is balanced. The estimate supports the answer.

**2**  Ordered: 0.25 g tab PO daily. Label: dose concentration 125 mg/ tab scored.

  **a.** Metric conversion formula needed: _____

  **b.** Estimated dose: _____

  **c.** Amount of tablets to administer:
     DA equation:

  **d.** Evaluation: _____

3  Ordered: 0.1 g tab PO daily. Label: dose concentration 0.05 g/ tab.
  **a.** Metric conversion formula needed: _____
  **b.** Estimated dose: _____
  **c.** Amount of tablets to administer:
     DA equation:

  **d.** Evaluation: _____

4  Ordered: 75 mcg tab PO daily. Label: dose concentration 50 mcg/ tab scored.
  **a.** Metric conversion formula needed: _____
  **b.** Estimated dose: _____
  **c.** Amount of tablets to administer:
     DA equation:

  **d.** Evaluation: _____

5  Ordered: 20 mEq tab PO bid. Label: dose concentration 10 mEq/ tab.
  **a.** Metric conversion formula needed: _____
  **b.** Estimated dose: _____
  **c.** Amount of tablets to administer:
     DA equation:

  **d.** Evaluation: _____

6  Ordered: 0.2 g cap PO at bedtime. Label: dose concentration 100 mg/ cap.
  **a.** Metric conversion formula needed: _____
  **b.** Estimated dose: _____
  **c.** Amount of capsules to administer:
     DA equation:

  **d.** Evaluation: _____

7 Ordered: 250 mg cap PO at bedtime. Label: dose concentration 0.25 g/ cap.

   **a.** Metric conversion formula needed: _____

   **b.** Estimated dose: _____

   **c.** Amount of capsules to administer:
   DA equation:


   **d.** Evaluation: _____


8 Ordered: 0.25 g cap PO tid. Label: dose concentration 125 mg/ cap.

   **a.** Metric conversion formula needed: _____

   **b.** Estimated dose: _____

   **c.** Amount of capsules to administer:
   DA equation:


   **d.** Evaluation: _____


9 Ordered: 0.175 mg tab PO daily. Label: dose concentration 350 mcg/ tab scored.

   **a.** Metric conversion formula needed: _____

   **b.** Estimated dose: _____

   **c.** Amount of tablets to administer:
   DA equation:


   **d.** Evaluation: _____


10 Ordered: 0.1 mg tab PO daily. Label: dose concentration 50 mcg/ tab.

   **a.** Metric conversion formula needed: _____

   **b.** Estimated dose: _____

   **c.** Amount of tablets to administer:
   DA equation:


   **d.** Evaluation: _____


1   What are the two pieces of information obtained from the order and label that must be entered in every dose calculation?

_____

**Q** *Ask Yourself*

**A** *My Answer*

# Converting Grams to Micrograms and Micrograms to Grams by Moving Decimal Places

When a problem calls for converting micrograms to grams or grams to micrograms, beginners enter *two* conversion formulas in a DA equation: micrograms to milligrams and milligrams to grams, or grams to milligrams and milligrams to micrograms.

Microgram-milligram conversions are frequently encountered in dose calculations. Microgram-gram conversions are occasionally needed in calculations of intravenous doses. Medication errors can occur when the prescriber writes an order in micrograms and the nurse mistakes it for milligrams or vice versa.

Microgram-gram conversions can be reduced to one step if desired by using the conversion formula 1,000,000 mcg = 1 g, since *micro-* means one millionth of the base unit.

| | |
|---|---|
| **EXAMPLES** | Conversion formula: 1,000,000 mcg = 1 g. |

➤ To convert grams to micrograms, move the decimal place 6 places to the right.
➤ To convert micrograms to grams, move the decimal place 6 places to the left.

| Ordered | | Equivalent | Decimal Movement |
|---|---|---|---|
| 0.5 g | = | 500,000 mcg | decimal moved six places to the right |
| 250,000 mcg | = | 0.250000 g | implied decimal moved six places to the left |
| 0.004 g | = | 4000 mcg | decimal moved six places to the right |

**Tip:** If you are comfortable with milligram conversions (milligrams to micrograms and milligrams to grams), use a stepped approach for microgram-gram conversions. First, change the ordered amount to milligrams by moving the decimal point *3 places* to the left or right. Then, insert *3 more* decimal places to the left or right.

Moving decimals carefully is a great timesaver.

➤ Converting micrograms to grams and grams to micrograms involves two steps—1000 mcg = 1 mg, and 1000 mg = 1 g—for a total of 6 decimal place movements. It is expedient to study the relationships among the mcg/mg/g conversions at one time.

## RAPID PRACTICE 5-4 Moving Decimal Places for Microgram-Gram Conversions

**Estimated completion time: 5-10 minutes**   Answers on page **526**

**Directions:** *Convert the units ordered to micrograms (mental arithmetic) and then the desired units using decimal place movement.*

| Ordered | Milligrams | Micrograms or Grams |
|---|---|---|
| **1** 0.3 g | 300 mg | 300,000 mcg |
| **2** 0.1 g | _____ | _____ mcg |
| **3** 8000 mcg | _____ | _____ g |
| **4** 25,000 mcg | _____ | _____ g |
| **5** 300,000 mcg | _____ | _____ g |

## RAPID PRACTICE 5-5  Decimal Conversions Using 1 or 2 Conversion Formulas

**Estimated completion time: 10-15 minutes**   Answers on page **526**

**Directions:** *Make the units equivalent. Examine the example in problem 1. Complete problems 2-10 in the same manner.*

| Needed Conversion | Number of Decimal Places to Be Moved | Direction to Move Decimal Place (**R**ight or **L**eft) | Answer |
|---|---|---|---|
| 1  0.3 g = ? mg | 3 | R | 300 mg |
| 2  200 mcg = ? mg | | | |
| 3  0.5 mg = ? mcg | | | |
| 4  15,000 mcg = ? g | | | |
| 5  0.004 g = ? mcg | | | |
| 6  2200 mg = ? g | | | |
| 7  350 mcg = ? mg | | | |
| 8  5000 mcg = ? g | | | |
| 9  0.05 g = ? mg | | | |
| 10  50 mg = ? g | | | |

## RAPID PRACTICE 5-6  Metric Oral Medication Calculation Practice

**Estimated completion time: 30 minutes**   Answers on page **526**

**Directions:** *Study the medication order and the unit dose supplied. Estimate the answer and verify it with a DA equation. Evaluate the answer. Is the equation balanced? Does the estimate support the answer?*

➤  The desired answer unit is always to be found in the available unit dose concentration. How is the ordered drug supplied: in tablets, capsules, or milliliters? That unit will be the desired answer unit.

1  Ordered: codeine sulfate 30 mg.

**a.** Estimated dose: _____

**b.** Actual dose: _____
    DA equation:




**c.** Evaluation:_____

**2** Ordered: Ativan 1 mg.

**a.** Estimated dose: _____

**b.** Actual dose: _____
   DA equation:

**c.** Evaluation: _____

**3** Ordered: Biaxin 0.25 g.

**a.** Estimated dose: _____

**b.** Actual dose: _____
   DA equation:

**c.** Evaluation: _____

**4** Ordered: Lopressor 0.1 g.

NDC 0028-0051-10          FSC 3602
6505-01-071-6557

**Lopressor® 50** mg

**metoprolol tartrate USP**

EXP
LOT

**1000 tablets**

Keep this and all drugs out
of the reach of children.

Dispense in tight, light-resistant
container (USP).

**Caution:** Federal law prohibits
dispensing without prescription.

**Geigy**

PHARMACIST: Container closure is not child-resistant.
Dosage: See package insert.
Store between 59°- 86°F (15°- 30°C).
Protect from moisture.

Ciba-Geigy Corporation
Pharmaceuticals Division
Summit, NJ 07901

645120

N 3  0028-0051-10  6

**a.** Estimated dose: _____

**b.** Actual dose: _____
   DA equation:

**c.** Evaluation: _____

5  Ordered: Cogentin 1 mg.

a. Estimated dose: _____

b. Actual dose: _____
   DA equation:

c. Evaluation: _____

## RAPID PRACTICE 5-7 Metric Oral Medication Calculation Practice

**Estimated completion time: 20 minutes**   Answers on page **527**

**Directions:** *Estimate answer and verify with DA equation. Evaluate the answer. Supply needed conversion formulas.*

1  Ordered: alprazolam 0.5 mg PO q12h.

a. Estimated dose: _____
   DA equation:

b. Evaluation: _____

2  Ordered: sulfisoxazole 1000 mg PO tid.

a. Estimated dose: _____
   DA equation:

b. Evaluation: _____

3  Ordered: digitoxin 100 mcg PO daily.

a. Estimated dose: _____
   DA equation:

b. Evaluation: _____

4  Ordered: zidovudine capsules 0.1 g PO tid.

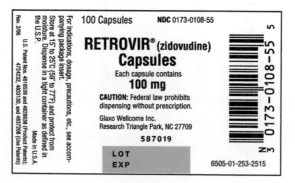

a. Estimated dose: _____
   DA equation:

b. Evaluation:_____

**5**  Ordered: diltiazem HCl 0.12 g PO daily.

NDC 0088-1792-47          6505-01-259-2914

120 mg | **Hoechst Marion Roussel**

**CARDIZEM®**
(diltiazem HCl)

**120 mg**

**100 Tablets**

EXP.: B6     50007212

**a.** Estimated dose: _____
   DA equation:

**b.** Evaluation:_____

## Analyzing Liquid Dose Orders

Liquids may be supplied in a variety of containers. As with all dose calculations, the ordered dose and the drug concentration noted on the label must be included in the calculation. Liquid medications *ordered* and *supplied* in milligrams may require a calculation if the dose is supplied in more than 1 mL of solution. The estimate of the answer can be made right away if the metric units are matched.

### Estimating Liquid Doses

| | |
|---|---|
| Ordered: 350 mg PO daily.<br><br>Available: dose concentration supplied: 250 mg/ 5 mL.<br><br>The dose ordered and the drug supplied are in the same terms (milligrams). It is easy to see that the dose *ordered* (350 mg) will be *more than one* but *less than two* times the drug concentration supplied (250 mg in 5 mL, less than $2 \times 5$ mL). | **EXAMPLES** |

### Misinterpretation

Loss of focus may cause the nurse to reverse the order with the concentration supplied.

➤ Avoid distractions. Focus on the order in relation to the strength on hand.

### Rounding Numbers to Simplify Estimated Liquid Dose

➤ Rounding up helps the estimation in some instances.

| | |
|---|---|
| Ordered: 300 mg.<br><br>Available: 75 mg in 1 mL of liquid<br><br>It is obvious that the order calls for *much more* than the dose per milliliter supplied. The nurse might approximate the dose by rounding the 75 up to 100 for easier division, giving a rough estimate of around 3 or more unit doses. This calculation would require a DA equation. | **EXAMPLES** |

EXAMPLES

Examine the following order:

Ordered: 200 mg liquid.

Available: 80 mg/ 5 mL concentration.

The terms are the same: milligrams. It is obvious that the order for 200 mg exceeds two times the dose (80 mg) per volume on hand. Thus, *the estimate is that more than 10 mL will be given.* Follow the estimate with an exact calculation in a DA equation. Compare the result with the estimate.

## RAPID PRACTICE 5-8 Metric Conversions and Estimating Answers for Liquid Medications

**Estimated completion time: 10 minutes**  Answers on page **528**

**Directions:** *Examine the order and the label concentration. Follow the example in problem 1 to estimate the dose to be administered to the nearest milliliter or number of tablets.*

| Dose Ordered | Concentration Available | Conversion | Give Same, More, or Less of Available Dose per Volume | Estimated Amount |
|---|---|---|---|---|
| 1  0.25 g | 250 mg/ mL | 0.25 g = 250 mg | Same | 1 mL |
| 2  5000 mcg | 2.5 mg/ mL | | | |
| 3  0.1 g | 300 mg/ mL | | | |
| 4  750 mg | 0.5 g/ mL | | | |
| 5  200 mg | 0.1 g/ mL | | | |

**Clinical Relevance**

Liquid unit dose concentrations are often written with a slash (e.g., 100 mg/2 mL). The slash mark (/) appears in printed drug literature for drug concentration. It should *not be handwritten* in a patient's medical record. The slash can be misinterpreted as the number 1 if it occurs next to a number. For example, 100 mg/5 mL could be read as 100 mg per 15 mL instead of 5 mL. Write *per* instead of using the slash: 100 mg *per* 5 mL. The slash is clearly seen in printed materials.

➤ If you use a slash in your personal note-taking, be sure to follow the metric notation requirement of leaving a space between numbers and metric measurements, as in 100 mg/ 5 mL. Without spaces (i.e., 100mg/5mL), such expressions can lead to serious calculation errors.

➤ With oral liquid metric measurements, the final question is usually: How many milliliters should be given?

## Setting Up DA-Style Equations for Liquid Dose Calculations

**Review:** The process required is to multiply a known quantity by one or more conversion formulas to solve an equation. The process is the same for a liquid as for a solid.

- The known quantity in medication calculations is the *prescribed order.*
- The first conversion formula is the *dose concentration on the label with the desired answer in the numerator.*

# When Ordered Dose and Available Unit Concentration Match

Ordered: Valium 10 mg.
Available concentration (on label): Valium 20 mg/ 5 mL.

| Step 1: Desired Answer Units | Step 2: Conversion Formulas (Dose Concentration) | Step 3: Original Factors to Be Converted (Ordered Dose) | Step 4: Estimate, Multiply, and Evaluate |
|---|---|---|---|
| | | ➤ Cancel unwanted units. | |
| | | Stop: Are all unwanted units cancelled? | Estimate: will give about ½ of dose per milliliter supplied. |
| ➤ mL = | $\dfrac{5 \text{ mL}}{\cancel{20 \text{ mg}}\atop 2}$ | $\times \overset{1}{\cancel{10 \text{ mg}}} =$ | $\dfrac{5}{2} = 2.5$ mL (answer) |
| Liquids are administered in milliliters. | Milligrams will be in next numerator. | Ordered dose. | Evaluation: Estimate supports answer. The equation is balanced. |

Set up equations as shown below:

$$mL = \frac{5 \text{ mL}}{\cancel{20 \text{ mg}}\atop 2} \times \overset{1}{\cancel{10 \text{ mg}}} = 2.5 \text{ mL (answer)}$$

- Identify and place all the elements carefully.
- If another conversion is necessary, make room for it in *step 2* before entering the ordered dose.
- Remember to cancel all the unwanted units before doing the math.

**FAQ** | *What is the most common error seen with liquid dose calculations?*

**ANSWER:** Sometimes the amount of drug is confused with the amount of solution. For example, *10 mg/ 5 mL* means there are 10 mg of drug in *each 5 mL* of solution. The nurse needs to stay focused when doing the math.

Remember to cancel all unwanted units before doing the math.

## When the Ordered Units Do Not Match the Available Units

A metric equivalent conversion formula is necessary when the ordered units do not match the available dose concentration. If another conversion is necessary, make room for it before entering the ordered dose.

Ordered: 1 mg of a drug.

Available: dose concentration 500 mcg/ 2 mL.

Conversion formula: 1000 mcg = 1 mg.

How many milliliters will you give?

| Step 1 | Step 2 | Step 2A | Step 3 | Step 4 |
|---|---|---|---|---|
| mL = | $\dfrac{2 \text{ mL}}{\cancel{500 \text{ mcg}}\atop 1}$ | $\times \dfrac{\overset{2}{\cancel{1000 \text{ mcg}}}}{1 \text{ mg}\atop 1}$ | $\times \dfrac{\overset{1}{\cancel{1 \text{ mg}}}}{}$ | $=$ 4 mL (answer) |

**Review:** It can be seen that the *only* desired answer unit is milliliters. Milligrams and micrograms need to be canceled. The milliliter data is entered *first*, with its accompanying dose strength: 500 mcg. The next entry needs to cancel the micrograms. The conversion formula is positioned to do that with micrograms in the numerator. The milligrams in the denominator will be canceled by the milligrams in the order. All of the entries *proceed* automatically from the desired answer entry. A known quantity ordered, 1 mg, was multiplied by the dose concentration available and a conversion formula to arrive at a solution to the problem.

Q: *Ask Yourself*

A: *My Answer*

1   As you look at the previous example, which *three* key pieces of data are entered in the equation?

_____

2   If the units supplied and the units ordered were in the same measurement terms, milligrams, which entry in step 3 could be eliminated?

_____

# Usual Unit Doses

➤   Most solid doses ordered are ½ to 2 times the available unit dose, such as ½ to 2 tablets or 1 to 2 capsules.
➤   With liquids, check current drug references for the usual dose; the amount can vary.

**Clinical Relevance**   Sometimes a very frail person—a baby or an adult with a very low weight, or a person with a very serious illness—will receive a fractional dose (a very small amount of the unit dose), or because an illness is so aggressive or the person is larger than average, an unusually large dose will be ordered.

➤   Hold the medication and promptly clarify unusual doses with the prescriber to be on the safe side.

**FAQ** | *Why are DA equations required when the answer can be calculated more simply?*

**ANSWER:** Safe dose calculations require that the nurse have two methods of calculating the dose. Mental arithmetic is fine in most instances, but a solid backup method for verification and for more complex problems must be available. With repetition and practice, the nurse will find it easy to quickly and independently confirm calculations. It is unsafe to rely on peers who may make a calculation error.

➤   The nurse who administers the medication is legally responsible for that medication even if the order was incorrect.

**RAPID PRACTICE 5-9**  Calculating Oral Liquid Doses Using DA

**Estimated completion time: 20-30 minutes**  Answers on page **528**

**Directions:** *Estimate, calculate, and evaluate the following ordered doses using DA.*

1 Ordered: chlorpromazine HCl syrup 25 mg PO tid.

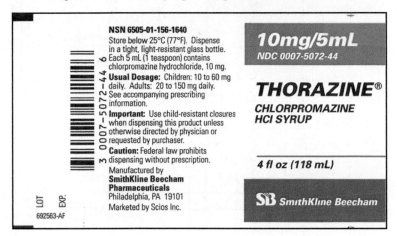

  **a.** Estimated dose: _____
    DA equation:

  **b.** Evaluation: _____

2 Ordered: prochlorperazine syrup 8 mg PO stat.

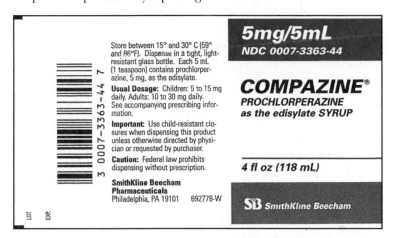

  **a.** Estimated dose: _____
    DA equation:

  **b.** Evaluation: _____

**3** Ordered: Benadryl Elixir 15 mg PO at bedtime.

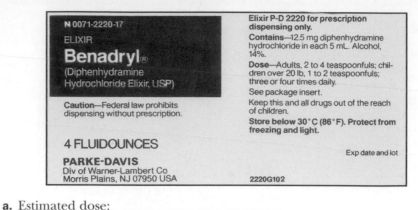

**a.** Estimated dose: _____

DA equation:

**b.** Evaluation: _____

**4** Ordered: digoxin elixir pediatric 25 mcg PO daily in AM.

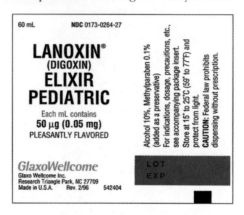

**a.** Estimated dose: _____

DA equation:

**b.** Evaluation: _____

**5** Ordered: ondansetron hydrochloride oral sol 6 mg PO.

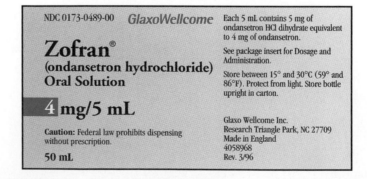

**a.** Estimated dose: _____

DA equation:

**b.** Evaluation: _____

## Equipment for Administering Oral Liquid Doses

Depending on the medication, a 30-mL calibrated medicine cup, a special medicine teaspoon (5 mL), a calibrated dropper, a calibrated tablespoon, an oral syringe, or a needleless syringe may be selected if the agency does not have oral syringes.

### Selecting the Implement for Oral Liquid Medications

The implement used to deliver an oral liquid unit dose is selected according to

1  The amount of liquid to be administered
2  The ability of the patient to drink from a nipple or cup or to swallow from a medication spoon or dropper

Choosing the appropriate implement is not always age-related. Often, the medication is packaged with the equipment to be used, such as a medicine cup, a calibrated dropper, a teaspoon, or an oral syringe.

Many oral liquid medications are delivered in units of 5 mL (1 medication teaspoon) or 15 mL (1 medication tablespoon; Figure 5-1). Medication cups may be used for 5 to 30 mL (1 oz).

*Sterile* oral liquid medications may be prepared for infants, babies, immunosuppressed patients, and other at-risk populations. The nurse should check agency policies on the use of sterile oral liquid medications.

➤ Nurses do not use household implements because they vary greatly in capacity. Patients must be instructed to use calibrated measuring devices if they will be discharged on liquid oral medications.

Figure 5-1. Medication cups. **A,** Filled to 5 mL. **B,** Filled to 15 mL.

## Measuring Liquids

### Measuring Oral Milliliter Doses That Call for More or Less Than the Calibrated Lines on the Cup

Measuring oral doses may require the use of a syringe for more precise dosing if the dose is not a multiple of 5 mL. The metric measurements on the medication cups are calibrated in multiples of 5 mL (see Figure 5-1).

## Reading Syringe Calibrations

➤ The exact amount ordered to the nearest tenth of a mL should be poured. The nurse selects the syringe (Figure 5-2):

Follow these steps to read syringe calibrations on these two syringes:

➤ Identify the 1-mL marking if present.
➤ Count the number of lines within 1 mL (10 lines in 1 mL on the 3-mL syringe and 5 lines in 1 mL on the 5-mL syringe):

10 lines in 1 mL mean each line is worth 0.1 mL (the 3-mL syringe).

5 lines in 1 mL mean each line is worth 0.2 mL (the 5-mL syringe).

➤ The amount is read at the ring closest to the opening in the syringe (Figure 5-3).
➤ Locate the amount desired.

**A**

**B**

Figure 5-2. **A,** 3-mL syringe calibrated in 0.1-mL increments. **B,** 5-mL syringe calibrated in 0.2-mL increments.

Figure 5-3. Reading measured amount of medication in a syringe. (From Potter PA, Perry AG: Fundamentals of nursing, ed. 6, St. Louis, 2005, Mosby.)

**EXAMPLES**

Amount to give: Prepare 17.5 mL.

Procedure: Pour to 15 mL and add 2.5 mL with a syringe (Figure 5-4).

Figure 5-4. Total dose will be 17.5 mL: 15 mL prepared in medicine cup and 2.5 mL precise remainder added to syringe.

Figure 5-5 shows medication being withdrawn from a cup with a syringe.

Figure **5-5**. Using a needleless syringe to withdraw liquid medication for oral administration. (Modified from Clayton BD, Stock YN: Basic pharmacology for nurses, ed. 13, St. Louis, 2004, Mosby.)

**EXAMPLES**

Amount to give: 12.4 mL.

Procedure: Pour to 10-mL calibration and add 2.4 mL with a 3-mL syringe.

Amount to give: 19 mL.

Procedure: Pour to 15-mL calibration and add 4 mL with a 5-mL syringe.

**Review the steps:**

➤ Pour the nearest measurable dose in a 30-mL medicine cup; when the dose is *not* a multiple of 5, pour the liquid to the *nearest* 5-mL calibration that is *less* than the dose.

➤ *Add* the precise additional amount needed to the *nearest tenth* of a milliliter with a syringe. The top center of the fluid is read at eye level (Figure 5-6).

Figure **5-6**. Measuring liquid medication. (In Lilley LL, Harrington S, Snyder JS: Pharmacology and the nursing process, ed. 4, 2005, Mosby. From Rick Brady, Riva, MD.)

> **FAQ** | *May the whole dose be prepared in a syringe and inserted in the cup?*
>
> **ANSWER:** Yes, the dose needs to be drawn to the nearest tenth of a milliliter. Larger syringes do not have 0.1-mL calibrations. Select the syringe that will provide the nearest measurable dose.

**Clinical Relevance**

➤ It is best not to get into the habit of returning medications to containers. Avoid drawing excess amounts. Sterile medications should not be returned to containers.

## RAPID PRACTICE 5-10 Measuring Liquid Doses with 30-mL Medicine Cup and Syringe

**Estimated completion time: 10 minutes**   Answers on page **528**

**Directions:** *Given the amount to prepare, state the nearest measurable amount to place in the 30-mL medicine cup and the amount to place in the syringe, and state whether a 3-mL or a 5-mL syringe is needed.*

✳ **Communication**

"I have 250 mg of Diuril, the diuretic water pill your doctor prescribed for your leg swelling. Have you taken this medicine before?" Listen to the answer and follow up any concerns with the prescriber promptly, withholding the medication if necessary. Document and report.

| Amount to Prepare | Amount to Place in Cup | Amount to Place in Syringe | Syringe Size (3-mL or 5-mL) |
|---|---|---|---|
| 1  6.5 mL | _____ | _____ | _____ |
| 2  14 mL | _____ | _____ | _____ |
| 3  9 mL | _____ | _____ | _____ |
| 4  17 mL | _____ | _____ | _____ |
| 5  27.4 mL | _____ | _____ | _____ |

**Clinical Relevance**

**Patient Safety: Seven Ways to Avoid Calculation Errors:**
1. Know the metric conversions, and keep current on the DA setup.
2. Focus strictly on the situation at hand. Screen out distractions.
3. Make a habit of estimating a reasonable answer, if possible, before performing final calculations.
4. Write neatly and watch placement of decimals.
5. Evaluate equation and answers using a systematic method.
6. Consult an *appropriate* source for assistance when needed.
7. Keep the patient and/or family informed about the medication and the dose that you plan to administer. They may provide the final protection from an error.

## RAPID PRACTICE 5-11 Liquid Doses

**Estimated completion time: 20-30 minutes**   Answers on page **529**

**Directions:** *Estimate, calculate, and evaluate the liquid dose problems to the nearest tenth of a milliliter.*

1 Ordered: 75 mg. Supplied dose concentration: 50 mg/ mL.

   **a.** Estimated dose: _____
      DA equation:

   **b.** Evaluation: _____

**2** Ordered: 20 mg. Supplied dose concentration: 5 mg/ 5 mL.

   **a.** Estimated dose: _____
      DA equation:

   **b.** Evaluation: _____

**3** Ordered: 35 mg. Supplied dose concentration: 15 mg/ 2 mL.

   **a.** Estimated dose: _____
      DA equation:

   **b.** Evaluation: _____

**4** Ordered: 125 mg. Supplied dose concentration: 75 mg/ 8 mL.

   **a.** Estimated dose: _____
      DA equation:

   **b.** Evaluation: _____

**5** Ordered: 45 mg. Supplied dose concentration: 25 mg/ 10 mL.

   **a.** Estimated dose: _____
      DA equation:

   **b.** Evaluation: _____

---

## RAPID PRACTICE 5-12   Calculating and Measuring Liquid Dose Orders

**Estimated completion time: 30 minutes**   **Answers on page 529**

**Directions:** *Identify and enter all the required elements in the DA equation. Estimate the answer, solve to the nearest tenth of a milliliter, and evaluate the equation. Shade in the medicine cup to the nearest 5 mL, and draw a vertical line through the calibrated line of the syringe for the remainder of the dose.*

**1** Ordered: phenobarbital elixir 25 mg PO at bedtime stat.

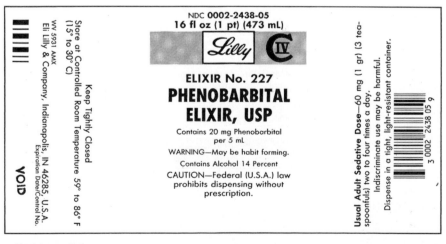

   **a.** Estimated dose: _____
      DA equation:

   **b.** Evaluation: _____

Shade in the dose in mL for the medicine cup and draw a vertical line through the calibrated line of the syringe.

2 Ordered: potassium chloride 25 mEq PO daily 20% sugar-free solution.

**a.** Estimated dose: _____

DA equation:

**b.** Evaluation: _____

Shade in the dose in mL for the medicine cup and draw a vertical line through the calibrated line of the syringe.

**3** Ordered: Mellaril oral solution 50 mg tid PO daily.

**a.** Estimated dose: _____
   DA equation:

**b.** Evaluation: _____

Draw a vertical line through the calibrated line of the syringe.

This medication will be measured in a syringe and served in a *needleless* syringe, a teaspoon, or a 30-mL measuring cup.

4  Ordered: chlorpromazine sol 25 mg PO for preoperative agitation.

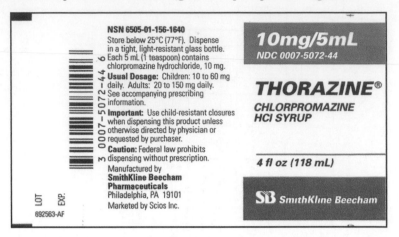

**a.** Estimated dose: _____
   DA equation:

**b.** Evaluation: _____

Shade in the dose in mL for the medicine cup and draw a vertical line through
the calibrated line of the syringe.

5 Ordered: lithium citrate 0.6 g PO tid.

**NDC 0054-3527-63**

**500 mL**

**LITHIUM**
**Citrate**
**Syrup USP**

**8 mEq per 5 mL**

Each 5 mL contains: 8 mEq of LITHIUM ION
(Equivalent to 300 mg of Lithium Carbonate
per 5 mL), Alcohol 0.3% v/v.
**SUGAR FREE**
**FOR ORAL ADMINISTRATION ONLY**
**Usual Adult Dose:** 5 or 10 mL, 1 or 2
teaspoonfuls, (8 or 16 mEq of Lithium)
three times a day.
Dispense in tight container as defined in the USP/NF.
Store at Controlled Room
Temperature 15°-30°C (59°-86°F)
See Package Insert for Complete Prescribing Information.
**Caution:** Federal law prohibits dispensing
without prescription.

LITHIUM CITRATE SYRUP USP, 8 mEq per 5 mL
Store at Controlled Room Temperature 15°-30°C (59°-86°F)

**LOT**
**EXP.**

NSN 6505-
01-168-0537

**Roxane**
Laboratories, Inc.
Columbus, Ohio 43216

4121000
033
© RLI, 1993

**a.** Estimated dose: _____

DA equation:

**b.** Evaluation: _____

Shade in the dose in mL for the medicine cup and draw a vertical line through the calibrated line of the syringe.

2 TBSP —— 30 ML
—— 25 ML
—— 20 ML
1 TBSP —— 15 ML
2 TSP —— 10 ML
1 TSP —— 5 ML
1/2 TSP ——

➤ If you are administering the oral medication with an injectable syringe, re-move the needle.

# Safe Dose Ranges

Verifying SDRs for medications and estimating doses for all medications are two techniques that protect patients and nurses from medication dose calculation errors.

## Calculating Safe Dose Ranges

Medications are approved by the FDA with guidelines for the safe amount to administer to the target audience, for example, "For adult use, 20 mg per day" or "Safe dose range 10-20 mg per day." The safe dose range may be even more specific for powerful drugs, for drugs that are supplied in various dose strengths or for intravenous routes, and for at-risk populations, such as infants, children, and frail adults (e.g., 1-2 mg/ kg body weight per day).

The nurse must compare the prescribed order with the SDR in current pharmacologic references or drug package inserts to be sure that the order is within the SDR for a given dose and target population.

The SDR guidelines are usually for a 24-hour day. If the total dose cannot safely be administered on a once-a-day basis, the recommendation will include the *frequency schedule:* the number of times at which the total daily dose should be *divided* into individual doses.

The arithmetic to calculate the SDR is very simple:

- Calculate the low safe dose.
- Calculate the high safe dose.
- Evaluate the order in relation to the SDR and frequency schedule.
- Decision: *Hold* the medication and contact the prescriber because the order is not within the safe dose range or frequency, or *give* the medication because the order is within the safe dose range and frequency.

Three kinds of SDRs are commonly seen:

1 Simple range
2 Divided doses
3 Simple or divided based on weight

### SDR with Simple Ranges

| EXAMPLES | Ordered: Drug X 10 mg tid. SDR: 10-30 mg/ day. |
|---|---|
| | Order: 10 mg × 3 doses = 30 mg/ day |

10 mg is the *low safe dose* for 24 hours. 30 mg is the *maximum safe dose* for 24 hours.

Evaluation: It can be seen at a glance that this order is within the SDR for the total daily dose.

➤ Take care to avoid confusing the SDR amount with the ordered amount. It is easier to avoid error if the SDR is placed above the order, as illustrated in the previous example.

### SDR with Divided Doses

| EXAMPLES | Ordered: Drug X 10 mg tid. SDR: 30 mg/ day in 2-3 divided doses. |
|---|---|

The phrase *divided doses* indicates that the entire daily dose cannot be given safely at one time. 30 mg/ day must be divided into two servings:

$$\frac{30}{2} = 15 \text{ mg/ dose}$$

or into 3 servings: $\frac{30}{3} = 10 \text{ mg/dose}$

*Continued from previous page.*

SDR: 30 mg/ day in 2-3 divided doses.

Order: 10 × 3 or 30 mg a day total in 3 divided doses.

Evaluation: The order falls within SDR for both total daily dose and frequency.

## Safe and Unsafe Orders

| Safe Order | Unsafe Order |
|---|---|
| Ordered: Drug X 75 mg/ day | Drug X 200 mg/ day |
| SDR: 50-100 mg/ day | SDR 50-100 mg/ day |
| Order: 75 mg/ day | Order: 200 mg/ day |
| Evaluation: Safe to give. | Evaluation: Hold medication and contact prescriber promptly. Order exceeds maximum. |

EXAMPLES

## SDR with Range Based on Weight

EXAMPLES

Ordered: Drug X 150 mg four times daily.

Patient's weight: 88 lb.

SDR: 10-20 mg/ kg/ day in 3-4 divided doses.

**1.** Find weight in kilograms:

Conversion formula: 2.2 lb = 1 kg. Estimated weight: 44 kg (88 ÷ 2).

$$\text{DA equation: kg} = \frac{1 \text{ kg}}{\cancel{2.2 \text{ lb}}} \times \overset{40}{\cancel{88.0 \text{ lb}}} = 40 \qquad \text{Actual weight: 40 kg}$$

**2.** Multiply the low and high safe doses in milligrams by the weight in kilograms to obtain the SDR:

$$10 \text{ mg} \times 40 \text{ kg} = 400 \text{ mg} = \textit{low} \text{ safe dose}$$

$$20 \text{ mg} \times 40 \text{ kg} = 800 \text{ mg} = \textit{highest} \text{ safe dose}$$

**3.** Compare the order with the SDR:

SDR: 400 mg − 800 mg/ day in 3-4 divided doses.

Order: 600 mg/ day in 4 doses of 150 mg.

**4.** Evaluation: The order falls within the SDR of 400-800 mg/ day and matches the frequency. It is safe to prepare.

The exact weight in kilograms must be calculated to the *nearest t*enth for drug doses. Estimating the conversion of pounds to kilograms is a good way to double check calculations.

➤ Note that after the doses are multiplied by the kilogram weight, the answer is in milligrams.

➤ It is suggested that the nurse write the SDR *above* the order for easy comparison. By doing this, the nurse can see whether the order falls within the SDR, as shown in the previous example.

➤ Compare the order and SDR for total *daily dose and frequency* to be given. The frequency or divided dose schedule is as important for the patient's safety as is the total dose. Giving too much of a medicine at one time can be toxic, damage kidneys, and exceed the body's ability to metabolize the drug.

**RAPID PRACTICE 5-13** Safe Dose Range and Milligrams
per Kilogram of Body Weight

**Estimated completion time: 30-45 minutes**   Answers on page **531**

**Directions:** *Fill in the estimated weight, actual weight, and SDR in the spaces provided. Follow the example given for problem 1. Move decimal places to change the metric units to milligrams if necessary. Use a calculator to convert pounds to kilograms and calculate the SDR.*

| SDR | Patient's Weight (lb) | Estimated Weight (kg) to the Nearest Whole Number | Actual Weight (kg) to the Nearest Tenth | Total SDR to Nearest Tenth |
|---|---|---|---|---|
| 1  10 - 20 mg/ kg/ day | 66 | 33 | 30 | 10 × 30 = 300 mg/ day<br>20 × 30 = 600 mg/ day<br>SDR = 300-600 mg/ day |
| 2  100 - 200 mcg/ kg/ day | 40 | _____ | _____ | _____ |
| 3  0.2 - 0.5 g/ kg/ day | 44 | _____ | _____ | _____ |
| 4  0.25 - 1.5 mg/ kg/ day | 150 | _____ | _____ | _____ |
| 5  2 - 5 mcg/ kg/ day | 180 | _____ | _____ | _____ |
| 6  0.1 - 0.2 g/ kg/ day | 95 | _____ | _____ | _____ |
| 7  5 - 10 mcg/ kg/ day | 88 | _____ | _____ | _____ |

| SDR | Patient's Weight (lb) | Estimated Weight (kg) to the Nearest Whole Number | Actual Weight (kg) to the Nearest Tenth | Total SDR to Nearest Tenth |
|---|---|---|---|---|
| 8  10 - 20 mg/ kg/ day in 3 divided doses | 200 | _____ | _____ | _____ |
| 9  1 - 5 mcg/ kg/ day | 30 | _____ | _____ | _____ |
| 10  0.05 - 0.1 g/ day in 4 divided doses | 150 | _____ | _____ | _____ |

The SDR is particularly needed for unfamiliar medications and medications that represent a fraction of the unit dose or more than two times the unit dose. SDR checks are also needed for frail patients, immunocompromised patients, patients in the intensive care unit, and pediatric populations.

**Clinical Relevance**

## RAPID PRACTICE 5-14 Evaluation of Medication Orders According to SDR

**Estimated completion time: 25 minutes**  Answers on page **532**

**Directions:** *Examine the example given for problem 1. Compare the frequency, total daily dose, and total daily dose ordered with the SDR guidelines for problems 2-5. Evaluate the findings and make a decision to hold the medication, clarify the order promptly with the prescriber and document the clarification, or give the medication because the order is a safe dose. Use a calculator to calculate the SDR.*

1 **Ordered:** Drug X 0.5 g tid PO.

   **SDR:** 25-50 mg/ kg/ day in 3 divided doses.
   a. Patient's weight: 100 lb. Estimated kilograms: 50 (nearest whole number). Actual kilograms: 45.5 (nearest tenth).
   b. SDR low and high dose based on actual kilogram weight.

   25 mg × 45.5 kg = 1137.5 mg/ day = low safe dose

   50 mg ÷ 45.5 kg = 2 × 1137.5, or 2275 mg/ day = high (maximum) safe dose

   Conversion of order using decimal movement: 0.5 g = 500 mg tid = 1500 mg ordered per day

   **SDR:** 1137.5-2275 mg/ day

   c. Daily dose ordered: 1500 mg
   d. Evaluation: Within SDR and recommended frequency (circle one)? (Yes) or *No*.
   e. Decision: Order is within SDR and safe to give.

**2 Ordered:** Drug X 50 mg q4h.

   **SDR:** 1-2 mg/ kg/ day in 4-6 divided doses.

   **a.** Patient's weight: 160 lb. Estimated weight in kilograms: _____. Actual weight in kilograms: _____.

   **b.** SDR low and high dose based on actual kilogram weight:

   _____

   **c.** Daily dose ordered: _____

   **d.** Evaluation: Within SDR and recommended frequency (circle one)? *Yes* or *No.*

   **e.** Decision: _____

**3 Ordered:** Drug X 50 mg/ day q6h.

   **SDR:** 2-4 mg/ kg/ day in 4 divided doses.

   **a.** Patient's weight: 120 lb. Estimated weight in kilograms: _____. Actual weight in kilograms: _____.

   **b.** SDR low and high dose based on actual kilogram weight:

   _____

   **c.** Daily dose ordered: _____

   **d.** Evaluation: Within SDR and recommended frequency (circle one)? *Yes* or *No.*

   **e.** Decision: _____

**4 Ordered:** Drug X 0.25 g tid.

   **SDR:** 10-20 mg/ kg/ day in 2-3 divided doses.

   **a.** Patient's weight: 100 lb. Estimated weight in kilograms: _____. Actual weight in kilograms: _____.

   **b.** SDR low and high dose based on actual kilogram weight: _____

   **c.** Daily dose ordered: _____

   **d.** Evaluation: Within SDR and recommended frequency (circle one)? *Yes* or *No.*

   **e.** Decision: _____

**5 Ordered:** Drug X: 25 mg bid.

   **SDR:** 5-10 mg/ kg/ day in 2-3 divided doses.

   **a.** Patient's weight: 60 lb. Estimated weight in kilograms: _____. Actual weight in kilograms: _____.

   **b.** SDR low and high dose based on actual kilogram weight:

   _____

   **c.** Daily dose ordered: _____

   **d.** Evaluation: Within SDR and recommended frequency (circle one)? *Yes* or *No.*

   **e.** Decision: _____

---

**Q:** *Ask Yourself*

**A:** *My Answer*

**1**  What are three instances in which the medication ordered needs to be clarified with the prescriber?

_____

**2**  Why is documentation of the clarification important for the patient and the nurse?

_____

**FAQ** | *Are low or high doses outside of the SDR ever administered?*

**ANSWER:** ➤ Yes, but only the prescriber can make the decision. Beginning practitioners should hold the medication and clarify the order with the prescriber promptly. They should research the reason why the dose might be so low as to seem nontherapeutic or so high as to seem toxic. Always recheck the order and the label first. Document and report contacts with the prescriber and actions promptly.

Even if the medication order falls within safe dose range guidelines in the literature, the nursing assessments of the patient's record and of the patient may generate a decision to hold the medication pending clarification with the prescriber. Medication-related nursing assessments may disclose that one or more medications are unsafe for the patient at that point in time. For example, a change in the patient's mental status may render the patient unable to swallow food or fluids. This condition would necessitate a new order for a changed route of administration. Nausea and vomiting are also good reasons to withhold oral medications. If the medication is a critical one, such as a heart medication, the prescriber needs to be informed immediately.

**Clinical Relevance**

➤ Interactions cited in the literature with one or more drugs already being administered would be another reason to hold the medication and clarify the order with the prescriber.

**FAQ** | *How do I know whom to contact when there is a question about a medication order?*

**ANSWER:** The decision comes with experience. There are three good sources: the prescriber, the pharmacist, and a recent drug reference or drug information insert. The source to select depends upon the nature of the question. Here are some general guidelines:

➤ If the medication order is illegible, unclear, or incomplete, contact the prescriber.
➤ If the problem is with the amount of the *dose,* check a drug reference first and then the prescriber if necessary.
➤ If the medication *supplied is* in question, contact the pharmacist.
➤ Students should hold the medication, analyze the problem, use the references to determine the SDR and/or contact the pharmacist if appropriate, determine independently which action would be best, and promptly contact the instructor to confer regarding the decision, particularly if the prescriber is to be contacted.

**RAPID PRACTICE 5-15** Calculating Safe Doses with DA Verification

**Estimated completion time: 25 minutes**   Answers on page **532**

**Directions:** *Examine and analyze the example in problem 1. Then complete problems 2-5, working out each step of the problem in order. If the decision is to hold the medication, stop calculations.*

1 **Ordered:** Digoxin (Lanoxin) pediatric elixir 0.1 mg po daily for an adult patient with heart failure.

**SDR:** *adult maintenance* 50 mcg-300 mcg/ day.

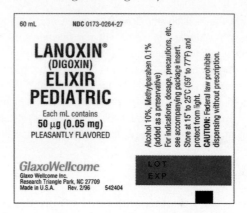

➤ Note that the label uses *μg* for *mcg*. It is safer for the nurse to write mcg.

  **a.** Unit dose available: 50 mcg/ mL, or 0.05 mg/ mL

  **b.** Conversion needed: mg/ mcg to compare order to SDR. Decimal change needed: 0.1 mg = 100 mcg.

  **c.** Order within SDR (circle one)? (Yes) or *No*. The answer is yes, since the SDR is 50-300 mcg/ day and the order is 100 mcg (0.1 mg).

  **d.** Decision (circle one): Safe to (Give) or *Hold*.

  **e.** Estimated dose to be given to nearest whole number: 0.1 mg ordered, 0.05 mg/0.1 mL available. More than 1 mL would be given, two times the unit dose.

  **f.** Actual dose to be given to nearest *tenth* of a milliliter: 2 mL
    DA equation:

$$? \text{ mL} = \frac{1 \text{ mL}}{\cancel{0.05 \text{ mg}}} \times \cancel{1 \text{ mg}}^{\,2} = 2 \text{ mL (answer)}$$

  No conversion is required to calculate the dose because the units are the same (mg/ mg).

  **g.** Evaluation: The estimate supports the answer. The answer is 2 mL. The equation is balanced. If the calculations resulted in an answer greater than 2 mL, the nurse would revisit the problem and the setup.

**2 Ordered:** lithium carbonate, 0.6 g bid daily for a patient with a bipolar disorder.

**SDR:** 900-1200 mg daily in 2-3 divided doses.

a. Unit dose available in mg/ mL: _____

b. Conversion needed: _____

c. Order within SDR (circle one)? *Yes* or *No.*

d. Decision (circle one): *Give* or *Hold.*

e. Estimated dose to be given to the nearest tenth of a milliliter: _____

f. How many milliliters will you prepare? _____

DA equation:




g. Evaluation: _____

Shade in the dose in mL for the medicine cup and draw a vertical line through the calibrated line of the syringe as applicable:

Remember that the estimate usually cannot be made until the measurement units are *the same.*

**3 Ordered:** loperamide hydrochloride sol. 2 mg PO after each loose stool up to six times daily.

**SDR:** 4 mg initially, then 2 mg after each loose stool, not to exceed 16 mg/ day.

**a.** Conversion needed: _____

**b.** Order within SDR (circle one)? *Yes* or *No*.

**c.** Decision (circle one): Safe to *Give* or *Hold*.

**d.** Estimated dose to be given to the nearest tenth of a milliliter: _____

**e.** How many milliliters will you prepare? _____
DA equation:


**f.** Evaluation: _____

Shade in the dose in mL for the medicine cup and draw a vertical line through the calibrated line of the syringe as applicable:

**4** **Ordered:** Kaon-Cl liquid 45 mEq PO stat for a patient with hypokalemia.

SDR for adult for potassium depletion: 40 mEq - 100 mEq/ day PO.

NDC 0013-3113-51

# KAON-CL 20%®
(POTASSIUM CHLORIDE)

**40 mEq/15 ml**

**CHERRY**

Sugar-Free

Each 15 ml (tablespoonful) supplies 40 mEq each of potassium and chloride (as potassium chloride, 3 g), with saccharin and alcohol 5%.

**CAUTION:** Federal law prohibits dispensing without prescription.

**ONE PINT**

〈Adria〉®

**a.** Conversion needed: _____

**b.** Order within SDR (circle one)? *Yes* or *No.*

**c.** Decision (circle one): Safe to *Give* or *Hold.*

**d.** Estimated dose to be given to the nearest tenth of a milliliter: _____

**e.** How many milliliters will you prepare? _____

DA equation:

**f.** Evaluation: _____

Shade in the dose in mL for the medicine cup and draw a vertical line through the calibrated line of the syringe as applicable:

2 TBSP —— 30 ML
—— 25 ML
—— 20 ML
1 TBSP —— 15 ML
2 TSP —— 10 ML
1 TSP —— 5 ML
1/2 TSP ——

Potassium is a medication with high risk for error and high potential for harm if an error occurs. Refer to www.ismp.org for more information.

Check carefully for dilution directions.

**5 Ordered:** dyphylline elixir 120 mg for a child who needs sedation.

**SDR** for sedation of a child: 3-6 mg/ kg/ day in 3 divided doses.

Child's weight: 44 lb. Estimated weight in kilograms (nearest whole number): _____. Actual weight in kilograms (nearest tenth): _____.

**a.** Conversion needed: _____

**b.** Order within SDR (circle one)? *Yes* or *No*.

**c.** Decision (circle one): Safe to *Give* or *Hold*.

**d.** Estimated dose to be given to the nearest tenth of a milliliter: _____

**e.** How many milliliters will you prepare? _____
DA equation:

**f.** Evaluation: _____

Shade in the dose in mL for the medicine cup and draw a vertical line through the calibrated line of the syringe as applicable:

## CHAPTER 5 MULTIPLE-CHOICE REVIEW

**Answers on page 534**

**Directions:** *Select the best answer.*

**1** One of the most important safety nets a nurse can use for catching calculation errors is

  **1.** Performing metric conversions
  **2.** Estimating answers
  **3.** Using a calculator
  **4.** Carrying a math text to clinical

**2** Which of the following pairs of units will need to have the decimal moved 6 places?

  **1.** Grams to micrograms
  **2.** Grams to milligrams
  **3.** Micrograms to milligrams
  **4.** Milliequivalents to milliliters

**3** Which is the correct conversion for 50 mg to grams?

  **1.** 0.005 g
  **2.** 0.05 g
  **3.** 0.5 g
  **4.** 500 g

**4** Which is the correct conversion for 25,000 mcg to grams?

  **1.** 250 g
  **2.** 25 g
  **3.** 0.25 g
  **4.** 0.025 g

**5** The recommended way to write large numbers in the metric system for ease of reading, as in one hundred thousand micrograms, is

  **1.** With commas: 100,000
  **2.** With decimal points: 100.000
  **3.** With spaces: 100 000
  **4.** Without spaces or inserts: 100000

6 If 25 mg/ kg/ day is ordered in 2 divided doses and kg = 10, what will be the unit dose?

**1.** 50 mg

**2.** 100 mg

**3.** 125 mg

**4.** 250 mg

7 The SDR for 10-30 mg/ kg/ day for a patient weighing 44 lb is

**1.** 300 mg/ day

**2.** 440 mg-1320 mg/ day

**3.** 200-600 mg/ kg/ day

**4.** 200-600 mg/ day

8 Milligram-gram conversions require movement of how many decimal places?

**1.** 3 places

**2.** 5 places

**3.** 6 places

**4.** 1 million places

9 Select the appropriate measuring device and volumes when preparing an oral medication of 24 mL to be administered in a 30-mL calibrated medicine cup.

**1.** Pour to 25 mL in the measuring cup and remove 1 mL.

**2.** Pour to 20 mL in the measuring cup and administer 4 mL with a 3-mL syringe.

**3.** Pour to approximately 24 mL, just short of the 25-mL line.

**4.** Pour to 20 mL in the cup and administer 4 mL with a 5-mL syringe.

10 Which of the following conversions is correct?

**1.** 0.5 g = 50 mg

**2.** 10 000 mcg = 20 mg

**3.** 0.05 g = 50,000 mcg

**4.** 120 mg = 1.2 g

## CHAPTER 5 FINAL PRACTICE

Answers on page **534**

**Directions:** *Evaluate the order and SDR. If safe to give, estimate and approximate dose. Verify the estimate with a DA style equation. Evaluate the answer. Use a calculator to determine kg weights and SDR. Write the answers in the space provided.*

1 **Ordered:** aspirin 0.65g PO q4h prn for a 22-year-old patient with a painful sprained ankle.

**SDR** (adult): (Consult label.)

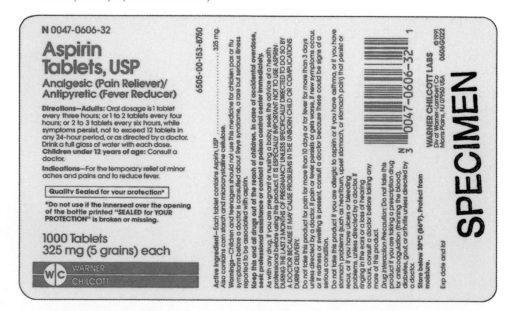

**a.** SDR comparison with order: _____

**b.** Decision: _____

**c.** Estimate of number of tablets to be given: _____ More or less than unit dose? _____

**d.** Actual number of tablets to be given: _____
DA equation:

**e.** Evaluation: _____

➤ Note that the drug label has "5 grains" after "325 mg." This unit of measure is derived from the outdated apothecary system. Use the ordered metric (mg) unit of measurement for calculations.

2 **Ordered:** acetaminophen liquid 0.65 g PO q6h for a patient with a fever.

**SDR** (Adult): 325-650 mg q4-6h up to 4 g/ day.

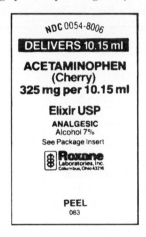

NDC 0054-8006
**DELIVERS 10.15 ml**
**ACETAMINOPHEN**
**(Cherry)**
**325 mg per 10.15 ml**
**Elixir USP**
ANALGESIC
Alcohol 7%
See Package Insert
**Roxane**
Laboratories, Inc.
Columbus, Ohio 43216
**PEEL**
083

**a.** SDR comparison with order: _____

**b.** Decision: _____

**c.** Estimated dose: _____

**d.** Amount to give: _____

**e.** Evaluation: _____

Shade in the dose in mL for the medicine cup and draw a vertical line through the calibrated line of the syringe as applicable:

2 TBSP —— 30 ML
—— 25 ML
—— 20 ML
1 TBSP —— 15 ML
2 TSP —— 10 ML
1 TSP —— 5 ML
1/2 TSP —

**3 Ordered:** raloxifene HCl 0.06 g bid PO daily for an adult patient with osteoporosis.

**SDR** (adult): 60 mg once a day.

a. SDR comparison with order: _____

b. Decision: _____

c. Estimate: _____

d. Amount to give: _____

DA equation:

e. Evaluation: _____

**4 Ordered:** potassium chloride elixir 30 mEq PO daily for a patient on diuretics.

**SDR:** 20-40 mEq/ day.

a. SDR comparison with order: _____

b. Decision: _____

c. Estimate: _____

d. Amount to give: _____

DA equation:

e. Evaluation: _____

Shade in the dose in mL for the medicine cup and draw a vertical line
through the calibrated line of the syringe as applicable

5 **Ordered:** thioridazine HCL solution 0.05 g tid PO for a patient with severe
psychosis.

**SDR:** 10-50 mg 3-4 times daily.

Directions: Immediately before use, dilute the medication with distilled water,
acidified tap water, or juice.

**a.** SDR comparison with order: _____

**b.** Decision: _____

**c.** Estimate: _____

**d.** Amount to give: _____
   DA equation:

**e.** Evaluation: _____

Draw a vertical line through the calibrated line of the syringe as applicable.

6 **Ordered:** phenobarbital tablets 0.09 g bid PO for a patient with seizures.

   **SDR:** 100-300 mg/ day in divided doses or at bedtime.

   **a.** SDR comparison with order: _____

   **b.** Decision: _____

   **c.** Estimate: _____

   **d.** Amount to give: _____

   DA equation:

   **e.** Evaluation: _____

7 **Ordered:** carbamazepine 0.2 g bid PO for a patient with *initial* treatment for seizures.

   **SDR:** 200 mg bid to start; may be increased by 200 mg/ day in divided doses.

   **a.** SDR comparison with order: _____

   **b.** Decision: _____

   **c.** Estimate: _____

   **d.** Amount to give: _____

   DA equation:

   **e.** Evaluation: _____

CHAPTER 5

**8 Ordered:** Synthroid 0.1 mg PO daily for a patient with hypothyroidism.

**Maintenance:** 75-125 mcg/ day.

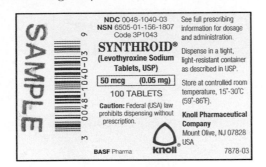

**a.** SDR comparison with order: _____

**b.** Decision: _____

**c.** Estimate: _____

**d.** Amount to give: _____

DA equation:



**e.** Evaluation: _____

**9 Ordered:** dyphylline elixir 75 mg AM and bedtime for a patient with a cough weighing 50 lb.

**SDR:** 5 mg/ kg in 2-3 divided doses per day.

**a.** SDR comparison with order: _____

**b.** Decision: _____

**c.** Estimate: _____

**d.** Amount to give: _____

DA equation:



**e.** Evaluation: _____

Shade in the dose in mL for the medicine cup and draw a vertical line through the calibrated line of the syringe as applicable.

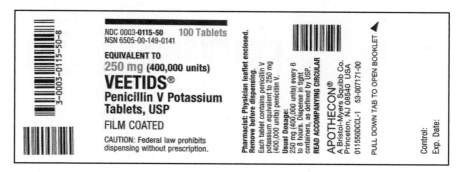

**10 Ordered:** penicillin V potassium tabs 0.25 g PO q8h × 10 days for a patient with streptococcal infection.

**SDR:** 125-250 mg q6-8h × 10 days.

**a.** SDR comparison with order: _____

**b.** Decision: _____

**c.** Estimate: _____

**d.** Amount to give: _____
  DA equation:

**e.** Evaluation: _____

## Suggestions for Further Reading

Clayton BD, Stock YN: Basic pharmacology for nurses, ed. 13, St. Louis, 2004, Mosby.

Pagana KD, Pagana TJ: Mosby's diagnostic and laboratory test reference, ed. 7, St. Louis, 2005, Mosby.

PDR Nurse's Handbook, Montvale NJ, 2003, Medical Economics Co.

Skidmore-Roth L: Mosby's drug guide for nurses, ed. 6, St. Louis, 2007, Mosby.

www.ampainsoc.org/advocacy/pdf/range.pd

www.drhull.com/EncyMaster/M/measurement.html

 Additional practice problems can be found in the Calculating by Dimensional Analysis and Basic Calculations sections on the enclosed companion CD.

Chapter 6 covers syringe measurements in preparation for measuring injectable medication doses.

# PART III
## RECONSTITUTED MEDICATIONS

> *"A thing is obvious mathematically after you see it."*
> —R.D. CARMICHAEL

# SYRINGE MEASUREMENTS

## Objectives

- State the total volume capacity for various syringes.
- Differentiate the calibrations for various syringe sizes per milliliter.
- State the lowest and nearest measurable dose for syringes.
- Select the appropriate syringe size for stated volumes.
- Draw a vertical line through an accurate dose on a syringe.
- Select the appropriate syringe for selected purposes.
- Identify safety principles related to syringes and needles.
- Define needle gauge and three criteria for needle selection.

## Essential Prior Knowledge

Mastery of Chapters 1-5

## Equipment

- Basic syringe measurements can be learned from the chapter practice. Learning will be expedited if actual syringes are on hand.

## Estimated Time To Complete Chapter

- 30 minutes to 1 hour

## Introduction

Liquid doses in mL for oral medications have been covered in Chapter 4 as well as an introduction to measuring syringe volumes with the 3 mL and the 5 mL syringe. Sufficient drawings and practice will be offered in this chapter so that syringe volume measurements for any syringes can be identified for providing the nearest measurable dose.

Examining and handling a variety of syringes and needles in the laboratory will be necessary to obtain a more comprehensive view and competence in the use of the equipment.

## ESSENTIAL Vocabulary

| | |
|---|---|
| **Hypodermic** | General term used to describe injectables under the skin. |
| **Insulin Syringe** | Small syringe, with a 1-mL capacity *or less*, calibrated for specific insulin mixtures in standardized units. |

| Intradermal (ID) | Shallow injection to be given just under the skin between the dermis and the epidermis. Used mainly for skin tests. Not used to deliver medications. *0.1 mL* is the usual volume of skin test injections. |
| Intramuscular (IM) | Into the muscle. The muscle is able to accept more irritating substances than other injectable routes. |
| Intravenous (IV) | Into the vein. These injections provide *instant* drug access to the circulation. |
| Needle Gauge | Diameter (thickness) of the needle shaft. The lower the gauge number, the larger the diameter of the needle. |
| Parenteral Medications | Injectable medications. Excludes oral, nasogastric, gastric, and intestinal routes. |
| Prefilled Syringe | Syringe prefilled with specific frequently ordered doses of medication by manufacturer or pharmacy. This method is thought to reduce dose measurement errors. |
| Safety Syringe | Syringe designed with a variety of locking sheath covers to protect needle sterility and prevent accidental injury during and after disposal. |
| Subcutaneous | Under the skin into the fatty layer. Used for less irritating substances than are intramuscular injections. Insulin and heparin are given subcutaneously. |
| Syringe Holder | Specially designed device to be used only with an inserted prefilled medication cartridge. |
| Tuberculin Syringe | Small-volume syringe, with a 1-mL capacity, used for intradermal skin tests and small-volume injections of less than 1 mL in frail at-risk populations |
| Viscosity | Ability to flow; thickness of a solution. A solution that is viscous may have directions for dilution. Blood is viscous, as are some reconstituted medications. Viscous solutions require larger-gauge needles. |

## RAPID PRACTICE 6-1 Vocabulary Review

**Estimated completion time: 5-10 minutes**   Answers on page **536**

**Directions:** *Review the vocabulary list and fill in the definitions with one- or two-word phrases.*

1 The marked lines on a syringe that indicate the capacity are called _____

2 The route that is used for skin tests is called _____, and the syringe used for that route has a _____-mL capacity.

3 Injectable medications are given through various routes called _____, as opposed to the oral route.

4 The size of a needle diameter is called _____

5 Do needles that have a larger gauge number have a larger or smaller diameter? _____,

# Syringe Sizes

## 20-mL, 10-mL, 5-mL, 3-mL, and 1-mL Syringes

Syringes are available in many sizes, ranging from *0.3-mL* to *60-mL* capacity. The decision to use a specific syringe is based on the volume of medication to be administered and the route of administration.

Intravenous medications may be given with a 20-mL syringe, which is selected for doses of 20 mL or less (Figure 6-1).

Intravenous medications may be also given with a 10-mL syringe, selected for doses of 10 mL or less (Figure 6-2).

Intramuscular and intravenous injections may be given with a 5-mL syringe. It is used for doses of 5 mL or less (Figure 6-3)

Many subcutaneous, intramuscular, and intravenous injections are given with a 3-mL syringe, used for doses of 3 mL or less (Figure 6-4).

A 1-mL syringe is used for skin tests and vaccines and may be used for infants' injections and for very small doses. It is selected for doses of 1 mL or less (Figure 6-5).

Figure **6-1**. 20-mL syringe with 1-mL calibrations.

Figure **6-2**. 10-mL syringe with 0.2-mL calibrations.

Figure **6-3**. 5-mL syringe with 0.2-mL calibrations.

Figure **6-4**. 3-mL syringe with 0.1-mL calibrations.

Figure **6-5.** 1-mL tuberculin syringe.

Figure **6-6.** Insulin syringes. **A,** 100 units (1 mL). **B,** 50 units (0.5 mL). **C,** 30 units (0.3 mL).

Figure **6-7. A,** 1-mL tuberculin syringe. **B,** 100-unit 1-mL insulin syringe. (From Potter PA, Perry AG: Fundamentals of nursing, ed. 6, St. Louis, 2005, Mosby.)

## Insulin Syringes

Insulin syringes are sized in 100 units, 50 units, and 30 units (Figure 6-6). A 100-unit insulin syringe is selected for insulin doses up to 100 units.

A 50-unit insulin syringe is selected for better visualization of insulin doses up to 50 units. A 30-unit insulin syringe is selected for better visualization of insulin doses up to 30 units.

➤ Do not use insulin syringes for medications ordered in milliliters. Insulin doses are ordered in units. Avoid confusing insulin syringes with tuberculin syringes.
➤ All used syringes as well as used needles must be placed in hazardous waste containers immediately after use. They may not be thrown in trash baskets.
➤ Do not confuse 1-mL syringes or tuberculin syringes marked in milliliters (or cubic centimeters) with 1-mL *insulin* syringes, which are marked with the word *insulin* and calibrated in *units* (Figure 6-7).

## Parts of the Syringe

Figure 6-8 shows the parts of a syringe. Syringes are supplied without needles or with attached needles. Supervised clinical practice is required in order to learn safe handling of syringes and needles.

Figure **6-9.** 3-mL syringe showing 0.5-mL and the 1-mL markings.

0.5 mL   1 mL

Figure **6-8.** Parts of a syringe. (From Potter PA, Perry AG: Fundamentals of nursing, ed. 6, St. Louis, 2005, Mosby.)

The 3-mL syringe is the most commonly used syringe for subcutaneous and intramuscular injections. The arrows illustrate the location of the 1- and 0.5-mL markings (Figure 6-9).

## Total Capacity and Lowest Measurable Dose

Finding the total capacity and the lowest measurable dose involves the same process for all syringes. Syringe size selection is based on the total volume and nearest *measurable* dose on the syringe. Examine the empty 3-mL syringe shown in Figure 6-9 for a review:

- The total capacity is 3 mL.
- Look for two adjacent darker lines.
- There are 5 lines between the 0 and $\frac{1}{2}$ (0.5) dark milliliter line and 10 lines between the 0 and the dark 1-mL mark near the needle end of the syringe.
- Therefore, each line represents 0.1 mL (1 mL ÷ 10 lines, or 0.5 mL ÷ 5 lines).
- The lowest measurable dose is 0.1 mL.
- Medications for these syringes can be given to the *nearest tenth of a milliliter* (e.g., 2.2 mL, 2.3 mL, etc.) because that is the *lowest measurable dose.*
- The calibrations are slightly more prominent for the *whole*-milliliter marks.
- It is sometimes easier to count the lines to a whole number, if present, such as 0 to 1 mL, or between whole numbers, such as 1 and 2 mL. Keep in mind that smaller syringes may not have whole numbers. Examine the 1-mL syringe illustrated in Figure 6-5. It has 100 calibrations between 0 and 1 mL. In this case, the line count is more easily read between 0.1 and 0.2 mL.

**EXAMPLES**

$$\frac{1 \text{ mL}}{10 \text{ calibrations}} = 0.1 \text{ mL lowest measurable dose}$$

$$\frac{1 \text{ mL}}{5 \text{ calibrations}} = 0.2 \text{ mL lowest measurable dose}$$

**FAQ** | *Why do I need to look at the total volume and the 1-mL markings?*

**ANSWER:** The total dose cannot exceed the volume ordered. To avoid reading errors, you need to know the precise measurements. After the dose is calculated, select a syringe that will contain the total number of milliliters that you need to give. You would not select a 3-mL syringe if you had to give 4.5 mL. The patient would not appreciate two injections instead of one. The best way to avoid making a syringe measurement error is to locate the 1-, 0.5-, or other major mL mark if available and then to observe the value of each calibration. Larger syringes will not have all the smaller calibrations. Misreading *1.5 mL* for *0.5 mL* is a major error. Nevertheless, it has occurred.

**Figure 6-10.** 20-mL syringe illustrating a 12-mL measurement reading at the upper ring of the plunger. (From Macklin D, Chernecky C, Infortuna H: Math for clinical practice, St. Louis, 2005, Mosby.)

# Where to Measure the Dose on Syringes

The dose in syringes is measured at the upper flat ring of the plunger, the ring closest to the needle end. For practice measurements, the plunger will not be shown (Figure 6-10).

## RAPID PRACTICE 6-2 Measuring Syringe Capacities

**Estimated completion time: 10-15 minutes**   Answers on page **537**

**Directions:** *Examine the numbers and calibrations on the syringe, and provide the answer in the space provided.*

1 What is the total capacity of this syringe in milliliters? _____

2 How many calibrations are there between 0 and 5 mL? _____

3 What is the smallest measurable dose (the first space up to the first line) on the syringe? _____

4 Draw a vertical line through the syringe below at 1 mL.

**5** Draw a vertical line through the syringe below at 14 mL.

Problems 6 to 8 pertain to the syringe below:

**6** What is the total capacity of the syringe in milliliters? _____

**7** How many calibrations are there between 0 and 1 mL? _____

**8** What is the smallest measurable dose on the syringe? _____

**9** Draw a vertical line through the syringe below at 5.6 mL.

**10** Draw a vertical line through the syringe below at 8.8 mL.

**Q** *Ask Yourself*

**A** *My Answer*

**1** How do the lowest measurable doses on the 10- and 20-mL syringe shown in the text differ from the lowest measurable doses on the 3- and 5-mL syringe?

_____

**RAPID PRACTICE 6-3** Measuring Syringe Capacities

**Estimated completion time: 10 minutes**    Answers on page **538**

**Directions:** *Examine the numbers and calibrations on the syringe and provide the answers in the space provided.*

1 What is the total capacity of the syringe above in milliliters? _____

2 How many calibrations are there between 0 and 1 mL? _____

3 What is the smallest measurable dose on the syringe? _____

4 Draw a vertical line through the syringe below at 0.6 mL. (Note: There are also 5-mL syringes that have 10 calibrations per milliliter.)

5 Draw a vertical line through the syringe below at 3.4 mL.

6 What is the total capacity of the syringe below in milliliters? _____

7 How many calibrations are there between 0 and 0.1 mL? _____

8 What is the smallest measurable dose on the syringe? _____

9 Draw a vertical line through the syringe below at 0.05 mL.

10 Draw a vertical line through the syringe below at 0.1 mL.

➤ Pay special attention to the decimal place in the doses for the 1-mL syringe.

**Q:** *Ask Yourself*

1 What are the two most commonly used sizes of syringes?

**A:** *My Answer*

_____

## RAPID PRACTICE 6-4 Measuring Syringe Capacities

**Estimated completion time: 5 minutes**   Answers on page **539**

**Directions:** *Examine the numbers and calibrations on the syringe and provide the answers in the space provided or by putting a line on the syringe drawing.*

1 What is the total capacity of the syringe in milliliters? _____

2 What is the smallest measurable dose on the syringe? _____

**3** Draw a vertical line through the syringe at 2.7 mL.

**4** Draw a vertical line through the syringe at 1.6 mL.

**5** Draw a vertical line through the syringe at 0.9 mL.

The 3- and 5-mL syringes are the most commonly used. However, nurses must know how to distinguish the differences in calibrations in the other sizes to avoid a dose measurement error.

**1**  What is the difference in the lowest measurable dose between the 3-mL and the 5-mL syringe shown in this text?

_____

**2**  Of the 3- and the 5-mL syringe shown in this text, which one can accommodate a 2.7-mL ordered dose?

_____

QAsk Yourself

AMy Answer

# Examining the Calculated Doses for Correct Syringe Selection

- If the amount ordered is a whole number (e.g., 3 mL) or in tenths of a milliliter (e.g., 2.8 or 0.8 mL), the 3-mL syringe would be appropriate.
- If the amount to be given is 0.08 mL, the 3-mL syringe would not be used because it is not calibrated in hundredths of a milliliter. A 1-mL (tuberculin) syringe would be selected.
- If the amount to be given is 3.6 mL, the 3-mL syringe would not be used because the patient would have to receive two injections. A 5-mL syringe would be selected.

**RAPID PRACTICE 6-5** Identifying the Syringe for the Dose Ordered

**Estimated completion time: 10-15 minutes** Answers on page **539**

**Directions:** *State the preferred syringe size in mL that provides the nearest measurable dose for the dose ordered. Note that a TB syringe is a 1-mL syringe.*

| Ordered Dose Volume | Syringe Size |
|---|---|
| 1  2.8 mL | _____ |
| 2  3.2 mL | _____ |
| 3  6.4 mL | _____ |
| 4  0.08 mL | _____ |
| 5  1.7 mL | _____ |
| 6  9.6 mL | _____ |
| 7  12.6 mL | _____ |
| 8  0.6 mL | _____ |
| 9  1.5 mL | _____ |
| 10  0.1 mL | _____ |

**RAPID PRACTICE 6-6** Syringe Selections and Disposal

**Estimated completion time: 5 minutes** Answers on page **539**

**Directions:** *Refer to the preceding text and syringe photographs that follow to answer the following questions.*

1 What is the main criterion for selection of syringe size? _____

2 Can used syringes without needles be placed in ordinary trash containers? ____

3 If a nurse prepares 0.06 mL of a medication, which size syringe should the nurse select? _____

4 If a nurse calculates a dose of 3.19 mL of a medication, which size syringe should the nurse select? _____What will be the nearest measurable dose on the syringe?____

5 If a nurse calculates a dose of 5.79 mL of a medication, which size syringe should the nurse select? _____How much medication will be drawn up in the syringe for the nearest measurable dose? _____

## Oral Syringes

Oral syringes have milliliter marks on one side, and some have household *teaspoon* mark on the other (Figure 6-11). Their tips may be off center. Some of them are capped (Figure 6-12).

Figure **6-11.** Oral syringes. **A,** 5-mL. **B,** 10-mL. From Clayton BD, Stock YN: Basic pharmacology for nurses, ed. 13, St. Louis, 2004, Mosby.

Figure **6-12.** Prefilled, capped oral syringe. From Brown M, Mulholland J: Drug calculations: process and problems for clinical practice, ed. 7, St. Louis, 2004, Mosby.

## Oral Syringes Versus Injectable Syringes

Empty and prefilled oral syringes are not usually available in all clinical facilities. Nurses may measure and administer oral medications with a regular syringe with the needle removed. They may also transfer the medication to a medicine cup or a nipple.

| | |
|---|---|
| **Clinical Relevance** | ➤ Oral syringes are not to be used for injections. Do not confuse oral syringes with parenteral syringes. Oral syringes have milliliter calibrations and may have teaspoon or tablespoon marks as well. Their tips do not fit needles. They are *not sterile*. Errors have been caused by jamming needles onto oral syringes. The needles do not fit properly and can fall off during "injection." |

## Prefilled Injectable Syringes

Prefilled injectable syringes contain a single-dose of medication. They have a needle attached and are disposable (Figure 6-13). If the order calls for less than the supplied amount, the nurse adjusts the dose by discarding unneeded amounts into

Figure 6-13. Prefilled syringes. **A,** 10-mL Emergency Syringe (Lifeshield® Ansyr®) containing 10% calcium chloride. **B,** Prefilled Hepatitis B Vaccine (Recombinant) Engerix-B 20 mcg/mL syringe. (**A** from Hospira Inc., Lake Forest, IL; **B** from Macklin D, Chernecky C, Infortuna H: Math for clinical practice, ed. 1, St. Louis, 2005, Mosby.)

a sink before administration. Check agency protocols for discard of controlled substances.

➤ Many prefilled syringe medications look similar. The nurse must check all the information on the syringe to avoid giving the wrong medicine or dose.

## Prefilled Medication Cartridges for Injection

Injectables may be supplied in a cartridge with an attached needle. The cartridge containing the medicine is to be locked in the plastic holder for injection of the medication (Figure 6-14).

Dexterity with this equipment requires *intermittent* practice sessions for insertion, locking, unlocking, and needle safety techniques (Figure 6-15). The cartridges usually have 0.1 or 0.2 mL extra medication in case of loss. The label and calibrations must be read and compared with the order *before* the cartridge is inserted. The cartridge can be rotated so that the calibrations are in view for adjusting the dose.

➤ Be especially careful to examine prefilled syringes and cartridge calibrations before administering them. Rotate the cartridge after placement in the holder so that the amounts and calibrations can be clearly seen (Figure 6-16).

Figure **6-14.** Carpuject cartridge and holder. (From Hospira, Inc., Lake Forest, IL.)

**A**

**B**

**C**

Figure **6-15. A,** Carpuject syringe and prefilled sterile cartridge with needle. **B,** Assembling the Carpuject. **C,** Cartridge locks at needle end. Plunger screws into opposite end. (From Potter PA, Perry AG: Fundamentals of nursing, ed. 6, St. Louis, 2005, Mosby.)

Figure 6-16. **A,** Cartridge and holder assembled. **B,** Prefilled sterile medication cartridge with calibrations. (From Macklin D, Chernecky C, Infortuna H: Math for clinical practice, ed. 1, St. Louis, 2005, Mosby.)

# Needle Sizes

*Needle size* refers to length and gauge. There are many options available (Figure 6-17). Supervised laboratory and clinical experience is needed to master needle size selection, dexterity, and safe handling.

Needle lengths are as follows:

- Intramuscular: 1 to 2 inches

- Subcutaneous: $\frac{3}{8}$ to $\frac{5}{8}$ inch

- Intradermal: $\frac{3}{8}$ to $\frac{1}{2}$ inch

Figure 6-17. Needles of various gauges and lengths. (In Lilley LL, Harrington S, Snyder JS: Pharmacology and the nursing process, ed. 4, St. Louis, 2005, Mosby. From Rick Brady, Riva, MD.)

| TABLE 6-1 | Usual Needle Sizes and Purposes |
| --- | --- |
| **Usual Needle Size*** | **Purpose** |
| 27-29 gauge | Intradermal skin tests, subcutaneous insulin administration |
| 25-27 gauge | Subcutaneous injections, heparin administration |
| 22 gauge | Spinal canal insertion |
| 20-23 gauge | Intramuscular injections |
| 16- 20 gauge | Intravenous injections |
| 18 gauge | Preferred for blood administration because blood is viscous |

*Check your agency supply and protocols. There are other sizes available.

## Basics of Needle Selection

Needle selection, length, and gauge depend on three criteria:

1  Purpose and route of the injection
2  Size and skin integrity of the patient
3  Viscosity of the solution

Intramuscular injections require longer needles than do intradermal and sub-cutaneous injections. Irritating substances are not injected into *subcutaneous* tissue because they are not absorbed as quickly into the circulation. The muscle would be a better alternative for such a substance because it has a better circulation supply. A larger-than-average adult requires a longer needle than does a frail adult or a child. The shortest needles are reserved for intradermal use. See Table 6-1 for usual needle sizes and their purposes. In addition to altering needle size, the angle of injection is altered for different-sized patients. This is learned in supervised clinical practice.

> ☀ **Mnemonic**
>
> LL: **L**ower gauge number, **L**arger needle.

1  If you were going to have an intramuscular injection, which gauge would you prefer for the injection, provided your body size was appropriate for any of them: 20, 21, 22, or 23?

> Q: *Ask Yourself*
>
> A: *My Answer*

_____

2  If a solution is viscous, might you need a lower or higher gauge needle?

_____

## Safety Syringes

> ➤ The greatest risks for needle-stick injury are during the handling and disposal of used needles *after* injection. Risks of needle-stick injury include transmission of blood-borne pathogens such as hepatitis B and C and AIDS.

**Clinical Relevance**

There is a trend to provide prepared medicines and needles with safety features to prevent needle-stick injuries. Many syringes are supplied with a variety of sheaths and sliding or retracting devices to cover the needle as soon as it is withdrawn from the patient to prevent needle-stick injuries. See Figures 6-18 and 6-19 for examples.

Figure 6-18. **A,** BD Safety-Lok™ 3-mL syringe. **B,** BD SafetyGlide™ tuberculin syringe. **C,** BD Monovial™ IV. (Used with permission from Becton, Dickinson, and Company, copyright 2003.)

Figure 6-19. Needle with plastic guard to prevent needle-sticks. **A,** Position of guard before injection. **B,** After injection, the guard locks in place, covering the needle. (From Potter PA, Perry AG: Fundamentals of nursing, ed. 6, St. Louis, 2005, Mosby.)

## Safety Issues and Disposal of Sharps

Used syringes and needles must be disposed *of immediately* in special hazardous waste sharps containers (Figure 6-20).

| **Clinical Relevance** | Do not recap used needles. |
| --- | --- |
| | Beware of needles projecting from overfilled containers. |
| | Beware of human traffic when crossing a room or exiting a curtained area with an exposed contaminated needle. The needle needs to be pointed away from the carrier and toward the floor (not angled toward the ceiling). |
| | Sharps containers need to be replaced when they are $\frac{2}{3}$ full. |
| | Do not attempt to push a syringe into a filled sharps container. Your hand may be stuck by an upright needle in the container. |
| | Be very careful if a bedside treatment that included an injection (e.g., a spinal tap) has been performed. A used needle inadvertently dropped in the bedding poses a needle-stick risk. |

Figure **6-20.** Never recap a used needle! Always dispose of uncapped needles in the appropriate sharps container. (In Lilley LL, Harrington S, Snyder JS: Pharmacology and the nursing process, ed 4, 2005, Mosby. From Rick Brady, Riva, MD.)

➤ During orientation to any new clinical agency, nurses need to familiarize themselves with the types and uses of syringes and needles, the needleless equipment available, and the location of sharps disposal containers. Agency policies pertaining to handling of the equipment must also be checked.

**Clinical Relevance**

## RAPID PRACTICE 6-7 Reading Syringe Volumes

**Estimated completion time: 10 minutes**   Answers on page **540**

**Directions:** *Examine the calibrations of the syringes pictured to answer the questions. Follow these three steps to rapidly interpret syringe calibrations:*

• Identify the total capacity.

• Note the volume and number of calibrations between two adjacent dark lines.

• Calculate the smallest measurable dose (specific volume ÷ number of calibrations).

1

    **a.** Total volume of this syringe: _____

    **b.** Number of calibrations between 0 and 1 mL: _____

    **c.** Value of each calibration (smallest measurable dose): _____

    **d.** What is the amount marked on the syringe? _____

2

**a.** Total volume of this syringe: _____

**b.** Number of calibrations between 0 and 0.1 mL: _____

**c.** The value of each calibration (smallest measurable dose): _____

**d.** What is the amount marked on the syringe? _____

3

**a.** Total volume of this syringe: _____

**b.** Number of calibrations between 0 and 1 mL: _____

**c.** The value of each calibration (smallest measurable dose): _____

**d.** What is the amount marked on the syringe? _____

4

**a.** Total volume of this syringe: _____

**b.** Number of calibrations between 0 and 1 mL: _____

**c.** The value of each calibration (smallest measurable dose): _____

**d.** What is the amount marked on the syringe? _____

5

**a.** Total volume of this syringe. _____

**b.** Number of calibrations between 0 and 1 mL. _____

**c.** The value of each calibration (smallest measurable dose) _____

**d.** What is the amount marked on the syringe? _____

**RAPID PRACTICE 6-8** Measuring Syringe Volumes in 5- and 10-mL Syringes

**Estimated completion time: 5 minutes** Answers on page **540**

**Directions:** *Draw a vertical line through the calibrated line for the requested volume on each syringe.*

**1** 3.8 mL

**2** 4.2 mL

**3** 8.2 mL

**4** 4.6 mL

**5** 7.2 mL

## RAPID PRACTICE 6-9   1-mL Syringe Measurements

**Estimated completion time: 5-10 minutes**   Answers on page **541**

**Directions:** *Draw a vertical line through the calibrated line of each syringe for the dose to be given. The top ring of the plunger,* closest to the needle, *must rest on that calibrated line of the dose in milliliters when the medication is drawn into the syringe.*

**1** Draw a line through the 0.24-mL calibration.

**2** Draw a line through the 0.86-mL calibration.

**3** Draw a line through the 0.55-mL calibration.

**4** Draw a line through the 0.3-mL calibration.

**5** Shade in 0.1 mL, the volume used for most skin tests, such as that for tuberculosis

**RAPID PRACTICE 6-10** 3-mL Syringe Measurements

**Estimated completion time: 5-10 minutes**   Answers on page **542**

**Directions:** *Draw a vertical line through the calibrated line of each syringe for the dose to be given.*

**1** Draw a vertical line through the 1.4-mL calibration.

**2** Draw a vertical line through the 1.8-mL calibration.

**3** Draw a vertical line through the 0.6-mL calibration.

**4** Draw a vertical line through the 2.8-mL calibration.

**5** Draw a vertical line through the 0.7-mL calibration.

**RAPID PRACTICE 6-11** Syringe Measurement Review

**Estimated completion time: 15 minutes** Answers on page **542**

**Directions:** *Draw a vertical line or arrow through the calibrated line for the dose to be given.*

**1**

a. Total capacity of the syringe: _____

b. This syringe would be used for dose volumes greater than _____ mL.

c. Capacity of each calibration in milliliters: _____

d. Draw an arrow pointing to the 4.2-mL calibration.

**2**

a. Total capacity of the syringe: _____

b. Draw an arrow pointing to the 0.05-mL calibration.

c. Capacity of each calibration in milliliters: _____

d. Draw a vertical line intersecting the 0.1-mL calibration.

**3**

a. Total capacity of the syringe:

b. Draw a line through the 1-mL calibration.

c. Capacity of each calibration in milliliters: _____

d. Draw an arrow pointing to the 17-mL calibration.

**4**

a. Total capacity of the syringe: _____

b. Draw an arrow pointing to the 1 mL line.

c. Capacity of each calibration in milliliters: _____

d. Draw a vertical line intersecting the 7.2-mL calibration.

**5**

a. Total capacity of the syringe: _____

b. Draw lines at the 0.5- and the 1-mL lines.

c. Capacity of each calibration in milliliters. _____

d. Draw an arrow pointing to the 1.8-mL calibration.

---

**1**  When you read and check volumes on a syringe, why is it advisable to have the calibrations at eye level and eyeglasses on hand?

Q *Ask Yourself*

A *My Answer*

# Recommended Fluid Volume for Selected Sites

An excess of injected fluid volume into tissue is not absorbed within a reasonable amount of time, and it causes discomfort for the patient. The recommended fluid volumes for selected sites are as follows:

- 0.1 mL for intradermal skin tests
- 0.5-1 mL for subcutaneous injections at a single site
- Up to 3 mL for intramuscular injections at a single site
- 1-60 mL for intravenous injections

➤ Assuming the correct syringe is selected, the nurse rounds the number of milliliters of medication to the *nearest measurable dose* on the syringe. If the syringe is calibrated in *tenths* of a milliliter, the medication is prepared to the *nearest tenth*. If the syringe is calibrated in *hundredths* of a milliliter, the medication prepared to the *nearest hundredth*.

➤ Do *not* round up to whole numbers, such as from 0.8 to 1 mL or from 0.5 to 1 mL on a syringe. For a review of rounding instructions, see p. 20.

## CHAPTER 6 MULTIPLE-CHOICE REVIEW

**Estimated completion time: 10-15 minutes**    Answers on page **544**

**Directions:**  If necessary, *review the syringe measurements presented in this chapter. Then circle the correct syringe measurement for the information supplied.*

**1**  A 1-mL syringe is calibrated in which of the following increments?

   **1.** Hundredths of a milliliter        **3.** 0.2 mL
   **2.** Tenths of a milliliter            **4.** 1 mL

**2**  A 3-mL syringe is calibrated in which of the following increments?

   **1.** Hundredths of a milliliter        **3.** 0.2 mL
   **2.** Tenths of a milliliter            **4.** 1 mL

**3**  The most commonly used size of syringe for adult intramuscular injections is

   **1.** 1 mL                             **3.** 5 mL
   **2.** 3 mL                             **4.** 10 mL

**4**  The *syringe* size and amount used for skin tests is

   **1.** 1-mL size, 0.1-mL amount         **3.** 5-mL size, 0.2-mL amount
   **2.** 3-mL, size, 1-mL amount          **4.** 10-mL size, 1-mL amount

5  Which of the following is the major criterion in *syringe* selection?

    **1.** Volume of medication to be given

    **2.** Route of administration specified by prescriber

    **3.** Trade and generic names of the drug

    **4.** Size of the patient in lb or kg

6  When do most needlestick injuries occur?

    **1.** During medication preparation     **3.** After medication administration

    **2.** During medication administration     **4.** When the patient self-administers

7  Which of the following are the main criteria for selection of needle size?

    **1.** Medication viscosity, medication route, size of patient, and skin condition of patient

    **2.** Volume of fluid to be administered and number of milligrams of medication to be administered

    **3.** Frequency of medication administration

    **4.** Gauge and length of needle

8  Which of the following statements pertaining to needle gauge is true?

    **1.** The highest-gauge needles have the smallest diameters.

    **2.** An 18-gauge needle is narrower than a 23-gauge needle.

    **3.** The needles with the smallest gauges are used for intradermal skin tests.

    **4.** The needles with the largest gauges are used for intramuscular tests.

9  If the dose ordered is 2.54 mL, to be administered with a 3-mL syringe, how many milliliters should the nurse administer?

    **1.** 2.5 mL                  **3.** 2.6 mL

    **2.** 2.54 mL              **4.** 3 mL

10  If the dose ordered is 0.88 mL, to be administered with a 1-mL syringe, how many milliliters should the nurse administer?

    **1.** 0.8 mL                  **3.** 0.88 mL

    **2.** 0.85 mL              **4.** 0.9 mL

## CHAPTER 6 FINAL PRACTICE

**Estimated completion time: 1 hour**    Answers on page **544**

**Directions:** *Estimate and calculate the dose using mental arithmetic and DA verification when requested. Evaluate the answer. Does the estimate support the answer? Draw a vertical line through the calibrated line of each syringe to indicate the dose to be given.*

1  Ordered: 200 mg of Drug X. Available: 100 mg/ mL.

    **a.** Estimated dose: Will you need to give *more or less* than the unit mL dose available? (Circle one.)

    **b.** How many mL will you give? (Use mental arithmetic.) _____

    **c.** Evaluation: _____

Draw a vertical line through the nearest measurable amount on the 3-mL syringe shown.

**2** Ordered: 15 mg of Drug X. Available: 30 mg/ mL.

    **a.** Estimated dose: Will you need to give *more or less* than the unit mL dose available? (Circle one.)

    **b.** How many mL will you give? (Use mental arithmetic.) _____

    **c.** Evaluation: _____

Draw a vertical line through the nearest measurable amount on the 3-mL syringe shown.

**3** Ordered: 320 mg of Drug X. Available: 50 mg/ mL.

    **a.** Estimated dose: Will you need to give *more or less* than the unit mL dose available? (Circle one.)

    **b.** How many mL will you give?

    DA equation:

    **c.** Evaluation: _____

Draw a vertical line through the nearest measurable amount on the 10-mL syringe shown.

**4** Ordered: 80 mg of Drug X. Available: 75 mg/ mL.

    **a.** Estimated dose: Will you need to give *more or less* than the unit mL dose available? (Circle one.)

    **b.** How many mL will you give?

    DA equation:

    **c.** Evaluation: _____

Draw a vertical line through the nearest measurable amount on the 3-mL syringe shown.

5 Ordered: 50 mg of Drug X. Available: 10 mg/ mL.

   **a.** Estimated dose: Will you need to give *more or less* than the unit mL dose available? (Circle one.)

   **b.** How many mL will you give? (Use mental arithmetic.) _____

   **c.** Evaluation: _____

Draw a vertical line through the nearest measurable amount on the 5-mL syringe shown.

6 Ordered: 40 mg of Drug X. Available 50 mg/ mL.

   **a.** Examine the ordered dose and the dose available. Estimate your dose calculation. Will you need to give *more or less* than the unit mL dose available? (Circle one.)

   **b.** How many mL will you give?

   DA equation:

   **c.** Evaluation: _____

Draw a vertical line through the nearest measurable amount on the 3-mL syringe shown.

7 Ordered: 120 mg of Drug X. Available: 100 mg/ mL.

   **a.** Examine the ordered dose and the dose available. Estimate your dose calculation. Will you need to give *more or less* than the unit mL dose available? (Circle one.)

   **b.** How many mL will you give?

   DA equation:

   **c.** Evaluation: _____

Draw a vertical line through the nearest measurable amount on the 3-mL syringe shown.

8  Ordered: 15 mg of Drug X. Available: 100 mg/ mL.

   **a.** Examine the ordered dose and the dose available. Estimate your dose calculation. Will you need to give *more or less* than the unit mL dose available? (Circle one.)

   **b.** How many mL will you give for the nearest measurable dose on the syringe provided?

   DA equation:

   **c.** Evaluation: _____

   Draw a vertical line through the nearest measurable amount on the 1-mL syringe provided.

9  **a.** What is the most important criterion for syringe selection in relation to the ordered dose? _____

   **b.** Should you select the syringe *before* or *after* calculating the dose volume in mL?

   _____

10 **a.** List two special precautions that must be taken when disposing of used and/or contaminated needles? _____

   _____

   **b.** Name two diseases mentioned in the chapter that can be acquired through needle-stick injuries. _____

## Suggestions for Further Reading

Perry AG, Potter PA: Clinical nursing skills and techniques, ed. 5, St. Louis, 2004, Mosby.
www.bd.com
www.cdc.gov/niosh/2000-108.html
www.fda.gov/cder/drug/MedErrors
www.ismp.org
www.usp.org/patientSafety

 Additional information can be found in the Safety in Medication Administration section on the enclosed companion CD.

Chapter 7 covers the calculations for reconstitution of powder and liquid medications. Syringes are often used to reconstitute medications. DA equations will be needed to calculate a variety of doses.

*"Each problem that I solved became a rule which served afterwards to solve other problems."*

—RENÉ DESCARTES

# RECONSTITUTION OF POWDERS AND LIQUIDS

## Objectives

- Distinguish routes of drugs for reconstitution.
- Interpret directions for dilution of reconstituted medications.
- Select the appropriate concentration to prepare for the ordered dose.
- Calculate doses for reconstituted medications using DA equations.
- Measure the appropriate dose using a medicine cup and a syringe.
- Identify appropriate notation on reconstituted multidose medication labels.
- Interpret directions for safe storage of reconstituted medications.
- Calculate ratio dilutions for partial-strength solutions.

## Essential Prior Knowledge

Mastery of Chapters 1-6

## Equipment

- The mathematics can be mastered without equipment, but eventually supervised clinical laboratory experience with vials, syringes, and powders will be necessary.

## Estimated Time To Complete Chapter

- 1-2 hours

## Introduction

Campers who have reconstituted dried food and care-givers who have mixed powdered baby formula with water to prepare a bottle have applied the technique of reconstitution of dry products. Some medications are supplied in the form of powders or crystals to which a liquid must be added for reconstitution shortly before use.

The medications are supplied in dry form because the product can be stored for a long time in dry form but becomes unstable and deteriorates in solution within a relatively short time. Such solutions are said to have a "short shelf life." The equipment used to reconstitute medications must be calibrated for the medicines being dispensed. The capacity of syringes, medicine droppers, and "medication teaspoons" is precise, while that of household equipment varies greatly from spoon to spoon and cup to cup.

224

## ESSENTIAL Vocabulary

| | |
|---|---|
| **Diluent** | Fluid that makes a mixture less concentrated or viscous. The fluid dilutes the mixture. It is also used to convert a dry form of a substance to a liquid form. For example, water is used to liquefy a dry form of baby formula. When reconstituting medications, read the directions to find out which diluent needs to be used. Water or normal saline (NS) solution is often used to dilute medicines and to liquefy dry, powdered forms of medicines. |
| **Dilution** | Extent to which the concentration of a mixture is reduced. |
| **Dilution Ratio** | Special ratio indicating the number of parts of an active ingredient to the number of parts of inactive ingredients in a solution. For example, a 1:4 dilution ratio means that, out of 5 total parts, 1 part is active and 4 parts are inactive. Adding 4 parts water to 1 part powdered milk would provide a dilution ratio of 1:4. |
| **Displacement** | Process that increases the volume of a fluid when a liquid is added to another liquid or a solid, such as a powder. |
| **Reconstitution** | Process of combining the dry form of a mixture with a fluid to achieve a usable state. Process of diluting a liquid concentrate to achieve a usable state. |
| **Solution Concentration (Strength)** | Amount of drug in a quantity of solution expressed as a ratio (e.g., 100 mg/ 100 mL, or 1:1) or as a fraction or a percentage (e.g., $\frac{1}{2}$ strength, or 50% solution). |
| **Suspension** | Liquid in which fine particles are dispersed throughout a fluid, where they are supported by the buoyancy of shaking or stirring. If a suspension is left standing, the solid particles settle. Antibiotics are often supplied as oral suspensions. |
| **SW** | Sterile water. |
| **Bacteriostatic SW** | Sterile water with an antimicrobial agent, such as benzyl alcohol. |
| | Sterile water and bacteriostatic sterile water cannot be used interchangeably with each other or with tap water. The product label specifies the diluent. |
| **Unit** | Standardized laboratory measure of the therapeutic strength, as opposed to the weight or volume, of a drug. Often used as a standard of measure for medications that are derived from plants and animals and that have components with variable strengths. Substances, such as hormones and penicillin, that are partially derived from animal and plant sources are easily broken down to an unstable state of diminished effectiveness. The term *units* is also used to describe metric units of measurement. |
| **Unstable** | Easily broken down to a state of diminished effectiveness. Breakdown can occur rapidly with reconstituted solutions. Foods, solutions, and certain medications that are unstable, such as reconstituted medications, have a short shelf life. They must be discarded if they are not used in a timely fashion. |

## RAPID PRACTICE 7-1 Vocabulary Review

**Estimated completion time: 5 minutes**   **Answers on page 547**

**Directions:** *Circle the correct definition for the following.*

1  The amount of drug in a quantity of solution expressed as a ratio is called

    **1.** An emulsion             **3.** A suspension

    **2.** The concentration       **4.** A diluent

2  The solution used to reconstitute powders and crystals from a dry form of medicine to a liquid form is called

    **1.** An emulsion             **3.** A suspension

    **2.** An elixir               **4.** A diluent

3 Solutions that deteriorate rapidly in liquid form are considered to have a short shelf life and are described as:

1. Crystals
2. Unstable

3. Bacteriostatic
4. Diluents

4 The process of combining a liquid with a solid form of medication so that the medication can be used is called

1. Reconstitution
2. Dilution

3. Calibration
4. Concentration

5 Accurate measurement of liquid medications requires which type of equipment?

1. Household teaspoons and tablespoons
2. Metric equipment with calibrations
3. Household droppers and cups
4. A syringe and needle

# Reconstituted Medications

Some medicines are very unstable in liquid form. Therefore, they are supplied in a dry form to which an inactive diluent is added just before use. The information about the specific type and amount of diluent to be added to achieve specific concentrations is provided on the label. The nurse selects the amount of diluent that will provide the concentration closest to the dose ordered.

## Interpreting Orders and Reading Labels for Reconstituted Medications

Examine the following order: Augmentin suspension 125 mg tid PO × 5 days. The order includes the form, oral *suspension,* but does *not* mention that the drug requires reconstitution or describe how to prepare it. The nurse must read the medication label and insert to determine how to prepare the medication.

**Reading Labels** Directions on the label state the precise amount and type of liquid diluent to add in order to achieve specific dilutions or concentrations of the drug per milliliter. The directions always state conditions and time limits for storage after reconstitution to liquid form. Some products must be discarded immediately, while others may be refrigerated for several hours so that they can be used for additional doses.

There is a lot of information on the label, but most of it is self-explanatory once you have read one or two types of labels. Examine the directions on the following label for an oral suspension to be reconstituted:

➤ The route is oral. This is important to note because there are injectable antibiotics and other drugs with similar names made specifically for intramuscular or intravenous routes.

➤ The type of *diluent* is water. Most oral suspension diluents use tap water unless otherwise specified. Pediatric patients and immunocompromised patients may need SW.

➤ The total *amount of diluent* to be added is 90 mL, added in two parts: 60 mL for the first mix and 30 mL for the second. If you have ever made pan gravy, the same principle applies: you do not add all the water at once because it is harder to get the lumps out.

➤ After reconstitution, the drug *concentration* will be 125 mg/ 5 mL water. The total amount of medication will be 100 mL, although only 90 mL of water was added. This discrepancy is due to displacement of liquid by the powder. Both ingredients occupy space. Discard after 10 days.

| | |
|---|---|
| It is critical to communicate the date and time of preparation and the specific concentration of reconstituted solutions to nursing staff on subsequent shifts with a *clearly marked added label*. | **Clinical Relevance** |

## Marking the Label for Reconstituted Medications

The label is marked by the nurse only under the following conditions:

**1** The drug label states that the medication may be used more than once after reconstitution.

**2** The patient is eligible to receive another dose before the drug must be discarded.

➤ The label for reconstituted medications must contain the patient's name, the date and time of preparation, the diluent type and amount added, the concentration per milliliter after dilution, and the nurse's initials or name, according to agency policy. Discard date and time are added according to agency policy.

| | |
|---|---|
| Note the following example:<br>RECONSTITUTED AUGMENTIN ORAL SUSPENSION BOTTLE<br>Patient: John B. Doe<br>01/05/06 1800: 90 mL SW added; 125 mg/ 5 mL, jm, RN<br>Discard date and time*:<br>_____<br>*Check institutional policies for specific agency requirements, especially discard date requirements. Some agencies require that the nurse add the discard date and *time* for the prepared reconstituted drug to the label. Other agencies prefer that the expiration or discard date and time be redetermined from the reconstitution date and label directions by *each* nurse administering the medication. | **EXAMPLES** |

| | |
|---|---|
| ➤ Reconstituted medications for multidose use are the one exception to the rule, "Never give a medication prepared by someone else."<br>➤ The exception may be made only if the label is clearly marked with all the required data.<br>➤ Reconstituted medications with labels that are not annotated with all the required data must be discarded to avoid giving an ineffective drug or a spoiled liquid. | **Clinical Relevance** |

## Expired Reconstituted Drugs

Single-dose preparations cannot be stored. They must be discarded if they are not used by the expiration date and time. Only multidose preparations may be stored according to label directions and hospital policy.

| Clinical Relevance | Because of the cost and short shelf life of reconstituted medications, it is appropriate that the nurse review the patient's records and recent orders to be sure that the medication order has not expired before preparing the medication. |
|---|---|

**RAPID PRACTICE 7-2**  Interpreting Labels for Reconstituted Medications

**Estimated completion time: 25 minutes**   Answers on page 547

**Directions:** *Read the labels for the medications to be reconstituted, and fill in the spaces with the required information for preparation and storage. Use brief phrases.*

1

**TO PATIENT:**
Shake well before using.
Keep tightly closed. Store in refrigerator and discard unused portion after ten days. Oversize bottle provides shake space.
**TO THE PHARMACIST:**
When prepared as directed, each 5 mL teaspoonful contains erythromycin ethylsuccinate equivalent to 200 mg of erythromycin in a cherry-flavored suspension.
Bottle contains erythromycin ethylsuccinate equivalent to 8 g of erythromycin.
**Usual Dose:** See package outsert.
Store at room temperature in dry form.
Child-Resistant closure not required; Reference: Federal Register Vol.39 No.29.
**DIRECTIONS FOR PREPARATION:** Slowly add 140 mL of water and shake vigorously to make 200 mL of suspension.
**BARR LABORATORIES, INC.**
Pomona, NY 10970
R11-90

BARR LABORATORIES, INC.

**Erythromycin Ethylsuccinate**
for Oral Suspension, USP

**200 mg of erythromycin activity per 5 mL reconstituted**

Caution: Federal law prohibits dispensing without prescription.

**200 mL** (when mixed)

NDC 0555-0215-23
NSN 6505-00-080-0653

0555-0215-23  3

SAMPLE

Exp. Date:
Lot No.:

a. Form and route of medication: _____

b. Type of diluent to be used: _____

c. Amount of diluent to add to bottle: _____

d. Mixing directions: _____

e. Unit dose concentration after reconstitution: _____

f. Unit dose or multidose container: _____

g. Total volume in container after reconstitution: _____

h. Number of unit doses in container after reconstitution: _____

i. Storage location in dry form: _____

j. Storage location after reconstituted: _____

k. Expiration, or discard, time after reconstitution: _____

2

**AMOXIL®**
125mg/5mL

**Directions for mixing:** Tap bottle until all powder flows freely. Add approximately 1/3 total amount of water for reconstitution (total=78 mL); shake vigorously to wet powder. Add remaining water; again shake vigorously. Each 5 mL (1 teaspoonful) will contain amoxicillin trihydrate equivalent to 125 mg amoxicillin.
**Usual Adult Dosage:** 250 to 500 mg every 8 hours.
**Usual Child Dosage:** 20 to 40 mg/kg/day in divided doses every 8 hours, depending on age, weight and infection severity. See accompanying prescribing information.

*Keep tightly closed.
Shake well before using.
Refrigeration preferable but not required.
Discard suspension after 14 days.*

**125mg/5mL**
NDC 0029-6008-23

**AMOXIL®**
AMOXICILLIN
FOR ORAL
SUSPENSION

**100mL**
(when reconstituted)

**SB** SmithKline Beecham

NSN 6505-01-153-3862
**Net contents:** Equivalent to 2.5 grams amoxicillin.
Store dry powder at room temperature.
**Caution:** Federal law prohibits dispensing without prescription.
**SmithKline Beecham Pharmaceuticals**
Philadelphia, PA 19101

3  0029-6008-23  1

LOT
EXP.
9405793-E

a. Form and route of medication: _____

b. Type of diluent to be used: _____

c. Total amount of diluent to add to bottle: _____

**d.** Mixing directions: _____

**e.** Unit dose concentration after reconstitution: _____

**f.** Usual adult dose: _____

**g.** Usual child dose: _____

**h.** Unit dose or multidose container: _____

**i.** Expiration, or discard time, after reconstitution: _____

If a slash (/) is used on a drug label or in a drug order, be careful to avoid reading it as the number 1.

Compare and contrast the contents and directions in the label in problem 1 with those in the label in problem 2. It is easy to see why the labels must be scrutinized. The information on both labels is easy to follow but very different in content.

3

**a.** Form and route of medication: _____

**b.** Type and amount of diluent to be used: _____

**c.** Total volume in container after reconstitution: _____

**d.** Unit dose concentration after reconstitution: _____

**e.** Storage directions: _____

**f.** Mixing directions after reconstitution: _____

**g.** Discard directions: _____

Note that the labels in problems 2 and 3 are for the same medication but contain different unit dose concentrations per 5 mL (1 medication teaspoon). Remember to use special calibrated medication teaspoons and/or droppers if those implements are needed. Use a syringe without a needle for measurement if the implements are not provided.

4

| PREPARATION OF CLAFORAN STERILE | | | |
|---|---|---|---|

Claforan for IM or IV administration should be reconstituted as follows:

| Strength | Diluent (mL) | Withdrawable Volume (mL) | Approximate Concentration (mg/mL) |
|---|---|---|---|
| 1g vial (IM)* | 3 | 3.4 | 300 |
| 2g vial (IM)* | 5 | 6.0 | 330 |
| 1g vial (IV)* | 10 | 10.4 | 95 |
| 2g vial (IV)* | 10 | 11.0 | 180 |
| 1g infusion | 50-100 | 50-100 | 20-10 |
| 2g infusion | 50-100 | 50-100 | 40-20 |
| 10g bottle | 47 | 52.0 | 200 |
| 10g bottle | 97 | 102.0 | 100 |

*in conventional vials

Shake to dissolve; inspect for particulate matter and discoloration prior to use. Solutions of Claforan range from very pale yellow to light amber, depending on concentration, diluent used, and length and condition of storage.

This label is included to illustrate medications that need to be reconstituted for routes other than oral and that offer *multiple options for dilution*. If the label permits several choices of dilution in order to obtain different unit dose strengths, the nurse must take special care to focus on the appropriate dilution. Several choices of dilution are more likely to be found with reconstituted parenteral drugs.

**a.** What are the amounts of diluent recommended for the 1 gram reconstituted intramuscular preparation and for the 1 gram intravenous preparation? _____

**b.** What will be the concentration of the 1 gram reconstituted intramuscular preparation and the 1 gram intravenous preparation? _____
_____

If you require reading glasses, keep them handy for reading the reconstitution directions.

5

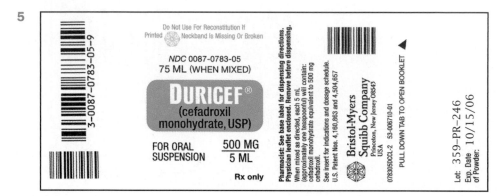

**a.** Trade name: _____
**b.** Generic name: _____
**c.** Form and route: _____
**d.** Unit dose concentration after reconstitution: _____
**e.** Lot number: _____
**f.** Expiration date (in dry form): _____

Many antibiotics come in both oral and injectable forms as noted on the labels.

## RAPID PRACTICE 7-3 Reconstituting, Calculating, and Measuring Doses

**Estimated completion time: 30 minutes**   Answers on page **548**

**Directions:** *Read the order and the label, estimate the dose, calculate the nearest measurable dose for a 3-mL syringe using a DA equation, and evaluate the answer.*

**1** Ordered: cefaclor for oral susp 0.3 g PO bid for a patient with sinusitis.

**a.** Amount and type of diluent to be added: _____

**b.** Estimate: *more than* or *less than* unit dose after reconstitution? (Circle one.)

**c.** How many milliliters will you prepare? _____

DA verification:

**d.** Evaluation: _____

Shade in the dose in mL on the medicine cup and draw a vertical line through the calibrated line of the syringe as applicable.*

---

*\*Throughout,* shade in the medicine cup in multiples of 5 mL as applicable; place the balance of the dose in the syringe.

**2** Ordered: Augmentin oral susp 0.25 g q8h PO for a patient with otitis media.

**a.** Amount and type of diluent to be added: _____

**b.** Estimate: *more than* or *less than* unit dose after reconstitution? (Circle one.)

**c.** How many milliliters will you prepare? _____

DA verification:

**d.** Evaluation: _____

Shade in the dose in mL on the medicine cup and draw a vertical line through the calibrated line of the syringe as applicable.

**3** Ordered: amoxicillin oral susp 0.2 g PO q8h for a patient with an infection.

**a.** Estimate: *more than* or *less than* unit dose after reconstitution? (Circle one.)

**b.** How many milliliters will you prepare? _____

DA verification:

**c.** Evaluation: _____

Shade in the dose in mL on the medicine cup and draw a vertical line through the calibrated line of the syringe as applicable.

**4** Ordered: fluconazole oral susp 0.03 g PO daily for a patient with oral candidiasis.

**a.** Amount and type of diluent to be added: _____

**b.** Estimate: *more than* or *less than* unit dose after reconstitution? (Circle one.)

**c.** How many milliliters will you prepare? _____

　　DA verification:

**d.** Evaluation: _____

Draw a vertical line through the calibrated line of the syringe as applicable.

**5** Ordered: penicillin V potassium for oral sol 75 mg PO tid for a patient with an infection.

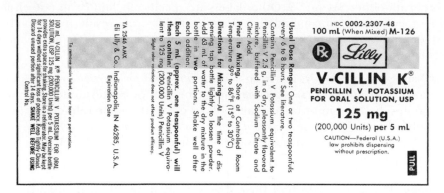

**a.** Amount and type of diluent to be added: _____

**b.** Estimate: *more than* or *less than* unit dose after reconstitution? (Circle one.)

**c.** How many milliliters will you prepare? _____

    DA verification:


**d.** Evaluation: _____

Shade in the dose in mL on the medicine cup and draw a vertical line through the calibrated line of the syringe as applicable.

# Reconstituted Parenteral Drugs

➤ Parenteral medications must be sterile and have a much shorter shelf life than do drugs administered by other routes.

## Diluents

Whereas tap water may be used for oral reconstituted medications, sterile diluents must be used for parenteral medications.

Sterile water *for injection* and sterile NS solution are the most commonly used diluents. Occasionally, custom diluents or dextrose solutions are required. Some labels permit either SW or NS. Other labels are specifically limited to one choice of diluent because of incompatibility. Incompatibility can result in crystallization and/or clumping of the drug in solution and can cause a problem in the tissue or circulation of the patient.

➤ Distinguish *SW for injection* from *bacteriostatic water for injection* on diluent directions. The latter contains a *preservative*. One cannot be substituted for the other. The label must be read and followed exactly. Some references use the abbreviation *SW* for *sterile water for injection* and *NS* for *sterile normal saline solution for injection*. Bacteriostatic water is spelled out in the dilution directions on the label.

**Selecting the Appropriate Unit Dose Concentration based on Dilution Directions When More Than One Dilution Is Offered** If a 1:100 concentration of sugar water was needed for your hummingbird feeder and you had on hand a 1:30 solution, a 1:50 solution, and a 1:100 solution, you would select the more dilute 1:100 concentration for the feeder. Giving the more concentrated solutions would overdose the hummingbirds with sugar. Similarly, with medications the nurse prepares the strength that provides the dose needed and the most convenient volume for the route ordered.

In selecting the appropriate amount of diluent, the nurse considers the relevant factors in the following sequence when reading the label:

- Route ordered
- Dose ordered and amount needed
- Drug concentrations and volumes available that are close in amount to the ordered dose for that route

Based on the ordered amount, the nurse examines the label to make critical decisions. For example, consider an order of Drug X 200 mg IM. The label dilution directions state:

**For IM injection,**
Add 1.8 mL SW for injection to obtain 200 mg/ mL.
Add 3.6 mL SW for injection to obtain 100 mg/ mL.
Add 5.2 mL SW for injection to obtain 75 mg/ mL.
**For IV injection,**
Add 8.4 mL SW for injection to obtain 50 mg/ mL.

According to the label, three concentrations are safe to inject into the muscle. The nurse chooses a concentration based on the order. In this example, one intramuscular option allows the patient to receive the smaller injected *volume* of 200 mg/ mL.

**Q:** *Ask Yourself*

**A:** *My Answer*

1 Which is the more concentrated solution after reconstitution according to the reconstitution directions cited above for Drug X?

_____

2 Can I use SW, NS, and bacteriostatic water interchangeably to dilute medicines? (Refer to Essential Vocabulary.)

_____

**RAPID PRACTICE 7-4** Selecting Diluents to Calculate Doses

**Estimated completion time: 20-30 minutes** Answers on page **550**

**Directions:** *Examine the following reconstitution directions and the example in problem 1. Select the appropriate dilution for problems 2-5 using the reconstitution directions provided. Evaluate your equations for problems 3-5.*

**Reconstitution directions for Drug X for IM administration:**

| Diluent SW | Total Volume | Solution Concentration |
| --- | --- | --- |
| 1 mL | 1.4 mL | 480 mg/ mL |
| 2 mL | 3 mL | 250 mg/ mL |
| 4 mL | 5.8 mL | 100 mg/ mL |
| **For IV administration:** | | |
| 12 mL | 15.8 mL | 50 mg/ mL |

➤ The more diluent added, the weaker the concentration of the solution.

> ➤ Keep in mind that the average-sized adult should receive no more than 3 mL in one intramuscular site and that the nurse should select a dilution that permits at least 0.5 mL of intramuscular injection.
>
> **Clinical Relevance**

Select the dilution from the list above that is closest to the unit dose you need and that meets the foregoing criteria. Calculate doses to the *nearest tenth of a milliliter*. Examine the routes first. Then compare the order to the concentrations to find a reasonable low-volume dose. Verify the answer with a DA equation where requested.

1  Ordered: Drug X 50 mg IM.

   **a.** How much diluent will you add? 4 mL
   **b.** What will be the unit dose concentration? 100 mg/ mL
   **c.** How many milliliters will you give? 0.5 mL

2  Ordered: Drug X 0.1 g IM.

   **a.** How much diluent will you add? _____
   **b.** What will be the unit dose concentration? _____
   **c.** How many milliliters will you give? _____

3  Ordered: Drug X 0.25 g IM.

   **a.** How much diluent will you add? _____
   **b.** What will be the unit dose concentration? _____
   **c.** How many milliliters will you give? _____

4  Ordered: Drug X 0.3 g IM.

   **a.** How much diluent will you add? _____
   **b.** What will be the unit dose concentration? _____
   **c.** How many milliliters will you give? _____

   DA equation:

   **d.** Evaluation: _____

5  Ordered: Drug X 0.5 g IV.

   **a.** How much diluent will you add? _____
   **b.** What will be the unit dose concentration? _____
   **c.** How many milliliters will you give? _____

   DA equation:

   **d.** Evaluation: _____

**1**   If you were to receive 150 mg of an intramuscular injection and the directions for reconstitution of the medicine specified (a) add 20 mL to obtain 50 mg/ mL or (b) add 10 mL to obtain 100 mg/ mL, which concentration would you select for reconstitution?

# Reconstituted Drug Prefilled Containers

Some parenteral medications for reconstitution are supplied with diluents that are in prefilled syringe cartridges, ampules, or vials. Others are attached to the vial (Figure 7-1) and can be mixed by depressing the stopper without opening the vials. There is less chance for contamination of the contents when the ingredients are not exposed to air.

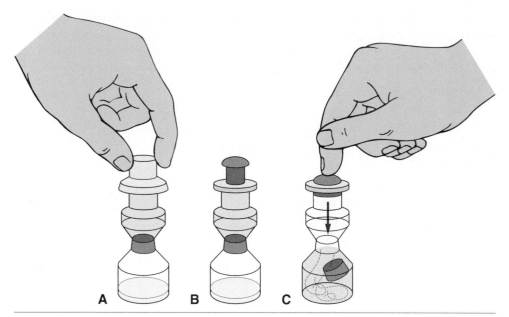

**A**   **B**   **C**

Figure **7-1.** Mix-o-vial. (From Clayton BD, Stock YN: Basic pharmacology for nurses, ed. 13, St. Louis, 2004, Mosby.)

## Reconstituting Injectable Medications Using Two Vials

Some reconstituted parenteral drugs are supplied in two vials: one with the dry drug and one with the diluent. Using sterile technique, both vials are cleaned with an alcohol swab. The amount in milliliters of diluent for the desired concentrate is withdrawn with a syringe and placed in the dry drug vial. The mixture is rotated until it is thoroughly mixed. This technique requires some clinical practice with the actual equipment. It is not complicated.

**RAPID PRACTICE 7-5**   Interpreting Directions and Calculating
Reconstituted Injectables

**Estimated completion time: 30 minutes**   Answers on page **550**

**Directions:** *Examine the worked-out problem 1. Read the labels to answer the questions for problems 2-5. Calculate doses to the nearest measurable dose on the syringe provided.*

**1** Ordered: ceftazidime 0.5 g IM, an antibiotic, for a patient with an infection.

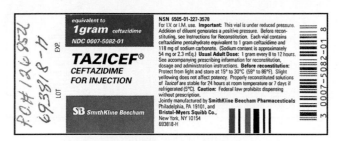

**RECONSTITUTION**

**Single Dose Vials:**
For I.M. injection, I.V. direct (bolus) injection, or I.V. infusion, reconstitute with Sterile Water for injection according to the following table. The vacuum may assist entry of the diluent. SHAKE WELL.

**Table 5**

| Vial Size | Diluent to Be Added | Approx. Avail. Volume | Approx. Avg. Concentration |
|---|---|---|---|
| **Intramuscular or Intravenous Direct (bolus) Injection** | | | |
| 1 gram | 3.0 ml. | 3.6 ml. | 280 mg./ml. |
| **Intravenous Infusion** | | | |
| 1 gram | 10 ml. | 10.6 ml. | 95 mg./ml. |
| 2 gram | 10 ml. | 11.2 ml. | 180 mg./ml. |

Withdraw the total volume of solution into the syringe (the pressure in the vial may aid withdrawal). The withdrawn solution may contain some bubbles of carbon dioxide.

**NOTE: As with the administration of all parenteral products, accumulated gases should be expressed from the syringe immediately before injection of 'Tazicef'.**

These solutions of 'Tazicef' are stable for 18 hours at room temperature or seven days if refrigerated (5°C.). Slight yellowing does not affect potency.

For I.V. infusion, dilute reconstituted solution in 50 to 100 ml. of one of the parenteral fluids listed under COMPATIBILITY AND STABILITY.

**a.** What kind of diluent is specified? <u>SW for injection</u>
**b.** How much diluent will you add? <u>3 mL</u>
**c.** What will the total volume in milliliters be after the diluent is added? <u>3.6 mL</u>
**d.** Unit dose concentration after dilution: <u>280 mg/ mL</u>
**e.** Is the dose ordered (after you move decimal places) (more) or *less* than the unit dose after dilution? <u>0.5 g = 500 mg, which is more than 280 mg</u>
**f.** Estimated dose in milliliters: <u>A little less than 2 mL</u>
**g.** Actual dose in milliliters calculated with a DA equation to the nearest measurable dose on a 3-mL syringe: _____

$$? \text{ mL} = \frac{\text{mL}}{\cancel{280 \text{ mg}}_{14}} \times \cancel{500 \text{ mg}}^{25} = \frac{25}{14} = 1.78 \text{ rounded to } 1.8 \text{ mL for the 3-mL syringe}$$

**h.** Evaluation: <u>Estimate supports answer. Equation is balanced.</u> If satisfactory, draw a vertical line through the calibrated line of the exact dose on the syringe.

**i.** How will you mark label? <u>Patient: John Doe, 2/01/06 1800, 3 mL sterile H₂O added, 280 mg/ mL, jm reeze, RN</u>
**j.** Storage and/or discard directions: <u>Stable 18 hours at room temperature or 7 days if refrigerated (5° C)</u>

2 Ordered: oxacillin 200 mg IM, an antibiotic, for a patient with an infection.

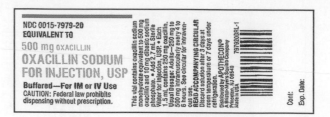

**a.** What kind of diluent or diluents are specified? _____

**b.** How much diluent will you add? _____

**c.** Unit dose concentration after dilution: _____

**d.** Estimated dose: Is the dose ordered (after you move decimal places) *more* or *less* than the unit dose after dilution? (Circle one.)

**e.** Actual dose in milliliters calculated with a DA equation to the nearest measurable dose on the syringe below:

DA equation:

**f.** Evaluation: _____

If satisfactory, draw a vertical line through the calibrated line of the exact dose on the syringe.

3 Ordered: Ancef 0.4 g IM, an antibiotic, for a patient with an infection

**a.** What kind of diluent or diluents are specified? _____

**b.** How much diluent will you add? _____

**c.** Unit dose concentration after dilution: _____

**d.** Estimated dose: Is the dose ordered (after you move decimal places) *more* or *less* than the unit dose after dilution? (Circle one.)

**e.** Actual dose in milliliters calculated with a DA equation to the nearest measurable dose on the syringe on p. 241.

DA equation:

**f.** Evaluation: _____

If satisfactory, draw a vertical line through the calibrated line of the exact dose on the syringe.

4 Ordered: cephapirin 0.5 g IM, an antibiotic, for a patient with an infection.

**a.** What kind of diluent or diluents are specified? _____

**b.** How much diluent will you add? _____

**c.** Unit dose concentration after dilution: _____

**d.** Estimated dose: Is the dose ordered (after you move decimal places) *more* or *less* than the unit dose after dilution? (Circle one.)

**e.** Estimated dose in milliliters? _____

**f.** Actual dose in milliliters calculated with a DA equation to the nearest measurable dose on the syringe below:

DA equation:



**g.** Evaluation: _____

If satisfactory, draw a vertical line through the calibrated line of the exact dose on the syringe.

**h.** Storage and/or discard directions: _____

5 Ordered: Geopen 0.8 g IM, an antibiotic, for a patient with an infection.

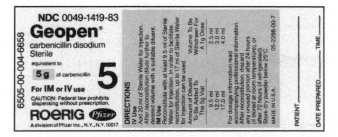

**a.** Total number of grams and milligrams in vial? _____

**b.** Using the 9.5 mL of diluent for the 5-g vial, what will the unit-dose concentration be? _____

**c.** Estimated dose: Is the dose ordered (after you move decimal places) *more* or *less* than the unit dose after dilution? (Circle one.)

**d.** Actual dose in milliliters to *nearest measurable dose* on the syringe on p. 242.

DA equation:

**e.** Evaluation: _____

If satisfactory, draw a vertical line through the calibrated line of the exact dose on syringe.

**f.** Storage and/or discard directions: _____

---

| Clinical Relevance | Many of the medications for reconstitution are antibiotics. They may be supplied in several forms and a variety of concentrations for oral, topical, intramuscular, or intravenous routes. Some have similar-sounding generic and trade names. Take care when comparing the order to the label. |
|---|---|

| Generic Name | Trade Name |
|---|---|
| cefaclor | Ceclor |
| cefprozil | Cefzil |
| cefuroxime | Ceftin |
| cephalexin | Keflex |
| cephazolin | Kefzol |
| ciprofloxacin | Cipro |
|  | Cipro XR |
| gatifloxacin | Tequin |
| gemifloxacin | Factive |
| sulfamethoxazole + trimethoprim | Bactrim DS |
|  | Septra DS |

**✳ Communication**

"Good morning, Mr. Smith. How are you today? Any changes since yesterday?" (Wait for an answer and respond.) "I have an antibiotic, Cefzil 500 mg for your infection. Have you had problems with antibiotics?"

| Clinical Relevance | Some patients are allergic to certain antibiotics and need a reminder. Assess lung sounds for wheezes and the skin for rashes, and ask the patient if there have been any bowel changes (e.g., diarrhea). These are the most common symptoms of allergic reactions. A skin rash may precede more serious symptoms. |
|---|---|

# Liquid Concentrates: Diluting Liquids

The pharmacy usually dilutes medication solutions to the ordered strength. Occasionally, the nurse will need to dilute a medication, nutritional beverage supplement, or irrigation solution based on a dilution ratio or percent concentration. Dilution is done to protect the patient from side effects of an overly strong concentration.

➤ Always look for dilution instructions when you see the word *concentrate* on a medication label. Failure to do so could result in serious injury to the patient.

Liquids administered through feeding tubes full strength may cause gastrointestinal distress. Solutions for irrigation treatments may need to be diluted to avoid tissue injury.

Orders may be written in one of three ways to indicate the strength or concentration of a solution:

| Order | Meaning |
|---|---|
| Percentage | *Percent* means "per 100." For example, *50% strength* denotes a solution that contains 50% active ingredient (the drug) plus 50% inactive ingredient (the diluent). |
| Fraction | For example, $\frac{1}{2}$ or "half strength" indicates that 1 part out of a total of 2 parts is the active ingredient and the other part is the inactive ingredient. The *denominator* of the fraction denotes the total number of parts. |
| Ratio | For example, 1:1 denotes 2 total parts: 1 part active ingredient *added to* 1 part inactive ingredient. The left number is the active ingredient, or the drug. The right number is the inactive ingredient, or the diluent. |

➤ Drug concentrations are expressed as ratios.

## Inactive Ingredients Used for Dilutions

Water or normal saline (NS) is often the *inactive* ingredient used for dilution. Check the order and label for the diluent. Sterile water may be indicated for wound irrigations, pediatric formulas, or immunocompromised patients. Normal saline solution is supplied as a sterile solution. Read the label and check agency protocols. Order the supplies from the pharmacy or central supply, according to agency guidelines.

Percent or fractional strengths are written more frequently for dilution than are ratios.

➤ The two sides of a ratio need to be added to obtain the total number of parts.
➤ The nurse must be able to interpret any of the three ways the order may be written.

The order may read as follows:

"Ensure $\frac{1}{2}$ strength, for 3 days PO,"
"Irrigate abdominal wound with 20% hydrogen peroxide ($H_2O_2$) and NS bid," or
"Baby formula 60 mL 1:3 sol q2h. If tolerated, increase to 1:2 sol tomorrow."

## Converting Dilution Ratios to Fractions and Percentages

➤ To convert a ratio to a fraction, add the *total number of parts* to create a *denominator*. Place the number of active-ingredient parts in the numerator.
➤ To convert a fraction to a percentage, multiply the fraction by 100 and add a percent sign.
➤ To convert a percentage to a fraction, divide the percentage by 100, remove the percent sign, and reduce the fraction.

**EXAMPLES**

1 Ordered: 120 mL q2h Ensure 50%. Preparation: 60 mL Ensure; 60 mL water to make a 1:1 ratio, $\frac{1}{2}$ strength, or 50% solution. 1:1 = 1 part active ingredient per, to, or plus 1 part inactive ingredient (ratio of Ensure to water). Total parts = 2 = $\frac{1}{2}$ strength = 50% solution ($\frac{1}{2} \times 100$).

2 Ordered: Irrigation with peroxide solution: 1:4. 1:4 = 1 part active ingredient (peroxide) per, to, or plus 4 parts inactive ingredient (water). Total parts = 5, $\frac{1}{5}$, or 20% solution. Use 1 part active ingredient, and add 4 parts diluent.

➤ Note that the dilution ratio 1:4 does not convert to the fraction $\frac{1}{4}$.
➤ Think of the dilution ratio 1:4 as 1 part added to 4 parts (1 + 4 =5 total parts).
➤ Read the fraction as 1 part out of 5 total parts, or $\frac{1}{5}$.
➤ Read 20% strength as 20 parts per 100 parts, or $\frac{1}{5}$.

Recall from Chapter 1, Essential Math Review, that the denominator of a fraction indicates the *number of total parts* and that *percent* means "per 100." Read $\frac{1}{5}$-strength concentration as 20%.

# Using a DA Equation to Calculate the Amount of Concentrate

Most dilution orders can be solved with mental arithmetic or simple arithmetic. The nurse needs to know the concentration and the total amount to be given in order to calculate the amount of active ingredients per the amount of inactive ingredients in milliliters.

➤ Simple DA-style equations are solved using fraction forms. Change the percentage in the order to a fraction.

---

**EXAMPLES**

Ordered: 120 mL of 25% formula per feeding tube q2h for 12 hours/ day. $25\% = \dfrac{25}{100} = \dfrac{1}{4}$. The desired answer is the amount in milliliters of the *active ingredient:*

| ? mL active ingredient = Total mL | × | fraction | = answer |
|---|---|---|---|
| 120 mL | × | $\dfrac{1}{4}$ | = 30 mL *active ingredient* |

120 mL total −30 mL active ingredient (NaCl) = 90 mL *diluent (SW)*

Evaluation: 30 is 25%, or $\dfrac{1}{4}$, of 120. 30 + 90 = 120 = 1:3 ratio. Both sides of the equation balance mathematically.

---

➤ When in doubt about dilutions, consult the agency pharmacist.

## RAPID PRACTICE 7-6 Interpreting Dilution Orders

**Estimated Completion Time: 25 minutes**  **Answers on page 552**

**Directions:** *Fill in the dilution tables from left to right with the correct equivalent terms and solution amounts, as shown in the first row of the table that follows.*

| | Fractional Strength | Ratio of Active to Inactive Ingredients | Percent | Order | Amount of Active Ingredient | Amount of Diluent (Inactive Ingredient) |
|---|---|---|---|---|---|---|
| 1 | $\dfrac{1}{4}$ | 1:3 | 25% | 100 mL q1h | 25 mL | 75 mL |
| 2 | | | 60% | 60 mL tid | | |
| 3 | | | 75% | 1000 mL q8h | | |
| 4 | | | 20% | 240 mL four times daily | | |
| 5 | | | 10% | 50 mL once a day | | |

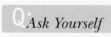

**Q** *Ask Yourself*

**A** *My Answer*

1  What is the difference between a dilution ratio and a fraction? How will I remember? Which one is easier (one less step) to convert to a percentage: the ratio or the fractional strength?

_____

## CHAPTER 7 MULTIPLE-CHOICE REVIEW

**Estimated completion time: 20-30 minutes**  **Answers on page 552**

**Directions:** *Circle the correct answer for the following.*

1  Which of the following statements defines *displacement?*

   **1.** Liquid oral medications are prepared using clean technique and nonsterile equipment.

**2.** The diluent for oral liquid medications is usually water.

**3.** The volume after reconstitution exceeds the amount of liquid diluent added.

**4.** Oral liquid medications are usually prepared to the nearest tenth of a milliliter for adults.

**2** Which of the following statements can lead to medication calculation errors?

**1.** Suspensions must be combined with a precise amount of diluent and thoroughly mixed.

**2.** Elixirs are solutions that contain alcohol.

**3.** Extracts are solutions that are concentrated.

**4.** It is acceptable to use household teaspoons and tablespoons to measure liquids.

**3** Plastic medication cups have the following milliliter calibrations:

**1.** Multiples of 5               **3.** Multiples of 15
**2.** Multiples of 10              **4.** Multiples of 30

**4** If a liquid medication order calls for 13 mL, how will the nurse prepare it?

**1.** Pour at eye level to just below the 15 mL line

**2.** Pour to 10 mL at eye level and add 3 mL with a needleless syringe.

**3.** Pour to 15 mL, remove 2 mL, and return the 2 mL to the medication bottle.

**4.** Draw 20 mL in a 20-mL syringe and discard 7 mL.

**5** If a liquid medication order calls for 7.5 mL, how will the nurse prepare it?

**1.** Pour at eye level to 5 mL and add 2.5 mL with a needleless syringe.

**2.** Pour to 10 mL, remove 2.5 mL, and return the 2.5 mL to the medication bottle.

**3.** Withdraw 7.5 mL in a 10-mL syringe and place it in the medication cup.

**4.** Give $1\frac{1}{2}$ medication teaspoonsful.

**6** One of the most important ways to eliminate errors in the dose calculations is to

**1.** Estimate the answer.

**2.** Pour oral medications to the nearest tenth of a milliliter.

**3.** Move decimal places to obtain equivalent measurements.

**4.** Check your calculations with another nurse.

**7** Which conversion is most commonly used in medication problems?

**1.** 2.2 lb = 1 kg              **3.** 1,000,000 mcg = 1 g
**2.** 1000 mg = 1 g             **4.** 1000 mL = 1 L

**8** The usual adult dose for oral liquid medications is measured to the

**1.** Nearest tenth of a milliliter       **3.** Nearest 0.5 mL
**2.** Nearest hundredth of a milliliter   **4.** Nearest whole milliliter

**9** What is the advantage of converting metric units by moving decimal places?

**1.** It reinforces multiples, base units, and powers of 10.

**2.** It simplifies the math and often permits mental calculation of the dose.

**3.** It eliminates the need to compare answers with estimates.

**4.** It eliminates the need to analyze the equation setup.

**10** An order calls for hydrogen peroxide 20% irrigation of 150 mL with NS diluent. The nurse prepares 150 mL of total irrigation. How many milliliters of hydrogen peroxide will be prepared?

**1.** 15                       **3.** 100
**2.** 30                       **4.** 120

**Estimated completion time: 1 hour**   **Answers on page 552**

**Directions:** *Examine the labels, change the units to equivalents by moving decimal places, estimate the answer, calculate the dose to the nearest tenth of a milliliter, and evaluate your answer. Then shade in the dose on the medicine cup and draw a vertical line through the calibrated line of each syringe for the dose to be given.*

1  Ordered: amoxicillin clavulanate potassium oral susp 0.3 g q8h.

This drug is a combination drug.

**a.** Estimated dose: _____

**b.** Calculated dose with equation to the nearest tenth of a milliliter:

   DA equation:



**c.** Evaluation: _____

Shade in the dose in mL on the medicine cup and draw a vertical line through the calibrated line of the syringe as applicable.

**2** Order: amoxicillin 0.2 g PO q8h.

**AMOXIL®**
**250mg/5mL**

**250mg/5mL**
NDC 0029-6009-21

**Directions for mixing:** Tap bottle until all powder flows freely. Add approximately 1/3 total amount of water for reconstitution (total=59 mL); shake vigorously to wet powder. Add remaining water; again shake vigorously. Each 5 mL (1 teaspoonful) will contain amoxicillin trihydrate equivalent to 250 mg amoxicillin.
**Usual Adult Dosage:** 250 to 500 mg every 8 hours.
**Usual Child Dosage:** 20 to 40 mg/kg/day in divided doses every 8 hours, depending on age, weight and infection severity. See accompanying prescribing information.

**Keep tightly closed.**
**Shake well before using.**
**Refrigeration preferable but not required.**
**Discard suspension after 14 days.**

**AMOXIL®**
AMOXICILLIN
FOR ORAL
SUSPENSION

**80mL** *(when reconstituted)*

**SB** SmithKline Beecham

NSN 6505-01-153-3442
**Net contents:** Equivalent to 4.0 grams amoxicillin.
Store dry powder at room temperature.
**Caution:** Federal law prohibits dispensing without prescription.
**SmithKline Beecham**
Pharmaceuticals
Philadelphia, PA 19101

3 0029-6009-21 4

LOT

EXP.

9405783-E

**a.** Estimated dose: _____

**b.** Calculated dose with equation to nearest tenth of a milliliter:

DA equation:

**c.** Evaluation: _____

Shade in the dose in mL on the medicine cup and draw a vertical line through the calibrated line of the syringe as applicable.

2 TBSP — 30 ML
— 25 ML
— 20 ML
1 TBSP — 15 ML
2 TSP — 10 ML
1 TSP — 5 ML
1/2 TSP —

**3** Ordered: Erythromycin ethylsuccinate susp 0.25 g PO q8h.

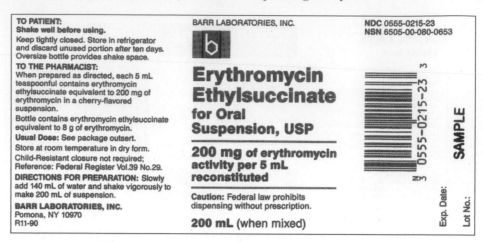

**a.** Estimated dose: _____

**b.** Calculated dose with equation to nearest tenth of a milliliter:

DA equation:

**c.** Evaluation: _____

Shade in the dose in mL on the medicine cup and draw a vertical line through the calibrated line of the syringe as applicable.

4 Ordered: cefaclor 0.2 g mg PO q8h.

**a.** Estimated dose: _____

**b.** Calculated dose with equation to nearest tenth of a milliliter:

DA equation:

**c.** Evaluation: _____

Shade in the dose in mL on the medicine cup and draw a vertical line through the calibrated line of the syringe as applicable.

**5** Ordered: clarithromycin oral susp 0.15 g. Note the form of this oral solid drug before reconstitution.

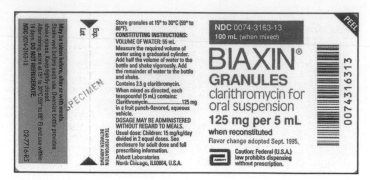

**a.** Estimated dose: _____

**b.** Calculated dose with equation to nearest tenth of a milliliter:

DA equation:

**c.** Evaluation: _____

Shade in the dose in mL on the medicine cup and draw a vertical line through the calibrated line of the syringe as applicable.

**6** Ordered: Ensure food supplement 200 mL 25% strength q8h for 3 days.

**a.** What will be the ratio of Ensure to the water diluent? _____

**b.** How would the 25% concentration be expressed as a fraction? _____

**c.** How many milliliters of Ensure will be used for the dose? _____

**d.** How many milliliters of water will be added? _____

7 Ordered: Baby formula $\frac{1}{3}$ strength, 30 mL/ hr to be diluted with SW.

   **a.** What is the equivalent percent concentration to the nearest whole number? _____

   **b.** What is the equivalent ratio of active to inactive ingredients? _____

   **c.** How much formula will the nurse pour? _____

   **d.** How much diluent will the nurse add? _____

8 The baby in problem 7 tolerated the $\frac{1}{3}$ strength formula without vomiting or diarrhea. The prescriber changed the order 48 hours later to, "Increase formula to 1:1 concentration."

   **a.** What is the equivalent percent concentration of this order? _____

   **b.** What is the equivalent fractional concentration of this order? _____

   **c.** How much formula will the nurse place in the bottle? _____

   **d.** How much SW will the nurse add? _____

9 An NS solution has a concentration of sodium chloride (NaCl) 0.9%. NaCl is supplied in grams. The diluent is SW.

   **a.** Is the concentration more or less than a 1% solution? _____

   **b.** How many grams of solute (NaCl is the concentrate) are contained in 100 mL of NS? _____

   **c.** How many grams of solute are contained in 1000 mL (1 L) of NS? _____

10 A wound irrigation order calls for 50 mL $\frac{1}{2}$ strength NS irrigations tid. The nurse needs to prepare the irrigation from full-strength NS by adding SW.

   **a.** What will be the ratio of NS solution to SW? _____

   **b.** How much NS solution will the nurse pour? _____

   **c.** How much SW will the nurse add? _____

## Suggested References

Mosby's medical dictionary of medicine, nursing and health professions, ed. 7, St. Louis, 2006, Mosby.

www.emea.eu.int/html/vet/presub/q11.htm

www.niaid.nih.gov/publications/allergies.htm

www.rxmed.com

www.vh.org/navigation/vh/topics/adult_provider_pharmacy_services.html

 Additional practice problems can be found in the Basic Calculations section on the enclosed companion CD.

Chapter 8 provides a variety of practice problems for subcutaneous and intramuscular dose calculations.

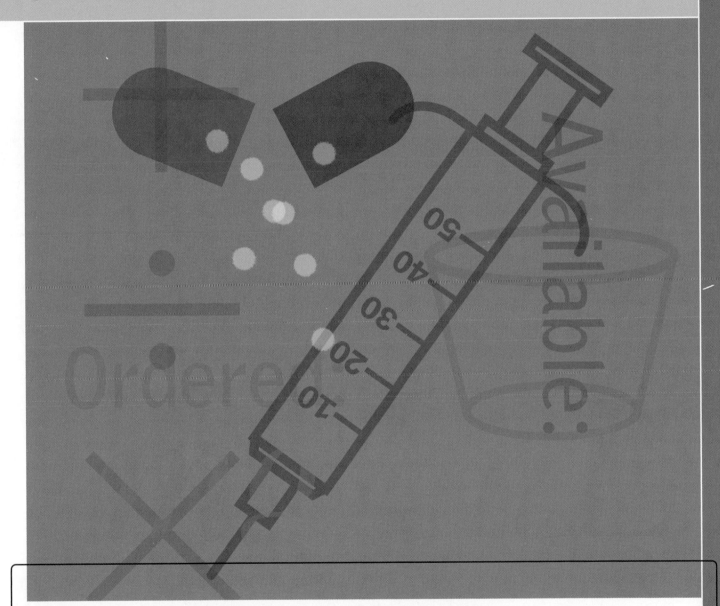

# PART IV
# PARENTERAL MEDICATION CALCULATIONS

> *"What I hear, I forget, What I see, I remember,*
> *What I do, I understand."*

—KUNG FU TZU (CONFUCIUS), 555-470 BC

# INJECTABLE MEDICATION CALCULATIONS

## Objectives

- Calculate and measure intradermal, subcutaneous, and intramuscular doses.
- Calculate and combine doses for two medications to be mixed in one syringe to the nearest measurable dose.
- Identify safety hazards of injectable medications.

## Essential Prior Knowledge

Mastery of Chapters 1-7

## Equipment

- No special equipment is required. It would be helpful to have a 3-mL syringe on hand and some food coloring for practice injection mixes. If two separate colors are used for two simulated liquid medicines, it will be easy to see if any contamination takes place when drawing up the second "medication."

## Estimated Time To Complete Chapter

- 1-2 hours

## Introduction

This chapter offers a variety of practice problems involving subcutaneous and intramuscular dose calculations. Work out all the problems. This practice will speed your calculations in the clinical setting so that you can focus on injection technique. Selected injectable drugs are mixed in one syringe to spare the patient two injections. Technical competence in preparing parenteral medications requires supervised clinical practice.

## ESSENTIAL Vocabulary

| | |
|---|---|
| **Drug Incompatibilities** | Consider all drugs incompatible unless compatibility is stated. Compatibility is affected by several factors, including pH, temperature, strength, and composition, to name a few. Compatibility data are listed in drug package inserts and current drug references. This information includes the choice of diluents, such as SW or sterile NS solution. One may be compatible with a drug and the other may not. With increasing numbers of drugs, the need to check for drug interactions and incompatibilities becomes more urgent. |
| | ➤ When in doubt, check with the pharmacist and document the finding. |
| **Hypodermic** | General term used for injections "under the skin." |

| Intradermal (ID) Injection | Injection into the dermal layer, just under the epidermis, as for skin tests. |
| Intramuscular (IM) Injection | Injection into a muscle. |
| Parenteral | Medications given outside the gastrointestinal (GI) tract. Includes medications delivered via a needle. |
| Parenteral Mix | Two or more compatible liquid medications combined in one syringe for injection. Medication combinations may include a narcotic and an anticholinergic agent to reduce nausea or dry secretions. Mixes relieve the patient from having to receive two separate intramuscular injections. |
| Subcutaneous (Subcut) Injection | Injection into loose connective tissue, or fatty layer, underlying the dermis. |

## RAPID PRACTICE 8-1   Vocabulary Review

**Estimated completion time: 5 minutes**   Answers on page **555**

**Directions:** *Study the essential vocabulary and select the correct injection-related definition.*

1  An injection into the fatty layer beneath the dermis is called _____

   **1.** Subcutaneous          **3.** Intravenous
   **2.** Intramuscular          **4.** Intradermal

2  Medications administered outside the GI tract, including those administered with a needle, are called _____

   **1.** Subcutaneous          **3.** Intradermal
   **2.** Parenteral            **4.** Intramuscular

3  When two or more medications, such as a narcotic and an anticholinergic agent, are combined in a single syringe, they are referred to as _____

   **1.** Intramuscular          **3.** Parenteral mix
   **2.** Therapeutic           **4.** Hypodermic

4  The route used to administer skin tests is called _____

   **1.** Subcutaneous          **3.** Hypodermic
   **2.** Intramuscular          **4.** Intradermal

5  Medications that, when combined, cause an undesired change in the effect or composition of one or both of the individual medications are referred to as _____

   **1.** Hypodermic            **3.** Incompatible
   **2.** Parenteral            **4.** Diluted

## Intradermal Injections

Small-volume injections usually administered as skin tests are injected intradermally just under the epidermis at a very shallow angle. A small fluid-filled wheal or bleb like a mosquito bite forms. The area is examined daily for a few days to see if there is an antibody reaction to the antigen injected. The observations are measured and documented.

Medications are not delivered via the ID route because this route offers poor absorption capability.

0.1 mL is the usual dose for a skin test administered with a 1-mL syringe and a 26- to 29-gauge needle (Figure 8-1). Up to 0.5 mL of a vaccine may be administered in one site intradermally.

Many patients are afraid of "needles." When giving vaccines and administering skin tests, the nurse can reassure patients about ID injections by showing them how little medicine will be given and how small and fine the needle is, if the patient is willing to take a look. Do not give false reassurances, such as, "Oh, you won't feel a thing." Prepare the patient for some discomfort even though there usually is minimal pain with these types of injections: "Mrs. Brown, most people dislike injections. This is just a drop or two of medicine. This will just feel like a little mosquito bite."

**Figure 8-1.** During intradermal injection, note the formation of small bleb on the skin surface. (From Potter PA, Perry AG: Fundamentals of nursing, ed. 6, St. Louis, 2005, Mosby.)

# Subcutaneous Injections

Nonirritating substances up to 1 mL may be injected into subcutaneous fatty tissue sites, usually with a 25- to 29-gauge needle. Insulin and anticoagulants, such as heparin and Fragmin, are medications that are delivered through the subcutaneous route. The fluid volume needle gauge, needle length (average ½ inch), and angle of injection depend on the patient's size, skin thickness, and condition.

The most common sites for subcutaneous injection are the subcutaneous fatty areas of the upper posterior arm, the abdomen, and the anterior thigh (Figure 8-2). A 2-inch zone around the umbilicus is to be avoided. As with all injections, the sites must be rotated systematically to avoid tissue injury.

**Figure 8-2.** Sites recommended for subcutaneous injections. (From Potter PA, Perry AG: Fundamentals of nursing, ed. 6, St. Louis, 2005, Mosby.)

➤ It is best to write out *subcutaneous* or *subcut* on medical records to avoid misinterpretation. *Subq* and *subc* can be misinterpreted. Printed materials do use abbreviations such as *subc* or *subQ* but are less likely to be misinterpreted than is handwriting.

## Intramuscular Injections

Intramuscular injection sites are selected to deliver medications for faster absorption and tolerate more concentrated substances than do subcutaneous sites. Solutions up to 3 mL may be injected with a 20- to 23-gauge needle into a single muscle site, depending on the patient's skin integrity and muscle size. The volume of fluid and the length, gauge, and angle of needle are scaled down for smaller adults, children, and infants.

The most common sites for intramuscular injection are the deltoid, the dorsogluteal area (upper outer quadrant of the buttock), the rectus femoris, the ventrogluteal muscle, and the vastus lateralis (Figure 8-3).

➤ Check workplace policies and procedures for injection sites.

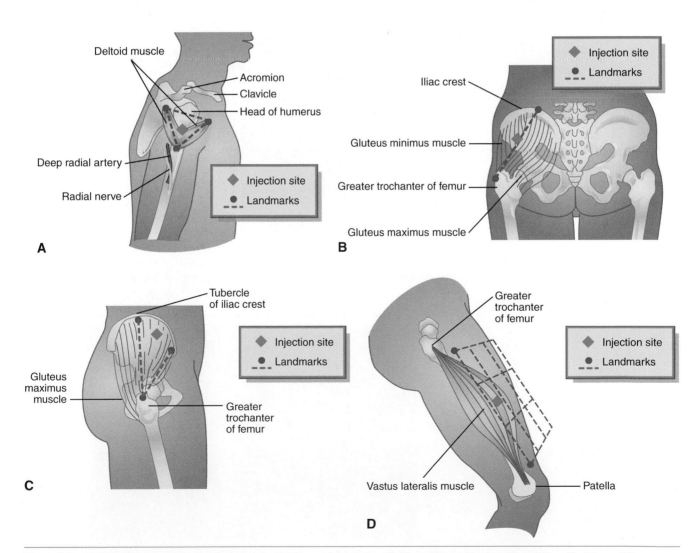

Figure 8-3. **A,** Deltoid site. **B,** Dorsogluteal site. **C,** Ventrogluteal site. **D,** Vastus lateralis site. (From Kee JL, Hayes ER, McCuiston LE: Pharmacology: a nursing process approach, ed. 5, St. Louis, 2006, Mosby.)

# Administering Injections

Mastery of the technique of delivering injections to the correct layer of tissue requires supervised laboratory and clinical practice with anatomical models and variety of different-sized patients (Figure 8-4).

Medications for subcutaneous and intramuscular injections are administered with a variety of equipment, including vials, ampules, prefilled syringes, and syringe cartridges, as illustrated below. Ampules are single-dose glass containers containing liquid medications and solutions. Vials are supplied as single-dose or multidose glass containers and may contain liquid or dry medication forms (Figure 8-5).

Prefilled syringes reduce the chance of contamination during preparation of the medication. However, they do not entirely eliminate that risk because dose adjustments may be required with prefilled syringes. They contain 0.1-0.2 mL of medication in case of loss during preparation.

Most syringes supplied need to have needles attached. There is a trend to supply needleless syringes to reduce the chance of needle-stick injury. Some types of prefilled syringes are supplied with needles.

The medication calculations for subcutaneous and intramuscular injections are the same as for oral liquid medications. The dose is usually calculated to the nearest tenth of a milliliter. The syringe that can deliver the nearest measurable dose should be selected. The 3-mL syringe is most commonly used.

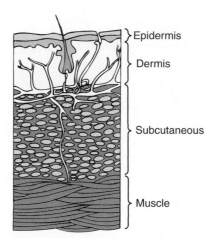

Figure 8-4. Layers of tissue for intradermal, subcutaneous, and intramuscular injections. (From Clayton BD, Stock YN: Basic pharmacology for nurses, ed. 13, St. Louis, 2004, Mosby.)

Figure 8-5. Assorted ampules and vials. (From Perry AG, Potter PA: Clinical nursing skills and techniques, ed. 6, St. Louis, 2006, Mosby.)

CHAPTER 8

| TABLE 8-1 | Usual Syringes and Doses for Average-Sized Patient | | | |
|---|---|---|---|---|
| Route | Usual Syringe Size | Needle Size | Average/Usual Amount | Maximum Amount |
| Intradermal* | 1-mL syringe | $\frac{1}{2}$ inch or less | 0.1-mL injection | 0.5 mL* |
| Subcutaneous | 1- to 3-mL syringe | $\frac{1}{2}$ to 1 inch | 0.5 mL | 1 mL |
| Intramuscular | 3-mL syringe | 1 to 2 inches | 2 mL | 3 mL |

\* The intradermal route is not used for medication administration. Skin test amounts are usually 0.1 mL. Vaccines may be up to 0.5 mL.

**FAQ** | *What is the quickest way to learn selection of syringe and needle sizes?*

**ANSWER:** There is no substitute for supervised and, later, independent experience, but learning can be greatly expedited. Assuming that you have learned to identify syringe capacities and calibration amounts (covered in Chapter 6), focus on a commonly used syringe size for each route and an approximate needle size and amount for an *average-sized adult*. Try to learn syringe and needle size selection in sequential order from the intradermal to intramuscular or vice versa (Table 8-1). Then, in the clinical setting, modifications and the selection of needles and the appropriate angle of injection for specific-sized patients can be added to the body of knowledge.

➤ There are many variations on the sizes and amounts shown in Table 8-1. These figures are just averages.
➤ Note that the 3-mL syringe for intramuscular injections corresponds to the maximum 3-mL amount preferred for intramuscular injections in one site.
➤ Remember: Never recap a used needle.

## RAPID PRACTICE 8-2  Parenteral Dose Calculations

**Estimated completion time: 20-30 minutes**    Answers on page **555**

**Directions:** *Estimate the dose, verify it with a DA-style equation to the nearest tenth of a mL, and evaluate. Draw a vertical line through the calibrated line of each syringe for the dose to be given.*

**1** Ordered: nafcillin 0.45 g mg IM q4h, an antibiotic, for a patient with infection.

  **a.** Drug concentration after reconstitution: _____
  **b.** Estimated dose: _____
  **c.** How many mL will you prepare?

    DA equation:

  **d.** Evaluation: _____

Draw a vertical line through the nearest measurable amount on the syringe provided.

**2** Ordered: Cogentin 1500 mcg IM bid, a specific anti-Parkinson disease anticholinergic, for a patient with Parkinson's disease.

NDC 0006-3275
2 mL INJECTION
**COGENTIN®**
(BENZTROPINE MESYLATE)
2 mg per 2 mL
Dist. by:
◆ MERCK & CO., INC.
West Point, PA 19486, USA

USUAL ADULT DOSAGE:
See accompanying circular.
9113907
Lot
Exp.

**a.** Drug concentration: _____

**b.** Estimated dose: _____

**c.** How many mL will you prepare?

   DA equation:

**d.** Evaluation: _____

Draw a vertical line through the nearest measurable amount on the syringe provided.

**3** Ordered: morphine sulfate 9 mg IM stat, an opioid narcotic, for a patient in pain.

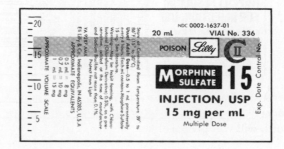

NDC 0002-1637-01
20 mL          VIAL No. 336
POISON *Lilly* **CII**
**M ORPHINE**
**SULFATE** **15**
INJECTION, USP
**15 mg per mL**
Multiple Dose

**a.** Drug concentration: _____

**b.** Estimated dose: _____

**c.** How many mL will you prepare?

DA equation:

**d.** Evaluation: _____

Draw a vertical line through the nearest measurable dose on the syringe provided.

➤ Note the *CII* on the morphine label. It means that the drug is a federally controlled substance, Schedule II, a category of drugs with strong potential for abuse as well as useful medical purposes. Morphine is an opium-derived narcotic. There are strict record-keeping requirements for controlled drugs as well as limitations on the number of doses that can be prescribed before a renewal is required.

➤ Assess the patient for respiratory depression before giving an opioid and thereafter until the drug effect has diminished. There are several visual analog scales (VAS) available for assessing current pain levels. The patient identifies the current level on a "no pain" to "worst pain" or "severest pain" subjective rating. Find out which scale your agency prefers. This practice may reduce the risk of overmedication.

**Clinical Relevance**

**4** Ordered: lorazepam 2 mg bid IM stat, a sedative and anti-anxiety agent, for an agitated elderly patient.

**a.** Drug concentration: _____
**b.** Estimated dose: _____
**c.** How many mL will you prepare?

DA equation:

**d.** Evaluation: _____

Draw a vertical line through the nearest measurable dose on the syringe provided.

Note that Ativan (lorazepam) is labeled *CIV* (i.e., controlled substance Schedule IV). Drugs in this category have *less* potential for abuse or addiction than do Schedule I, II, or III drugs. Schedule IV drugs include phenobarbital and certain other anti-anxiety agents.

**5** Ordered: digoxin 0.125 mg IM daily, for a patient with heart failure.

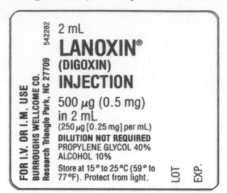

**a.** Drug concentration: _____

**b.** Estimated dose: _____

**c.** How many mL will you prepare?

DA equation:

**d.** Evaluation: _____

Draw a vertical line through the nearest measurable dose on the syringe provided.

| **Clinical Relevance** | ➤ Focus intently on decimals when they appear in medication orders or drug labels. Review decimal calculations in Chapter 1 as needed to ensure that you are comfortable with decimal addition, division, and multiplication. Dose calculation errors are large if a decimal point is misplaced. Write neatly and make decimal points prominent. |
|---|---|

| **Q:** *Ask Yourself*<br><br>**A:** *My Answer* | **1**  How many times does 0.05 go into 0.1? How many times does 0.25 go into 0.5? How many times does 0.5 go into 1? How many times does 0.025 go into 0.05? |
|---|---|

**RAPID PRACTICE 8-3**  More Parenteral Dose Calculation Practice

**Estimated completion time: 20-30 minutes**   Answers on page 556

**Directions:** *Examine the order and calculate the dose. Recalculate if the estimate does not support the answer.*

**1** Ordered: codeine 0.02 g IM q3-4h prn for pain, a narcotic analgesic, for a patient in pain.

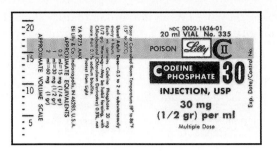

a. Estimated dose: _____

b. How many milliliters will you prepare for this syringe?

   DA equation:


c. Evaluation: _____

Draw a vertical line through the nearest measurable amount on the syringe provided.

2  Ordered: furosemide 38 mg IM, a diuretic, for a patient with edema.

a. Estimated dose: _____

b. How many milliliters will you prepare for this syringe?

   DA equation:


c. Evaluation: _____

Draw a vertical line through the nearest measurable amount on the syringe provided.

d. What is the smallest measurable dose in a 5-mL syringe?

**3** Ordered: Solu-Cortef 0.3 g IM, an anti-inflammatory steroid, for a patient with severe inflammatory response.

**a.** Estimated dose: _____

**b.** How many milliliters will you prepare for this syringe?

DA equation:

**c.** Evaluation: _____

Draw a vertical line through the nearest measurable amount on the syringe provided.

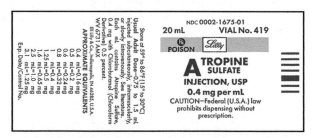

**4** Ordered: atropine 0.3 mg IM on call to OR, an anticholinergic for a preoperative patient.

**a.** Estimated dose: _____

**b.** How many milliliters will you prepare for the 1-mL syringe?

DA equation:

**c.** Evaluation: _____

Draw a vertical line through the nearest measurable amount on the syringe provided.

**5** Ordered: tuberculin skin test ID for an adult patient. The volume for this skin test is 0.1 mL.

Draw a vertical line through the nearest measurable dose on the syringe provided.

**1** Why is it important to make a habit of evaluating the equations and comparing the answers to the estimates? What are the risks if this step is skipped?

**Q:** *Ask Yourself*

**A:** *My Answer*

# Parenteral Mixes

When two medications are administered together in one syringe, the order is bracketed:

morphine 5 mg IM ⎫
⎬ on call to OR
atropine 0.2 mg IM ⎭

Compatibility between medications to be mixed must be checked in a current drug reference. Many drug references have compatibility charts. Note the example shown in Table 8-2.

➤ When in doubt about drug compatibility, call the pharmacy. Consider all drugs incompatible unless otherwise documented.

**Example of parenteral mix order**

Ordered:

meperidine 75 mg ⎫
⎬ IM q4h prn pain
Vistaril 25 mg ⎭

| TABLE 8-2 | **Drug Compatibility Chart (Excerpt)** |
|---|---|

| | Atropine | Buprenorphine | Butorphanol | Chlorpromazine | Codeine | Diazepam | Dimenhydrinate | Diphenhydramine | Droperidol | Fentanyl | Glycopyrrolate | Heparin | Hydroxyzine | Meperidine | Metoclopramide | Midazolam | Morphine |
|---|---|---|---|---|---|---|---|---|---|---|---|---|---|---|---|---|---|
| Atropine | | | C | C | | I | C | C | C | C | C | | C | C | C | C | C |
| Buprenorphine | | | | | | | | | | | | | | | | | |
| Butorphanol | C | | | C | | I | I | C | C | C | | | C | C | C | C | C |
| Chlorpromazine | C | | C | | | I | I | C | C | C | C | C | C | C | C | C | C |

*C*, compatible; *I*, incompatible

Excerpt from Skidmore-Roth L: Mosby's Drug Guide for Nurses, ed 6, St. Louis, 2005, Mosby.

Sometimes the order states "mix" after the route.

➤ The nurse cannot legally continue to administer any drug after the expiration date, be it automatic or written out. The prescriber must be contacted promptly if the medication is still perceived to be needed. By giving an expired drug, the nurse becomes a prescriber without the license to prescribe, an illegal practice. When medications expire, the medication must be renewed by the prescriber.

The use of parenteral mixes spares the patient the discomfort of two separate injections. The mixes usually consist of a narcotic and an anticholinergic type of medication that extends the action of the narcotic and decreases nausea, a common side effect of narcotics, or dries respiratory secretions for patients who are to receive general anesthesia.

## Mixing Two Medications in One Syringe

Mixtures may be combinations of vial, ampule, prefilled syringe, and/or prefilled cartridge medications. The first medication is drawn up to the precise dose, followed by the draw from the second container (Figures 8-6 to 8-8). This technique requires supervised clinical practice.

## Calculating the Dose for a Parenteral Mix

Calculate each dose separately to the nearest tenth of a milliliter. Add them together. Round the dose to the nearest tenth of a milliliter, for example,

morphine sulfate    0.4 mL

atropine sulfate    +0.2 mL

0.6 mL total volume for syringe

A                                    B

Figure 8-6. **A,** Medication aspirated with ampule inverted. **B,** Medication aspirated with ampule on a flat surface. (From Potter PA, Perry AG: Fundamentals of nursing, ed. 6, St. Louis, 2005, Mosby.)

**A          B          C**

Figure 8-7. **A,** Insert the adapter through the center of the vial diaphragm (with vial flat on the table). **B,** Withdraw fluid with the vial inverted. **C,** Hold the syringe upright, tap the barrel to dislodge air bubbles. (From Potter PA, Perry AG: Fundamentals of nursing, ed. 6, St. Louis, 2005, Mosby.)

Figure 8-8. Mixing medications from a vial. **A,** Injecting air into a vial. **B,** Injecting air into vial B and withdrawing dose. **C,** Withdrawing medication from vial A.

| *Containers:* | First | Second | Third |
|---|---|---|---|
| *Steps:* | Air in | Air in & Medicine Out | Medicine Out |

Medications are now mixed. (From Potter PA, Perry AG: Fundamentals of nursing, ed. 6, St. Louis, 2005, Mosby.)

## RAPID PRACTICE 8-4  Calculating Parenteral Mix Doses

**Estimated completion time: 10-15 minutes**   Answers on page **558**

**Directions:** *Examine the order and the labels. Estimate the ordered doses. Calculate the two individual doses to the nearest tenth of a milliliter using DA-style equations. Evaluate the equation. Is the equation balanced? Does the estimate support the answer? Draw a vertical line through the* total *desired amount to the nearest measurable dose on the syringe. Follow the example given in problem 1. The order of the questions for each problem suggests the order to follow to solve these problems.*

**1** Ordered: meperidine hydrochloride 75 mg ⎫ IM q4–6h prn pain
        hydroxyzine hydrochloride 25 mg ⎭

*Meperidine*

**a.** Estimate: Does the order call for *more* or ⟨*less*⟩ than the unit dose available?
Less. Estimated dose: about $\frac{3}{4}$ mL.

**b.** How many mL will you prepare?

DA equation:

$$? \text{ mL} = \frac{1 \text{ mL}}{\underset{4}{100 \text{ mg}}} \times \overset{3}{\cancel{75 \text{ mg}}} = \underline{0.75 \text{ mL rounded to } 0.8 \text{ mL meperidine}}$$

**c.** Evaluation: Is the equation balanced? Yes. Does the estimate support the answer? Yes.

*Hydroxyzine*

**d.** Estimate: Does the order call for *more* or ⟨*less*⟩ than the dose available?
Less. Estimated dose: about $\frac{1}{2}$ of 1 mL.

**e.** How many mL will you prepare?
DA equation:

$$? \text{ mL} = \frac{1 \text{ mL}}{\underset{2}{50 \text{ mg}}} \times \overset{1}{\cancel{25 \text{ mg}}} = \underline{0.5 \text{ mL hydroxyzine}}$$

**f.** Evaluation: Is the equation balanced? Yes. Does the estimate support the answer? Yes.

*Total Dose*

**g.** *Total combined volume* in milliliters *to nearest tenth:* 0.8 + 0.5 mL = 1.3 mL

Draw a vertical line through the nearest measurable amount for the total dose on the syringe.

The only difference between this calculation and other calculations of liquid doses learned earlier is the addition of the two doses together.

**2** Ordered: hydromorphone HCL 1.5 mg  ⎤ IM at 0800
  atropine 0.4 mg  ⎦

*Dilaudid*

**a.** Estimated dose: _____

**b.** How many mL will you prepare?

  DA equation:

**c.** Evaluation: Is the equation balanced? Does the estimate support the answer?

  _____

*Atropine*

**d.** Estimated dose: _____

**e.** How many mL will you prepare?

  DA equation:

**f.** Evaluation: Is the equation balanced? Does the estimate support the answer?

  _____

*Total Dose*

**g.** Total combined volume: _____

Draw a vertical line through the nearest measurable amount for the total dose on the syringe provided.

➤ Do not confuse morphine and hydromorphone (Dilaudid). Hydromorphone is considerably more powerful than morphine.

**3** Ordered: morphine sulfate 8 mg ⎫ IM stat.
⠀⠀⠀⠀⠀⠀ atropine 0.6 mg ⎭

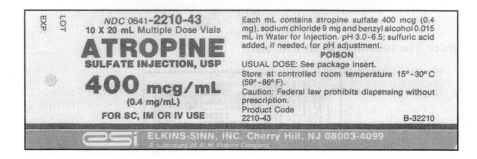

*Morphine*

**a.** Estimated dose: _____

**b.** How many mL will you prepare?

⠀⠀ DA equation:

**c.** Evaluation: Is the equation balanced? Does the estimate support the answer?
⠀⠀ _____

*Atropine*

**d.** Estimated dose: _____

**e.** How many mL will you prepare?

⠀⠀ DA equation:

**f.** Evaluation: Is the equation balanced? Does the estimate support the answer?
⠀⠀ _____

*Total Dose*

**g.** Total combined volume: _____

Draw a vertical line through the nearest measurable amount for the total dose on the syringe provided.

4  Ordered: hydromorphone HCl 3 mg ⎫ IM stat
        Compazine 8 mg ⎭

*Dilaudid*

**a.** Estimated dose: _____

**b.** How many mL will be prepared?

DA equation:

**c.** Evaluation: Is the equation balanced? Does the estimate support the answer?
_____

*Compazine*

**d.** Estimated dose: _____

**e.** How many mL will you prepare?

DA equation:

**f.** Evaluation: Is the equation balanced? Does the estimate support the answer?
_____

*Total Dose*

**g.** Total combined volume: _____

Draw a vertical line through the nearest measurable amount for the total dose on the syringe provided.

**5** Ordered: morphine 15 mg ⎫ IM q6h prn pain
hydroxyzine 35 mg ⎭

*Morphine*

**a.** Estimated dose: _____

**b.** How many mL will you prepare?

DA equation:

**c.** Evaluation: Is the equation balanced? Does the estimate support the answer?
_____

*Vistaril*

**d.** Estimated dose: _____

**e.** How many mL will you prepare?

DA equation:

**f.** Evaluation: Is the equation balanced? Does the estimate support the answer?
_____

*Total Dose*

**g.** Total dose in milliliters to nearest tenth: _____

Draw a vertical line through the nearest measurable amount for the total dose on the syringe provided.

# Medicines Supplied in Units

Medicines that are supplied in units and also may be administered via the subcutaneous route are covered in Chapters 11 and 12.

## CHAPTER 8 MULTIPLE-CHOICE REVIEW

**Estimated completion time: 30 minutes to 1 hour**    Answers on page **559**

**Directions:** *Place a circle around the letter of the correct answer. Select reconstituted drugs for an IM injection with a 3-mL syringe.*

**1** Ordered: Dilaudid 4 mg ⎫ IM stat
       Vistaril 35 mg ⎬

How many total milliliters will you administer?

| | |
|---|---|
| **1.** 1.1 | **3.** 1.3 |
| **2.** 1.2 | **4.** 1.7 |

**2** Skin tests are administered via which route?

| | |
|---|---|
| **1.** Subcutaneous | **3.** Intramuscular |
| **2.** Intradermal | **4.** Intravenous |

**3** The most commonly used syringe size for intramuscular injections is

| | |
|---|---|
| **1.** 1 mL | **3.** 3 mL |
| **2.** 2 mL | **4.** 5 mL |

**4** Parenteral mixes most often include which types of medications?

**1.** A narcotic and another medication, for example, to control nausea
**2.** Potassium and bacteriostatic sterile water for injection
**3.** Two different kinds of antibiotics
**4.** An intravenous medication and an intramuscular medication

**5** The maximum amount of fluid that is recommended for one site for average-sized adult intramuscular injections is

| | |
|---|---|
| **1.** 1 mL | **3.** 3 mL |
| **2.** 2 mL | **4.** 5 mL |

**6** Ordered: morphine sulfate 6 mg. Available: morphine sulfate 10 mg/ mL. What is the estimated dose?

| | |
|---|---|
| **1.** 0.06 mL | **3.** 1.2 mL |
| **2.** 0.6 mL | **4.** 6 mL |

7 Examine the following dose concentrations. Which dilution would be most appropriate for a 10-mg IM dose? (Consider the volume to be administered.)

**1.** Add 20 mL to make 1 mg/ mL
**2.** Add 10 mL to make 2 mg/ mL
**3.** Add 5 mL to make 5 mg/ mL
**4.** Add 1 mL to make 40 mg/ mL

8 Examine the following dose concentrations. Which dilution would be appropriate for a 50-mg IM dose?

**1.** Add 10 mL to make 5 mg/ mL
**2.** Add 8 mL to make 10 mg/ mL
**3.** Add 5.6 mL to make 12 mg/ mL
**4.** Add 3 mL to make 25 mg/ mL

9 Identify the difference between SW and bacteriostatic water, if any.

**1.** Bacteriostatic water contains a preservative and may be used as a diluent only if the medication label so states.
**2.** Both solutions are sterile and may be used interchangeably.
**3.** SW may be used in place of bacteriostatic water.
**4.** Both are bacteriostatic.

10 What is the first step the nurse must take after reading an order for a parenteral mix?

**1.** Estimate the doses.
**2.** Prepare each medication separately, maintaining sterile technique.
**3.** Evaluate the DA dose calculation against the estimated dose.
**4.** Check current drug literature for drug compatibility.

## CHAPTER 8 FINAL PRACTICE

**Estimated completion time: 1 hour**   Answers on page **560**

**Directions:** *Analyze the problems. Estimate and calculate the requested doses to the nearest tenth of a mL. Use a calculator for long division and multiplication. Evaluate your equations and answers on your own.*

1 Ordered: hydromorphone 3 mg ⎱ IM for postoperative pain and nausea
    hydroxyzine 40 mg ⎰

*Dilaudid*

**a.** Estimated dose: _____
**b.** How many mL will be prepared?

DA equation:

Evaluation: _____

*Vistaril*

**c.** Estimated dose: _____

**d.** How many mL will be prepared?

DA equation:

Evaluation: _____

*Total Combined Dose*

**e.** Total dose in mL to nearest tenth: _____

Draw a vertical line through the nearest measurable amount on the syringe provided.

**2** Ordered: meperidine hydrochloride 35 mg ⎫ IM for postoperative discomfort
prochlorperazine 10 mg ⎬

*Meperidine*

**a.** Estimated dose: _____

**b.** How many mL will be prepared?

DA equation:

Evaluation: _____

*Compazine*

**c.** Estimated dose: _____
**d.** How many mL will be prepared?

DA equation:

Evaluation: _____

*Total Combined Dose*

**e.** Total dose in mL to nearest tenth: _____

Draw a vertical line through the nearest measurable amount on the syringe provided.

**3** Ordered: morphine 12 mg
glycopyrrolate 0.3 mg } IM, a narcotic and an anticholinergic, on call to OR

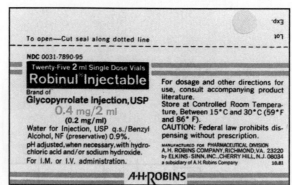

*Morphine*

**a.** Estimated dose: _____
**b.** How many mL will be prepared?

DA equation:


Evaluation: _____

*Robinul*

**c.** Estimated dose: _____
**d.** How many mL will be prepared?

   DA equation:



Evaluation: _____

*Total Combined Dose*

**e.** Total dose in milliliters to nearest tenth: _____

Draw a vertical line through the nearest measurable amount on the syringe
provided.

**4** Ordered: codeine 10 mg IM stat, for a child with complaints of pain.

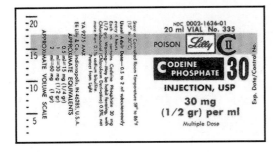

**a.** Estimated dose: _____
**b.** How many mL will be prepared?

   DA equation:




Evaluation: _____

If estimated dose is confirmed, draw a vertical line through the nearest measurable amount on the syringe provided.

**1** What is the apothecary equivalent of codeine 30 mg? (Refer to label on p. 277.)

_____

**5** Ordered: nafcillin sodium 0.4 g IM, an antibiotic, for a patient with an infection.

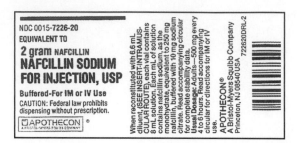

**a.** Total dose in vial: _____

**b.** Amount of diluent needed:

_____

**c.** Dose concentration after reconstitution: _____

**d.** Estimated dose: _____

**e.** How many mL will you prepare?

DA equation:




Evaluation: _____

Draw a vertical line through the nearest measurable amount on the syringe provided.

**6** Ordered: ampicillin 0.2 g IM q6h, an antibiotic, for a patient with an infection.

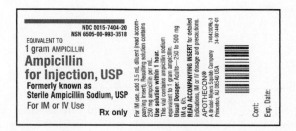

**a.** Total dose in vial: _____

**b.** Amount of diluent needed:

_____

**c.** Dose concentration after reconstitution: _____

**d.** Estimated dose: _____

**e.** How many mL will you prepare?

DA equation:

Evaluation: _____

Draw a vertical line through the nearest measurable amount on the syringe provided.

**7** Ordered: phenobarbital sodium 0.1 g IM, a barbiturate, for a patient who needs sedation.

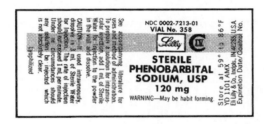

**a.** Total dose in vial: _____

**b.** Amount of diluent needed:

_____

**c.** Dose concentration after reconstitution: _____

**d.** Estimated dose: _____

**e.** How many mL will you prepare?

DA equation:

Evaluation: _____

Draw a vertical line through the nearest measurable amount on the syringe provided.

8 Ordered: penicillin G potassium IM 400,000 units q6h, an antibiotic, for a patient with infection.

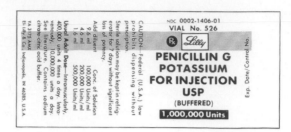

a. Total number of units in vial: _____

b. Amount of diluent that would yield closest to a 2-mL dose: _____

c. Dose concentration after reconstitution: _____

d. Estimated dose: _____

e. How many mL will you prepare?

DA equation:




Evaluation: _____

Draw a vertical line through the nearest measurable amount on the syringe provided.

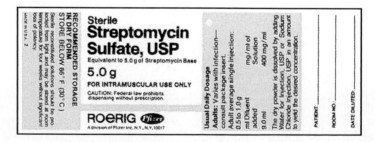

9 Ordered: streptomycin 0.3 g IM bid, an antibiotic, for a patient with an infection.

a. Total dose in vial: _____

b. Dose concentration after reconstitution: _____

c. Estimated dose: _____

d. How many mL will you prepare?

DA equation:




Evaluation: _____

Draw a vertical line through the nearest measurable amount on the syringe provided.

**10** Ordered: atropine 0.2 mg IM stat, for a preoperative child.

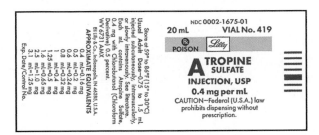

**a.** Dose concentration in micrograms and milligrams: _____

**b.** Estimated dose: _____

**c.** How many mL will you prepare?

DA equation:

Evaluation: _____

Draw a vertical line through the nearest measurable amount on the syringe provided.

## Suggestions for Further Reading

Clayton BD, Stock YN: Basic pharmacology for nurses, ed. 13, St. Louis, 2004, Mosby.

Lilley LL, Harrington S, Snyder JS: Pharmacology and the nursing process, ed. 4, St. Louis, 2005, Mosby.

Perry AG, Potter PA: Clinical nursing skills and techniques, ed. 6, St. Louis, 2006, Mosby.

Potter PA, Perry AG: Fundamentals of nursing, ed. 6, St. Louis, 2005, Mosby.

Skidmore-Roth L: Mosby's drug guide for nurses, ed. 6, St. Louis, 2005, Mosby.

http://opioids.com/hydromorphone/hydromorphine.html

www.jcipatientsafety.org

www.medtronic.com/neuro/paintherapies/pain_treatment_ladder/drug_infusion/patient_management/drug_pat_mgmt_strat.html

www.nysna.org/departments/communications/publications/report/2006/mar/research.htm

Additional practice problems can be found in the Basic Calculations section on the enclosed companion CD.

Chapter 9 introduces basic intravenous dose and rate calculations. These calculations are used on a daily basis in clinical agencies. Much of the mathematics needed to solve intravenous dose and rate problems has been covered and can be applied to the intravenous route with some modifications.

*"The only thing we have to fear is fear itself."*
—**FRANKLIN DELANO ROOSEVELT**

# BASIC INTRAVENOUS CALCULATIONS

## Objectives

- Interpret basic intravenous (IV) solution orders for peripheral infusion.
- Identify contents of commonly ordered IV fluids.
- Identify average flow rates for adults who are NPO and the general rationale for variations.
- Estimate, calculate, and verify flow rates for intermittent and continuous IV solutions on gravity and electronic devices.
- Calculate grams of dextrose and sodium in IV fluids.
- Estimate and calculate the duration of flow for IV solutions in hours and minutes.
- Identify patient safety assessments related to IV solution therapy.

## Essential Prior Knowledge

Mastery of Chapters 1-8

## Equipment

- Calculations can be taught without equipment. Referring to the illustrations will be helpful.
- The student will benefit from an examination of equipment for similarities, differences, and labels either in a clinical laboratory or agency setting.

## Estimated Time To Complete Chapter

- 2-3 hours

## Introduction

Most patients receive at least one IV solution during hospitalization. Students often care for patients with IV lines before learning to prepare and give oral and injectable medications. Monitoring the site and flow rate is a basic skill. Reporting concerns to the primary nurse is appropriate to protect the patient from fluid drug overload or underdose as well as to protect the site from tissue damage due to a displaced venous access cannula or needle. Additional IV therapy skills and theory can take place later and will progress faster because of the experience gained with the orders, site, and flow rate.

Basic IV calculations require only the simplest arithmetic once the nurse knows how to analyze the order and has an overall understanding of the names and types of equipment available. Examining each piece of IV equipment encountered in the laboratory and clinical agency and noting the key features, functions, similarities, and differences will expedite understanding.

➤ Patients may have some ability to monitor their therapy with oral medications because they may have knowledge and experience with them at home. However, patients are totally dependent on the nurse for safe IV administration. Hazards from improper IV administration occur more rapidly than from other, slower routes of absorption and may not be reversible.

**283**

| | |
|---|---|
| **Bolus** | Concentrated medication solution given by IV route over a relatively brief period of time. Equipment used to deliver varies, depending on existing IV lines, volume, and time to be infused. Often given by direct injection into a vein (IV push). |
| **Continuous IV Infusion** | IV solution that flows continuously, as the name implies, and does not have a stop or discontinue date or time (e.g., dextrose 5% in water at 75 mL/ hr). Patients who are NPO and surgical patients are two of the many types of patients who receive continuous infusions. |
| **Drop Factor (DF)** | Number of drops per milliliter delivered through various sizes of IV tubing devices. The tubing diameter affects the size of the drop. The DF is used to calculate flow rates on gravity devices. DF is also known as tubing factor. |
| | The abbreviation *gtt(s)* is the apothecary term for *drop(s)*. It may be seen on some prescriber's orders. It is recommended that the word *drops* be written out. |
| **Electronic Infusion Devices (EIDs)** | Variety of devices that deliver IV fluids and medications at a preselected rate. |
| **1. Controllers (Nonvolumetric)** | Flow rate controllers that are *gravity* dependent use drop sensors and pinching action to regulate rate. They are used for many IV solutions in large clinical agencies. |
| **2. Pumps (Volumetric)** | Cassette pumps are not gravity dependent. They deliver fluids under positive pressure and are used for powerful drugs, high-risk patients, and more accurate controlled flow rates. |
| **Flow Rate** | Rate at which fluid is delivered by IV infusion devices, most often ordered in whole milliliters per hour (mL/ hr) (e.g., "Infuse [solution] at 100 mL/ hr"). |
| **Gravity Infusion Device** | IV delivery device with flow rate affected by the height of solution and the patient's position. The most elementary devices use a manually operated plastic slide or ball-roller clamp to control flow rate. |
| **Infusion Line, Primary** | Main IV line or lines connected to the patient. Also called primary tubing on the IV administration set label. A patient may have more than one primary line. The first one is usually "dedicated" to fluid delivery and maintenance. Additional primary and secondary lines are usually reserved for medications or medicated solutions that are incompatible with other fluids. Primary lines may be vented or nonvented. |
| **Infusion Line, Secondary** | Tubing that connects to ports on the primary line and permits a variety of additional medications and fluids to be added without disruption of the primary line. Use of a secondary infusion line spares the patient additional injections into the veins. Labels on the administration sets indicate "secondary." |
| | ➤ Compatibility must be carefully checked before "mixing" additional substances into the primary line. |
| **Injection Ports** | Latex or rubber ports located on IV lines and solution containers to permit access for injection of additional fluids or medications. A port adapter may also be attached directly to a cannula that is in a vein (also known as a heparin lock or intermittent IV infusion device). |
| **Intermittent Infusions** | Usually small-volume (up to 250-mL) medicated IV solutions delivered at intervals. A variety of devices and methods are available, the most common being IV piggyback equipment, syringe pumps, and calibrated volume-control burette chambers. |
| **IV Containers** | Variously sized plastic bags are the most common. Glass bottles are used for medications that cause plastic to deteriorate. |

| | |
|---|---|
| **IV Piggyback** | Small-volume infusions, usually 50 or 100 mL, infused through a short secondary tubing line that is "piggybacked" to a port on a primary line. Intermittent medicated infusions are delivered over 20-60 minutes, as specified by the pharmacy or manufacturer in drug references. |
| **IV Push** | IV concentrated, medicated, intermittent bolus dose of 1-50 mL, usually administered by manual direct injection with a syringe, sometimes via an infusion pump. It is occasionally written incorrectly as "IVP," which can be confused with the common abbreviation for the intravenous pyelogram (IVP) test. Also, do not confuse with IVPB (IV piggyback) |
| **Macrodrip** | Gravity IV infusion tubing set that has a wide diameter to deliver large drops (10-20 drops/ mL drop factor) and fast flow rates. |
| **Microdrip** | Gravity IV infusion tubing set that has a narrow diameter to deliver small drops (60 drops/ mL drop factor) and slower flow rates. Also known as pediatric tubing. |
| **Osmolality** | Solute concentration in solution. The unit of measurement is the osmol. The milliosmol (mOs) is the unit of measurement in *plasma* and is used as a basis for comparison with the contents of IV solutions. Plasma contains approximately 290 mOs/ L. *Isotonic* solutions, such as normal saline solution, 5% dextrose in water, and lactated Ringer's solution, approximate plasma osmolality. *Hyper*tonic solutions contain a higher number of milliosmols per liter and have higher tonicity. *Hypo*tonic solutions contain a lower number of milliosmols per liter and have lower tonicity. |
| **Patency** | State of being open and unblocked, such as a "patent IV site" or "patent airway." Sites are checked for patency during every visit to the bedside to ensure that the ordered fluids and medications are flowing into the vein and not into tissue. |
| **PCA Pump** | Patient-controlled analgesia pump. An electronic IV device with a syringe or narcotic injector vial programmed to dispense prescribed amounts of analgesic narcotics and other medications at pre-scribed intermittent intervals with intermittent lockout intervals. Patients self-administer boluses of medication in solution to control pain by remote push-button control.<br><br>**Mnemonic**: PC, Pain Control. |
| **Port** | Resealable *access* device that permits additional IV lines or medications to be added into or on primary (main) IV tubing without initiating another injection site or disrupting the main IV line. Ports may also be indwelling venous cannulas that can be capped and kept patent with a saline or heparin (lock) flush solution and accessed when needed. The latter type of port frees the patient of the need to have IV solutions and tubing connected continuously. |
| **TKO KVO** | "To keep open" or "Keep vein open," a flow rate order that may be given for gravity devices for the minimum rate that will keep the IV line patent and prevent coagulation. This order has mostly been replaced by the insertion of an indwelling access port. See "Port." Some institutions specify a TKO rate in their procedure manuals. The nurse needs to check the agency policy. EIDs can be pro-grammed for specific minimum rates. |
| **Volume-Control Burette Device** | Transparent, calibrated small-volume container, with a capacity of 100, 110, or 150 mL, that is manually connected to an IV line just below the main IV solution container. It is filled with only 1 or 2 hours' worth of IV fluid and/or smaller amounts of medicated solution at a time, depending on agency policy. As the name implies, it protects at-risk patients from fluid or med-ication overload by limiting the total amount of solution available in case of equipment or a rate failure incident. |

➤ This vocabulary is essential for interpreting IV solution orders. The calculations are dependent on the type of equipment used.

**RAPID PRACTICE 9-1**   Vocabulary Review

**Estimated completion time: 10-15 minutes    Answers on page 563**

**Directions:** *Examine the IV-related vocabulary to expedite comprehension of the material in this chapter. Fill in* very brief *descriptions of the vocabulary terms supplied.*

1  What is the difference between a continuous IV solution order and an intermittent IV order? _____

2  What is the difference between a primary and a secondary infusion line?

_____

3  **a.** What is a DF, and which kind of IV equipment requires the DF to determine flow rate?

_____

   **b.** Which type of administration set delivers the smallest drops and is used for low flow rates?

_____

4  What is the difference between a nonvolumetric and a volumetric EID?

_____

5  Flow rates for IV solutions are usually ordered in which measurement terms?

_____

# Overview of Intravenous Therapy

Oral medications and IV solutions that may be medicated are the two most common routes of medication administration. The nursing responsibilities related to the patient's safety during oral and IV medication therapy are paramount.

## Purpose of Intravenous Solutions

Intravenous solutions are ordered to

- Provide daily maintenance fluid therapy.
- Replace prior deficits.
- Replace concurrent losses.

The fluids may consist of dextrose solutions, electrolytes, medications, or blood products. They may be *isotonic, hypotonic,* or *hypertonic,* based on the prescriber's assessment of current laboratory test results and the patient's clinical needs.

Intravenous solutions are ordered to be either *continuous* or *intermittent,* depending on the patient's fluid and medication needs and fluid intake status. They are administered through peripheral or larger-diameter central veins. They are supplied in *nonvented plastic* or *vented* and nonvented glass containers.

*Continuous* IV lines are placed on *primary infusion administration lines. Intermittent* infusions are administered in a variety of ways but are frequently connected (piggybacked) to a port on a primary line via a *secondary* tubing set.

**Q:** *Ask Yourself*

**A:** *My Answer*

1  What are the three general purposes for ordering IV solutions? (Use one- or two-word answers.)

_____

## Maintenance Intravenous Flow Rates

The average-sized adult patient who is to be NPO for a short period of time but is otherwise well hydrated, with good heart, lung, and renal function, may have a *maintenance isotonic* continuous IV solution ordered at about *75-125 mL/ hr.* When an order calls for much less or more than this flow rate, the nurse needs to research the need for the variation. It is easier to keep in mind an average of about 1 L q8h or 2-3 L q24h for the hypothetical hydrated adult who is NPO for a limited period of time. Often, the reason for variation is clear.

A dehydrated patient will receive a higher-than-average volume and flow rate, depending on clinical tolerance. A patient with compromised heart, lung, or renal function or a baby will receive a lower-than-average flow rate. The more the patient is able to drink, the less the need for a high flow rate or a continuous IV infusion. Even if the patient is able to take 2-3 L of fluid a day by mouth, an IV access line is frequently established and "capped" in order to provide prompt access for IV medications or fluids if needed.

**Clinical Relevance**

1  What are examples of the patient-related criteria that the prescriber uses to make an informed decision about the flow rate for an IV order? (Give a brief answer.)

**Q:** *Ask Yourself*

**A:** *My Answer*

2  What are the main purposes of a primary line, a secondary line, and a port?

3  What is an average range of isotonic maintenance solution flow rates that might be ordered for a maintenance IV for an adult patient who is NPO and has good heart, lung, and renal function?

## RAPID PRACTICE 9-2  More Vocabulary Review

**Estimated completion time: 10-15 minutes**  Answers on page **563**

**Directions:** *Select the IV-related term or phrase that best completes the sentence.*

1  The name for the main infusion administration set is _____
   1. Intermittent
   2. Drop factor
   3. Primary
   4. Secondary

2  An IV solution that does not have a discontinue date or time is _____
   1. 5% dextrose in water
   2. Continuous
   3. Intermittent
   4. PCA

3  The term for the *calibrated container* that can be used to deliver intermittent infusions is _____
   1. Gravity infusion device
   2. Volume-control burette device
   3. Electronic infusion device
   4. IV piggyback

4  The term that describes undesired reactions that can result from a mixture of certain combinations of IV medications, diluents, and/or other solutions is _____
   1. Incompatibility
   2. IV push
   3. Constant
   4. KVO

**5** When a medication is manually injected directly into a vein by the nurse, the procedure is referred to as _____

   **1.** IV piggyback          **3.** IV push

   **2.** TKO                 **4.** PCA

# Basic Intravenous Equipment

The essential elements of infusion equipment are

- A prescribed unmedicated or medicated solution
- A pole or stand to hold the solution and delivery devices
- A rate controller or cassette pump or pumps as desired and available
- Infusion tubing of various sizes and types to connect the solution to the access device, needle, or needleless port
- Dressings and tape to protect and secure the injection site

| **Clinical Relevance** | Safety trends pertaining to IV equipment include increasing use of premixed medicated IV solutions supplied by the pharmacy or the manufacturer; needleless equipment; and sophisticated electronic devices that can handle up to four IV lines for one patient and have the capability of extensive programming of alarms, drug doses, and flow rates. |
|---|---|

# Types of Intravenous Solutions

There are many types of IV solutions. The contents depend on the purpose of the IV order, the condition of the patient as evidenced by laboratory test results, the hydration and fluid and electrolyte status of the patient, and compatible parenteral medications that need to be added to the solution.

The following are some of the most frequently ordered solutions to which medications can be added if necessary. Their names and abbreviations must be learned. Dextrose (D), normal saline (NS) solution, water (W), and lactated Ringer's (L/R) solution may contain varying percentages of dextrose or electrolytes. The nurse needs to focus on the percentage of contents ordered and match that with the label.

➤ A number indicates the % of grams of solute per 100 mL, for example, 5D = 5% dextrose or 5 grams of dextrose per *100 mL* of solution.

# Tonicity of Intravenous Solutions

➤ Examine and learn the names and contents of the isotonic solutions *first*. Then contrast the isotonic solution with the selected hypo- and hypertonic solutions.

| Hypotonic | Isotonic (290 mOs) | Hypertonic |
|---|---|---|
| 2.5% dextrose in water (2.5% DW) | 5% dextrose in water (D5W or 5DW) | 10% dextrose in water or (10DW) |
| 0.45% NaCl (sodium chloride) solution (0.45NS, $\frac{1}{2}$ NS, or $\frac{1}{2}$-strength NS) | Normal saline (NS) solution (0.9% NaCl solution) | 5DW in 0.45% NaCl solution or D5W in $\frac{1}{2}$ NS |
| | Lactated Ringer's solution (L/R, R/L, or LRS) | D5LR or D5RL solution |

**Figure 9-1.** Labels of isotonic solutions. **A,** 5% dextrose. **B,** 0.9% sodium chloride. **C,** Lactated Ringer's solution.

Additives such as vitamins, minerals, potassium chloride (KCl), and many other medications may be ordered for inclusion in these solutions. Figure 9-1 shows labels of selected isotonic solutions.

**1** Which type of solution most closely approximates the tonicity of plasma—hypotonic, isotonic, or hypertonic?

_____

**2** How does the percentage of solute in hypotonic and hypertonic solutions differ from that in isotonic solutions? (Give a brief answer.)

**Q:** *Ask Yourself*

**A:** *My Answer*

**FAQ** | *Why is $\frac{1}{2}$ NS labeled 0.45% rather than 0.5% NaCl?*

**ANSWER:** Because it contains half the NaCl content of NS solution. NS solution contains 0.9%, not 1%, NaCl.

➤ All IV solutions and medications must be checked for compatibility using a current drug reference before being administered. When in doubt, the nurse should consult the pharmacy. In some large agencies, the pharmacy has an IV telephone "hotline."

**1** What are five types of equipment needed for all IV infusions?

_____

**Q:** *Ask Yourself*

**A:** *My Answer*

## Intravenous Solution Volume

Volumes of solution per IV container are usually 500 or 1000 mL but can vary from less than 50 to more than 1000 mL. Some medicated solutions are provided in 100- and 250-mL containers. Volumes of 500 and 1000 mL are among the most frequently encountered for maintenance and continuous solutions.

If the order calls for a liter, the nurse selects a 1000-mL container. Often, the order for a continuous IV infusion states only the name of the solution and the flow rate per hour. The nurse selects the volume for the infusion that will last a reasonable amount of time.

➤ A superscript *o* may be seen on orders to designate *hour* (e.g., q8°). Do not use this notation. The *o* may be mistaken for a zero.

## Intravenous Solution Orders for Milliliters per Hour

➤ One calculation needed for *all* infusions is a determination of the number of milliliters per hour (mL/ hr).

The following are two typical orders for a *continuous* IV infusion:

| Order | Meaning |
|---|---|
| 1000 mL 5DW at 125 mL/ hr | 1 Liter of 5% dextrose in water to flow at a rate of 125 mL/ hour until further notice |
| 1 Liter L/R solution q8h | 1000 mL of lactated Ringer's solution every 8 hours |

• Identify the ordered flow rate in mL/ hr and any special instructions.
• Determine how long the IV solution will last.
  The calculations are usually very basic.
• If the prescriber orders D5W at 125 mL/ hr, the nurse administers a *continuous* flow rate of *125 mL/ hr* until the order is discontinued or changed. The equipment may vary and require further calculations, but the essential rate in mL/ hr must be known.
• If the prescriber orders 1 L D5W q8h, the flow rate is derived with a simple calculation:

$$\frac{mL}{hr} = \frac{1000\ mL}{8\ hr} = 125\ mL/\ hr$$

• Milliliters and hours are both desired in the answer. This distinguishes hours from minutes or other time frames that may be ordered. The *initial* entry in the equation setup is the matched units in the numerator (milliliters). Hours (hr) must be entered in a denominator.
• Round flow rates to the nearest whole number.

*Q: Ask Yourself*

*A: My Answer*

**1** What is the one calculation that is needed for all infusion rates?

_____

## Determining Infusion Durations

• If the order states *1 L q8h*, it is obvious that the IV infusion will require replacement in 8 hours. If the order states only the mL per hour, a simple calculation is required.

---

**EXAMPLES**

If the order states mL/ hr such as *120 mL/ hr,* and a Liter (1000 mL) will be supplied:

  **1** Determine the hours of duration first (total mL ÷ mL per hr)
  **2** Convert any remainder of hours to minutes using conversion formula: 60 minutes = 1 hr (60 × hr = minutes).

$$Hr = \frac{1\ hr}{120\ \cancel{mL}} \times 1000\ \cancel{mL} = 8.3\ hr$$

$$Minutes = \frac{60\ minutes}{1\ \cancel{hr}} \times 0.3\ \cancel{hr} = 18\ min$$

Total expected duration of 1000 mL flowing at 120/ hr = 8 hr and 18 min.

Experienced nurses use mental calculations and/or a calculator for this multiplication and division.

> Calculating the duration of an infusion helps the nurse to know when to prepare the subsequent infusion (i.e., *before* the current one runs dry) or when to discontinue the infusion. If an infusion runs dry, the site coagulates and the patient needs to have a new site established. This is very unpleasant for the patient and takes time that could be better spent on other nursing priorities.

**Clinical Relevance**

✶ **Communication**

After the nurse identifies the patient, she or he briefly explains the purpose for administering the IV solution: "Mr. Smith, your doctor has ordered some fluids and (name) medications in your vein to help your (state the condition)." It is better to say "help" than "prevent." Accentuate the positive. "Have you had an IV before? How did it go?" or "How did you do with them?" "Do you have any allergies to these medications or any other medications? What kind of reaction did you have?" *Listen carefully* to the patient's responses to these questions.

## Calculating Simple Milliliter per Hour (mL/ hr) Orders

Experienced nurses mentally calculate simple orders, such as 1 L q8h, by converting 1 L to 1000 mL and performing simple division, 1000 mL ÷ 8 (total volume of the container divided by hours), yields a flow rate of 125 mL/ hr.

> ➤ When the question is, How many mL/ hr, think of *per* as a *division line:* total milliliters ÷ total hours = $\frac{mL}{hr}$.

Check agency policy pertaining to IV solution, tubing, and needle replacement. Some solutions need to be changed every 24 hours, others every 48 hours. JCAHO regulations present replacement guidelines. The contents of solution are factors in the policies. The product label may indicate an expiration date.

**1** What are the abbreviations for three commonly ordered isotonic IV solutions?

_____

> ➤ With all patient communications it pays to *stop*, *look*, and *listen* and respond accordingly.

If you are comfortable with multiplication and division skills, use a calculator for multiplication and long division.

*Q:Ask Yourself*

*A:My Answer*

**RAPID PRACTICE 9-3**  Flow Rates and Infusion Times for Intravenous Solutions

**Estimated completion time: 15-20 minutes**  Answers on page **564**

**Directions:** *Using the flow rate supplied, fill in the abbreviations for the solution ordered, the flow rate in mL/ hr, the nearest whole number, and the infusion time in hours and minutes, if applicable. Use a calculator for long division and multiplication.*

| Order | Abbreviation(s) for Solution | Flow Rate (mL/ hr) | Infusion Time, Hours (and Minutes, If Applicable) |
|---|---|---|---|
| **1** Infuse 500 mL normal saline over 6 h | _____ | _____ | _____ |
| **2** 1000 mL 5% dextrose in water at 125 mL/ hr | _____ | _____ | _____ |
| **3** 1 L lactated Ringer's q10h | _____ | _____ | _____ |
| **4** 250 mL half-strength normal saline q4h | _____ | _____ | _____ |
| **5** 500 mL 5% dextrose in lactated Ringer's @40mL/ hr | _____ | _____ | _____ |

The commonly available solutions are packaged in amounts of 250, 500, and 1000 mL. Smaller amounts, including medicated solutions, are also supplied by the pharmacy. If the infusion is to last 8 hours and the flow rate is 100 mL/hr, 800 mL would be the minimum needed. The closest amount that can be selected would be a 1000 mL bag. If the solution is to infuse at 50 mL/hr continuously, most nurses will select a bag that contains at least enough to last for an 8- or 12-hour shift: 50 mL × 8 = 400 mL, or 50 mL × 12 = 600 mL. The nurse would probably select a 500 or 1000 mL bag even for the 50 mL/8 hr order, assuming that the IV infusion would be reordered.

## Intravenous Flow Rate Entries for Electronic Infusion Devices

When electronic controllers or pumps are used for IV infusion, the nurse must enter the ordered flow rate in mL/hr on the digital device. The LED screen displays the number of milliliters being infused per hour, the total number of milliliters that have been infused, and various other information, depending on the sophistication of the device (Figure 9-2).

For an order of 1000 mL q8h, the nurse would set up the equipment and enter a flow rate of 125 mL/hr. The volume already infused can be read on the LED screen, as shown in the photograph in Figure 9-3.

It is preferable to administer medicated solutions through EIDs. Critical care units do not usually use gravity infusions.

A                                    B

Figure 9-2. **A,** Single-channel electronic infusion pump. **B,** Dual-channel electronic infusion pump. (**A** from Perry AG, Potter PA: Clinical nursing skills and techniques, ed. 5 revised reprint, St. Louis, 2004, Mosby. **B** from Kee JL, Marshall SM: Clinical calculations: with applications to general and specialty areas, ed. 5, St. Louis, 2004, Saunders.)

Figure **9-3.** Plum A+® Medication Infusion System Pump. (From Hospira, Inc., Lake Forest, IL.)

# Gravity Infusions

Some agencies use simple gravity devices with manual rate controllers for temporary emergency purposes, for administering unmedicated solutions or less powerful medicated solutions, and for maintenance unmedicated IV therapy (Figure 9-4).

Figure **9-4.** Gravity IV infusion set. (From Clayton BD, Stock YN: Basic pharmacology for nurses, ed. 13, St. Louis, 2004, Mosby.)

Plastic bag

Primary port

Insertion spike

Macrodrip chamber

Roller clamp

Filter

Needle adapter and protective cap

Secondary port

Outpatient centers, emergency vehicles, outpatient recovery units, home-care settings, rehabilitation units, and long-term care units are examples of places where gravity devices may be encountered.

Gravity infusions are hung on a pole approximately 36 inches above heart level of the patient. The flow rate is dependent on the flow rate control clamp adjustment, positioning of the solution, tubing patency, and the patient's position.

## Intravenous Administration Sets

Intravenous tubing provides the connection between the IV solution and the patient. The nurse selects the tubing needed based on the order and the infusion equipment provided by the agency.

➤ The physician does not specify the equipment. Some tubing administration sets may be used interchangeably on infusion pumps and gravity devices. The tubing label describes the use. The containers are available in supply stations. The tubing is supplied in various widths to accommodate various flow rates and solution viscosities.

There are several types of specialized IV tubing. The main types include

- Primary (main) tubing for "main" and "maintenance" IV lines, EIDs, and gravity infusion devices
- Secondary, *shorter* tubing that connects to the primary tubing at a port to permit additional intermittent solutions to be added (piggybacked) without having to create a new injection site
- Blood administration sets with special filters and a Y connector for NS solution to prime the lines before and flush after blood transfusion or to use if the blood needs to be stopped or removed for any reason

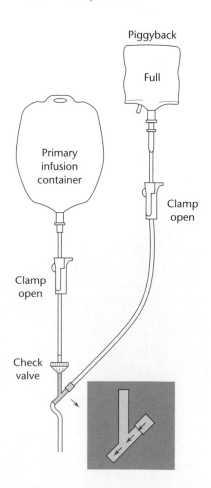

Figure 9-5. Primary and secondary administration set. The higher solution flows first. On gravity-dependent devices, the lower solution flows after the higher one is completed. (From Clayton BD, Stock YN: Basic pharmacology for nurses, ed. 13, St. Louis, 2004, Mosby.)

- Extension tubings that are used when more length is needed (e.g., for ambulation)

A needle adapter with a cap, tubing, a clamp to stop and start flow, a drip chamber, and an insertion spike are included in the administration sets (see Figure 9-4).

Figure 9-5 shows an example of a primary and a secondary administration set.

## Selection of Gravity Infusion Administration Sets

For gravity devices, the nurse selects the calibration of tubing needed based on the equipment available, the flow rate ordered, and the contents of the IV solution. The DF is available on the tubing administration set. Figure 9-6 illustrates a DF of 10 (10 drops/ mL).

*Macrodrip* (large-diameter) tubing, with a DF of 10, 15, or 20, is selected for unmedicated solutions, solutions requiring faster flow rates, and solutions that have less powerful medications (Figure 9-7, *A* and *B*).

*Microdrip* tubing (also known as pediatric tubing) has a DF of 60 and narrow tubing that delivers tiny drops from a *needle-like* projection to achieve 60 drops/ mL. Because of the projection, microdrip sets can be recognized at a glance without having to go to a supply room to check the DF (Figure 9-7, *C*).

Check agency policy for administration set selection protocols.

➤ Agency policies must be checked for regulations pertaining to choice of IV equipment. If a solution is medicated, it may be required to be on a volumetric pump.

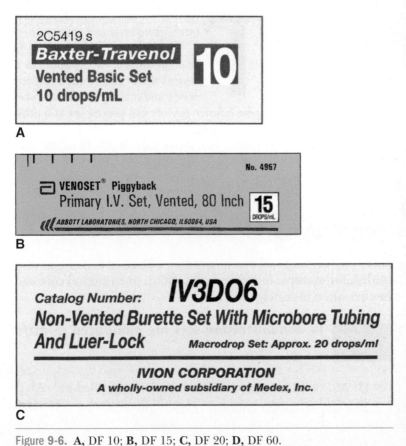

Figure 9-6. **A,** DF 10; **B,** DF 15; **C,** DF 20; **D,** DF 60.

**Figure 9-7.** Contrast the macrodrip chamber (**A-B**) with the microdrip chamber (**C**). (From Clayton BD, Stock YN: Basic pharmacology for nurses, ed. 13, St. Louis, 2004, Mosby.)

# Calculating Flow Rates for Gravity Infusion Devices

The flow rate for simple gravity devices that consist of only an IV solution and tubing is derived from the number of mL/hr ordered and is delivered in *drops per minute*. The drop-per-minute rate is calculated by the nurse. The nurse adjusts the flow rate with a hand-operated slide pinch or roller clamp (Figure 9-8).

To convert mL/hr to drops per minute, identify the following factors:

**1** Number of mL/hr ordered
**2** Calibration (DF, or drops per milliliter) of the selected tubing administration set, stated on the administration set package: 10, 15, 20, or 60.

When the drop-per-minute count is correct, the flow rate will deliver an *approximate equivalent* of the number of mL/hr ordered.

Figure 9-8. Nurse adjusting flow of IV infusion. (From Elkin MK, Perry AG, Potter PA: Nursing interventions and clinical skills, ed. 3, St. Louis, 2004, Mosby.)

Figure 9-9. Dial-a-Flo® extension set with pre-pierced Y site. (From Hospira, Inc., Lake Forest, IL.)

Some agencies provide a flow rate control device for gravity infusions such as the one shown in Figure 9-9. The Dial-a-Flo device is an example of an in-line apparatus that can be added to a gravity infusion set so that the number of *mL/hr* can be set on the dial and the number of drops per minute does not have to be calculated.

➤ Check calibrations on gravity flow rate devices. Dial-a-Flo provides a range from 5 to 250 mL/hr.

## Calculation of Gravity Infusion Rates

The key to rapid, accurate calculation of flow rates for gravity devices is to understand the underlying process. Once the method described in this section is thoroughly understood, faster methods will become apparent.

Ordered: IV D5W 1000 mL at 100 mL/ hr or 1 L D5W q10h. How many drops per minute will the nurse set on the gravity infusion set?

- Identify the *mL per hour* to be infused: D5W at 100 mL/ hr
- Identify the DF from the IV administration set.

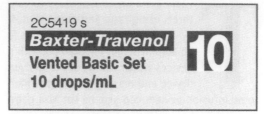

> Note that 10 drops/ mL × 100 mL/ hr ordered = 1000 drops/ hr. The nurse cannot count the drops for an hour to see if the rate is correct. The nurse wants to know the count for 1 minute that would result in the desired number of drops per hour.

- Enter the data in a DA equation along with an hr to min conversion.

All the data can be entered in *one* equation (when the number of mL/ hr is known) to obtain the number of drops per minute. Examine the example that follows.

## Calculation of Gravity Infusion Rates Using DA

Ordered: IV D5W 1000 mL at 100 mL/ hr, DF 10 (10 drops/ mL) on the tubing administration set. The nurse will set the flow rate for how many drops per minute?

| Step 1: Desired Answer Units | Step 2: DF Conversion Formula | Step 3: Original Factors to Convert (from the Order) | Step 4: Hours to Minutes Conversion Formula | Answer |
|---|---|---|---|---|
| $\dfrac{\text{drops}}{\text{min}}$ | $\dfrac{\overset{1}{\cancel{10}}\ \text{drops}}{1\ \text{mL}}$ | $\times\ \dfrac{100\ \text{mL}}{1\ \text{hr}}$ | $\times\ \dfrac{1\ \text{hr}}{\underset{6}{\cancel{60}}\ \text{min}}$ | $=\ \dfrac{100\ \text{drops}}{6\ \text{min}}$ |

$$= 16\tfrac{2}{3}\ \text{drops/ min, rounded to 17 drops/ min}$$

The completed equation looks like this:

$$\frac{\text{drops}}{\text{minute}} = \frac{\overset{1}{\cancel{10}}\ \text{drops}}{1\ \text{mL}} \times \frac{100\ \cancel{\text{mL}}}{1\ \cancel{\text{hr}}} \times \frac{1\ \cancel{\text{hr}}}{\underset{6}{\cancel{60}}\ \text{min}} = \frac{100}{6} = 16\tfrac{2}{3}\ \text{rounded to 17 drops/ min}$$

> Drops must be rounded to a whole number. They cannot be divided.

Evaluation: Equation is balanced. Only drops/ minute remain.

Analysis: First, drops must be entered in the equation from the DF to correspond to the desired answer units, with the accompanying denominator in milliliters. The ordered amount (mL/ hr) is entered and canceled. These calculations require an *hour* to *minute* conversion.

**Q**: *Ask Yourself*

**A**: *My Answer*

1   What are *abbreviations* for the entries for steps 2, 3, and 4 that can be obtained from the heading or the equation entries in the example shown above that will help me remember these steps?

**RAPID PRACTICE 9-4**   Calculating Flow Rates for Gravity Infusions Using
DA Equations

**Estimated completion time: 15 minutes**   Answers on page **564**

**Directions:** *Examine the example on p. 298 and the example in problem 1. For problems 2-5, identify the number of mL/ hr and the drop factor. Calculate the flow rates to the nearest whole drop per minute for the ordered solutions. Evaluate the equation. Use a calculator for long division and multiplication.*

➤   Remember that the DF is in drops per 1 mL. The DF and the number of mL/ hr ordered must be entered in the equation.

1   Ordered: IV 500 mL to infuse over 4 hours on a gravity infusion. Administration set DF: 15.

   **a.** How many mL/ hr are ordered? mL/ hr = 500 ÷ 4 = 125 mL/ hr
   **b.** How many drops per minute will be set?

   DA equation:

$$\frac{\text{drops}}{\text{minute}} = \frac{\overset{1}{\cancel{15}}\ \text{drops}}{1\ \cancel{mL}} \times \frac{125\ \cancel{mL}}{1\ \cancel{hour}} \times \frac{1\ \cancel{hour}}{\underset{4}{\cancel{60}}\ \text{min}} = 31.25,\ \text{rounded to 31 drops/ min}$$

   **c.** Evaluation: The equation is balanced. The desired answer units are the only ones remaining. (Milliliters and hours had to be entered twice in order to be canceled). All drops per minute equations use an hour-to-minutes conversion formula.

   ➤   Note that 500 mL was not needed in the equation because the mL/ hr was known.)

2   Ordered: IV 1000 mL q12h on a gravity infusion device. Administration set DF: 20.

   **a.** How many mL/ hr are ordered? _____
   **b.** How many drops per minute will be set? _____

   DA equation:


   **c.** Evaluation: _____

3   Ordered: IV 250 mL to infuse at 75 mL/ hr. Administration set DF: 10.

   **a.** How many mL/ hr are ordered? _____
   **b.** How many drops per minute will be set? _____

   DA equation:


   **c.** Evaluation: _____

4   Ordered: IV 500 mL to infuse over 6 hours. Administration set DF: 20.

   **a.** How many mL/ hr are ordered? _____
   **b.** How many drops per minute will be set? _____

   DA equation:


   **c.** Evaluation: _____

5 Ordered: IV 100 mL to infuse at 10 mL/ hr. The drop factor is 60.
  **a.** How many hours will it last? _____
  **b.** How many drops per minute will be set? _____
  DA equation:

  **c.** Evaluation: _____

## Estimating the Number of Drops per Minute for a Drop Factor of 60

Equations must be set up for DFs of 10, 15, and 20 and can be set up for DF 60.

➤ Drop factors of 60, for microdrip pediatric administration sets, do *not* require equations *when the number of mL/ hr is known.* Because a DF of 60 divided by 60 minutes provides a factor of 1, the number of mL/ hr = the number of drops per minute. Study the example that follows.

**EXAMPLES**

Ordered: IV 50 mL to infuse over 1 hour, with a DF of 60.

$$\frac{drops}{minute} = \frac{60 \ drops}{1 \ mL} \times \frac{50 \ mL}{1 \ hr} \times \frac{1 \ hr}{60 \ minutes} = 50 \ drops \ per \ minute$$

Note how the quantity 60 in the *numerator* and the quantity 60 in the *denominator* are canceled, leaving only the 50 mL/ hr. Thus, 50 mL/ hr = 50 drops/ min.

Microdrip (60 DF) flow rate in drops per minute = mL/ hr.

➤ 60 DF = mL/ hr applies only to *continuous infusions* or those that are to infuse for *60 minutes* or more

Study the explanations and equation above and the example worked out in Rapid Practice 9-4, Problem 1.

**Q: Ask Yourself**

1 How many drops per minute would I estimate if the infusion was ordered for 30 mL/ hr and the DF was 60?

**A: My Answer**

2 If the DF on the tubing administration is known to be 60 and the order is for 20 mL/ hr, how many drops per minute would I estimate for the gravity device?

➤ Microdrip tubing is used for low flow rates up to and including 60 drops/ min (60 mL/ hr). It is too difficult to count a faster drop flow than 1 drop/ sec, or 60 drops/ min.
➤ You will encounter the abbreviation gtts for the word drops in some written orders and printed literature.

**RAPID PRACTICE 9-5** Calculating Solution Flow Rates for EIDs and Macrodrip and Microdrip Gravity Devices Using DA-Style Equations

**Estimated completion time: 20-25 minutes**  Answers on page **565**

**Directions:** *Calculate the flow rate in mL/ hr or drops per minute. Use a calculator when needed. Round all mL/ hr and drops per minute to the nearest whole number. For credit, please label all answers in mL/ hr or drops per minute, as appropriate for the equipment available.*

1  Ordered: 600 mL NS q8h to be infused continuously on an EID.

   What flow rate will the nurse set? (Use simple arithmetic.) _____

2  Ordered: 500 mL D5W at 25 mL/ hr. Equipment: pediatric microdrip administration set for gravity infusion with a DF 60 (60 drops/ mL).

   **a.** What is the estimated flow rate? (Use mental calculation.) Label the answer.
   _____

   **b.** Calculated flow rate:

      DA equation:

   **c.** Evaluation: _____

3  Ordered: 1000 mL L/R at 80 mL/ hr. Equipment: gravity infusion with a DF of 10.

   **a.** Calculated flow rate:

      DA equation:

   **b.** Evaluation: _____
   **c.** Is the flow rate reasonable for counting drops per minute? (see p. 300)
      Yes or No? _____

4  Ordered: 250 mL 0.45NS at 25 mL/ hr. Equipment: gravity infusion set with macrodrip tubing, DF 15.

   **a.** Calculated flow rate:

      DA equation:

   **b.** Evaluation: _____
   **c.** Is the flow rate reasonable for counting drops per minute?
      Yes or No? _____

5  Ordered: 1000 mL 5LR at 100 mL/ hr. Equipment: gravity infusion set with macrodrip tubing, DF 20.

   **a.** Calculated flow rate:

      DA equation:

   **b.** Evaluation: _____
   **c.** Is the flow rate reasonable for counting drops per minute?
      Yes or No? _____

> **FAQ** | *What is the advantage of a Dial-a-Flo type rate control device (Figure 9-9, p. 297) over gravity infusion sets?*
>
> **ANSWER:** The nurse does not have to take time to calculate drops per minute. The Dial-a-Flo device takes care of that step when the precise mL/ hr from the order is entered. (These devices are not always supplied.)

➤ Remember that calculations of IV flow rates begin with examination of the prescriber's order to be able to determine milliliters for mL/ hr. IV calculations require this value, not just for further calculations, but also to evaluate flow rate at the bedside.

**Q:** *Ask Yourself*

**A:** *My Answer*

1 If a flow rate is 50 mL/ hr using a microdrip (pediatric) set, how many drops per minute will I set? (Use mental arithmetic.)

_____

2 Noting that the DF denotes the number of drops per milliliter, which of three *macrodrip* sets—10, 15, and 20—would deliver the largest drop and therefore be suitable for a fastest rate of flow or more viscous fluids, such as blood products?

_____

➤ Remember that the microdrip set is selected for flow rates up to 60 drops/ min.

## Counting Drops per Minute at the Bedside

The nurse counts the drops at eye level for 15 or 30 seconds or 1 minute, if it is a very slow rate, to ensure that the IV solution is flowing at the appropriate rate (Figure 9-10).

Figure **9-10.** IV sites, flow rates, and volume infused need to be assessed during each visit to the bedside. (From Perry AG, Potter PA: Clinical nursing skills and techniques, ed. 6, St. Louis, 2006, Mosby.)

**RAPID PRACTICE 9-6** Gravity Infusion Rates and DA Equations

**Estimated completion time: 20-25 minutes**  Answers on page **565**

**Directions:** *Use DA equations to calculate the flow rates. Remember that gravity infusion calculations include an "hour-to-minute" conversion. Use a calculator for long division and multiplication to solve the equations. Use mental calculations for continuous microdrip calculations. Refer to p. 300 for an explanation.*

1  Ordered: IV D5W (continuous) at 10 mL/ hr, DF 60.

   **a.** What flow rate will the nurse set? (Use mental calculation.) _____
   **b.** Is this a macrodrip or microdrip tubing factor? _____
   **c.** How can the nurse tell at a glance if a tubing factor is macro- or microdrip when it is infusing? _____

2  Ordered: IV D5NS at 100 mL/ hr, DF 10 administration set selected.

   **a.** Flow rate will be set at_____

   DA equation:

   **b.** Evaluation: _____

3  Ordered: IV LRS at 125 mL/ hr, DF 15 administration set selected.

   **a.** Flow rate will be set at _____

   DA equation:

   **b.** Evaluation: _____

4  Ordered: IV D10W at 75 mL/ hr, DF 20 administration set selected.

   **a.** Flow rate will be set at _____

   DA equation:

   **b.** Evaluation: _____

5  Ordered: IV 0.45% NaCl sol at 120 mL/ hr, DF 10 administration set selected.

   **a.** Flow rate will be set at _____

   DA equation:

   **b.** Evaluation: _____

1  What does the DF on the gravity tubing mean exactly in terms of a milliliter?

   _____

2  Which is the DF of the narrowest tubing that delivers the smallest drops and therefore delivers the greatest number of drops per milliliter?

   _____

**Q:** *Ask Yourself*

**A:** *My Answer*

**RAPID PRACTICE 9-7**   Gravity Infusion Rates for Continuous IV Infusions

**Estimated completion time: 15 minutes**   Answers on page **566**

**Directions:** *Calculate the IV flow rates. Use the simplified method for pediatric (microdrip) tubing if minutes equal 60. Verify with a DA equation.*

➤ Use the hourly volume or less to calculate the flow rate.

1 Ordered: 1000 mL D5W at 125 mL/ hr, DF 10.

   **a.** Flow rate: _____

    DA equation:

   **b.** Evaluation: _____

2 Ordered: 500 mL NS at 50 mL/ hr, DF 15.

   **a.** Flow rate: _____

    DA equation:

   **b.** Evaluation: _____

3 Ordered: 5RL 500 mL at 50 mL/ hr, DF 20.

   **a.** Flow rate: _____

    DA equation:

   **b.** Evaluation: _____

4 Ordered: 10DW 500 mL at 75 mL/ hr, DF 10.

   **a.** Flow rate: _____

    DA equation:

   **b.** Evaluation: _____

5 Ordered: 5LRS 250 mL at 40 mL/ hr, DF 60.

   **a.** Flow rate: _____

    DA equation:

   **b.** Evaluation: _____

# Intravenous Piggyback Solutions

For intermittent use, medicated piggyback solutions are often prepared in the pharmacy and supplied in small volumes of 50 or 100 mL to be administered through a secondary line for 20, 30, or 60 minutes (Figure 9-11). These solutions

**Figure 9-11.** Fifty milliliters of solution for IVPB infusion. (From Brown M, Mulholland JL: Drug calculations: process and problems for clinical practice, ed. 7, St. Louis, 2004, Mosby.)

frequently contain antibiotics that may be infused intermittently (e.g., q4h or q6h) to maintain therapeutic blood levels of the medication.

They are connected (piggybacked) to a primary line port through a shorter secondary tubing set. Most intermittent infusions will be administered over 30 or 60 minutes. However, the nurse must be prepared to know the math for 20- and 40-minute infusions.

## Calculating Flow Rates in Milliliters per Hour (mL/ hr) for Intravenous Piggyback Infusions to Infuse in Less than 1 Hour

EXAMPLES

Ordered: IVPB antibiotic 50 mL in 30 minutes. How many mL/ hr will be set on the EID? The equation will require a conversion formula from minutes to hours.

DA equation:

$$\frac{mL}{hr} = \frac{50\ mL}{\underset{1}{\cancel{30}\ min}} \times \frac{\overset{2}{\cancel{60}\ min}}{1\ hr} = 100\ mL/\ hr$$

Evaluation: The equation is balanced. It is logical that, to infuse 50 mL in 30 minutes, the rate would have to be set at 100 mL/ hr (60 min). The 60 min = 1 hr conversion is needed to convert the 30-min order to an hourly rate.

## Increasing Your Understanding of Calculations for Intermittent Small-Volume Intravenous Flow Rates on Electronic Infusion Devices

The flow rate for piggyback solutions is set in *mL/ hr* for EIDs.

1   If I drink 60 mL in 60 minutes, how much fluid will I have consumed in *30 minutes* if I had been sipping at the same rate for the entire time?

*Q: Ask Yourself*

*A: My Answer*

**2** If an IV antibiotic label states, "Infuse at 60 mL/ hr for 30 minutes," what volume will have been completed in an hour if the infusion "continued" for the hour?

**3** If an IV is to infuse at 20 mL/ hr for 30 minutes, how much fluid should infuse in *30 minutes?*

## Simplified Piggyback Calculations for Milliliter-per-Hour Settings

Because small-volume intermittent piggyback infusions are usually administered over 20, 30, or 60 minutes on a secondary IV line, the nurse can perform mental calculations to obtain the flow rate in mL/ hr. A simple DA equation can be employed for verification. No arithmetic is required for a 60-minute infusion.

➤ For 60-minute infusions, volume = milliliter-per-hour rate.
➤ For 30-minute infusions, *double* the amount of milliliters ordered for 30 minutes to obtain the 60-mL (hourly) rate
➤ For 20-minute infusions, *triple* the milliliter volume ordered for 20 minutes to obtain the 60-mL (hourly) rate.

Do not forget to check the infusion to be sure that the main IV line restarts after the 20-, 30-, or 60-minute period is completed. On some EIDs, each line is programmed separately. The nurse needs to confirm that the programming is accurate for both the primary and secondary solutions.

The IV infusion will be completed in the ordered time period. The nurse then ensures that the primary IV line resumes at its ordered rate.

➤ The flow rate for the IVPB line is set at what would have been the volume for 1 hour. That rate is often different from and may be faster than the primary IV infusion rate.

---

**EXAMPLES**

Primary rate: D5W continuous IV at 75 mL/ hr.

Piggyback rate: 50 mL over 20 minutes, or 150 mL/ hr.

Adjust the rate from 150 down to 75 mL/ hr when the piggybacked solution is finished. With some EID equipment, there are separate control devices for flow rates for primary and secondary lines.

---

**FAQ** | *Why are IVPB solutions given at different rates than the primary IV infusion?*

**ANSWER:** Effective treatment of resistant or acute conditions, such as acute infections or tumors, requires heavily concentrated infusions of drugs at periodic intervals to maintain therapeutic blood levels of the medication around the clock. These infusions must be given on time and are ordered at a specific rate to deliver the amount of drug for maximum effectiveness. It is important to change the flow rate for the medication if the order so indicates and to change the rate back to the primary rate when the intermittent infusion is completed. To do less imperils the patient's recovery. If the intermittent medicated solution is to be administered quickly and the primary solution is a maintenance IV infusion, failure to adjust the rates as required can result in fluid or medication underload or overload.

➤ The nurse's responsibility to adjust IV infusion flow rates is time-consuming and requires a variety of nursing skills: comprehension, calculation, organization, prioritization, vigilance, and focus.

## RAPID PRACTICE 9-8   Estimated Piggyback Flow Rate for Milliliters per Hour with DA Verification

**Estimated completion time: 30 minutes**   Answers on page **567**

**Directions:** *Examine the examples on p. 305 and in problem 1 below. For problems 2-5, use mental calculations to calculate the milliliters-per-hour setting on an EID for the piggybacked solution. Verify the calculation with a DA equation.*

**1** Ordered: 100 mL (IVPB) antibiotic over 30 minutes.

   **a.** Estimated flow rate in mL/ hr: <u>100 mL × 2, or 200 mL/ hr for 30 minutes</u>
   **b.** DA verification:

$$mL/ hr = \frac{100\ mL}{\underset{1}{\cancel{30\ min}}} \times \frac{\overset{2}{\cancel{60\ min}}}{1\ hour} = 200\ mL/ hr$$

   **c.** Evaluation: <u>The equation is balanced. The estimate supports the answer.</u>

**2** Ordered: 80 mL anti-cancer drug (IVPB) over 30 minutes.

   **a.** Estimated flow rate in mL/ hr: _____
   **b.** DA verification:



   **c.** Evaluation: _____

**3** Ordered: 50 mL antibiotic (IVPB) over 20 minutes.

   **a.** Estimated flow rate in mL/ hr: _____
   **h.** DA verification:



   **c.** Evaluation: _____

**4** Ordered: 30 mL antibiotic (IVPB) over 20 minutes.

   **a.** Estimated flow rate in mL/ hr: _____
   **b.** DA verification:



   **c.** Evaluation: _____

**5** Ordered: 25 mL anti-cancer drug (IVPB) over 30 minutes.

   **a.** Estimated flow rate in mL/ hr: _____
   **b.** DA verification:



   **c.** Evaluation: _____

**FAQ** | *Why is the DA verification needed if we can mentally calculate the flow rate for the IVPB solution?*

**ANSWER:** As with all other calculations, the nurse must be proficient in setting up the DA equation as a backup method in case an odd number of minutes is ordered, which would make a mental calculation difficult. Applying the DA setup to a variety of problems now and reviewing it periodically is necessary to *maintain* proficiency.

### Calculating Flow Rates for Piggyback Gravity Infusions in Drops per Minute to Infuse in Less than 1 Hour

Equations used to calculate IVPB infusions on *gravity* devices are very simple and *different* from other infusion equations: they do not use a milliliter-per-hour calculation.

If an IVPB order is for 50 mL over 30 minutes with a DF administration set of 10, the question to be solved by a DA equation is: *How many drops per minute will be set?*

EXAMPLES

$$\frac{\text{drops}}{\text{min}} = \frac{\overset{1}{\cancel{10}}\text{ drops}}{1\text{ }\cancel{mL}} \times \frac{50\text{ }\cancel{mL}}{\underset{3}{\cancel{30}}\text{ min}} = 16.6\text{, rounded to }17\text{ drops/ min}$$

Analysis: The desired answer units are drops per minute. Enter the drop factor with its accompanying milliliter unit first to match the desired answer numerator. The order to be converted is 50 mL over 30 minutes. There is *no need to enter hours* in the equation. The answer will *not* be in mL/ hr. Entry of the minutes unit is postponed until the entry of the denominator of the second fraction. Seventeen drops per minute will deliver 50 mL in 30 minutes.

## RAPID PRACTICE 9-9  IVPB Flow Rates Practice in Milliliters per Hour and Drops per Minute for Gravity Devices

**Estimated completion time: 15-25 minutes**    **Answers on page 567**

**Directions:** *Estimate the flow rate in mL per hour. Calculate the flow rate in drops/ minute to the nearest whole number for gravity devices. Use a calculator for long division and multiplication to solve the equations. Label answers.*

1  Ordered: IVPB antibiotic 50 mL over 20 minutes, DF 10.

   **a.** Estimated flow rate in mL/ hr: _____

   **b.** Flow rate in drops per minute: _____

    DA equation:

   **c.** Evaluation: _____

2  Ordered: IVPB antibiotic 100 mL over 30 minutes, DF 15.

   **a.** Estimated flow rate in mL/ hr: _____

   **b.** Flow rate in drops per minute: _____

    DA equation:

   **c.** Evaluation: _____

3  Ordered: IVPB anti-cancer drug 75 mL over 60 minutes, DF 20.

   **a.** Estimated flow rate in mL/ hr: _____

   **b.** Flow rate in drops per minute: _____

    DA equation:

   **c.** Evaluation: _____

4  Ordered: IVPB anti-infective drug 30 mL over 30 minutes, DF 60.

   **a.** Estimated flow rate in mL/ hr: _____

   **b.** Flow rate in drops per minute: _____

DA equation:

c. Evaluation: _____

5  Ordered: IVPB cortisone product 50 mL over 20 minutes, DF 10.

a. Estimated flow rate in mL/ hr: _____
b. Flow rate in drops per minute: _____

DA equation:

c. Evaluation: _____

# Regulating and Positioning Gravity Infusion Devices

Note the positioning of the primary and secondary IVPB solutions in Figure 9-12. The higher IV solution is currently infusing. When it is empty, the lower solution will resume infusing. At this point, the nurse will change the flow rate back to the primary flow rate if the secondary rate is different.

Figure 9-12. Gravity-flow IVPB. The IVPB is elevated above the existing IV solution, allowing it to infuse by gravity. (In Lilley LL, Harrington S, Snyder JS: Pharmacology and the nursing process, ed. 4, St. Louis, 2005, Mosby. From Rick Brady, Riva, MD.)

Solutions for gravity flow devices need to be 3 feet above the patient's heart level. The solution that is on "hold" is lowered *below* the solution that is to flow. A simple hanger extender device is used to accomplish this.

**RAPID PRACTICE 9-10**   Calculating IVPB Flow Rates for EID and Gravity Devices

**Estimated completion time: 15 minutes**   Answers on page **568**

**Directions:** *Fill in the following IVPB flow rate table with the needed flow rates in the spaces provided. Examine the example provided for the first entry. Label all answers in mL/ hr or drops/ minute, as needed.*

| IVPB Order and Equipment | Estimated Flow Rate (mL per hour) | Flow Rate Equation (in mL/ hr or drops/ min as needed) |
|---|---|---|
| **1** 50 mL antibiotic solution to infuse over 30 minutes on EID | 100 mL/ hr | $\dfrac{50 \text{ mL}}{\underset{1}{\cancel{30 \text{ min}}}} \times \dfrac{\overset{2}{\cancel{60 \text{ min}}}}{1 \text{ hr}} = 100 \text{ mL/ hr}$ |
| **2** 30 mL anti-cancer medication to infuse over 20 minutes on EID | _____ | _____ |
| **3** 20 mL antibiotic solution to infuse over 30 minutes on gravity infusion device DF 60 | _____ | _____ |
| **4** 60 mL antibiotic solution to infuse over 40 minutes on EID | _____ | _____ |
| **5** 25 mL antibiotic solution over 20 minutes on gravity infusion device DF 20 | _____ | _____ |

**RAPID PRACTICE 9-11**   Intravenous Infusion Practice

**Estimated completion time: 15 minutes**   Answers on page **569**

**Directions:** *Read the IV order and equipment available, and supply the infusion information in the spaces provided.*

| Order | Equipment Available | Continuous or Intermittent | Flow Rate Equation (Label Answer) |
|---|---|---|---|
| **1** 1000 mL D5W q10h | IV administration set DF 10 | _____ | _____ |
| **2** 50 mL antibiotic solution to infuse over 20 minutes | Volumetric pump | _____ | _____ |

| Order | Equipment Available | Continuous or Intermittent | Flow Rate Equation (Label Answer) |
|---|---|---|---|
| 3 250 mL D5W every 4 hr | Electronic rate controller | _____ | _____ |
| 4 500 mL NS every 6 hr | IV administration set DF 15 | _____ | _____ |
| 5 30 mL antibiotic solution to infuse over 30 minutes | Pediatric microdrip administration set | _____ | _____ |

The nurse always needs to know the ordered flow rate and must be able to verify that rate at the bedside, whether it is being administered on a volumetric pump or any other kind of equipment.

The prescriber orders mL/ hr, not drops per minute.

# Flow Rate Errors

Flow rates can get behind or ahead of schedule for many reasons:

- Positional dislodgement of the needle
- Movement of the patient
- Occlusion of the entry site
- Incorrect flow rate entry
- Administration of other fluids on a secondary line
- Incorrect positioning of the IV solutions
- Equipment failure
- Temporary discontinuance for travel to the x-ray or other department
- A change in flow rate orders by the prescriber since the nurse last checked for new orders

# Monitoring the Flow Rate on Infusion Devices

The nurse verifies the *ordered flow rate* by

- Reading the entry on the infusion pump
- Checking the rate controller on a gravity device
- Counting the drops on a gravity device and converting to mL/ hr
- Examining the timed tape, if present, on the solution container

**Clinical Relevance**

The patient and family need to be given a call bell, advised that the nurse will be checking in on them, and advised to call the nurse if an alarm device becomes activated. "There will be an alarm to warn us when the solution gets low," "Here is the call light," or "Call me if the solution stops dripping." It is a bad shift when an IV has to be restarted in another site because of coagulation from running dry. It is also a bad shift when the nurse finds that an IV that was supposed to infuse in 8 hours has infused in 2 hours. There is no need to warn the patient of all the malfunctions that can cause an alarm, such as air in the line and the like. If the patient has orders to leave the bed for any reason, tell the patient to call for assistance before getting out of bed until there is assurance the patient can move independently with the equipment. Remember that IV fluids will increase the need to urinate. Do not forget to ask, "Do you have any questions?"

➤ Each hour and during visits to the bedside, the IV site is examined and the solution is examined to ensure that the site is patent, the appropriate volume has been infused to date, and the rate is correct. Previous caretakers may have set incorrect rates. The nurse also needs to be aware that orders may be changed frequently by the prescriber.

## Timed Tapes

Timed tapes are placed on full IV solution containers by the nurse. The top calibration on the top of the tape is placed opposite the hanging fluid level, with the current time written next to it (Figure 9-13).

The nurse writes in the anticipated time the solution should reach the major volume calibrations based on the rate ordered. Examining a few timed tapes at the bedside provides a quick understanding of the information to be entered and the placement of the tape.

➤ A timed tape should be placed on all IV solution containers, both with electronic devices and with gravity devices, to further ensure that the volume infused matches the hourly ordered rate. The timed tape is very helpful but only if it is checked frequently as a rough gauge of fluid infused. Flow rate devices can fail. Check agency policies for timed tapes.

| **Clinical Relevance** | ➤ The nurse must be aware of the following *warnings about flow rate adjustments.* If the flow is deemed to be infusing too slowly or quickly, beware of "catching-up." There are no hard and fast rules about how much a flow rate can be adjusted to catch up to the ordered rate. The |

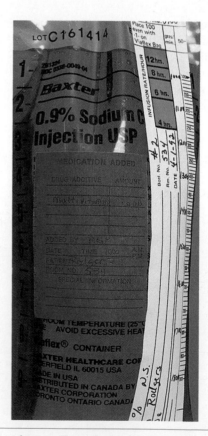

Figure **9-13.** IV bag with timed tape. (From Potter PA, Perry AG: Fundamentals of nursing, ed. 6, St. Louis, 2005, Mosby.)

safety of such adjustments depends on the patient's condition and the contents of the IV solution. Guessing is dangerous. Flow rates affect major organ function. Medicated IV solutions are prescribed to deliver drugs at a therapeutic rate. It may seem safe to lower an IV rate, but if there is a medication included, slowing the infusion may cause the patient to suffer from abrupt withdrawal. Check with the prescriber about any adjustments.

➤ The best way to keep IV flow rates on target is through knowledge of the ordered IV infusion rate and frequent monitoring, every hour and every visit.

➤ Check with the prescriber before speeding up an IV flow rate. Increasing the flow rate should be done gradually to ensure that the patient's condition does not suffer adverse effects.

➤ Never open up an IV line to full flow to catch up.

➤ Gravity flow rates are not stable. The tubing may become pinched; the clamp that regulates the flow may slip; or a positional change may cause a flow rate to increase, decrease, or halt. Educate the patient and family, if possible, to call for assistance if the flow rate stops or seems to be infusing too quickly. Volumetric pumps are more reliable than gravity infusion devices but not 100% reliable.

There have been incidents in which a patient or family member changed the setting on an EID. Also, staff on the previous shift may have entered the wrong setting.

## Calculating Milliliters per Hour from Drops per Minute on Gravity Devices at the Bedside

As mentioned before, the *ordered* flow rate is in mL/ hr, not drops/ minute.

When caring for patients whose IV infusions have been initiated by someone else—a previous caretaker—the currently assigned nurse must verify during each visit that the flow rate is as ordered. For example, a nurse visits the bedside and notes that a gravity device has been used. She or he will count the current drop-per-minute flow rate. At that point, the nurse has two choices for verifying that *ordered flow rate* is infusing:

1  Calculate the derived flow rate in drops/ minute from the mL/ hr order and compare it to the current drops-per-minute flow rate.
2  Calculate the milliliters-per-hour flow rate from the current flow.

The nurse must be able to perform both calculations. A prescriber may ask at the bedside, "What is the current flow rate?," and will want the answer in mL/ hr.

By counting the current flow rate in drops/ minute, the nurse can verify the flow rate in mL/ hr.

---

**EXAMPLES**

An IV is infusing at 30 drops/ min. The DF is 20. How many mL/ hr are being infused at this rate?

$$\frac{mL}{hr} = \frac{1\ mL}{\underset{2}{\cancel{20\ drops}}} \times \frac{\overset{3}{\cancel{30\ drops}}}{1\ min} \times \frac{60\ \cancel{min}}{1\ hr} = \frac{180}{2} = 90\ mL/\ hr$$

Evaluation: The equation is balanced. Only mL per hr remains.

Analysis: The number of drops per minute and the DF are the known data. (Most agencies buy one brand of administration sets in bulk. The nurse learns the DFs for the main equipment used in the agency during orientation and initial observation of the tubing set labels.) The DF must be entered in the DA equation along with the number of drops per minute. If *hour* is needed in the *answer*, the conversion *60 minutes = 1 hour* is required in the equation to convert minutes to hours.

**RAPID PRACTICE 9-12** Calculating Flow Rates in Milliliters per Hour for Gravity Infusions

**Estimated completion time: 20-30 minutes** Answers on page **569**

**Directions:** *Calculate mL/ hr from the drops per minute flowing on the gravity device. Use a calculator for long division and multiplication to solve the equations. Label all answers.*

| Drops/Sec Counted at Bedside | Drops/ Min (Mental Calculation) | Administration Set DF | Flow Rate Equation |
|---|---|---|---|
| 10 drops/ 15 sec | 40 (10 × 4) | 20 | $\dfrac{mL}{hr} = \dfrac{1\ mL}{\cancel{20\ drops}_{1}} \times \dfrac{40\ \cancel{drops}}{1\ \cancel{min}} \times \dfrac{\cancel{60\ min}^{3}}{1\ hr} = 120\ mL/\ hr$ |
| 8 drops/ 30 sec | _____ | 10 | |
| 6 drops/ 15 sec | _____ | 60 | |
| 12 drops/ 30 sec | _____ | 15 | |
| 15 drops/ 30 sec | _____ | 60 | |

# Setting the Alarm for Intravenous Equipment

EIDs have a variety of safety alarm settings, depending on the sophistication of the device. In addition to setting the flow rate in mL/ hr, the nurse programs the volume that will generate an alarm to give notice that the current infusion is almost finished. This warning serves several functions:

- The nurse has warning time to prepare a subsequent solution, if ordered.
- The IV line is prevented from running dry.
- The entry site will maintain patency and will not become coagulated.
- The patient will not have to be subjected to another injection for a new site because of clot formation.
- Medications and fluids will be delivered at the scheduled time.

Maintaining patency means safety and comfort for the patient, on-time delivery of fluids and medications, and time saved for the nurse.

# Calculating the Volume for a "Volume to be Infused" Alarm

Setting the advance warning alarm time is simple. Usually, the nurse programs the alarm to sound based on three criteria:

How many hours will the IV solution be infused and at what rate?
How much notice does the nurse need or want in order bring the next infusion container and equipment, such as new tubing, that may be needed?
How many milliliters will have been infused by the time the nurse wants the alarm to sound?

➤ The nurse does not enter the entire volume to be infused. That would prevent advance warning time.

A rough guideline for determining the volume at which the alarm should sound is to subtract 50 mL from the total volume in the bag for faster infusion rates and 25 mL for slower flow rates. This guideline should be adjusted for other volumes, for low volumes or very slow volumes, or for very rapid rates. Experience, preference, and work load help the nurse to determine how much warning is needed.

**EXAMPLES**

For a total IV infusion volume of 1000 mL,

| Infusion Rate | Amount to Subtract from Total Volume | Volume to Be Infused for Alarm to Sound |
|---|---|---|
| 150 mL/ hr | 50 mL | 950 mL |
| 75 mL/ hr | 25 mL | 975 mL |

✳ **Communication**

"Mr. and Mrs. Smith, I have set an alarm to let me know when the IV needs replacement. Please use the call bell to reach me if you have any concerns about the solution running out or if the flow stops or your arm hurts."

➤ With or without an alarm, the nurse needs to develop a reminder for the anticipated time at which to prepare the next container. Some nurses tune out alarms because they sound too often from various rooms.

1 If the flow rate was very rapid, would I want the alarm to sound earlier or later than average?

Q: *Ask Yourself*

A: *My Answer*

➤ Disposal of IV tubing, needles, and sponges according to the guidelines and policies of the clinical agency and the federal Occupational Safety and Health Administration is a critical safety issue. Special hazardous waste containers must be used, and special care must be taken to avoid leaving any contaminated equipment at or in the bedside furnishings. Doing so could cause a needle-stick injury or bodily fluid exposure to a staff member at bedside or during transport for disposal.

## RAPID PRACTICE 9-13    Intravenous Infusion Review

**Estimated completion time: 10-20 minutes**    Answers on page **570**

**Directions:** *Study the previous material and supply the requested information pertaining to basic IV infusions:*

1 Intravenous flow rates are usually ordered in which of the following terms:

_____

**1.** Drops per minute
**2.** mL/ hr

**3.** Liters per minute
**4.** Liters per hour

2 How does the nurse determine the number of drops per milliliter for a gravity IV infusion line? _____

    **1.** Refer to relevant IV pharmacology references.
    **2.** Call the agency pharmacist or consult a wall chart on the unit.
    **3.** Ask an experienced nurse on the unit.
    **4.** Read the DF on the IV administration set container.

3 An example of an order indicating that a continuous IV infusion solution is to be started on a patient would be _____

    **1.** Ampicillin 2 g IVPB q6h     **3.** 5DW 1 L q8h at 50 mL/ hr
    **2.** Pantoprazole 40 mg IV push daily     **4.** Lorazepam 1 mg IV push

4 An IV device that permits the patient to control and administer an intermittent medicated (analgesic) solution for pain relief is called _____

    **1.** IV push     **3.** IV Piggyback
    **2.** PCA     **4.** TKO

5 A reasonable short-term IV maintenance rate for an NPO adult patient in good health would be _____

    **1.** 300 mL/ hr     **3.** 75-125 mL/ hr
    **2.** 150-200 mL/ hr     **4.** 10-20 mL/ hr

---

**RAPID PRACTICE 9-14**    Gravity Device Flow Rate Practice

**Estimated completion time: 20-25 minutes**    Answers on page **570**

**Directions:** *Assume that all the continuous IV infusions ordered in problems 1-5 are to be administered with gravity equipment. Calculate the flow rates as requested. Use a calculator for long division and multiplication.*

1 Ordered: IV D5W 1000 mL at 150 mL/ hr

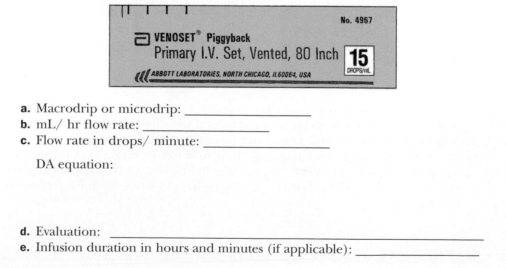

    **a.** Macrodrip or microdrip: _____
    **b.** mL/ hr flow rate: _____
    **c.** Flow rate in drops/ minute: _____

    DA equation:

    **d.** Evaluation: _____
    **e.** Infusion duration in hours and minutes (if applicable): _____

**2** Ordered: IV (D5LR) 500 mL q10h

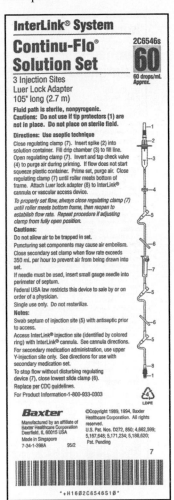

**a.** Macrodrip or microdrip: _____

**b.** Estimated flow rate in drops/ minute: _____

DA equation:

**c.** Evaluation: _____

**3** Ordered: IV D5NS 1000 mL q8h

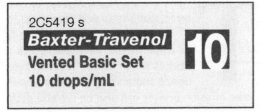

**a.** Macrodrip or microdrip: _____

**b.** Flow rate in drops/ minute: _____

DA equation:

**c.** Evaluation: _____

**4** Ordered: IVPB of 40 mL to infuse in 1 hour (an intermittent IV)

**a.** Macrodrip or microdrip: _____

**b.** Flow rate in drops/ minute: _____

DA equation:

**c.** Evaluation: _____

**5** Ordered: IV of 100 mL to infuse in 1 hour

Catalog Number: **IV3DO6**
**Non-Vented Burette Set With Microbore Tubing And Luer-Lock**    Macrodrop Set: Approx. 20 drops/ml

**IVION CORPORATION**
**A wholly-owned subsidiary of Medex, Inc.**

**a.** Macrodrip or microdrip: _____

**b.** Flow rate in drops/ minute: _____

DA equation:

**c.** Evaluation: _____

1   Can I write the four drop factors for gravity infusions, starting with the microdrip?

_____

**RAPID PRACTICE 9-15**    Distinguishing Flow Rates for Infusion Pumps and Microdrip-Macrodrip Gravity Infusion Devices

**Estimated completion time: 25 minutes**   Answers on page **571**

**Directions:** _Read the type of equipment that will be used: pump or gravity infusion device. Determine whether the flow rate will be set and monitored in mL/ hr or drops per minute. Determine the flow rate in mL/ hr. Calculate the flow rate in drops per minute if necessary. Round the answer to nearest whole number. Label all answers in mL/ hr or drops per minute, as appropriate._

1   Ordered: 1000 mL D5LR q12h. Equipment: gravity device with tubing DF 15.

   **a.** The nurse will set and monitor the flow rate at _____

   DA equation:



   **b.** Evaluation:  _____

2   Ordered: 500 mL L/R q4h. Equipment: infusion pump.

   **a.** The nurse will set and monitor the flow rate at _____

   DA equation:



   **b.** Evaluation:  _____

3   Ordered: 1000 mL D5W q8h. Equipment: gravity device with tubing DF 10 and Dial-a-Flo device.

   **a.** The nurse will set and monitor the flow rate in mL per hr at _____

   DA equation:



   **b.** Evaluation:  _____

4   Ordered: 250 mL NS q6h. Equipment: gravity device with tubing DF 20.

   **a.** The nurse will set and monitor the flow rate at _____

   DA equation:



   **b.** Evaluation:  _____

5   Ordered 1 L $\frac{1}{2}$ NS q24h. Equipment: gravity device with tubing DF 60.

   **a.** The nurse will set and monitor the flow rate at _____

   DA equation:



   **b.** Evaluation:  _____

**RAPID PRACTICE 9-16** Estimating Flow Rates in Milliliters per Hour for Intermittent IVPB Infusions Review

**Estimated completion time: 10 minutes** Answers on page **571**

**Directions:** *Estimate the hourly flow rate in mL/ hr. Assume that all solutions will be infused on an infusion pump. Perform a DA calculation to verify problem 5. Refer to pp. 305-306 for examples.*

| IV Solution Volume and Ordered Duration | Estimated Flow Rate (mL/ hr) |
|---|---|
| 1  25 mL to infuse in 30 min | |
| 2  50 mL to infuse in 20 min | |
| 3  60 mL to infuse in 60 min | |
| 4  100 mL to infuse in 60 min | |
| 5  75 mL to infuse in 40 min (estimate 20-min rate and divide in half) | |

    **a.** DA equation verification for problem 5:

    **b.** Evaluation:

## "To Keep Open" Flow Rates

The order "To keep open" indicates the slowest rate that can be infused when the goal is to have a patent's line available for potential future use. More frequently, prescribers order an indwelling injection port known as a "lock" or "heplock." Infusions, syringes, and long, straight infusion lines can be connected to an indwelling capped cannula or needle only when needed. The lock is flushed with saline or heparin solution to prevent clotting. It is accessed for IV solutions when needed. The IV lock provides convenience and more mobility for the patient.

# Calculating Grams of Solute in Intravenous Solutions

➤ As stated in Chapter 1, % means "per 100."

Using 5% DW as an example, the percentage of dextrose in solution means 5 g dextrose per 100 mL.

## Calculating Total Grams of Solute in a Solution

➤ To determine total grams of solute in a solution, given the percentage, change the percentage value to grams per 100 mL and multiply that fraction form by the total volume in milliliters.

Formula: g in solution = number of $\dfrac{g}{100\ mL}$ × total volume in mL = g in total volume.

---

Question: How many grams of dextrose are in the following solution: 5% DW in 1000 mL?

$$g = \frac{5\ g}{\underline{100\ mL}} \times \overset{10}{\underline{1000\ mL}} = 50\ g\ dextrose$$

Evaluation: The equation is balanced. The equation eliminates milliliters so that only grams remain.

> **EXAMPLES**

---

Question: How many grams of sodium are in the following solution: 500 mL NS solution (0.9%NaCl)?

$$g - \frac{0.9\ g}{\underline{100\ mL}} \times \overset{5}{\underline{500\ mL}} = 0.9 \times 5 = 4.5\ g\ sodium$$

Evaluation: Equation is balanced. Only grams remain.

> **EXAMPLES**

---

➤ Remember to make the decimal points prominent so they are not missed in calculations.

## RAPID PRACTICE 9-17   Calculating Grams of Dextrose and Sodium in IV Solutions

**Estimated completion time: 10 minutes**   Answers on page **572**

**Directions:** *Calculate the total number of grams of solute in the IV solution supplied. Write a DA equation. Then verify your answer using a calculator.*

1 Solution: 1 L of 10% DW

    **a.** What is the total number of grams of dextrose? _____

      DA equation:

    **b.** Evaluation: _____

2 Solution: 1.5 L of 5% D/RL.
   a. What is the total number of grams of dextrose? _____

      DA equation:

   b. Evaluation: _____

3 Solution: 3 L 5% D/NS.
   a. What is the total number of grams of dextrose? _____

      DA equation:

   b. Evaluation: _____

4 Solution: 2 L 10% D/RL.
   a. What is the total number of grams of dextrose? _____

      DA equation:

   b. Evaluation: _____

5 Solution: 500 mL $\frac{1}{2}$ NS.
   a. What is the total number of grams of sodium chloride (NaCl)? _____

      DA equation:

   b. Evaluation: _____

**Q:** *Ask Yourself*

**A:** *My Answer*

1 Which one of the IV solutions in Rapid Practice 9-17 is a hypotonic solution?

_____

## A Word about Potassium Chloride

Potassium chloride (KCl) is ordered to be added to many primary IV solutions, particularly for patients who are NPO. It has been identified by the Institute for Safe Medication Practices as a high-risk medication, meaning that it has high potential to cause adverse effects. For safety reasons, many agencies do not carry KCl ampules on the units. The pharmacy prepares the solution, or a premixed (diluted) solution is used.

➤ Consult agency and JCAHO guidelines regarding IV potassium administration. Following are some of the key considerations the nurse should keep in mind:

   • The *amount* ordered
   • The *concentration* ordered
   • The *SDR* and *dilutions* recommended in the literature
   • The *rate* ordered and the *rate* recommended in the literature

- Results of the patient's most recent *serum potassium* levels
- Results and implications of the patient's most recent *renal function* tests, including serum creatinine and BUN
- Results and implications of physical assessment for side effects of too little (hypokalemia) or too much potassium (hyperkalemia)

Potassium is never administered undiluted in an IV. Even if it is to be added to a large-volume IV, measures must be taken to ensure that it is well mixed with the IV fluid before it gets into the tubing.

If added by the nurse, it is usually added to a full bag of the main IV solution after the main solution is *removed* from the IV pole with the tubing temporarily clamped. It is then thoroughly mixed with the main solution so that the KCI does not proceed undiluted into the IV tubing. Do not inject directly into a *hanging* solution. Monitor the flow rate very closely.

➤ If KCI is administered undiluted, it can cause tissue necrosis, vessel damage, and cardiac arrest. Too rapid a flow of diluted KCl can also cause cardiac arrest.

➤ Administering KCI preparations safely requires further study, supervision, and experience.

# Intravenous Intermittent Solution Delivery Systems

Intermittent solutions, usually medicated, may be delivered in five ways: (1) IV piggyback solutions, which have already been studied, (2) volume-control devices, (3) IV (direct) push with a syringe, (4) syringe pumps, or (5) PCA pumps.

There is a trend toward using more manufacturer-prepared IV medication systems. An example of a pre-prepared piggyback IV solution container and medication is the Hospira Add-Vantage® with a drug vial of vancomycin (Figure 9-14) and the Hospira Add-Vantage® System (Figure 9-15).

## Volume-Control Device (Calibrated Burette Chamber)

When there is a need to protect the patient from a possible *fluid or medication overload*, a simple volume-control device may be placed between the main IV container and the drip chamber (Figure 9-16). If the volume-control device is being used for medication administration, the solutions in the primary bag and the medication must be checked for compatibility.

*Continued on p. 325*

Figure **9-14.** Hospira ADD-Vantage® with a drug vial of vancomycin. (From Hospira, Inc., Lake Forest, IL.)

# ADD–Vantage® System
### As Easy as **1, 2, 3**

## 1 Assemble ———————— Use Aseptic Technique

Swing the pull ring over the top of the vial and pull down far enough to start the opening. Then pull straight up to remove the cap. Avoid touching the rubber stopper and vial threads.

Hold diluent container and gently grasp the tab on the pull ring. Pull up to break the tie membrane. Pull back to remove the cover. Avoid touching the inside of the vial port.

Screw the vial into the vial port until it will go no further. Recheck the vial to assure that it is tight. Label appropriately.

## 2 Activate ——— Pull Plug/Stopper to Mix Drug with Diluent

Hold the vial as shown. Push the drug vial down into container and grasp the inner cap of the vial through the walls of the container.

Pull the inner plug from the drug vial; allow drug to fall into diluent container for fast mixing. Do not force stopper by pushing on one side of inner cap at a time.

Verify that the plug and rubber stopper have been removed from the vial. The floating stopper is an indication that the system has been activated.

## 3 Mix and Administer ——— Within Specified Time

Mix container contents thoroughly to assure complete dissolution. Look through bottom of vial to verify complete mixing. Check for leaks by squeezing container firmly. If leaks are found, discard unit.

Pull up hanger on the vial.

Remove the white administration port cover and spike (pierce) the container with the piercing pin. Administer within the specified time.

For more information on Advancing Wellness with ADD-Vantage® family of devices, contact your Hospira representative at **1-877-9467(1-877-9Hospira)** or visit **www.Hospira.com**

©Hospira, Inc. - 275 North Field Drive, Lake Forest, IL 60045       6-131-1-Nov, 04

Figure **9-15.** Hospira ADD-Vantage® System. (From Hospira, Inc., Lake Forest, IL.)

Figure 9-16. Volume-control device. (From Perry AG, Potter PA: Clinical nursing skills and techniques, ed 6, St. Louis, 2006, Mosby.)

The calibrated chamber, which usually holds 100 to 150 mL, will be filled with a limited specific amount of the primary IV solution or with a medication. A *clamp above the chamber* to the main IV line *will be closed*. This system may be used for pediatric and other at-risk patients. Burettes have a DF of 60, so 1 mL = 1 drop.

➤ Agencies specify the *maximum amount* of fluid that may be placed in the burette at any one time: *1 to 2 hours' worth at the ordered flow rate*. Medications placed in the burette will need to be diluted according to the manufacturer's guidelines for IV infusion. Flushing procedures before and after administering medications with the device must be followed according to policy, and comprehensive labels stating date, time, medication contents, and flow rate need to be employed. The nurse opens the clamp to refill the calibrated chamber as needed.

➤ The nurse must have a system in place for the timing of the refill. If the chamber empties and the clamp to the primary bag is closed, the IV site will coagulate.

1 If the ordered flow rate is 15 mL/ hr for a baby and the agency policy is a limit of 2 hours' worth of volume in the volume-control device, what is the maximum number of milliliters that may be placed in the device?

**Q** *Ask Yourself*

**A** *My Answer*

## Intravenous (Direct) Push

IV push medications are very small-volume medications administered one time only or intermittently with a syringe directly into a vein or into an infusion line port closest to a vein (Figure 9-17). Many of these medications must be diluted in a small volume of a specific diluent, and all must be administered at a controlled rate. In large agencies, the pharmacy will specify these instructions. If they are not available, the nurse must check with an appropriate pharmacology reference or the pharmacist for dilution and rate instructions. IV push calculations are covered in more detail in Chapter 10.

**Figure 9-17.** **A,** IV push with needleless syringe. **B,** Injection into port. (**A** from Elkin MK, Perry AG, Potter PA: Nursing interventions and clinical skills, ed. 3, St. Louis, 2004, Mosby. **B** from Potter PA, Perry AG: Fundamentals of nursing, ed. 6, St. Louis, 2005, Mosby.)

## Syringe Pump

Syringe pumps are electronic or battery-operated devices that use positive pressure and a plunger to deliver a specific programmed amount of a smaller-volume medicated or unmedicated IV solution over a specific period of time. Tubing from the syringe is connected to an access device, such as a port (Figure 9-18).

**Patient-Controlled Analgesia (PCA) Pump.** A PCA pump is an IV infusion syringe pump device connected to an indwelling line and programmed by the nurse to deliver pain medication in prescribed small increments at programmed intervals with lockout periods to prevent overdoses (Figure 9-19).

**Figure 9-18.** Freedom 60 syringe infusion pump system. (From Repro-Med Systems, Inc., Chester, NY.)

**Figure 9-19.** LifeCare® PCA 3 Infusion System. (From Hospira, Inc., Lake Forest, IL.)

Figure **9-20.** The nurse instructs the patient on the use of a PCA pump remote control device. (From Lilley LL, Harrington S, Snyder JS: Pharmacology and the nursing process, ed. 4, St. Louis, 2005, Mosby.)

The patient pushes a button on a small remote control device that releases boluses of medication into the established I.V. line. A small basal (continuous) rate of the medication *may* be programmed to be administered continuously between boluses (Figure 9-20).

A sample order for a programmed dose regimen for a patient with pain would be:

> *Initial bolus: morphine 2 mg*
> *Incremental dose: morphine 1 mg*
> *Lockout (delay time) interval: 15 minutes*
> *Basal rate: 0 mg/hr*
> *One-hour limit: 4-6 mg (permits prn bolus)*
> *PRN bolus: 2 mg q4h*

The pharmacy provides a prefilled syringe with the analgesic. The nurse places the pump on an established continuous-flow IV line with a compatible solution, inserts the syringe in the pump, programs the orders, and monitors the use and effectiveness of the dose.

The PCA pump gives control of pain to the patient, relieves anxiety about having to wait for medication, provides a steadier degree of pain relief, and is thought to result in overall reduced total usage of analgesics. Assessments of the pump readouts of the number of attempts made, amounts used, and relief obtained are usually recorded hourly.

The nurse replaces the prefilled syringe cartridges as needed.

## Administration of Blood

- There are many steps in the protocols for blood administration. The agency procedures must be followed scrupulously by a registered nurse to avoid a potentially very serious adverse event.
- Blood is administered only after a primary line is established with NS solution on Y tubing with a blood administration set for a pump as shown in Figure 9-22 (or a gravity device) (Figures 9-21 and 9-22).

➤ The usual initial flow rate for a unit of blood is 2 mL/min for the first 15 to 30 minutes. Check agency policies. The nurse is required to be present for the initial part of the transfusion for a specified time period in case of adverse reaction.

Figure 9-21. Blood administration setup with Y-tubing. (From Perry AG, Potter PA: Clinical nursing skills and techniques, ed. 5, St. Louis, 2004, Mosby.)

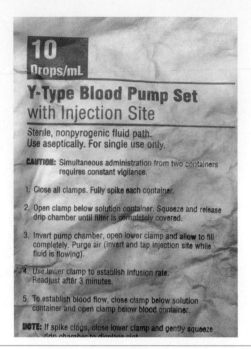

Figure 9-22. Y-type blood pump set,10 drops/ mL. (From Macklin D, Chernecky C, Infortuna H: Math for clinical practice, ed. 1, St. Louis, 2005, Mosby.)

A unit of whole blood is often administered without the plasma. Without plasma, the unit "packed cells" contains about 250 mL. With plasma, the amount will be closer to 500 mL.

➤ Agency protocols must be consulted for patient identification, patient care, blood storage and administration, disposal of used blood transfusion equipment, and actions to take should a suspected adverse event occur.

---

**FAQ** | *What should I do if ordered IV fluids are delayed, behind schedule, or have been infusing too fast?*

**ANSWER:** It takes a lot of nursing experience to make safe adjustments. Unfortunately, there is neither a simple answer nor a magic formula. Guidelines that state that the remaining fluid needs to be recalculated to make the IV finish on time are unsafe if taken at face value. IV infusions need to be monitored hourly or more often. Inexperienced nurses and those with any doubts should always consult with the prescriber.

---

| Question | Some Considerations |
|---|---|
| Is there medication in the solution? | Adjustments need to be made in consultation with the prescriber. There may be adverse consequences for underdose or sudden overdose and a need for remedial orders. |
| Has there been a significant drop or increase in percentage of IV infused? Over what time period? Was the ordered flow rate, slow or rapid? | Consult with the prescriber. When the ordered flow rate is particularly slow or rapid, there is a medical reason that will make it necessary to consult with the prescriber for adjustment. |
| How much time remains in the IV schedule? | Can a loss possibly be corrected gradually with the next infusion? |

| Question | Some Considerations |
|---|---|
| Is this an at-risk patient? Dehydrated, frail, poor heart, lung, or renal function? | Consult the prescriber. |
| When was volume infused last monitored? | A significant change over an unknown time period requires consultation with the prescriber. |
| What was the purpose of the solution? Maintenance? Replacement? | These issues affect urgency of corrective actions (e.g., hydration status of the patient). |
| Have intake and output been adversely affected? | Assess and then consult with the prescriber. |
| Is the site patent? | The line may have to be changed before any decision is made about fluid rate changes. |
| Is there a positional problem with a gravity infusion? | This can be adjusted and calls attention to the need for more frequent monitoring in addition to patient or family teaching, if applicable. |
| Is anyone tampering with the flow rate? | Not a frequent occurrence but can happen and will need to be documented and reported. |

Measures to prevent a flow rate error recurrence need to be put in place. The nurse cannot legally prescribe medications and flow rates unless the physician writes an order to titrate the drug.

➤ Above all, the nurse cannot "open up" the infusion line to try to catch up the flow rate in a few minutes at the bedside. This is a totally unsafe practice that has, unfortunately, been followed.

An adult patient with good cardiac, lung, and renal function receiving an unmedicated IV infusion of 75-125 mL/ hr can probably tolerate a small increase in rate without difficulty. If it is considered necessary by the prescriber to have the infusion complete on time, the calculation is very basic: Divide the remaining solution by the remaining number of hours as if it were a new IV infusion. Evaluate the difference in rate between the order and the new rate.

**EXAMPLES**

Ordered: 1000 mL D5W at 100 mL/ hr. Total duration: 10 hr. Start time: 1200. Scheduled end time: 2200.

| Remaining mL at 1800 | Remaining Hours | New Flow Rate |
|---|---|---|
| 600 mL | ÷ 4 hr | = 150 mL/ hr |

Do not forget to document the assessments and actions.

**Clinical Relevance**

Obtaining an order to change from 100 to 150 mL/ hr would be mandatory. Increases in rate need to be gradual to reduce physiological stress on the patient. Slowing down medicated IV infusions also often needs to be gradual. Remember the 75-125mL/ hr average figure cited at the beginning of the chapter. During the infusion and on completion, assess the patient for signs of fluid overload—shortness of breath, bounding pulse, moist lung sounds, and complaints of discomfort—and document the findings.

**RAPID PRACTICE 9-18** Calculating Catch-up Flow Rates

**Estimated completion time: 25 minutes**   Answers on page 572

**Directions:** *Calculate the new flow rate based on the remaining number of milliliters of infusion and the remaining hours to be infused. Assume that the solutions are unmedicated and that the prescriber has confirmed the catch-up or slowdown.*

**Note:** *The timed tape on the solution bag is useful.*

1  Started at 0700 hrs: 500 mL at 50 mL/ hr. Observed at 1000 hrs: 250 mL remains.

  **a.** Total hours to infuse: _____
  **b.** Hours elapsed: _____
  **c.** Amount infused: _____ Amount that should have infused: _____
  **d.** Ahead of schedule, behind, or on time: _____
  **e.** Hours remaining: _____ mL remaining: _____
  **f.** Adjusted flow rate: _____

2  Started at 1500 hrs: 1000 mL at 100 mL/ hr. Observed at 2200 hrs: 100 mL remains.

  **a.** Total hours to infuse: _____
  **b.** Hours elapsed: _____
  **c.** Amount infused: _____ Amount that should have infused: _____
  **d.** Ahead of schedule, behind, or on time: _____
  **e.** Hours remaining: _____ mL remaining: _____
  **f.** Adjusted flow rate: _____

3  Started at 2300 hrs: 250 mL NS at 50 mL/ hr. Observed at 0100 hrs: 200 mL remains.

  **a.** Total hours to infuse: _____
  **b.** Hours elapsed: _____
  **c.** Amount infused: _____ Amount that should have infused: _____
  **d.** Ahead of schedule, behind, or on time: _____
  **e.** Hours remaining: _____ mL remaining: _____
  **f.** Adjusted flow rate: _____

4  Started at 1100 hrs: 500 mL D5RL 125 mL / hr. Observed at 1300 hrs: 100 mL remains.

  **a.** Total hours to infuse: _____
  **b.** Hours elapsed: _____
  **c.** Amount infused: _____ Amount that should have infused: _____
  **d.** Ahead of schedule, behind, or on time: _____
  **e.** Hours remaining: _____ mL remaining: _____
  **f.** Adjusted flow rate: _____

5  Started at 1700 hrs: 250 mL RLS at 25 mL/ hr. Observed at 1900 hrs: 200 mL remains.

  **a.** Total hours to infuse: _____
  **b.** Hours elapsed: _____
  **c.** Amount infused: _____ Amount that should have infused: _____
  **d.** Ahead of schedule, behind, or on time: _____
  **e.** Hours remaining: _____ mL remaining: _____
  **f.** Adjusted flow rate: _____

## CHAPTER 9 MULTIPLE-CHOICE REVIEW

**Estimated completion time: 30 minutes**   **Answers on page 573**

**Directions:** *Analyze the IV-related questions and select the best answer:*

1 Ordered: 1000 mL D5W, an isotonic fluid maintenance solution, q12h. Equipment available: infusion pump. The nurse will set the flow rate at _____
   **1.** 80 mL/ hr          **3.** 84 ml/ hr
   **2.** 83 mL/ hr          **4.** 83 drops/ min

2 The average maintenance flow rate for a healthy adult who is NPO is _____
   **1.** 10-15 mL/ hr        **3.** 75-125 mL/ hr
   **2.** 25 mL/ hr           **4.** 150-250 mL/ hr

3 An isotonic electrolyte solution used for IV infusions is _____
   **1.** 5DW               **3.** RLS
   **2.** 10DW              **4.** 2.5% DW

4 Ordered: NS 500 mL q4h. Equipment available: gravity device with rate controller. The nurse will set the flow rate at _____
   **1.** 100 drops/ min     **3.** 125 mL/ hr
   **2.** 125 drops/ min     **4.** 150 mL/ hr

5 Ordered: RLS 1000 mL q8h. Equipment available: gravity device, DF 20. The nurse will set the flow rate at _____
   **1.** 20 mL/ hr          **3.** 42 mL/ hr
   **2.** 42 drops/ min      **4.** 125 mL/ hr

6 Ordered: 50 mL antibiotic IVPB q6h infused over 30 minutes. Equipment available: gravity device, DF 15. The nurse will set the flow rate at _____
   **1.** 25 drops/ min      **3.** 25 mL/ hr
   **2.** 12.5 drops/ min    **4.** 100 mL/ hr

7 Ordered: 30 mL antibiotic IVPB q4h infused over 30 minutes. Equipment available: infusion pump. The nurse will set the flow rate at _____
   **1.** 25 mL/ hr          **3.** 60 mL/ hr
   **2.** 50 drops/ min      **4.** 200 mL/ hr

8 Ordered: 1000 mL 5D/NS q24h. Equipment available: Pediatric microdrip administration set. The nurse will set the flow rate at _____
   **1.** 41 drops/ min           **3.** 42 drops/ min
   **2.** $41\frac{2}{3}$ mL/ hr   **4.** 42 mL/ hr

9 Ordered: 1 unit of blood (250 mL) to be infused over 2 hours. Equipment available: gravity blood administration set, DF 10. The nurse will set the flow rate at _____
   **1.** 13 drops/ min      **3.** 125 mL/ hr
   **2.** 21 drops/ min      **4.** 125 drops/ min

10 D10W 1000 mL contains how many grams of dextrose? _____
   **1.** 15                **3.** 50
   **2.** 25                **4.** 100

**Estimated completion time: 1 hour**   **Answers on page 573**

**Directions:** *Show work, label answers. Calculate with a DA equation when requested. Use a calculator for long division and multiplication. All flow rates must be labeled drops/ min or mL/ hr.*

1 Name the three purposes of IV therapy:

_____   _____   _____

2 State the names of three isotonic IV solutions commonly ordered:

_____

_____

_____

3 Select the type of administration set that would be selected for an IVPB solution: *primary* or *secondary?* (Circle one)

4 State the meaning of DF of 10 on a gravity infusion administration set.

_____

5 **a.** State the DF for a microdrip, or pediatric, infusion administration step.

_____

**b.** State the flow rate limit for infusions using microdrip sets. _____

6 Ordered: 250 mL NS q4h. Equipment available: gravity device with DF 10.

**a.** State the grams of sodium in the solution: _____

DA equation:

**b.** Evaluation: _____
**c.** State the flow rate that would be set: _____

DA equation:

**d.** Evaluation: _____

7 Ordered: 250 mL 5DW at 50 mL/ hr.

**a.** How long will the IV infusion last? _____
**b.** If an alarm is set for $\frac{1}{2}$ hour before the solution will be completely infused, how much volume to be infused would be entered for the alarm to sound?

_____

8 Ordered: 500 mL RLS q8h. Equipment available: EID

**a.** State the flow rate that would be set: _____
**b.** If the IV infusion started at 1200, at what time (military time) would the nurse prepare the next solution to have it at the bedside $\frac{1}{2}$ hour before the container would be empty? _____

9 What is a nursing responsibility pertaining to flow rate when a secondary infusion or IVPB has been completed and the primary IV resumes flow?

_____

**10** State the most serious adverse effect of an error with overdose or over-concentration during KCI IV administration: _____

**11** Ordered: whole blood to be infused initially at 2 mL/ min for the first 15 minutes. Equipment available: infusion pump for blood and blood administration pump set.

State the flow rate in mL/ hr that the nurse would set on the pump for the first 15 minutes: _____

**12** Ordered: 250 mL whole blood to be infused over 2 hours. Equipment available: gravity blood administration set, DF 10

  **a.** Calculate the flow rate with a DA equation:

  **b.** Evaluation: _____

**13** Ordered: 3 L D5RLS q24h. Equipment available: gravity administration set with DF 15.

  **a.** Calculate the flow rate with a DA equation:

  **b.** Evaluation: _____

**14** Ordered: 500 mL D5W q8h. Equipment available: gravity infusion device with DF 20.

  **a.** Calculate the flow rate with a DA equation:

  **b.** Evaluation: _____

**15** Ordered: 50 mL 50% dextrose solution for a diabetic patient in insulin shock.

  **a.** How many grams of dextrose are contained in the solution? _____

    DA equation:

  **b.** Evaluation: _____

**16 a.** What type of device would the nurse connect between an IV solution and tubing to protect a patient from a fluid or medication overload? _____

  **b.** What are the usual guidelines or criteria for the amount of fluid placed in this device? _____

**17** An IV of 1000 mL D5W at 100 mL/ hr is ordered and started at 0800. At 1200, the nurse observes that 600 mL remain. The prescriber wants the IV completed on time.

  **a.** Amount that should remain: _____
  **b.** Hour at which ordered IV should be completed: _____
  **c.** Remaining number of hours that ordered solution needs to be completed: _____

  **d.** Flow rate for remaining IV fluid on an infusion pump: _____

**18** An IVPB of 50 mL is ordered to be infused over 30 minutes. Estimate the flow rate on an infusion pump: _____

**19** An IVPB of 20 mL is ordered to be infused over 20 minutes.

    **a.** Estimate the flow rate on a microdrip device. _____

        DA equation:

    **b.** Evaluation: _____

**20** State five considerations that need to be kept in mind when an IV flow rate is behind schedule:

_____

_____

_____

_____

_____

_____

## Suggestions for Further Reading

Gahart B, Nazareno A: 2005 Intravenous medications, ed. 21, St. Louis, 2005, Mosby.
www.baxter.com/products/medication_management
www.cc.nih.gov/nursing/medfsyip.htmL
www.ismp.org
www.jcaho.org
www.jcipatientsafety.org

Additional practice problems can be found in the Intravenous Calculations section of the enclosed companion CD.

Chapter 10 covers advanced IV infusion calculations using this chapter as a foundation.

*"I have no great talent. I am just passionately curious."*
—ALBERT EINSTEIN

# ADVANCED INTRAVENOUS CALCULATIONS

## Objectives

- Calculate infusion flow rates for the following units of measurement: mg/ mL, mg/ hr, mg/ min, mcg/ mL, mcg/ hr, mcg/ min, mcg/ kg, mcg/ kg/ hr, mcg/ kg/ min, mg/ kg, mg/ kg/ hr, mg/ kg/ min, and mEq/ hr.
- Confirm IV medication orders with safe dose range (SDR) criteria.
- Calculate schedules for manual IV direct push medications.
- Calculate the parameters of flow rates for titrated IV infusions.
- State the difference between central venous lines and peripheral venous lines.
- Calculate the calories in selected IV solutions.
- State the general purpose and contents of hyperalimentation (TPN) formulas.
- Identify patient safety issues for the administration of IV medications.

## Essential Prior Knowledge

- Mastery of Chapters 1-9
- Review of Chapter 9, Basic Intravenous Calculations, highly recommended

## Equipment

- Calculator
- IV equipment for laboratory and clinical observation, when available

## Estimated Time to Complete Chapter

- 2-3 hours

## Introduction

Chapter 9 focused on prepared IV solutions that required simple flow rate calculations. This chapter emphasizes more complex dose-based flow rate calculations for a variety of medicated IV solutions for peripheral access sites. The principles of the equation setup are the same as in earlier chapters.

Although D5W, NS, and 5% L/R solutions are vehicles for many IV medications, certain medications require a specific solution. The nurse must always check for compatibilities *and incompatibilities* before mixing medications and solutions. It must be assumed that IV solutions and medications, including diluents, are incompatible unless the literature states otherwise. With the great increase in available medications, the responsibility to protect the patient increases.

Intravenous medications ordered for the treatment of at-risk patients, such as the acutely ill and frail young and elderly, may require calculation and adjustment of dosage (titration), depending on the patient's response to the medication. Many

**335**

of the math skills mastered in earlier chapters will be reviewed and employed: analysis of the problem, basic multiplication and division, conversion among metric units of measurement, calculation of weight in kilograms, DA-style equations setups, and flow rate calculations.

## ESSENTIAL Vocabulary

| | |
|---|---|
| **Filters** | Used in some IV medication lines to prevent contaminants, particles, and clots from reaching patient circulation. Liquids can pass through the filter. Specific guidelines for use and nonuse and filter size must be checked with agency and manufacturer guidelines prior to administration of medications. The smaller the size filter, the finer the filter. Blood administration sets are supplied with a clot filter, and other filters may be added for specific purposes, depending on the age of the blood product. Filters are not routinely used for IV infusions. |
| **Hyperalimentation, or Total Parenteral Nutrition (TPN) (Hyperal)** | IV caloric infusion of nutrients, vitamins, minerals, and electrolytes through a *central* or *peripheral venous line.* Contents and amounts are prescribed on an individual basis. |
| **Infusion Access Sites: Central and Peripheral Venous** | Central venous sites are large blood volume sites (such as the superior vena cava and right atrium) that can be accessed by catheter from large veins (such as the jugular) or surgically accessed chest veins. They can also be accessed from peripherally inserted central catheters (PICC), which are less invasive and threaded to the superior vena cava–right atrial junction from a peripheral vein. The central venous sites provide rapid dilution of concentrated solutions such as TPN and medications and are more suitable for longer term therapy and more concentrated solutions than smaller peripheral veins. |
| **IV Flush (SAS) (SASH)** | Technique that maintains patency of IV sites used before and after infusion of medications and for periodic maintenance. Saline solution and/or low-dose heparin solution is injected through infusion ports in accordance with agency protocols for milliliter amounts for each type of flush solution and the equipment being flushed. The longer the line, the more solution must be used. Also used to clear lines of solutions before administering a potentially incompatible solution. *SAS* means "saline, administer drug, saline flush." *SASH* means "saline, administer drug, saline, heparin flush." |
| **Kilocalorie (Kcal)** | Metric measurement, unit of energy, necessary to raise the temperature of 1 kg of water by 1°C. Commonly described as "calorie," even though there are 1000 calories in a *kilo*calorie, as the metric prefix indicates. The "calories" on food labels are actually kilocalories. |
| **Peak and Trough Levels** | Serum levels of drugs derived from blood samples drawn 30 minutes before the next dose is due (trough) and 30 minutes after administration (peak) for IV drugs and 1-2 hours after oral drugs (peak). Guides the prescriber for effective dosing and avoidance of toxicity or damage to renal function. Nurse must label specimen with peak or trough, exact time drawn, and time and dose of last medication infusion. Certain drugs, such as aminophylline, the IV bronchodilator used for severe asthma, have widely varying rates of individual absorption and necessitate peak and trough measurements. |
| **Titrated Medication** | Flexible drug dose order to achieve desired therapeutic result, such as a specific urinary output, systolic or diastolic blood pressure, or glucose level (e.g., "dobutamine 2-8 mg/ kg/ min IV infusion. Increase or lower by 1-2 mg every 30 minutes to achieve/maintain systolic pressure between 90 and 110 degrees). Administered and adjusted by experienced registered nurses. |
| **Vascular Implanted Devices** **Vascular Access Devices (VAD)** | Surgically implanted subcutaneous self-access sealing injection ports that can tolerate repeated injections with a special Huber needle. The port is attached to a catheter threaded to the target site, most commonly the subclavian vein. Saves the patient the discomfort of multiple injections |

## RAPID PRACTICE 10-1 Vocabulary Review

**Estimated completion time: 10 minutes**   Answers on page 575

**Directions:** *Read the introduction and the essential vocabulary. Identify the terms.*

1  Intravenous infusion access sites are generally divided into which two major areas: _____
   1. Hyperalimentation and IV push
   2. Peripheral and central
   3. Peaks and troughs
   4. Flushes and implantable vascular access ports

2  The term for IV nutritional infusions is _____
   1. Central venous line        3. Hyperalimentation
   2. Drug titrations            4. Kilocalories

3  Which of the following statements is true about infusion line filters? _____
   1. One size can be used for all infusions.
   2. All IV infusions must use filters.
   3. Blood administration sets are always supplied with a filter.
   4. The larger the filter size, the smaller the pores of the filter.

4  Flushes are used before and after administration of many medicated IV solutions for the following purpose: _____
   1. To prevent drug and solution incompatibility and site coagulation
   2. To provide a higher intake for the patient who may be dehydrated
   3. To test the patient's ability to tolerate an IV solution
   4. To provide medication before and after an infusion

5  An example of a titrated IV drug order would be _____
   1. Give clindamycin phosphate 1 g IV every 6 hours over 60 minutes.
   2. Give ampicillin 25 mg IV stat and q8h for 72 hours.
   3. Alternate 1000 mL D5W q8h with 1000 mL lactated Ringer's solution.
   4. Give nitroprusside sodium 0.1-5 mcg/ kg/ min to maintain systolic blood pressure below 160.

# Equation Setups for Advanced Intravenous Calculations

It will be helpful to practice a few exercises in preparation for setting up and understanding medicated IV calculations.

## RAPID PRACTICE 10-2 Basic Intravenous Calculations Review

**Estimated completion time: 20-25 minutes**   Answers on page 575

**Directions:** *Estimate and calculate the requested IV infusion as shown. Use a calculator for long division and multiplication to solve equations.*

1  Ordered: 2 mL/ min. Need to know: mL/ hr.
   a. Estimated answer: $2 \times 60 = 120$ mL/ hr.

   DA equation verification:

   $$\frac{mL}{hr} = \frac{2\ mL}{1\ \cancel{min}} \times \frac{60\ \cancel{min}}{1\ hr} = 120\ mL/\ hr$$

   b. Evaluation: Equation is balanced. Only mL/ hr remain.

2 Ordered: 120 mL/ hr. Need to know: mL/ min to nearest tenth of a mL.

   **a.** Estimated mL/ min: _____

      DA equation verification:

   **b.** Evaluation: _____

3 Ordered: 4 mg/ min. Need to know: mg/ hr.

   **a.** Estimated mg/ hr: _____

      DA equation verification:

   **b.** Evaluation: _____

4 Ordered: 60 mg/ hr. Need to know: mg/ min.

   **a.** Estimated mg/ min: _____

      DA equation verification:

   **b.** Evaluation: _____

5 Ordered: 2 mg/ kg/ min. Weight: 10 kg. Need to know: mg/ min.

   **a.** Estimated mg/ min: _____

      DA equation verification:

   **b.** Evaluation: _____

   **c.** Estimated mg/ hr: _____

      DA equation verification:

   **d.** Evaluation: _____

# Conversion Formulas that May Be Needed for Intravenous Infusion Calculations

One or more conversion formulas may be required to complete IV infusion calculations:

| Formulas | Purpose |
| --- | --- |
| 60 minutes = 1 hour | Often needed to obtain milliliters or medication dose per hour, this formula also may be needed to verify how much drug per minute or volume per minute is being infused. For example, |
| | Ordered: Drug Y 1 mg/ min. Question: How many milligrams or milliliters per hour will be infused? |
| 1000 mg = 1 g<br>1000 mcg = 1 mg | Needed for conversion when the drug units supplied do not match the drug units ordered. For example, |
| | Ordered: Drug Y 2 mcg/ min. Supplied: Drug Y 500 mg. |
| 1000 mL = 1 L | Needed to convert liters to milliliters for IV flow rate calculations. IV flow rates are delivered in milliliters. Ordered: 1 L q8h. 1 L = 1000 mL. 1000 mL ÷ 8 = 125 mL/ hr. |
| 2.2 lb = 1 kg | Occasionally needed to calculate the dose ordered when the dose is based on weight and the weight in pounds is known and that in kilograms is not. For example, |
| | Ordered: Drug Y 2 mg/ kg/ min. Weight: 50 lb. |

**1**   What are four conversion formulas that may be needed for IV infusion calculations? (Give a brief answer.)

**Q:** *Ask Yourself*

**A:** *My Answer*

# Calculating Medicated Intravenous Flow Rates That Require One Conversion Formula

Intravenous flow rates are usually calculated in milliliters per hour (mL/ hr) but may be ordered in units of a drug to be infused per hour or per minute. Following are some examples of how the amount of a drug to be given per a unit of time may be expressed in medication orders:

| | | |
|---|---|---|
| 2 mg/ min | 5 mcg/ min | 3 units/ min |
| 4 mg/ hr | 3 mcg/ hr | 10 mEq/ hr |
| 0.3 mg/ kg/ min | 1 mcg/ kg/ min | 0.5 milliUnits/ min |

Orders for powerful drugs may be written for a drug dose per minute or per hour. Following are some examples of drug concentrations supplied in IV solutions:

| | | |
|---|---|---|
| 250 mg drug/ 500 mL D5W | 500 mg drug/ 250 mL NS | 100 mg drug/ 250 mL D5W |
| 250 mg drug/ 1000 mL NS | 100 mg drug/ 50 mL NS | 1 g drug/ 1000 mL D5W |

---

**EXAMPLES**

Ordered: Drug Y 5 mg/ min. Available: Drug X 400 mg/ 200 mL. Question: The flow rate must be set at how many mL/ hr to deliver 5 mg/ min?

Three factors must be entered in the medication equation to determine mL per hour flow rates:

**1**  Available drug concentration
**2**  Ordered medication amount and time frame to be infused
**3**  Needed conversion formulas

Answer: mL/ hr are needed in the answer. In order to be in the answer, mL and hr must be entered in the equation. Minutes are not desired.

$$\frac{mL}{hr} = \frac{\overset{1}{\cancel{200}}\ mL}{\underset{\underset{1}{2}}{\cancel{400\ mg}}} \times \frac{5\ \cancel{mg}}{1\ \cancel{min}} \times \frac{\overset{30}{\cancel{60\ min}}}{1\ hr} = 150\ mL/\ hr$$

Evaluation: The equation is balanced. Only mL/ hr remain.

Analysis: The data with mL will be entered *in the first numerator.* The available liquid concentration will be in mL. Milligrams will need to be canceled. The order is in mg, and that quantity ordered is entered next to cancel the mg in the drug concentration. Hr is entered in last denominator with the required min to hr conversion. Note the progression for canceling undesired units from one denominator to the next numerator—mg /mg and min /min—as in prior DA equations.

---

➤  *One* conversion formula is needed. Because the drug ordered and the drug supplied are in the *same terms, milligrams*, a minutes to hours conversion is the *only* formula needed.
➤  If the drug was ordered in g and the amount supplied was also in g, the same principle would apply.
➤  If the drug ordered was ordered in mg, and the amount supplied in g, a conversion formula from mg to g would have to be entered.

**1** What are the three factors that need to be entered in the equation in order to calculate medicated IV infusion rates in mL/ hr? (Use one- or two-word answers.)

_____

_____

**RAPID PRACTICE 10-3** Converting IV Flow Rates from Milligrams per Minute to Milliliters per Hour

**Estimated completion time: 20 minutes**   Answers on page **575**

**Directions:** *For each problem, determine which conversion formula will be needed. Calculate the mL/ hr flow rate as shown in the preceding example. Cancel units before doing the math. Use a calculator for long division and multiplication. Label answers.*

**Test Tip:** After cancellation of units in the equation, it often simplifies the math to reduce the available drug concentration fraction if it can be reduced.

**1** Ordered: Drug Y 2 mg/ min. Available: 1000 mg Drug X in 1000 mL D5W.

  **a.** mL/ hr flow rate?

   DA equation:



  **b.** Evaluation: _____

**2** Ordered: Drug Y 1 mg/ min. Available: 500 mg Drug X in 1000 mL LRS.

  **a.** mL/ hr flow rate?

   DA equation:



  **b.** Evaluation: _____

**3** Ordered: Drug Y 0.5 mg/ min. Available: 500 mg/ 250 mL 0.45 NS.

  **a.** mL/ hr flow rate?

   DA equation:



  **b.** Evaluation: _____

**4** Ordered: Drug Y 0.2 mg/ min. Available: 100 mg/ 100 mL D5W.

  **a.** mL/ hr flow rate?

   DA equation:



  **b.** Evaluation: _____

**5** Ordered: Drug Y 0.4 mg/ min. Available: 250 mg in 1 L D5W.

  **a.** mL/ hr flow rate?

   DA equation:



  **b.** Evaluation: _____

# Calculating Intravenous Flow Rates That Require Two Conversion Formulas

A nurse who knows how to calculate flow rates no matter how they are ordered provides critical patient safety. The nurse is liable for any medication administration errors regardless of whether they may be computer, prescriber, or pharmacy errors.

➤ If a drug is ordered in mcg/ min but supplied in mg/ ml or ordered in mg/ min but supplied in g/ ml, two conversion formulas must be included in the equation:

  **1** mcg/ mg or mg/ g
  **2** min/ hr

➤ The drug ordered and the drug supplied must be converted to the same terms.

---

**EXAMPLES**

Ordered: Drug X 100 *mcg*/ min. Available: Drug X 400 *mg*/ 250 mL.

What flow rate will be set?

Conversion formulas available: 1000 mcg = 1 mg, 1000 mg = 1 g, 60 minutes = 1 hour, and 1000 mL = 1 L.

$$\frac{mL}{hr} = \frac{\overset{5}{\cancel{250}}\ mL}{\underset{8}{\cancel{400}\ mg}} \times \frac{1\ \cancel{mg}}{\underset{\underset{1}{10}}{\cancel{1000}\ \cancel{mcg}}} \times \frac{\overset{1}{\cancel{100}\ \cancel{mcg}}}{1\ \cancel{min}} \times \frac{\overset{6}{\cancel{60}\ \cancel{min}}}{1\ hr} = \frac{30}{8} = 3.75,\ \text{or}\ 4\ mL/\ hr$$

Evaluation: The equation is balanced. Only mL/ hr remain.

Analysis: Drug concentration was entered first because it contained mL for the desired answer. In addition to the drug order, two conversion formulas will be needed: mg to mcg to cancel mg in the first denominator and to cancel mcg in the drug order. Finally, the min to hr conversion formula was entered to provide hr for the desired answer. Stop before doing the math. Do only the desired answer units remain? Answer: Yes.

---

## RAPID PRACTICE 10-4   Calculating IV Flow Rates That Require Two Conversion Formulas

**Estimated completion time: 20-25 minutes**   Answers on page **576**

**Directions:** *Analyze the preceding example and worked-out problem 1. Determine how many conversion formulas are needed. Calculate using needed conversion formulas. Conversion formulas: 60 minutes = 1 hour, 1000 mcg = 1 mg, and 1000 mg = 1 g. Use a calculator for long division and multiplication.*

**1** Ordered: Drug X IV infusion 200 mcg/ min. Available: Drug X 250 mg/ 1000 mL D5W.

  **a.** What will the flow rate be in mL/ hr?

    DA equation:

$$\frac{mL}{hr} = \frac{\overset{4}{\cancel{1000}}\ mL}{\underset{1}{\cancel{250}\ mg}} \times \frac{1\ \cancel{mg}}{\underset{\underset{1}{5}}{\cancel{1000}\ \cancel{mcg}}} \times \frac{\overset{1}{\cancel{200}\ \cancel{mcg}}}{1\ \cancel{min}} \times \frac{\overset{12}{\cancel{60}\ \cancel{min}}}{1\ hr} = 48\ mL/\ hr$$

  **b.** Evaluation: Equation is balanced. Only mL/ hr remain.

**2** Ordered: Drug Y IV infusion 75 mcg/ min. Available: Drug Y 10 mg/ 100 mL NS.*

   **a.** What will the flow rate be in mL/ hr?

   DA equation:

   **b.** Evaluation: _____

**3** Ordered: Drug Y IV infusion 5 mg/ min: Available: Drug Y 1 g/ 200 mL LRS.

   **a.** What will the flow rate be in mL/ hr? _____

   DA equation:

   **b.** Evaluation: _____

**4** Ordered: Drug Y IV infusion 200 mcg/ min. Available: Drug Y 500 mg/ 250 mL D5W.

   **a.** What will the flow rate be in mL/ hr? _____

   DA equation:

   **b.** Evaluation: _____

**5** Ordered: Drug Y IV infusion 1.5 mg/ min. Available: Drug Y 2 g/ 200 mL NS.

   **a.** What will the flow rate be in mL/ hr? _____

   DA equation:

   **b.** Evaluation: _____

*Q: Ask Yourself*

*A: My Answer*

**1** Why are two conversion formulas needed in problems 1 and 2? Which formulas are they?

   _____

## Calculating Flow Rates for Weight-Based Doses

An order for a continuous IV infusion may read: dopamine 2 mcg/ kg/ min. The solution available may be: dopamine 200 mg/ 250 mL D5W. How many ml/ hr will be set? The patient weight today is 50 kg.

**1** Identify the desired answer units.
**2** Calculate the ordered dose based on the requested units of weight.
**3** Enter the drug concentration available, the ordered dose, and any needed conversion formulas in a DA equation to obtain the desired answer.

---

*NS solution is 0.9% NaCl solution. Refer to Chapter 9. Any concentration other than 0.9% is stated, e.g., 0.45% NaCl ($\frac{1}{2}$ NS).

As stated earlier, the dose ordered must always be entered in the medication equation along with the concentration available and the conversion factors.

➤ Step 2, calculating the ordered dose based on weight, is the only additional step compared to the problems in Rapid Practice 10-4.

➤ The desired answer is a ml/ hr flow rate.

## Calculating the Total Dose Ordered for Weight-Based Orders: Micrograms and Milligrams per Kilogram

Calculate the *total drug ordered* using the patient's body weight in kilograms.

Ordered: 2 mcg/ kg/ min. Patient's weight: 50 kg. Estimated dose in micrograms:
2 mg × 50 kg = 100 mcg total dose per minute. DA equation:

$$\text{total mcg} = \frac{2 \text{ mcg}}{1 \text{ kg}} \times 50 \text{ kg} =$$

100 mcg dose ordered per minute based on 50-kg weight $\left(\dfrac{100 \text{ mcg}}{1 \text{ min}}\right)$

If the patient's weight is 50 lb and the weight in kilograms is not known, enter the conversion formula for pounds to kilograms:

2.2 lb = 1 kg

$$\text{mcg} = \times \frac{2 \text{ mcg}}{1 \text{ kg}} \times \frac{1 \text{ kg}}{2.2 \text{ lb}} \times 50 \text{ lb} = \frac{100}{2.2} = 45.45, \text{ or } 45.5 \text{ mcg/ min}$$

**1** What is the difference in dose in micrograms per minute for 50 lb and 50 kg, as shown in the preceding two equations?

_____

**FAQ** | *Why are kilograms not retained in the answer for milligrams-per-kilogram problems?*

**ANSWER:** The desired answer is in *micrograms per minute*. The dose is *based on the patient's weight:* 2 mcg for *each* kilogram of weight. After factoring in the kilogram weight by multiplying micrograms by kilograms, the kilogram units *are eliminated* from the answer.

If you were asked how many cups of water you drink during the day, you might respond, "I drink about 1 cup *per hour,* so I drink 8 cups a day. The desired units in the answer are *cups per day.* Hours were only factored in to get the total amount, just as kilograms of body weight are factored in only to get a total amount of milligrams. Hours would be eliminated from the final answer, as are kilograms.

## Calculating the Flow Rate in Milliliters per Hour (mL/ hr) for Weight-Based Orders

Once the dose ordered has been calculated, it is inserted in the infusion equation with appropriate conversion formulas if needed, as earlier, to determine the flow rate in mL/ hr, as illustrated in the example that follows.

Ordered: dopamine 2 mcg/ kg/ min. Available: dopamine 500 mg/ 250 mL D5W. Patient's weight: 30 kg. What flow rate will be set?

Conversion formulas available: 60 minutes = 1 hour, 1000 mcg = 1 mg, 1000 mg = 1 g, and 1000 mL = 1 L. Estimated dose ordered: 2 mcg × 30 kg = 60 mcg/ min.

DA equation verification (two-step method):

*Step 1:* Total dose ordered in $\dfrac{mcg}{min} = \dfrac{2\ mcg}{1\ \cancel{kg}} \times \dfrac{30\ \cancel{kg}}{1\ min} = 60$ mcg/ min

*Step 2:* $\dfrac{mL}{hr} = \dfrac{\overset{\overset{1}{\cancel{2}}}{\cancel{500}\ mL}}{\underset{1}{250\ mg}} \times \dfrac{1\ mg}{\underset{500}{\cancel{1000\ mcg}}} \times \dfrac{60\ \cancel{mcg}}{1\ \cancel{min}} \times \dfrac{60\ \cancel{min}}{1\ hr} = \dfrac{3600}{500} = 7.2$ rounded to 7 mL/ hr

Two conversion factors are needed: one to change micrograms to milligrams and the other to change minutes to hours.

➤ Note that the math is simplified with reduction of the drug concentration fraction, the first fraction form in the equation.

**FAQ** | *Why do medication infusion orders sometimes specify a range for drug dose or flow rate?*

**ANSWER:** A range allows the nurse to titrate the drug dose or rate, starting with the lowest dose, until the desired response is achieved (e.g., a pulse over 60, to maintain a minimum urinary output, to maintain a safe blood pressure level, or to maintain a heart rate). Based on intervals of time and dose specified in the order, the rate or dose is increased at a specified interval or gradually until the desired response is achieved. This may require many adjustments if the patient's condition is unstable.

The order may read: Drug X at 10-20 mcg/ min to maintain a systolic pressure of 90-110 or a urinary output of 800 mL or more. May be increased by 2 mcg/ min every hour.

The calculations are performed separately for each amount in a range.

**FAQ** | *Can the weight-based ordered dose calculation be entered in the equation for mL/ hr, or must it be calculated separately ?*

**ANSWER:** You have the option of entering all of the data in one equation. It makes it a very long equation, as shown in the following example using the same information from the preceding example (Ordered: dopamine 2 mcg/ kg/ min. Available: dopamine 200 mg/ 500 mL D5W. Wt: 30 kg.) Another reason for calculating the dose ordered separately is that if the nurse is going to prepare the medicated IV solution, the dose ordered must be calculated first and independently of the flow rate. It then makes sense to simplify and shorten the DA equation by eliminating the mcg/ kg dose data entry as shown in the prior example.

$\dfrac{mL}{hr} = \dfrac{500\ mL}{250\ \cancel{mg}} \times \dfrac{1\ \cancel{mg}}{1000\ \cancel{mcg}} \times \dfrac{2\ \cancel{mcg}}{1\ \cancel{kg}} \times \dfrac{30\ \cancel{kg}}{1\ \cancel{min}} \times \dfrac{60\ \cancel{min}}{1\ hr} = \dfrac{3600}{500} = 7.2$ or 7 mL/ hr

Compare this example with the example above. Calculating the dose ordered separately shortens and simplifies the final equation. If the order is in kg and the weight is in lb, another conversion formula would also have to be entered to change lb to kg.

**RAPID PRACTICE 10-5** Calculating IV Infusion Rates for Weight-Based Orders

**Estimated completion time: 25 minutes** Answers on page **577**

**Directions:** *Study the preceding example and worked-out problem 1. Identify the desired answer units. Identify and calculate the dose ordered. Calculate the desired flow rate with a DA equation. Remember that reducing the drug concentration fraction after cancellation of units simplifies the math. Use a calculator for long division and multiplication.*

1 Ordered: dobutamine hydrochloride IV infusion 0.5 mcg/ kg/ min for 24 hours for a patient with cardiac decompensation. Available: dobutamine 250 mg/ 250 mL D5W. Patient's weight: 100 kg.

   **a.** Total dose ordered per minute based on weight: ___50 mcg/ min___

$$\frac{mcg}{min} = \frac{0.5\ mcg}{1\ mg} \times 100\ kg = 50\ mcg/\ min$$

   **b.** Number of conversion formulas needed to obtain a mL/ hr flow rate for the infusion equation: _2; mcg to mg; min to hr_
   **c.** DA equation to calculate mL/ hr:

$$\frac{mL}{hr} = \frac{\overset{1}{\cancel{250}}\ mL}{\underset{1}{\cancel{250}}\ mg} \times \frac{1\ \cancel{mg}}{\underset{20}{\cancel{1000}}\ \cancel{mcg}} \times \frac{\overset{1}{\cancel{50}}\ \cancel{mcg}}{1\ \cancel{min}} \times \frac{60\ \cancel{min}}{1\ hr} = \frac{60}{20} = 3\ mL/\ hr$$

   **d.** Evaluation: ___Equation is balanced. Only mL/ hr remain.___

2 Ordered: aminophylline IV infusion 0.5 mg/ kg/ hr for a patient with asthma. Available: aminophylline 500 mg in 250 mL D5W. Patient's weight: 80 kg.

   **a.** Total dose ordered per hour based on weight: _____
   **b.** Number of conversion formulas needed to obtain a mL/ hr flow rate for the infusion equation: _____
   **c.** DA equation to calculate mL/ hr:

   **d.** Evaluation: _____

3 Ordered: isoproterenol hydrochloride IV infusion 0.1 mcg/ kg/ min for 8 hours for a patient with severe asthma. Available: isoproterenol hydrochloride 1 mg in 250 mL D5W. Patient's weight: 88 lb.

   **a.** Total dose ordered per minute based on weight: _____
   **b.** Number of conversion formulas needed to obtain a mL/ hr flow rate for the infusion equation: _____
   **c.** DA equation to calculate mL/ hr:

   **d.** Evaluation: _____

4 Ordered: dopamine hydrochloride IV infusion 3 mcg/ kg/ min for 24 hours for a patient to maintain blood pressure. Available: dopamine hydrochloride 400 mg in 500 mL D5W. Patient's weight: 70 kg.

   **a.** Total dose ordered per minute based on weight: _____
   **b.** Number of conversion formulas needed to obtain a mL/ hr flow rate for the infusion equation: _____
   **c.** DA equation to calculate mL/ hr:

   **d.** Evaluation: _____

5 Ordered: bretylium tosylate IV infusion 2 mg/ min for a patient with a ventricular arrhythmia. Available: 1 g bretylium tosylate in 1 L NS.

**a.** Total dose ordered per minute: _____

**b.** Number of conversion formulas needed to obtain a mL/ hr flow rate for the infusion equation: _____

**c.** DA equation to calculate mL/ hr:


**d.** Evaluation: _____

# Equipment for Medicated Intravenous Solutions

The patient's safety is never more important than when administering IV medications. The trend of providing more prepackaged IV medications in a variety of doses and concentrations, needleless medication systems, and infusion pumps that calculate dose rates reflects the effort to reduce medication errors.

Remember that it is preferable to infuse medicated solutions on electronic volumetric pumps. EIDs can be very sophisticated. Figure 10-1 shows an example of an infusion pump used in intensive care units that can regulate four simultaneous infusions for one patient. This device frees space at the bedside. The nurse must ensure that each programmed rate is for the appropriate infusion solution.

This EID can be programmed by the nurse for the dose ordered, drug, concentration, and patient's weight. The pump calculates the flow rate. The nurse then confirms all the data (Figure 10-2).

➤ Remember that there is a 1000-fold difference between a microgram and a milligram. Be scrupulous about entering the correct units of measurement when programming doses. Errors have occurred from confusing the two units of measurement.

Figure 10-1. Omni-Flow® 4000 Plus Medication Management System 4-Channel IV Pump. (From Hospira, Inc., Lake Forest, IL.)

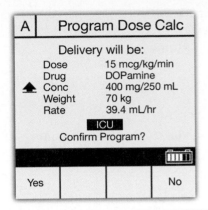

Figure **10-2.** Plum A+® Drug Confirmation Screen. (From Hospira, Inc., Lake Forest, IL.)

If an infusion pump is unavailable and a gravity device must be used, a microdrip pediatric set may be used for medicated infusions. The flow rate would be in drops per minute equal to the mL/ hr calculated flow rate. Review the material in Chapter 9 on microdrip gravity infusions, if needed.

➤ Powerful medications are often given at low flow rates. Careful attention must be given to dilution directions.

## RAPID PRACTICE 10-6  Calculating Flow Rates for Medicated Infusions

**Estimated completion time: 15-20 minutes**   Answers on page **578**

**Directions:** *Identify the desired answer units and conversion factors needed. Calculate the ordered dose if it is weight based. Enter the critical factors and cancel unwanted units so that only the desired answer units of mL/ hr remain. Use a calculator for long division and multiplication. Label answers.*

**1** Ordered: Infuse Drug Y at 1 mg/ min. Available: 200 mg Drug Y/ 250 mL NS.

  **a.** What flow rate should be set on the infusion pump?

    DA equation:

  **b.** Evaluation: _____

**2** Ordered: Infuse Drug Y at the rate of 2 mL/ min.

  **a.** What flow rate should be set on the infusion pump?

    DA equation:

  **b.** Evaluation: _____
  **c.** Would this flow rate be suitable for a gravity microdrip device? _____

**3** Ordered: Infuse Drug Y at 5 mg/ min. Available: Drug Y 1 g/ 250 mL D5W.

  **a.** What flow rate should be set on the infusion pump?

    DA equation:

  **b.** Evaluation: _____

4  Ordered: Titrate Drug Y at 8-10 mcg/ kg/ min to maintain a heart rate over 60.
   Available: Drug Y 500 mg/ 1 L LRS. Patient's weight: 44 kg.
   **a.** Initial total dose to be infused per minute:

   DA equation:


   **b.** What flow rate should be set on an infusion pump?

   DA equation:



   **c.** Evaluation: _____

5  Ordered: Increase the drug dose in problem 4 to 10 mcg/ kg/ min.
   **a.** Total dose to be infused per minute:

   DA equation:



   **b.** What flow rate should be set on the infusion pump?

   DA equation:



   **c.** Evaluation: _____

1  If the flow rate is 10 mL/ hr on a pump for a medicated infusion, what will
   the flow rate be if a microdrip pediatric set must be used?

   _____

# Calculating Milligrams per Milliliter (mg/ mL) from Available Drug Concentration

The nurse needs to be able to calculate the number of mg/ mL contained in any IV solution.

Some IV solutions offer multiple dilution directions. The concentration of mg/ mL will have specified limits for various routes, for example,

For IV infusion: do not exceed a concentration of 1 mg/ mL.
For IV push: do not exceed a concentration of 10 mg/ mL.

The *greater the amount* of drug per milliliter, the more concentrated the solution. (Think of 1 teaspoon of lemon juice in a glass of lemonade versus 10 teaspoons of lemon juice.) This is a very basic calculation: think of *per* as a division line.

➤  To obtain mg/ mL, divide the total number of milligrams of drug by the total number of mL of solution.

For example, if the available concentration is 500 mg of drug in a 250-mL solution, the number of mg/ mL is obtained as follows:

$$\frac{mg}{mL} = \frac{\overset{2}{\cancel{500}}\ mg}{\underset{1}{\cancel{250}}\ mL} = 2\ mg/\ mL$$

Evaluation: Equation is balanced. Only mg/ mL remain.

1    Which is *less* concentrated: Drug Y 100 mg/ mL or Drug Y 250 mg/ mL?

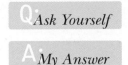

_____

## Deriving Infusion Dose from Existing Flow Rate and Available Solution

The nurse may be asked how many milligrams or micrograms of a drug a patient is currently receiving per minute at the existing flow rate.

An IV solution labeled Drug X 500 mg/ 250 mL is infusing at 15 mL/ hr. How many mg/ min are being delivered? The equation setup begins with the same rule as for other equations: identify the desired answer units.

**EXAMPLES**

Two factors are known:
  • Drug concentration ratio of the prepared solution: 500 mg/ 250 mL
  • Current flow rate: 15 mL/ hr

Milligrams are desired in the answer and in the numerator of the first fraction in the equation. Minutes are desired in the answer in a denominator. Hours must be converted to minutes.

$$\frac{mg}{min} = \frac{\overset{2}{\cancel{500}}\ mg}{\underset{1}{\cancel{250}\ mL}} \times \frac{\overset{1}{\cancel{15}\ mL}}{1\ \cancel{hr}} \times \frac{1\ \cancel{hr}}{\underset{4}{\cancel{60}}\ min} = \frac{2}{4} = 0.5\ mg/\ min\ (or\ 500\ mcg/\ min)$$

Evaluation: Equation is balanced. Only mg/ min remain.

Analysis: The three primary factors in IV infusion calculations are the dose ordered, the drug concentration, and the flow rate. When any two of the three are known, the third can be obtained. Earlier equations calculated the flow rate from the drug concentration and dose ordered. Any relevant conversion factors, such as minutes to hours or hours to minutes, must also be entered in the equation.

**RAPID PRACTICE 10-7** Calculating Infusion Rates in Milligrams per Minute and Micrograms per Minute

**Estimated completion time: 20-25 minutes**   Answers on page **579**

**Directions:** *Identify the desired answer units and conversion formulas. Calculate the number of milligrams per milliliter and milligrams per minute as shown in the preceding examples and problem 1. Evaluate the equation. Label answers. Use a calculator for long division and multiplication.*

**Test Tip:** Take a moment to decide which of the conversion formulas will be needed for the equation: metric and minutes/ hours.

1  Available: Drug X 500 mg/ 1000 mL. Existing flow rate: 20 mL/ hr.
   **a.** mg/ mL concentration: 0.5 mg/ 1 mL $(\frac{500\ mg}{1000\ mL})$
   **b.** mg/ min flow rate:

   DA equation:

   $$\frac{mg}{min} = \frac{\overset{1}{\cancel{500}}\ mg}{\underset{2}{\cancel{1000}\ mL}} \times \frac{\overset{1}{\cancel{20}\ mL}}{1\ \cancel{hr}} \times \frac{1\ \cancel{hr}}{\underset{3}{\cancel{60}}\ min} = \frac{1}{6} = 0.16\ mg/\ min$$

   **c.** Evaluation: Equation is balanced. Only mg/ min remain.

2 Available: Drug Y 250 mg/ 1000 mL. Existing flow rate: 30 mL/ hr.

   **a.** mg/ mL concentration: _____

   **b.** Micrograms/ min flow rate:

     DA equation:

   **c.** Evaluation: _____

3 Available: Drug Y 500 mg/ 250 mL. Existing flow rate: 25 mL/ hr.

   **a.** mg/ mL concentration: _____

   **b.** mg/ min flow rate: _____

     DA equation:

   **c.** Evaluation: _____

4 Available: Drug Y 1 g/ 250 mL. Existing flow rate: 10 mL/ hr.

   **a.** mg/ mL concentration: _____

   **b.** mg/ min flow rate: _____

     DA equation:

   **c.** Evaluation: _____

5 Available: Drug Y 500 mg/ 500 mL. Existing flow rate: 12 mL/ hr.

   **a.** mg/ mL concentration: _____

   **b.** mg/ min flow rate: _____

     DA equation:

   **c.** Evaluation: _____

# Dilutions: When the Nurse Prepares the Drug for the Intravenous Solution

If the pharmacy does not prepare the drug in solution and if it is not available pre- prepared by a manufacturer, the nurse must prepare the drug and add it to the appropriate IV infusion. For the initial drug dose ordered, preparation is exactly the same as for all injectables.

Medications for IV infusion often call for two dilutions:

- The first dilution is to reconstitute the drug with a specific diluent, such as SW or sterile saline solution, for injection. A small amount of diluent is added according to manufacturer directions, usually just enough so that the ordered dose can be withdrawn. This preparation is often too *concentrated* to administer to the patient.

- The second dilution, if required, provides a safe concentration for IV administration.

Ordered: ampicillin 1.2 g over 30 min. Available: ampicillin 500 mg powder. Directions: Each 500-mg ampule is to be reconstituted with 5 mL of SW for injection. May be further diluted in 50 mL or more of NS, D5W, or LR and given as an infusion over not more than 4 hours. Final concentration should not exceed 30 mg/ mL. May be added to the last 100 mL of a compatible IV solution.

1. *First dilution.* Prepare the drug so that the precise dose *ordered* may be withdrawn from the total amount in the vial. This is the same preparation as for any injectable. Three ampules will have to be reconstituted to have enough for 1200 mg of ampicillin. Fifteen milliliters of SW for injection will be used to reconstitute the 1500 mg. From that amount, the nurse will calculate the number of mL needed for the 1200 mg ordered.

$$? \text{ mL} = \frac{\overset{1}{\cancel{15} \text{ mL}}}{\underset{1}{\cancel{1500 \text{ mg}}}} \times 1200 \text{ } \cancel{mg} = 12 \text{ mL}$$

After reconstitution, there may be *more* than 12 mL because the powder will displace some of the solution. Read the label for that information.

Evaluation: Is the answer reasonable? Yes, because the answer has to be slightly less than 15 mL, which contained 1500 mg.

2. *Second dilution.* This dilution is for safe IV infusion. If 50 mL of IV solution is used, will the concentration be *less than* the 30 mg/ mL safe maximum limit stated on the label?

$$50 \text{ mL plus } 12 \text{ mL} = 62 \text{ mL}$$

$$\frac{\text{mg}}{\text{mL}} = \frac{1200 \text{ mg}}{62 \text{ mL}} = 19.35, \text{ or } 19 \text{ mg/ mL}$$

The 19 mg/ mL is *less* concentrated than 30 mg/ mL, so it is safe to use 50 mL of diluent. It also would be safe to dilute "to 50 mL" because the concentration would still be below 30 mg/ mL (1200/ 50 = 24 mg/ mL).

3. *Flow rate.* The order is to infuse 62 mL over 30 minutes. Calculate as for any infusion. Mental estimate: 62 mL over 30 minutes = 124 mL/ hr.

$$\frac{\text{mL}}{\text{hr}} = \frac{62 \text{ mL}}{\underset{1}{\cancel{30 \text{ min}}}} \times \frac{\overset{2}{\cancel{60 \text{ min}}}}{1 \text{ hr}} = 124 \text{ mL/ hr}$$

Evaluation: The equation is balanced. Only mL per hr remain.

Set the flow rate at 124 mL/ hr. The 62 mL will have infused in 30 minutes. The infusion pump is preferred for medicated solutions. Refer to p. 320 to review the math for small intermittent infusions.

**Clinical Relevance**

➤ The fact that more medications are being supplied in various concentrations imposes a greater burden for verification. Was a 10, 20, or 50% dextrose solution ordered? Was 100 mcg or 100 mg ordered? Was 10 mg given IV instead of 0.1 mg because a decimal was not seen? Was there a leading zero that indicated a decimal would follow? Was the medication supposed to be diluted once or twice?

➤ Always check the manufacturer's literature or a current IV drug reference for preparation including dilution directions. Don't hesitate to call pharmacy for assistance.

**FAQ** | *What is the difference between "dilute in" 100 mL and "dilute to" 100 mL?*

**ANSWER:** "Dilute in" means add the drug, whether it is powder or liquid, to the specified amount of diluent. This is often written for the *first* dilution of a drug so that the dose ordered may be withdrawn. Dilute 25 mg in 5 mL of SW means add the 25 mg to 5 mL water. This will result in more than 5 mL. The label will state the concentration after dilution.

*Continued*

> "Dilute to" means that the drug plus the diluent will add up to the specified amount. Dilute 25 mg of the drug to 5 mL (total) of SW or "further dilute" to 50 mL (total). This is often written when there is to be a second dilution of the medication in an IV infusion solution. The nurse can remove excess diluent before mixing the medication to obtain the desired total amount.

| **EXAMPLES** | Ordered: Drug Y 100 mg in IV infusion. Available: Drug Y 100 mg powder. Directions: Dilute each 100 mg in 3 mL of SW. Further dilute to 50 mL with IV solution. The nurse prepares the ordered amount first by reconstituting it with 3 mL SW. After that is gently and thoroughly mixed, it will be added to 47 mL of the IV solution. |
|---|---|

# Intravenous Direct Push Medications

IV push medications are usually diluted in 1 to 50 mL and may be administered into a vein. They may be administered over a minute to 30 minutes or more. A 5-mL minimum volume facilitates administration and titration rates.

The equipment selected depends on the amount of solution and duration of administration. If the injection is to be given through a distal port or an infusion line, agency flushing procedures must be followed. Current IV drug references must be consulted for safe dose ranges, dilutions, rates, and compatibility with the infusing solution.

Small amounts of some drugs usually are to be given over a period of 1-15 minutes and may be administered manually and slowly by the nurse with a syringe directly into a vein or port closest to the patient. Larger amounts of solutions to be administered over a longer period of time may be administered using a syringe pump or a volume-control device.

| **Clinical Relevance** | ➤ As with all IV medications—and this is even more urgent for patients receiving rapid concentrated doses—the patient needs to be assessed before, during, and after the medication is administered. The assessments include mental status, vital signs, and specific drug-related reactions and side effects. |
|---|---|

Many agencies now supply IV tubing with an adapter so that needles are unnecessary for direct IV injections. The syringe connects to the adapter. This prevents needle-stick injuries. Figures 10-3 and 10-4 show examples of medication being administered by IV push.

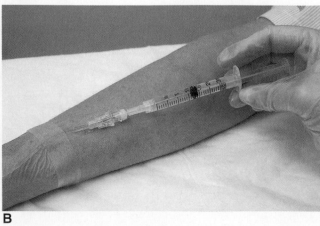

**A**        **B**

Figure **10-3.** IV push (bolus) into injection port. (From Perry AG, Potter PA: Clinical nursing skills and techniques, ed. 6, St. Louis, 2006, Mosby.)

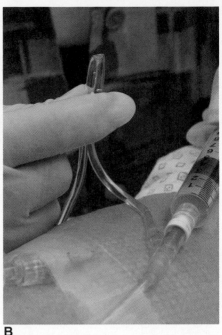

**A**    **B**

Figure 10-4. IV push (bolus) using blunt cannula needleless equipment into existing infusion line. (From Perry AG, Potter PA: Clinical skills and techniques, ed. 6, St. Louis, 2006, Mosby.)

# Direct Intravenous Push Calculations

Even though a direct IV push may be given over a very short period of time by the nurse, it is important to focus, use a watch, and record the time started and time to be finished so that the patient does not receive the medication too quickly. There are many distractions in the work place that may contribute to a rate error, and the medication is often concentrated and powerful.

The schedule is based on two factors:

1   Total number of mL in the *prepared* syringe after dilution
2   Total number of minutes and/or seconds to be injected

## Method 1: Milliliters per Minute

The drug is *first prepared* according to directions and then diluted according to current IV drug references for IV push medications and the manufacturer's guidelines. If the amount of mL/ min to be injected is a whole number, this method works easily.

---

Prepare the drug dose ordered, and then dilute according to directions. Determine the number of mL/ min (total mL in syringe ÷ total minutes to be given).

Treat "per" as a dividing line.

4 mL *prepared* to be given in 4 minutes: <u>1 mL/ min</u>

4 mL *prepared* to be given in 2 minutes: <u>2 mL/ min</u>

$$\frac{mL}{min} = \frac{4\ mL}{4\ min} = 1\ mL/\ min \qquad \frac{mL}{min} = \frac{\overset{2}{4}\ mL}{\underset{1}{2}\ min} = 2\ mL/\ min$$

**EXAMPLES**

---

Decide on a time to start and the exact stop time. Start when the second hand is on 12. Inject slowly and steadily. Avoid all distractions.

## Method 2: Seconds per Calibration

Two factors are needed to calculate the infusion rate of an IV push based on the number of seconds needed to inject a solution per calibration mark on a syringe:

1   Number of calibrations occupied by the *prepared, diluted* drug in solution
2   Number of total seconds the drug is to be administered

The syringe is examined for the number of calibrated lines the medication and diluent occupy. The total number of minutes for the injection is converted to seconds. How many seconds per calibration?

> **EXAMPLES**

Ordered: morphine 4 mg direct IV push. Available: morphine sulfate 10 mg/ mL. Literature: May be given undiluted, but it is appropriate to further *dilute to* 5 mL with SW, NS, or other compatible solutions. Administer over 5 minutes.

$$\text{mL prepared dose} = \underset{5}{\underset{10\ mg}{\underline{1\ mL}}} \times \overset{2}{4\ mg} = 0.4\ mL\ \text{to be administered}$$

Preparation: Withdraw ordered dose, 0.4 mL of morphine sulfate in a 5-mL syringe, and add 4.6 mL SW. This will make a total prepared volume of 5 mL.

$$\frac{\text{seconds}}{\text{calibration}} = \frac{60\ sec}{1\ min} \times \frac{\overset{1}{5\ min}}{\underset{5}{25\ \text{calibrations}}} = \frac{60}{5} = 12\ \text{sec per calibration}$$

Note that the calibrations replace the mL volume in this type of equation.

➤ Prepare the precise ordered dose before adding diluent. The total amount in the syringe is the prepared precise ordered dose plus the specified diluent. The total volume of the two solutions is used to calculate the schedule.

The nurse uses a watch to count 12 seconds while pushing each increment on the syringe. It is important *not to exceed* the prescribed rate of injection. The drugs may be powerful enough to cause severe adverse effects from too rapid injection (Figure 10-5).

**A**

**B**

Figure 10-5. IV (bolus) push into existing infusion line. (From Perry AG, Potter PA: Clinical nursing skills and techniques, ed. 5 revised reprint, St. Louis, 2004, Mosby.)

**1** When the seconds per calibration method is used to calculate rate of injection, why aren't the total mL needed in the equation? What data replace the total mL?

Q:
Ask Yourself

A:
My Answer

_____

Any site to be used for IV administration needs to first be checked for patency. If using a heparin lock-type device to administer the medication, patency can be assessed by slight withdrawal of the syringe plunger to observe a blood return, followed by a flush injection of a 2- or 3-mL of sterile NS solution, with observation for swelling or discomfort. Neither method guarantees patency.

**Clinical Relevance**

## RAPID PRACTICE 10-8 IV Push Calculations

**Estimated completion time: 20-25 minutes**   Answers on page **579**

**Directions:** _Calculate the medication dose. Using the directions for administration rate, examine the syringe for the calibrations occupied by the medication volume. Calculate the number of mL/ min and seconds per calibration. Use a calculator for long division and multiplication. Label answers. Evaluate your own equations._

**1** Atropine 0.8 mg IV, for bradyarrhythmia. Directions: Dilute in up to 10 mL of SW. The nurse adds enough SW to the prepared medication to make 5 mL. Inject 1 mg or less over 1 minute.

NDC 0641-**2210-43**
10 X 20 mL Multiple Dose Vials
**ATROPINE**
SULFATE INJECTION, USP
**400 mcg/mL**
(0.4 mg/mL)
FOR SC, IM OR IV USE

Each mL contains atropine sulfate 400 mcg (0.4 mg), sodium chloride 9 mg and benzyl alcohol 0.015 mL in Water for Injection. pH 3.0-6.5; sulfuric acid added, if needed, for pH adjustment.
**POISON**
USUAL DOSE: See package insert.
Store at controlled room temperature 15°-30° C (59°-86° F).
Caution: Federal law prohibits dispensing without prescription.
Product Code
2210-43                          B-32210

ELKINS-SINN, INC. Cherry Hill, NJ 08003-4099
A subsidiary of A. H. Robins Company

**a.** Total amount of prepared medication in mL:

DA equation:

**b.** Total amount of diluted medication in mL (if applicable): _____
**c.** Total minutes to administer: _____
**d.** mL/ min to be administered: _____
**e.** Total calibrations for the diluted medication: _____

**f.** Total seconds to administer: _____
**g.** seconds/calibration

DA equation:

**h.** Evaluation: _____

**2** Ordered: diazepam 10 mg IV push. Directions: Give undiluted directly into vein. Rate: Inject at rate of 5 mg/ min.

**a.** Total amount of prepared medication in mL:

DA equation:

**b.** Total amount of diluted medication in mL (if applicable): _____
**c.** Total minutes to administer: _____
**d.** mL/ min to be administered: _____
**e.** Total calibrations for the diluted medication: _____

**f.** Total seconds to administer: _____
**g.** seconds/ calibration

DA equation:

**h.** Evaluation: _____

**3** Ordered: phenobarbital 90 mg IV push, for a patient with seizures. Follow directions on label for dilution and rate of injection. For IV use, dilute to 3 mL of SW for injection. Do not exceed injection rate of 1 mL/ min. Do not use if solution is not clear.

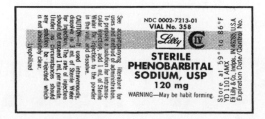

**a.** Total amount of prepared medication in mL *to the nearest tenth*:

DA equation:

**b.** Total amount of diluted medication in mL (if applicable): _____
**c.** Total minutes to administer: _____
**d.** mL/ min to be administered: _____

**e.** Total calibrations for the diluted medication: _____

**f.** Total seconds to administer: _____
**g.** seconds/ calibration

DA equation:

**h.** Evaluation: _____

4 Ordered: meperidine 50 mg IV push. Dilute to 5 mL of SW or NS. Give over
5 minutes.

**a.** Total amount of prepared medication in mL *to the nearest tenth*:

DA equation:

**b.** Total amount of diluted medication in mL (if applicable): _____
**c.** Total minutes to administer: _____
**d.** mL/ min to be administered: _____
**e.** Total calibrations for the diluted medication: _____

**f.** Total seconds to administer: _____
**g.** seconds/ calibration

DA equation:

**h.** Evaluation: _____

**5** Ordered: furosemide 40 mg IV push, for an anuric patient. Directions: Should be infused in anuric patients at a rate of 4 mg/ min. May be given undiluted.

**a.** Total amount of prepared medication in mL: _____

**b.** Total amount of diluted medication in mL (if applicable): _____

**c.** Total minutes to administer: _____

**d.** mL/ min to be administered: _____

**e.** Total calibrations for the medication: _____

**f.** Total seconds to administer: _____

**g.** seconds/ calibration

DA equation:

**h.** Evaluation: _____

---

*Ask Yourself*

*My Answer*

**1** Why is it suggested that the nurse start the push count with the second hand of the watch on the 12 o'clock mark?

_____

# Hyperalimentation: Total Parenteral Nutrition

Hyperalimentation (*hyperal*, for short) provides high-calorie IV nutrition. Also known as total parenteral nutrition (TPN), it can provide up to 1 Kcal/ mL with amino acids, dextrose, electrolytes, vitamins, and minerals to meet total nutritional needs. Ten or 20% lipid emulsions can also be delivered intravenously as part of the TPN order. Lipids may be added intermittently to provide needed calories (Figure 10-6).

When a patient is unable to ingest food or nutritional fluids through the gastrointestinal tract, ketosis, muscle wasting, and starvation will occur. Ordinary IV solutions cannot supply adequate nutritional needs.

The caloric contents of IV solutions are low:

- A maintenance solution of D5W, LRS, or NS contains 5 g dextrose per 100 mL of solution or 50 g dextrose per 1000 mL.
- A patient receiving 3 L/ day would receive 150 g/ day of dextrose.
- Carbohydrates contain 4 cal/ g (the dietary "calorie" is actually a kilocalorie, as mentioned under Essential Vocabulary). 150 g × 4 kcal/ g = 600 kcal/ day.
- 600 kcal/ day is inadequate for health maintenance.
- Adults usually consume between 1500 and 2500 kilocalories or more per day of protein, carbohydrate, and fat to meet energy and nutritional needs.

**1** How many calories of carbohydrate are contained in 1 L of D5W solution?

**Q:***Ask Yourself*

**A:***My Answer*

**A**      **B**

Figure 10-6. **A,** Amino acid. **B,** Liposyn. (**A** from Brown M, Mulholland JL: Drug calculations: process and problems for clinical practice, ed. 7, St. Louis, 2004, Mosby. **B** from Abbott Laboratories, Abbott Park, IL.)

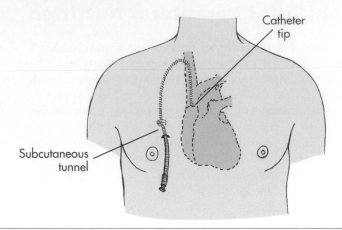

Figure **10-7.** Centrally inserted catheter. (From Perry AG, Potter PA: Clinical nursing skills and techniques, ed. 6, St. Louis, 2006, Mosby.)

Figure **10-8.** **A,** Implantable infusion port. **B,** Infusion port placed in subcutaneous pocket. **C,** Assortment of Huber needles. (From Perry AG, Potter PA: Clinical nursing skills and techniques, ed. 6, St. Louis, 2006, Mosby.)

Insulin may be added to the TPN solution as necessary to maintain normal blood glucose levels. The infusions may be given in the hospital and in the home health setting. If the patient's condition is stable, the TPN may be ordered for 12 hr/ day, as opposed to potentially 24 hr/ day for an insulin-dependent patient. The contents are customized according to the patient's weight, the length of time the infusion will be needed, whether the venous access site is central or peripheral, and current laboratory test results, including nitrogen balance, renal function, and glucose levels.

Because the solution is concentrated and irritating to the vein, it needs to be infused in a *large* vein. Central venous lines are preferred for long-term therapy because of rapid dilution in the superior vena cava (Figure 10-7). Vascular access devices (VADs), such as tunneled catheters and ports, are surgically implanted to provide central venous access. Lower concentrations may be administered for the peripheral access sites.

Vascular implanted ports for parenteral nutrition must be accessed with special non-coring Huber needles. Some ports permit up to 2000 punctures with this type of needle (Figure 10-8).

Peripherally inserted central catheters (PICC) can also be inserted in large peripheral veins, such as the antecubital, for shorter-term use. Small peripheral ports can be inserted in the forearm (Figure 10-9).

Peripheral parenteral nutrition (PPN) can be administered directly into a larger peripheral vein when necessary for short-term therapy. The concentration of the fluid will be less than that of central infusions.

- These life-sustaining venous access sites cannot be used for the administration of medications, blood, and other products.
- TPN and PPN are administered on an infusion pump.
- Strict protocols must be followed. Check agency and manufacturer's guidelines.
- TPN solutions' contents are customized by the prescriber and prepared by the pharmacist based on current laboratory test results. Orders may be changed daily. The prescriber's order needs to be compared in detail with the contents and percentage of contents of each TPN solution. Several concentrations of dextrose, amino acids, and lipids are available.

Figure **10-9.** Prepping PICC site. (From Perry AG, Potter PA: Clinical nursing skills and techniques, ed. 5 revised reprint, St. Louis, 2004, Mosby.)

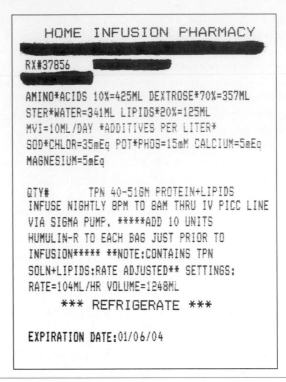

```
HOME INFUSION PHARMACY
████████████████████████████
RX#37856        ████████████
████████████

AMINO*ACIDS 10%=425ML DEXTROSE*70%=357ML
STER*WATER=341ML LIPIDS*20%=125ML
MVI=10ML/DAY *ADDITIVES PER LITER*
SOD*CHLOR=35mEq POT*PHOS=15mM CALCIUM=5mEq
MAGNESIUM=5mEq


QTY#        TPN 40-51GM PROTEIN+LIPIDS
INFUSE NIGHTLY 8PM TO 8AM THRU IV PICC LINE
VIA SIGMA PUMP. *****ADD 10 UNITS
HUMULIN-R TO EACH BAG JUST PRIOR TO
INFUSION***** **NOTE:CONTAINS TPN
SOLN+LIPIDS:RATE ADJUSTED** SETTINGS:
RATE=104ML/HR VOLUME=1248ML
        *** REFRIGERATE ***


EXPIRATION DATE:01/06/04
```

Figure **10-10.** TPN bag label for home infusion therapy. (From Brown M, Mulholland JL: Drug calculations: process and problems for clinical practice, ed. 7, St. Louis, 2004, Mosby.)

## CHAPTER 10 MULTIPLE-CHOICE REVIEW

**Estimated completion time: 30 minutes**   Answers on page **581**

**Directions:**  *Select the correct intravenous-related response. Verify answers with a DA equation. Use a calculator for long division and multiplication.*

1  An IV flow rate of 2 mL/ min of 5% L/R would be set at which flow rate on an infusion pump?

   **1.** 60 drops/ min                    **3.** 120 drops/ min
   **2.** 60 mL/ hr                        **4.** 120 mL/ hr

2  Ordered: IV of 500 mL D5 NS 40 mEq, for a patient with hypokalemia, at 10 mEq/ hr. Check serum potassium level when completed. Continue until serum potassium level greater than 4, then discontinue. The nurse will set the flow rate at:

   **1.** 10 mL/ hr for 4 hours            **3.** 50 mL/ hr for 4 hours
   **2.** 40 mL/ hr for 10 hours           **4.** 125 mL/ hr for 4 hours

   Direct injection of concentrated KCl can cause cardiac arrest.

**3** An available IV solution contains 1g in 250 mL. How many milligrams per milliliter are contained in the solution? (Use mental arithmetic.)

**1.** 4                                      **3.** 25
**2.** 0.25                                   **4.** 100

**4** How many kilocalories of dextrose are contained in a central TPN solution of 1 L that contains 25% dextrose? (Conversion formula: 4 kcal = 1 g of dextrose.)

**1.** 25                                     **3.** 250
**2.** 100                                    **4.** 1000

**5** Ordered: IVPB antibiotic of 30 mL to infuse in 30 minutes. What will the flow rate be set on a gravity device with a microdrip set? (Use mental arithmetic.)

**1.** 30 mL/ hr                             **3.** 90 drops/ min
**2.** 60 drops/ min                         **4.** 100 drops/ min

**6** Ordered: morphine sulfate 3 mg IV push, for a patient in pain. Drug reference directions for IV direct injection: Dilute to 5 mL with SW. Available: morphine sulfate 10 mg/ mL. Directions: Administer over 5 minutes. How many mL/ min will the medication deliver?

**1.** 1                                      **3.** 10
**2.** 5                                      **4.** 50

**7** The recommendation for adjusting medicated IV infusions that are behind the ordered schedule for the amount infused is

**1.** Adjust up to 25% more than the ordered rate.
**2.** Adjust up to 10% more than the ordered rate.
**3.** Let the IV infusion rate stay behind the ordered rate.
**4.** Assess the patient condition and consult with the licensed prescriber.

**8** An existing unmedicated IV solution is flowing at 100 mL/ hr when the nurse arrives to care for the patient. 500 out of 1000 mL have been infused in 5 hours. The order reads: 1000 mL q8h. The patient is NPO 1 day postoperatively and has good heart, lung, and renal function. The urinary output appears concentrated. The nurse's assessment is that it would be safe to adjust the IV to complete it on time. The adjustment would be:

**1.** The flow rate needs adjustment to 125 mL/ hr.
**2.** The flow rate needs adjustment to 167 mL/ hour.
**3.** The flow rate needs to be opened up until it is on target for the current time and then adjusted to 125mL/ hr.
**4.** The flow rate should be adjusted to 155 mL/ hr until completed.

**9** Which of the following is the most concentrated IV solution?

**1.** 250 mg/ 1000 mL                       **3.** 100 mg/ 100 mL
**2.** 250 mg/ 500 mL                        **4.** 50 mg/ 100 mL

**10** An order of 500 mg of a drug in 1000 mL is being infused at 10 mL/ hr. The hourly amount of drug infused is

**1.** 2 mg/ hr                              **3.** 10 mg/ hr
**2.** 5 mg/ hr                              **4.** 15 mg/ hr

**CHAPTER 10 FINAL PRACTICE**

**Estimated completion time: 1-2 hours**   **Answers on page 582**

**Directions:** *Calculate the advanced intravenous problems. Verify your answers with a DA equation. Label answers. Use a calculator for long division and multiplication. Evaluate your equations.*

1  Ordered: furosemide 30 mg IV push, for a patient with anuria, at 4 mg/ min. Directions: May be given undiluted.

**a.** Total mL to inject?

DA equation:

Evaluation: _____

**b.** Calibrations occupied by the medication:

**c.** Total seconds for injection:

DA equation:

Evaluation: _____

**d.** Seconds per calibration for injection:

DA equation:

Evaluation: _____

2 Ordered: aminophylline IV infusion for a patient with acute asthma. Titrate: 0.3 to 0.6 mg/ kg/ hr. Patient's weight: 75 kg. Directions: Dilute in 250 mL NS. Consult the label for drug amount placed in the IV. The nurse will withdraw 20 mL of NS before adding the aminophylline.

**a.** What flow rate will be set on the infusion pump for 0.3 mg/ kg/ hr?

DA equation:

Evaluation: _____

**b.** The patient's respiratory status does not improve. The theophylline serum levels are still within normal levels. The nurse increases the flow rate to 0.4/ mg/ kg/ hr. What will the flow rate be adjusted to?

DA equation (Refer to the 2-step example on p. 344.):

Evaluation: _____

3 Ordered: Nitropress IV infusion. Start at 0.3 mcg/ kg/ min, for a patient with severe hypertension. Titrate to keep systolic blood pressure below 160 and diastolic pressure below 90. Directions: Dilute 50 mg in 250 mL D5W. The nurse will use 250 mL as the total amount of solution for calculation purposes. Patient weight: 60 kg.

**a.** mg/ mL concentration in the final solution:

DA equation:

Evaluation: _____

**b.** The nurse will set the flow rate on the infusion pump at _____

DA equation (Refer to the 2-step example on p. 344.):

Evaluation: _____

**4** Ordered: dobutamine 2.5 mcg/ kg/ min. Directions: Dilute in 500 mL D5W. The nurse will withdraw 20 mL of the D5W, discard it, and use 480 mL of the D5W plus 20 mL of the dobutamine solution to make a 500-mL medicated solution. Patient weight: 64 kg.

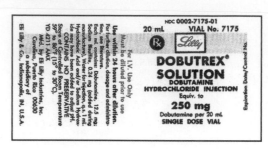

**a.** mg/ mL concentration in the final solution: _____

**b.** The nurse will set the flow rate on the infusion pump at _____

DA equation:

Evaluation: _____

**5** Ordered: KCl 10 mEq/ hr, for a patient with hypokalemia. Directions: Dilute in 500 mL D5 $\frac{1}{2}$ NS. Recheck serum potassium level in 4 hours and contact physician for orders if less than 3.5 mEq/ L. Available: KCl 40 mEq/ 500 mL D5 $\frac{1}{2}$ NS. The nurse will set the flow rate on the infusion pump at _____

DA equation:

Evaluation: _____

**6** Ordered: dopamine HCl infusion 3 mcg/ kg/ min. Patient's weight: 82 kg. Flow rate when the nurse begins the shift: dopamine HCl at 15 mL/ hr

**CHAPTER 10**

**a.** How many milligrams per hour are ordered?

DA equation:

Evaluation: _____

**b.** What is the ordered flow rate?

DA equation:

Evaluation: _____

**7** Ordered: atropine sulfate 1 mg bolus IV push, for a patient with bradyar-rhythmia. Directions: Dilute to 10 mL SW for injection (total amount) and give over 1 minute.

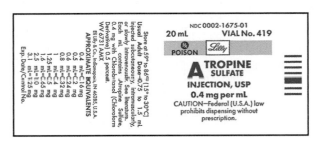

**a.** How many mL of atropine will the nurse prepare?

DA equation:

Evaluation: _____

**b.** After dilution, how many seconds/ mL will the atropine be injected?

DA equation:

Evaluation: _____

8 Ordered: naloxone infusion, to wean a patient with narcotic depression, to be infused over 6 hours at 0.03 mg/ hr. Directions: Dilute 2 mg in 500 mL NS or D5W.

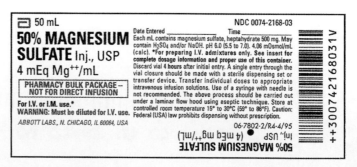

a. How many mL of naloxone will be added to the 500 mL?

DA equation:

Evaluation: _____

b. The nurse will set the flow rate on the infusion pump at (round to the nearest whole number):

DA equation:

Evaluation: _____

9 Ordered: magnesium sulfate 2.5 mL/ min IV infusion, for a patient with convulsions. Directions: Dilute 4 g in 250 mL of D5W. Read the label for mg/ mL and prepare 4 g.

a. How many mL of magnesium sulfate will the nurse prepare for the infusion?

DA equation:

Evaluation: _____

The nurse will remove an amount of D5W equal to the amount of medication being added so that the IV solution remains 250 mL.

**b.** Following the ordered rate, what will be the flow rate on the infusion pump?

DA equation:

Evaluation: _____

**c.** How many mg/ min will the patient receive? _____

DA equation:

Evaluation: _____

**10** Ordered: quinidine gluconate loading dose 15 mg/ kg over 4 hours' infusion, for a patient with *Plasmodium falciparum* malaria. Directions: Give in 250 mL NS. Patient's weight: 70 kg.

**a.** How many mL of quinidine gluconate will the nurse prepare and dilute in 250 mL NS?

DA equation:

Evaluation: _____

**b.** What flow rate will be set on the infusion pump? _____

DA equation:

Evaluation: _____

## Suggestions for Further Reading

Clayton BD, Stock YN: Basic pharmacology for nurses, ed. 13, St. Louis, 2004, Mosby.
Elkin MK, Perry AG, Potter PA: Nursing interventions and clinical skills, ed. 3, St. Louis, 2004, Mosby.
Gahart B, Nazareno A: 2005 Intravenous medications, ed. 21, St. Louis, 2005, Mosby.
Lilley LL, Harrington S, Snyder JS: Pharmacology and the nursing process, ed. 4, St. Louis, 2005, Mosby.

Potter PA, Perry AG: Fundamentals of nursing, ed. 6, St. Louis, 2005, Mosby.
www.Baxter.com
www.globalrph.com/tpn.htm
www.Hospira.com
www.safemedication.com/displaydrug.cfm?id=601166

 Additional practice problems can be found in the Advanced Intravenous Calculations section on the enclosed companion CD.

Now that you have mastered the principles and contents of this chapter, you will be on the road to safer practice and will also find Chapter 11, Antidiabetic Agents, and subsequent chapters relatively easy to learn.

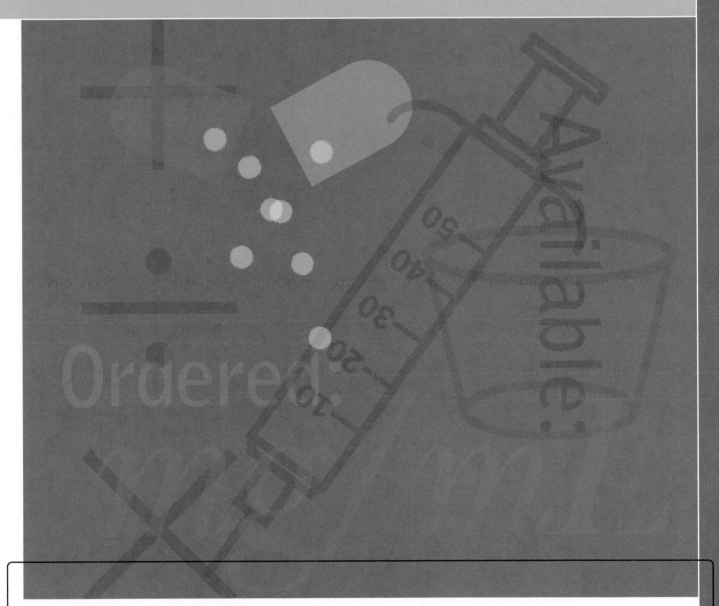

# PART V
## ORAL AND INJECTABLE HORMONE MEDICATIONS

CHAPTER 11    ANTIDIABETIC AGENTS

CHAPTER 12    ANTICOAGULANT AGENTS

> *"It is easier to change a person's religion than to change their diet."*
> —MARGARET MEAD

# ANTIDIABETIC AGENTS

## Objectives

- Define terms related to tests and treatment for patients receiving medications for type 1 and type 2 diabetes.
- Identify risks of look-alike generic oral antidiabetic products.
- Contrast the various insulin products by onset of activity.
- Calculate and titrate subcutaneous and IV insulin dosages based on blood glucose levels.
- Evaluate blood glucose levels for prescribed insulin administration.
- Select the appropriate syringe and measure syringe doses for subcutaneous insulin administration.
- Identify the most common adverse effect of insulin therapy.
- Define *hypoglycemia* and *hyperglycemia*.
- Identify causes of, risks of, and nutrients needed for hypoglycemia.
- Identify critical patient safety issues related to antidiabetic medications and blood glucose levels.

## Essential Prior Knowledge

Mastery of Chapters 1-10

## Equipment

- The learner will benefit from concurrent practice preparing and administering various types and mixtures of insulin under clinical supervision using insulin syringes.

## Estimated Time To Complete Chapter

- 2-2½ hours

# Introduction

Diabetes is an epidemic that is increasing at an alarming rate and has generated many new medicines for treatment. According to the International Diabetic Federation (IDF), the highest rate of diabetes prevalence in 2004 was in North America, where it was thought to be 7.9% of the population. Other estimates were higher, ranging from 8% to 10% for diabetes type 2. Worldwide prevalence of diabetes, if left untreated, was projected by the IDF to be 333 million cases by the year 2025.

Measuring an ordered insulin dose in a syringe for subcutaneous administration is a basic skill that does not require math. However, IV insulin administration does require math calculations. To administer antidiabetic agents safely, the nurse must understand frequently encountered terms, know how to interpret orders and labels, differentiate blood glucose laboratory levels, distinguish the

372

various pharmacological products ordered for treatment, identify manifestations of hypo- and hyperglycemia, understand emergency treatment for those manifestations, and know when to withhold medication and seek further orders. Insulin is a high risk medication meaning that it has higher than average potential to cause harm if used in error.* This chapter focuses on basic concepts related to safe administration of insulin.

Many new medications for diabetes have been developed to meet this epidemic and are commonly encountered in the patient care setting. The doses must be individualized based on frequent current test results.

The learner will need to consult pharmacology and pathophysioloy texts as well as nursing theory and skills texts for complete knowledge needed for the safe care of patients with diabetes.

## ESSENTIAL Vocabulary

| | |
|---|---|
| **Diabetes Mellitus (DM; see also DM types 1 and 2)** | An endocrine disorder of multiple causes affecting pancreatic insulin production and/or utilization, as well as carbohydrate, fat, and protein metabolism. Characterized by elevated blood glucose levels and associated with many serious complications. |
| **Diabetes Mellitus type 1 (DM type I)** | Characterized by little or no insulin production by beta ($\beta$) cells formed in the pancreatic islets of Langerhans. Usual onset in childhood, but not always. Treated with lifelong insulin hormone administration. DM type 1 occurs in less than 10% of cases. Causal factors theorized to be autoimmune, genetic, and/or environmental, among others. Formerly known as insulin-dependent diabetes mellitus or juvenile-onset diabetes. |
| **Diabetes Mellitus type 2 (DM type 2)** | Characterized by some insulin production but insufficient amount or resistance to insulin utilization. (See "Insulin Resistance.") If not controlled with dietary or lifestyle changes, treated with oral antidiabetics. Insulin may be added for better glucose control if diet and oral medications do not suffice to control blood glucose levels. Insulin may also be added intermittently for specific stressful events, such as infection and pregnancy. Several potential causal factors are associated with aging, genetics, obesity, diet, and sedentary lifestyle. Type 2 accounts for approximately 85%-95% of all cases in developed countries. Formerly was primarily adult onset, but presentation is increasingly seen in children, thought to be related to the growing obesity epidemic in children.<br><br>Patients may have the disease for several years before diagnosis. Formerly known as non–insulin-dependent diabetes or adult-onset diabetes. |
| **Diabetic Ketoacidosis (DKA)** | Emergency condition diagnosed by elevated blood glucose levels (>250 mg/ dL), blood pH <7.3, elevated ketones in blood and urine, and often coma. Requires hospitalization and insulin therapy as well as other medications. |
| **Hormones**<br>**Glucagon** | Blood glucose-*raising* hormone secreted by alpha ($\alpha$) cells in the pancreatic islets of Langerhans, released in response to a fall below normal in blood glucose levels. May be administered exogenously for severe hypoglycemia levels (e.g., blood glucose level <60 mg/ dL). |
| **Insulin** | Blood glucose-*lowering* hormone produced by the beta cells of the islets of Langerhans in the pancreas. It facilitates entry of glucose into muscle cells and other sites for storage as an energy source, thus lowering blood glucose levels.<br><br>**Mnemonic:** INsulin helps glucose get IN to cells. |
| **Hyperglycemia** | Elevated glucose level in blood. Levels vary for diabetes diagnosis, postprandial (after meal) norms, and treatment and control needs. Refer to agency laboratory norms. |

*continued*

---

*Refer to Institute for Safe Medication Practices (www.ismp.org).

| | |
|---|---|
| **Hypoglycemia** | Decreased level of glucose in blood (<70 mg/ dL). May be caused by several factors: *skipped or delayed meal after insulin and/or some oral antidiabetic agents,* or *insulin overdose.* Usually more severe in insulin-dependent patients. The major potential adverse effect of insulin administration. |
| | Symptoms are variable among individuals and range from mild confusion and irritability to impaired functioning to loss of consciousness and death. |
| | Brain function is dependent on glucose. Below *50 mg/ dL,* brain damage can occur. Symptoms depend on many factors, including *rate* of drop of blood glucose level. |
| | Should be treated early and promptly. |
| | All diabetics should carry some form of glucose, as well as medical information, on their persons. |
| **Incidence (see also "Prevalence")** | Number of *new* cases of a disease occurring within a specific time frame, usually a year. |
| **Insulin Resistance** | Diminished tissue ability to respond to insulin. Glucose levels continue to rise. Insulin production and levels then rise (hyperinsulinemia) in response, in an attempt to maintain normal glucose levels. Associated with DM type 2, obesity, and hypertension. |
| **Insulin "Shock"** | Urgent hypoglycemic condition (blood glucose <60 mg/ dL). May be caused by an overdose of insulin for current glucose level or as a result of taking usual dose of insulin followed by inadequate or delayed dietary intake. Must be treated promptly with immediate form of glucose administration, oral if the patient is conscious or IV if the patient is unconscious or unable to swallow, followed up by *complex carbohydrate* to cover possible hypoglycemic recurrence. Brain cells begin to be deprived of glucose when the blood glucose level falls below normal. (See "Hypoglycemia.") |
| **Prevalence (see also "Incidence")** | Total number of cases of a disease in existence at a certain time in a designated area. |
| **Units** | Standardized dose measurement of therapeutic effectiveness. Insulin is provided in units. |

# Laboratory Tests AND Terminology

| | |
|---|---|
| **Blood Glucose (BG)** | Laboratory serum venous blood glucose test. Prescribers may order this test to verify capillary BGM and SMBG test results. |
| **Blood Glucose Monitor (BGM)** | Blood capillary hand-held finger-stick device administered at the bedside by nurses or at home by patients. |
| **Self-Monitored Blood Glucose (SMBG)** | Administered by patients with the blood glucose monitor. The result is reported by the patient. |
| **Deciliter (dL)** | One-tenth of a liter. Used to report number of milligrams in blood glucose laboratory test results (e.g., 100 mg/ dL). |
| **Fasting Blood Sugar (FBS)** | Fasting (8-12 hr) reveals current blood glucose level (normal level, 70-100 mg/ dL).* |
| **Fructosamine** | Determines average blood glucose level over the *past 2 weeks.* |
| **Glycosylated Hemoglobin (A1c or HbA1c)** | Determines average blood glucose level over the *past 2-3 months* by measuring the amount of glucose attached to hemoglobin in the red blood cells. Helpful in assessing newly diagnosed patients, severity of disease, home maintenance in those being treated, and risk for complications. A normal HbA1c level is <7.0%.* |

*Normal values vary slightly from laboratory to laboratory. Glucose goal levels for diabetics may be slightly higher than for nondiabetics.

| Postprandial Glucose Test | "After-meals" blood glucose test. Usually performed 2 hr after meals to determine individual ability to metabolize glucose, and to evaluate treatment. Two-hour postprandial blood glucose level is usually normal in nondiabetics and elevated in diabetics.* |
|---|---|
| | *Normal values vary slightly from laboratory to laboratory. Glucose goal levels for diabetics may be slightly higher than for nondiabetics. |

➤ If blood glucose levels are reported by a laboratory in millimoles per liter, *multiply* by 18 to convert to milligrams per deciliter. Divide milligrams per deciliter by 18 to obtain the equivalent millimoles per liter.

## RAPID PRACTICE 11-1 Vocabulary Review

**Estimated completion time: 10-15 minutes**   Answers on page **584**

**Directions:** *Study the vocabulary and laboratory terminology. Answer the following questions with brief, one- or two-word answers.*

1 What are the main *differences* in measurement among the following tests: stat BG, FBS, 2-hour postprandial, fructosamine, and HbA1c?

_____

_____

_____

2 What four-letter *abbreviation* does a nurse write if the patient reports results of self-monitored sugar level? _____

3 What is a normal fasting blood sugar level range? _____

4 What does insulin do in the body to blood glucose? (State answer in a few words.)

_____

5 Contrast in one or two words the difference between insulin shock and diabetic ketoacidosis (DKA) in terms of blood glucose levels and the main drug administered for treatment.

Insulin shock _____

DKA _____

# Oral Antidiabetic Agents

Oral antidiabetic medications are a growing number of hypoglycemic agents with varying pharmacologic properties that target specific problems of glucose metabolism for patients with type 2 diabetes mellitus. Many are available in more than one concentration. The following are some of these agents:

Class: biguanide
    Metformin (glucophage, glucophage XR)

Class: meglitinides
    Prandin (repaglinide)
Class: sulfonylurea
    Diabeta (glyburide)
    Amaryl (glimepiride)
    Glucotrol (glipizide)
Class: thiazolidinedione
    Actos (pioglitazone)
    Avandia (rosiglitazone)

➤ Note carefully the similarities of generic names. Confusion of look-alike drug names has resulted in medication errors.

Some of these drugs are available in several doses. They may be combined with other drugs to enhance the effectiveness of treatment. For example, Avandamet is a combination of Avandia and Metformin, and Metaglip is a combination of glipizide and metformin.

➤ Match the prescriber's order, drug name, drug dose, and labels carefully. Do not try to guess the product contents from the name. The math is simple for the oral medications. The doses are available as ordered or in multiples of the amount ordered. They must be given at the prescribed time to control potential mealtime-generated elevations of glucose levels.

**EXAMPLES**

Following are some examples of prescribers' orders for oral antidiabetics, along with the drug labels:

*Glucophage 500 mg tid with meals*

*Prandin 1 mg tid 30 minutes ac*

CHAPTER 11

*Glucotrol XL 2.5 mg daily with breakfast*

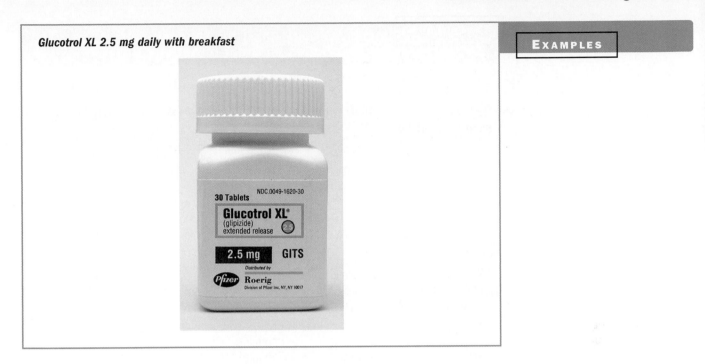

## Parenteral Antidiabetic Agents: Insulin Products

The hormone insulin is supplied in rapid-onset, intermediate-acting, and long-acting forms in standardized units.

- It is supplied in two concentrations: U 100 (100 units/ mL) and U 500 (500 units/ mL; Figure 11-1).
- U 100 is the most commonly ordered concentration.
- The U 500 concentration is ordered for the rare patient who needs very high doses.
- Insulin types are related to the product source as well as to the onset and duration of action. Recombinant DNA (rDNA) insulin, a highly purified version of human insulin, is similar in structure and function to human insulin.
- Insulin is most often prescribed and administered subcutaneously. The IV route is reserved for specific acute-care situations.

➤ Do not confuse U 100 with the total amount in the vial. U 100 refers to the concentration per milliliter (100 units/ mL).

➤ The most common adverse effect of insulin therapy is *hypoglycemia*.

➤ Spell out units even though the abbreviation U may be seen in some orders and preprinted MARs. It can be mistaken for zero and is on the "Do Not Use" list of the JCAHO.

Figure 11-1. **A,** U 100 (100 units/ mL) insulin. **B,** U 500 (500 units/ mL) insulin.

| TABLE 11-1 | Insulin Activity Chart for Subcutaneous Administration, in Order of Activity Onset | | | |
|---|---|---|---|---|
| Type | Brand name | Onset of subcutaneous route | Peak | Duration |
| **Short/rapid acting** | | | | |
| Insulin aspart | Novolog | 10-20 min | 1-3 hr | 3-5 hr |
| Insulin lispro | Humalog | 15 min | 1 hr | 3.5-4.5 hr |
| 70% insulin aspart protamine suspension + 30% insulin aspart (fixed premix) | Novolog Mix 70/30 | 10-20 min | 2.4 hr | 24 hr |
| 75% insulin lispro protamine + 25% insulin lispro (fixed premix) | Humalog Mix 75/25 | 15 min | 30-90 min | 24 hr |
| Insulin injection regular | Novolin R | 30 min | 2.5-5 hr | 8 hr |
| | Humulin R | 30 min | 2-4 hr | 6-8 hr |
| | Iletin II Regular (pork source) | 30 min | 2-4 hr | 4 hr |
| Insulin isophane suspension (NPH) + regular insulin combination | Novolin 70/30 | 30 min | 2-12 hr | 24 hr |
| | Humulin 70/30 | 30 min | 2-12 hr | 24 hr |
| | Humulin 50/50 | 30 min | 3-5 hr | 24 hr |
| **Intermediate acting** | | | | |
| Insulin isophane suspension (NPH) | Novolin N | 1.5 hr | 4-12 hr | Up to 24 hr |
| | Humulin N | 1-2 hr | 6-12 hr | 18-24 hr |
| **Long acting** | | | | |
| Insulin glargine | Lantus | 1 hr | None | 24 hr or more |
| Insulin zinc suspension (L) | | 1-3 hr | 6-12 hr | 18-26 hr |
| Insulin extended zinc suspension | | 4-6 hr | 8-20 hr | 24-48 hr |
| Insulin detenir | Levemir | 0.8-2 hr | None | 24 hr |

➤ Prescribed timing of insulin administration and timing of meals are linked to the time of onset of the insulin activity. *Hypoglycemic* reactions may occur at any time, but insulin onset and peak activity times warrant close observation for potential hypoglycemic reactions.

Examine the insulin activity chart in Table 11-1. Insulin fixed-combination mixes are supplied for patients who experience patterns of mealtime elevations. The mixes contain rapid-acting insulin mixed with longer-, slower-acting insulin, which reduces the fluctuations and elevations in blood glucose patterns. The intermediate- and longer-acting insulins contain additives that extend the action but render them unsuitable for IV administration.

Q: *Ask Yourself*

A: *My Answer*

1  What are the five column headings in Table 11-1 that reveal key pieces of information that the nurse must understand about each type of insulin?

**2**    Which type of insulin does not have a peak?

_____

> **FAQ** | *How are insulin types and amounts selected?*
>
> **ANSWER:** Types and amounts are selected on the basis of patterns in the patient's recent blood glucose levels, including the timing of elevations, particularly related to mealtime and activity patterns. The patient's motivation and compliance are also factored into insulin prescriptions.

**Clinical Relevance**

- If the patient is hospitalized with extremely high levels of blood glucose, a rapid-acting insulin may be administered subcutaneously or intravenously to stabilize the patient.
- Some patients exhibit elevations only after meals, some have nighttime or early-morning spikes, and others have constant elevations.
- For newly diagnosed patients, a small amount, a *basal* (slow, low, continuous release) dose of long-acting insulin, such as insulin glargine, may be ordered with weekly dose adjustments. This amount does not cover mealtime elevations. The dose will be low enough to avoid *hypo*glycemic reactions. *Bolus* (single, concentrated) doses of insulin aspart and lispro, or regular insulins, may be ordered and administered separately to cover mealtime and/or other elevations.
- When a pattern of blood glucose levels in relation to meals emerges, the type and amount of insulin can be customized.
- Insulin mixes may be ordered twice a day to cover a patient's basal needs and mealtime elevations when a pattern is known.
- Intermediate- and long-acting insulins are *not* used to treat *acute hyper*glycemia.

**Q:** *Ask Yourself*

**1**    What is a basal dose of insulin?

_____

**2**    What are two reasons that bolus doses would be added to basal doses?

**A:** *My Answer*

_____

## Insulin Labels

Take a few minutes to examine the insulin product labels and identify the following:

- Name
- Type
- Concentration: U 100 or U 500
- Product source: rDNA
- Storage directions: Insulin is kept cool. Bottles in use are refrigerated unless otherwise indicated on the label or product insert. The nurse writes the date opened on the label and discards the opened bottle according to manufacturer guidelines, usually a month after opening.
- Expiration date

**Clinical Relevance**

Teach the patient to place insulin in an insulated cooler for travel (not on dry ice) and to carry it on his or her person. If insulin is warm, it may develop particles or crystals, may become discolored, and will not be effective in lowering blood glucose levels.

# Short-, Rapid-Acting Insulins

There are several types and brands of short- or rapid-acting insulins on the market. Short-rapid acting insulins are administered to treat a current blood glucose elevation or an anticipated elevation in the near future, such as after the next meal. Figures 11-2 to 11-5 illustrate product labels of various short-acting insulins.

Humalog and Novolog insulin are to be given 10 to 15 minutes *before* a meal or with the meal, whereas Humulin R and Novolin R must be given 30 minutes before a meal (Figures 11-2 to 11-4).

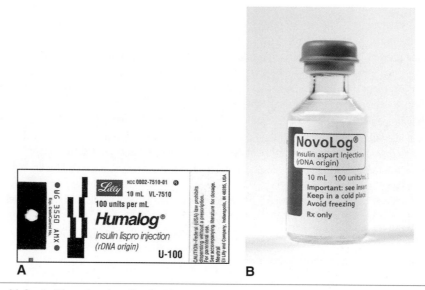

Figure 11-2. **A,** Humalog insulin. **B,** NovoLog insulin. (B, From NOVO Nordisk Inc., Princeton, NJ.)

Figure 11-3. Humulin R insulin.

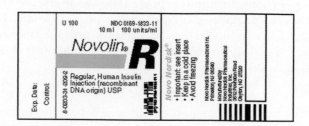

Figure 11-4. Novolin R insulin.

**A**   **B**

Figure **11-5. A,** Humalog insulin should always look clear. **B,** Insulin at the bottom of the bottle. Do not use if insulin stays on the bottom of the bottle after gentle rolling. (©Copyright Eli Lilly and Company. All rights reserved. Used with permission.)

> ☀ **Mnemonic**
>
> Humalog and Novolog, described as "mealtime" insulins, are analogs of human insulin and, when administered, "log" in faster than regular rapid-acting insulins on the market.

➤ If there is any chance that mealtime may be delayed, such as might occur in a hospital, do *not* give Humalog or Novolog until the meal arrives.

1 What does U 100 on the label of the insulin vial mean?

_____

2 What is the most common adverse effect of insulin therapy?

_____

Q **Ask Yourself**

A **My Answer**

➤ Avoid giving diet beverages or artificially sweetened foods, such as sugar alcohols and aspartame, for suspected *hypo*glycemic reactions. Follow prescriber and agency policies for insulin reactions. *Dextrose* is the ingredient needed to raise the blood glucose level promptly. Dextrose administration is usually followed by a complex carbohydrate-containing meal to sustain a higher blood glucose level.

**RAPID PRACTICE 11-2** Rapid- and Short-Acting Insulin Label Interpretation

**Estimated completion time: 10-15 minutes**   Answers on page **584**

**Directions:** *Read the information presented in the previous sections, examine the short-acting insulin labels on p. 380, and answer the questions briefly.*

1 If there is a chance that a meal will be delayed, which two of the fast-acting insulins should be held and given *with* the meal?

_____

2 **a.** What is the concentration of insulin on the labels? _____

 **b.** How many total units of insulin are contained in each vial? _____

3 What is the name of the ingredient needed to raise blood sugar levels promptly? _____

4 If the patient is experiencing a *hypo*glycemic episode, why should diet beverages and sugar alcohols not be given?

_____

_____

**5** Which two of these insulins are the fastest acting and must be given closest to mealtime?

  **a.** Novolin R           **c.** Humulin R

  **b.** Novolog             **d.** Humalog

---

➤ Only short-acting insulin products with Regular insulin and insulin lispro (Humalog) can be administered *intravenously as well as subcutaneously*. They must be clear, without precipitates, for IV administration. They do not need to be shaken because they are not suspensions (Figure 11-5).

➤ Novolog *cannot* be given intravenously. Always check the label for the permitted routes of administration.

As with all multiuse vials, the nurse needs to write the *date and time opened* and her or his initials on the label. Discard the opened vial according to the product insert directions, after approximately a month. Consult product labels and inserts for more detailed information about storage, activity, expiration dates, and incompatibilities.

➤ Some of the labels say "Human Insulin" injection. They are not made from human pancreas. They are identical in structure to human insulin but are of rDNA origin.

➤ Do not confuse the capital letter *R* for *Regular* insulin with the small superscript ® indicating a registered product.

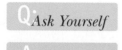
**Q**: *Ask Yourself*

**A**: *My Answer*

**1** What would be expected to happen to the patient's blood sugar levels if Humulin R, Novolin R, Insulin lispro, or Insulin aspart were given and the meal was delayed?

---

## Intermediate-Acting Insulins

Usually patients receiving intermediate-acting products, including mixes, receive *two* injections a day—one in the morning and one in the evening—plus a bed-time snack of complex carbohydrate, such as a half a cheese sandwich or milk, to cover a potential hypoglycemic reaction from overlapping duration. Mixes are usually prescribed for specified periods of time before breakfast and dinner because of the rapid-acting component. Some are ordered AM and PM without time specification.

➤ Clarify AM and PM orders with the prescriber as to precise time desired.

Isophane Insulin Human (abbreviated as NPH or N) is a modified insulin suspension that provides delayed basal insulin release. It has a longer duration than the short-acting insulins. The additives that extend the action make the solutions cloudy, rendering them inappropriate for IV administration. Suspension label directions call for either rolling or gentle shaking of the vial to mix the ingredients before drawing up in a syringe. Read the manufacturer label.

They then must be given promptly. The additives extend the duration of coverage up to 26 hours, depending on the preparation (Figure 11-6).

 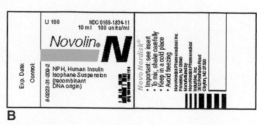

Figure **11-6.** Intermediate-acting modified insulin suspensions.

1  What would happen to the solution in the syringe if there were a delay between drawing up the suspension and administering it?

_____

2  Why might people whose employment regularly or irregularly requires second- or third-shift hours need special assistance with their antidiabetic medication schedule?

_____

## RAPID PRACTICE 11-3  Intermediate-Acting Insulin Suspensions

**Estimated completion time: 5-10 minutes**   Answers on page **585**

**Directions:**  *Read the foregoing material pertaining to intermediate-acting insulin products and answer the questions with brief phrases:*

1  How many injections of intermediate-acting insulins per day do people usually receive?_____

2  Can a suspension be administered intravenously in an emergency?

_____

3  What is the units/ mL concentration on each intermediate product label in Table 11-6 on p. 382?

_____

4  Would these intermediate-acting products be clear or cloudy?

_____

5  Why do patients on insulin mixes and bedtime short-acting insulins require a bedtime snack of a complex carbohydrate? What potential adverse effect are they trying to avoid?

_____

_____

_____

# Long-Acting Insulins

Long-acting insulin contains additives that cause it to be released more slowly than the fast- and intermediate-acting insulins. Long-acting insulin products are administered *subcutaneously* to patients with type 1 or 2 diabetes whose blood glucose levels are unresponsive to intermediate-acting insulins, such as patients with early-morning fasting elevations, and/or to patients who cannot tolerate more than one injection per day (Figure 11-7).

➤  Long-acting insulins cannot be given IV because they contain additives to extend the action. These additives are not suitable for IV use.

Insulin glargine (Lantus) and insulin detemir (Levemir) are clear. They do *not* have a peak. They provide a steady release of insulin throughout the duration of 24-26 hours. For this reason, they are known as basal long-acting insulins.

➤  Insulin glargine and insulin detemir *cannot* be mixed with any other insulin even though they are clear solutions. They may be given at any hour but must be given at the *same* time each day to provide a steady release of basal (low-dose) insulin for 24 hours without a peak. If additional short-acting insulin is needed, it is administered subcutaneously as a bolus in a *separate* syringe.

**✳ Mnemonic**

Lantus begins with an L and has a Long duration.

Figure **11-7.** Lantus insulin.

> It is safest to assume that insulin products cannot *be mixed* until you read the drug literature for each order. New products are emerging on the market. Some may be mixed, and others may not. Nurses who frequently work with diabetic patients can integrate the capabilities of new products. Nurses who do not regularly work with diabetic patients cannot rely on memory. It is best to make a habit of always checking compatibilities with current drug literature and/or the pharmacy.

> Patients on evening fast-acting or any intermediate- or long-acting insulin should have a bedtime snack.

> There are no intermediate- or long-acting forms of Humalog or Novolog.

**Q:** *Ask Yourself*

**A:** *My Answer*

1 What does the U-100 mean on the Lantus (insulin glargine) label in Figure 11-7?

_____

2 Which is the term for the most common adverse effect of insulin therapy: hypoglycemia or hyperglycemia?

_____

---

**RAPID PRACTICE 11-4** Long-Acting Insulin

**Estimated completion time: 5-10 minutes**   Answers on page **585**

**Directions:** *Read the foregoing information about long-acting insulin products and answer the following questions in two- or three-word phrases.*

1 What is the generic name for Lantus insulin? _____

2 What is a unique feature of insulin glargine and insulin detemir?

_____

3 Can long-acting insulins be administered intravenously? _____

4 What is the concentration of the insulin glargine label shown above?

_____

5 Can insulin glargine or insulin detemir be mixed with any other insulin?

_____

# Steps to Prepare Doses for Insulin Syringes

- Obtain and/or interpret the current blood glucose value. Follow the prescriber's directions for blood glucose values. Withhold insulin if the blood glucose level is low according to the prescriber's directions and agency policy. Contact the prescriber promptly if directions for low values are not written in the orders, and document the verification.
- Read the order for name, type, dose, time, and route. If you are using an opened bottle, check the discard date, as with all multidose vials.
- Select the appropriate insulin and an insulin syringe that is calibrated for the *same* concentration (e.g., 100 units/ mL).
- Examine all medication vials for clumps and precipitates. Insulin may develop precipitates if the temperature is too warm, if the vial has been contaminated, or if it has passed the expiration date.
- If the insulin is a suspension, *gently roll or* shake it to disperse the contents, according to the manufacturer's current recommendations. Rough shaking will cause air bubbles, which will alter the dose. Draw the appropriate amount of units in the insulin syringe using the technique learned for withdrawal of injectables from a vial.

  Calculations are not needed for insulin doses.

> ➤ Some agencies require two nurses for the *entire* preparation of all insulin orders. They must cosign the MAR indicating that each step of the preparation of the ordered insulin dose is correct. Check agency policy.

> ▲ **Cultural Note**
>
> In many countries, insulin preparations and syringe types vary. Remind patients to carry a generous supply of their own equipment in a small cooler for travel in their carry-on luggage.

# Matching Insulin Concentration and Syringes

➤ The insulin syringe matches the number of units/ mL on the label of the insulin bottle, for example, U 100 and 100 units/ mL on the insulin bottle label and 100 units/ mL on the syringe label. This is the most commonly used concentration in the United States.

Examine the following order: Give Novolin R 10 units subcut stat.

Examine the label. What is the brand name? *Novolin* R

What is the type (action)? *Short-acting*

Are there any terms not understood? Check current references and call the pharmacy if necessary.

How many total milliliters are there in the vial? *10 mL*

What is the concentration of drug to solution? *100 units/ mL (U 100)*

How many total units in the vial? *10 mL × 100 units = 1000 units, a multidose vial*

Does this type of insulin need to be mixed or rolled? *No, because it is not a suspension.*

➤ Prepare insulin with an insulin syringe only.

**A**

**B**

Figure 11-8. **A,** 100-unit insulin syringe marked at 12 units. **B,** 100-unit insulin syringe marked at 36 units.

## Reading Units on Insulin Syringes

Insulin is manufactured, prescribed, and administered in units. The insulin syringe is calibrated in units.

Examine the syringes in Figure 11-8. The calibrations are for even amounts of insulin. Always note the total capacity of the syringe (1 mL, 100 units for this syringe), then ensure that the syringe calibrations are units, and finally note the number of calibrations between the markings. Reading the calibrated units on the insulin syringe is straightforward.

Each calibration represents *two* units on these 100 unit/ 1 mL syringes.

## Even- and Odd-Numbered Scales on Insulin Syringes

Syringes are available with calibrations in even numbers on one side and odd numbers on the other. There are also syringes available with either even or odd calibrations (Figure 11-9).

The dose administered must be in the *precise* number of units ordered. Each calibration is worth *2* units on the even- and on the odd-numbered scale.

➤ The standard insulin syringe calibrated in units, designed for a concentration of 100 units/ mL, must be distinguished from the tuberculin syringe, which is also a 1-mL syringe calibrated in 0.01 mL (Figure 11-10).

**A**      100 units/ mL odd numbers

**B**      100 units/ mL even numbers

Figure 11-9. **A,** Insulin syringe calibrated in 100 units/ mL with odd-number markings up to 95 units. **B,** Insulin syringe calibrated in 100 units/ mL with even-number markings up to 100 units. (Used with permission from Becton, Dickinson, and Company, copyright 2003.)

**A**

**B**

Figure 11-10. **A,** 1-mL tuberculin syringe calibrated in hundredths of a milliliter with 0.1-mL markings up to 1 mL. **B,** 1-mL 100-U/ mL insulin syringe calibrated in 2-unit increments.

1    How will you know the difference between an insulin syringe and a tuberculin syringe?

Q:Ask Yourself

A:My Answer

_____

Several drugs, but not all, must be given at very precise times.

➤ Insulin is one of those drugs that must be *prioritized* to be given on time. Check insulin orders one or two times per shift. The orders change rapidly with the patient's response to treatment. Always know the patient's most recent blood glucose level.

**Clinical Relevance**

# Lo-Dose Syringes

Aging populations and patients with complications of diabetes often have diminished vision. Lo-Dose syringes are designed for persons with special visual needs. They allow for better visualization of the smaller doses.

➤ The Lo-Dose syringe is calibrated in 1-unit increments.

The syringe volume occupies 30 or 50 units and can be used by patients who are taking up to 30 or 50 units of insulin per dose (Figure 11-11).

50 unit

**A**

30 unit

**B**

Figure 11-11. **A,** 50-unit Lo-Dose insulin syringe. **B,** 30-unit Lo-Dose insulin syringe. (Used with permission from Becton, Dickinson, and Company, copyright 2003.)

**A**

**B**

**C**

Figure **11-12.** **A,** 30 units marked in a U-100 100-unit insulin syringe. **B,** 30 units marked in a U-100 50-unit Lo-Dose insulin syringe. **C,** 30 units marked in a U-100 30-unit Lo-Dose insulin syringe.

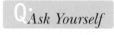
**Q:***Ask Yourself*

**1** What is the difference between the calibration of units on the 1-mL insulin syringe and that on the Lo-Dose syringe?

**A:***My Answer*

Note the difference in visualization of 30 units of insulin drawn in each of the following syringes (Figure 11-12).

## RAPID PRACTICE 11-5 Reading Units on an Insulin Syringe

**Estimated completion time: 10 minutes**   Answers on page **585**

**Directions:** *Read the syringe dose measurement in units and write the number of units in the space supplied for problems 1 and 2. For problems 3-5, mark the syringe with the ordered number of units.*

**1** _____ units

**2** _____ units

3 Ordered: Humulin R insulin 7 units subcut ac breakfast. Mark the dose ordered.

4 Ordered: Humulin N insulin 28 units subcut AM and PM. Mark the dose ordered.

5 Ordered: Insulin glargine 32 units at bedtime daily. Mark the dose ordered.

# Sites for Insulin Injection

Insulin may be administered subcutaneously in the fatty tissue of the abdomen in a radius 2 *inches away from the umbilicus*, in the thigh, in the fatty tissue of the posterior upper arm, or in the fatty tissue of the buttocks.

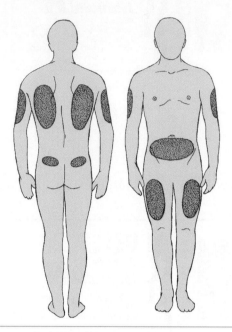

**Figure 11-13.** Sites recommended for subcutaneous injections. (From Potter PA, Perry AG: Fundamentals of nursing, ed. 6, St. Louis, 2005, Mosby.)

# Sliding-Scale Insulin

Sliding-scale short-acting insulins are titrated to *patients' current blood glucose* levels. They are usually ordered q6h for hospitalized patients on continuous liquid gastrointestinal tube feedings, or TPN.

They may also be ordered ac and bedtime to cover meal and bedtime glucose elevations for newly diagnosed patients until the patient can be stabilized on longer-acting insulins. The insulin dose "slides," or changes, with the most recent glucose levels. The scale is customized for each patient. Patterns of glucose elevations usually emerge.

Patients who experience difficult control of blood glucose levels may continue to cover elevated levels at mealtime on a sliding scale with bolus doses of short-acting insulin orders at home in addition to the longer-acting variety. The term *brittle diabetic* has been used to describe a patient who experiences poorly controlled blood glucose levels despite insulin therapy.

Examples of hand-held glucose monitors for bedside and home finger-stick draws of capillary blood are shown in Figure 11-14.

The patient may draw blood under the supervision of an experienced nurse or may self-monitor and report the result to the nurse (SMBG). The correct sliding scale amount is drawn promptly after the blood glucose level is obtained.

**Clinical Relevance**

Recheck a very low or high blood glucose level with a different monitoring device before acting on the reading. Examine the insulin bottle for discoloration if the product is supposed to be clear, and check it for particles. Ensure that a bottle that is supposed to be clear (Regular, insulin detemir, or insulin glargine) is clear, not cloudy. Suspensions will be cloudy.

There have been some cases where hospitalized patients who self-administered insulin had inexplicable elevations of blood glucose and were finally observed to be discarding the insulin rather than taking it. Observe patients' technique when they are self-administering.

Examine the following sample sliding scale for a hospitalized patient.

Ordered: Humulin R subcut per sliding scale q6h, for a patient on TPN.

### Sliding Scale for Subcutaneous Short-Acting Insulin Administration

| Blood Sugar (mg/ dL) | Insulin Amount |
|---|---|
| 70-150 | 0 units |
| 151-200 | 4 units |
| 201-250 | 6 units |
| 251-300 | 10 units |
| 301-350 | 12 units (Recheck blood glucose level 1 hr after administration.) |
| 351-400 | 15 units (Recheck blood glucose level 1 hr after administration.) |
| >400 | Call physician and draw plasma blood glucose. |

Monitor the results. Blood glucose levels are checked by the nurse with the handheld device at the bedside unless a serum blood glucose lab test is ordered. This may be done to verify abnormal BG levels.

➤ Note the *small amounts* of fast-acting insulin to be given.

**✳ Communication**

"Mr. Y, your blood glucose is 180. Your physician has ordered 2 units of Novalin R for this blood glucose level." Always keep your patient informed about BG levels and type and dose of insulin. This is not only a teaching mechanism, it may prevent administration of a type or dose with which the patient has had an adverse event.

Figure 11-14. Hand-held glucose monitors for bedside and home finger-stick draws of capillary blood. (From Elkin MK, Perry AG, Potter PA: Nursing interventions and clinical skills, ed. 3, St. Louis, 2004, Mosby.)

**RAPID PRACTICE 11-6** Interpreting Sliding Scale Orders

**Estimated completion time: 10 minutes** **Answers on page 586**

**Directions:** *Read the sliding scale in the previous example (p. 391) and answer the questions with brief phrases.*

1 If a morning capillary BGM test reveals a level of 300 mg/ dL, place an arrow on the syringe with the pointer touching the line for the amount of insulin you would prepare.

2 If the bedtime capillary BGM level was 330 mg/ dL, what two actions would you take?*

_____

_____

3 If a BGM test before dinner indicated a blood glucose level >400 mg/ dL, what two actions would you take?

_____

_____

4 What might be a reason that a plasma blood glucose test would be ordered from the laboratory instead of another capillary blood glucose test using the monitor at the bedside?

_____

5 If the sliding-scale blood glucose level was 140 mg/ mL, what would the nurse do?

_____

_____

**Q** *Ask Yourself*

**A** *My Answer*

1 If the sliding scale was written 70-150, 150-200, 201-250, 250-300, 300-350, how much insulin would you give if the patient's blood glucose level was 150 mg/ dL? With whom would you clarify this entire scale?

_____

_____

*➤ Take care if the abbreviation HS (bedtime) is encountered. It has been mistaken for half strength.

| **TABLE 11-2** | **Subcutaneous Insulin Administration Flow Sheet** |
| --- | --- |

### GENERAL HOSPITAL

**John Doe**
**#528995**

| Date | Test time | Test result | Type of test (BGM; SMBG; serum) | Insulin Type: dose | Route/location | Signature Title |
| --- | --- | --- | --- | --- | --- | --- |
| 1/1/06 | 0630 | 195 | BGM | Novolog 4 units | subcut LA | Mark Smith, RN |
| 1/1/06 | 1100 | 95 | SMBG | 0 | N/A | Mark Smith, RN |
| 1/1/06 | 1700 | 210 | BGM | Novolog 5 units | subcut RA | Jan Carter, RN |
| 1/1/06 | 2100 | 90 | BGM | 0 | N/A | Jan Carter, RN |
| 1/2/06 | 0630 | 200 | Serum FBS | Novolog 4 units | LT | Cal Pace, RN |

**FAQ** | *Why is insulin not given for all blood glucose levels that are above normal?*

**ANSWER:** Smaller elevations may not be treated with insulin to avoid hypoglycemic reactions. Dietary and lifestyle adjustments may be ordered to control lower elevations.

➤ Separate flow sheets are usually maintained on the MAR for insulin administration. Table 11-2 provides examples of the information that may be contained on such a record.

## RAPID PRACTICE 11-7 Interpreting Insulin Orders

**Estimated completion time: 10-15 minutes**   **Answers on page 586**

**Directions:** *Examine the answers given to problem 1. Read and interpret the insulin orders in problems 2-5 as requested. Refer to the vocabulary list and the insulin activity chart in Table 11-1 if needed. Mark the syringes with the dose ordered if appropriate.*

1 Ordered: Humalog insulin lispro 6 units subcut tid 15 minutes ac for a patient with DM type 1.

   **a.** What is the recommended time to administer this dose in the hospital?
   <u>With the arrival of the meals.</u>
   **b.** Why is this time recommended? <u>Because it is difficult to ensure the meal delivery within a 15-minute time frame.</u>
   **c.** What is the concentration of the product as shown on the label?
   <u>U-100, 100 units/ mL.</u>

**d.** Will the solution be clear or cloudy? <u>Clear.</u>
**e.** Which of the following syringes is shaded to the correct amount? <u>Syringe number 1.</u>

**1.**

**2.**

2  Ordered: Humulin N (NPH) 28 units subcut in AM daily for a patient with DM type 1.

**a.** Is this a rapid- or intermediate-acting product? _____
**b.** Is it clear, or is it a suspension? _____
**c.** Does it need to be mixed before being withdrawn from the vial? _____
**d.** In how many hours will it peak? _____
**e.** By what route will it be administered? _____
**f.** Mark the syringe with the ordered dose.

3  Ordered: Novolin R 10 units tid subcut ac, for a patient with a severe infection who has type 2 diabetes and poor vision. The nurse plans to assess the patient's ability to visualize the calibrations on a Lo-Dose syringe.

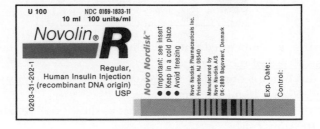

a. How long after administration will the action of this insulin action begin (onset)? _____
b. When will the action peak? _____
c. How long will it last? _____
d. Mark the syringe with the ordered dose.

4 A patient with DM type 1 who has a history of high, unstable blood glucose levels is taking Humulin R before meals and at bedtime.

a. According to the label, how many total units of insulin are contained in the vial? _____
b. Is this a rapid- or intermediate-acting product? _____
c. What is the concentration? _____

5 Ordered: Novolin N 42 units subcut AM daily for a patient with DM type 1 maintenance.

a. What route will be used to administer this order?
b. Mark the syringe with the ordered amount.

# Mixing Insulins: Short Fast-Acting and Slower-Acting Intermediate Mixes

Mixed insulins provide blood glucose coverage for meals with a small amount of short-acting insulin and between-meal coverage with an added amount of slower-release, intermediate-acting insulin. They are administered subcutaneously. Insulin mixes may be ordered twice a day for patients until their blood glucose pattern is established or to provide additional coverage for postprandial blood glucose elevations.

As with all insulins, initial orders for intermediate mixes are conservative to prevent hypoglycemic episodes.

The trend is to prescribe one of the *fixed premixed* combinations available on the market.

## Fixed Premixed Intermediate- and Short-Acting Combination Insulins

The *first* number of a fixed combination insulin mix indicates the *percentage* of slower-, *intermediate*-acting insulin. The second number indicates the *percentage* of short-, or *rapid*-acting insulin. The product label in Figure 11-15 illustrates this information.

Figure **11-15.** Humulin 70/ 30 insulin.

➤ If the order is for *10* units, 7 units (70% of 10 units) would contain NPH, the intermediate-acting insulin, and 3 units (30% of 10 units) would contain the fast-acting Humulin.

These mixes are offered as a safe and convenient method for patients who would have difficulty drawing up injectable mixtures in a syringe. The amounts are small, and an error of even 1 unit can make a difference. In addition to ease of preparation, the premixed combinations reduce chance of error and save time. Most patients receive a larger amount of intermediate-acting insulin and a smaller amount of short-, rapid-acting insulin. Some patients need a 50/ 50 mix because of very high mealtime blood glucose elevations.

A premix order specifies the number of units based on the patient's need for each type. For example:

Humulin Mix 50/50, 10 units subcut 30 minutes ac breakfast and dinner.

Novolin Mix 70/30, 18 units subcut 30 minutes ac breakfast and dinner.

➤ Note that the order for a mix is in *total* number of units.

1    If you were giving 8 units of Humulin 50/50 insulin, how many units would contain intermediate-acting NPH insulin and how many units would contain fast-acting insulin?

**Q** *Ask Yourself*

**A** *My Answer*

## When the Mix Must Be Prepared by the Nurse

Occasionally, the nurse must prepare an insulin mix, drawing up two different insulins in one syringe. Regular and intermediate-acting insulins are the most common combination. They are bracketed or designated "Mix" in the order:

Humulin R 6 units  
Humulin N 20 units ⎬ subcut bid AM and PM 30 minutes ac

Read both product labels to be sure they are compatible. Not all insulin brands can be mixed with others.

➤ Do not confuse Humulin products with Humalog.

Like the intermediate suspensions, the mixes need to be rolled or shaken gently but adequately until well mixed, according to the manufacturer's directions. Too vigorous shaking will result in extensive air bubble formation, making the dose inaccurate. The dose is less than 1 mL.

## Technique for Preparing Insulin Mixes

The technique for preparing a mix requires practice and supervision under the direction of an instructor or experienced nurse. Prepare a mix according to the following text:

Check the order and compatibility of the two types of insulin.

1    Identify the vials, verify the orders, and place them in a meaningful order in front of you. Shake the intermediate suspension gently. Clean the tops of each vial with an alcohol swab.

2    Measure and insert air *equal* to the amount of ordered insulin into each vial, the intermediate-acting insulin *first*, followed by the short-acting insulin, with the syringe to be used for administration. Keep the bottles on the counter to insert the air into the air at the top of the vial. Inserting air into the liquid will create air bubbles.

3    Always withdraw the clear, short-acting insulin *first* to protect the vial from contamination. A very small amount of intermediate-acting insulin can alter the action of the short-acting insulin. Verify the amount.

4  After withdrawing the ordered amount of regular insulin, gently mix the suspension according to label directions and withdraw exactly the amount ordered. Gently tap out any air bubbles and verify the precise combined amount. If the total amount is incorrect, discard the syringe and start over. One extra unit is 1 unit too much.

➤ Protect the short-acting insulin vials from contamination by withdrawing from them first. Do not allow distractions during this procedure (Figure 11-16).

In addition to verifying labels, it may be helpful to remember the sequence with the following table, keeping in mind that *cloudy* refers to intermediate suspension preparations and *clear* refers to short-acting preparations:

| Step 1 | Step 2 | Step 3 | Step 4 |
|--------|--------|--------|--------|
| Air in | Air in | Withdraw short-acting | Withdraw intermediate-acting |
| Cloudy | Clear | Clear | Cloudy |

This sequence permits the nurse to proceed from step 2 to step 3 with the short-acting preparation without removing the needle from the vial.

The following is an example of a mixture of 24 units of Humulin N plus 6 units of Humulin R, for a total dose of 30 units.

Total insulin dosage = 30 units

24 units
NPH U-100
Insulin

6 units
Regular
U-100 Insulin

**FAQ** | *How can I remember which insulin products can be mixed and which cannot?*

**ANSWER:** ➤ Always read the product label and inserts. Consult the pharmacy if necessary. Do not rely solely on the prescriber's order. In general, remember that a mix consists of a short-acting and an intermediate-acting insulin of the same brand and that the long-acting insulin glargine and insulin detemir cannot be mixed with any other insulin.

**A**

**B**

Figure 11-16. **A,** Vials of intermediate- or long-acting insulin and rapid- or short-acting insulin and syringe with air aspirated. **B,** Withdrawal of regular insulin. Always withdraw the regular insulin first after the vials have been prepared. (From Perry AG, Potter PA: Clinical nursing skills and techniques, ed. 6, St. Louis, 2006, Mosby.)

**RAPID PRACTICE 11-8**   Short-Acting and Intermediate-Acting Insulin Mixes

**Estimated completion time: 15 minutes**   Answers on page **587**

**Directions:** *Read the explanation of short-acting and intermediate-acting insulin mixes on p. 396 and study the illustrations. Examine the answers provided for problem 1 and complete problems 2-5 in a similar manner.*

**1** Ordered: Novolin R 6 units and Novolin N 20 units subcut bid AM and PM. Mark the syringe with the total amount. Place an arrow touching the intermediate-acting dose calibration.

**2** Ordered: Humulin N 30 units and Humulin R 4 units subcut bid AM and PM. Mark the syringe with the total amount. Place an arrow touching the intermediate-acting dose calibration.

**3** Ordered: Novolin R 2 units and Novolin N 16 units subcut AM and PM. Mark the syringe with the total amount. Place an arrow touching the intermediate-acting dose calibration.

**4** Ordered: Novolin R 10 units and Novolin N 42 units subcut 30 min ac breakfast and dinner. Mark the syringe with the total amount. Place an arrow touching the intermediate-acting dose calibration.

**5** Ordered: Humulin R 8 units and Humulin N 24 units subcut 30 minutes ac breakfast and dinner. Mark the syringe with the total amount. Place an arrow touching the intermediate-acting dose calibration.

---

**1** How many units/ mL are supplied in the labels shown above?

---

**2** How many units per milliliter are supplied in the label below?

---

A few patients with severe DM type 1 who must have very large amounts of insulin, over 100 units per dose, may be prescribed U-500 insulin (500 units/ mL) to reduce the volume of the injections and spare the injection sites. This is not a common order and is usually administered only in the hospital.

## Intravenous Insulin Infusions

Insulin infusions are administered in the hospital for acute hyperglycemia. Many agencies publish their own standard for the concentration of an insulin infusion, either 1 unit/ mL or 0.5 unit/ mL, in 0.9% NaCl solution.

➤ Use a fresh, unopened bottle of Regular or Humalog insulin, whichever is ordered, to prepare the infusion.

A label with the number of units and concentration needs to be attached to the IV solution, as with all other medicated IV solutions. Insulin should be administered on its own separate line.

When the concentration is 100 units in 100 mL of 0.9% NaCl (1 unit/ mL) or 50 units in 100 mL of 0.9% NaCl (0.5 unit/ mL), it is *very helpful* to estimate the flow rate in milliliters per hour using mental arithmetic. Remember that the flow rate cannot be calculated until the concentration of the solution in units per milliliter is known. Verify the estimate with a DA equation.

**EXAMPLES**

| Infuse | Concentration | Flow Rate |
|---|---|---|
| 0.5 units/ hr | 100 units/ 100 mL, or 1 unit/ 1 mL | 0.5 mL/ hr |
| 3 units/ hr | 100 units/ 100 mL, or 1 unit/ 1 mL | 3 mL/ hr |
| 1 unit/ hr | 50 units/ 100 mL, or 0.5 unit/ 1 mL | 2 mL/ hr |
| 3 units/ hr | 50 units/100 mL, or 0.5 unit/ 1 mL | 6 mL/ hr |

➤ Note that 100 mL of solution will last a long time because the orders are for very small amounts of insulin per hour. The flow rates are very low, and with a 1:1 (1 unit to 1 mL, or 100 units to 100 mL) concentration, the number of units ordered per hour is equal to the mL/ hr flow rate.

**EXAMPLES**

Ordered: Humulin R IV infusion 5 units/ hr, recheck BG 1 hr and call office.

$$mL/\ hr = \frac{100\ mL}{100\ units} \times \frac{5\ units}{1\ hr} = 5\ mL/\ hr$$

**Clinical Relevance**

➤ Check orders frequently for changes. Changes are common in acute-care situations. Monitor blood glucose levels at least every hour or more often, according to agency protocol. Report low and high blood glucose levels and unusual changes promptly. Follow the prescriber's and agency's directions for treatment. Document the instructions. Know where a 50% dextrose injection and/or a glucagon injection is available for hypoglycemic emergencies (Figure 11-17).

Figure 11-17. **A,** Glucagon emergency kit. **B,** Dextrose 50%. (**A** copyright Eli Lilly and Company. All rights reserved. Used with permission.)

## RAPID PRACTICE 11-9 IV Infusions

**Estimated completion time: 20 minutes**   Answers on page **587**

**Directions:** *Study the foregoing examples. Calculate the flow rate with mental arithmetic if possible and verify with a written DA equation. Use a calculator for long division and multiplication. Label answers.*

1 Ordered: Humulin R insulin IV at 3 units/ hr. Available: Humulin R insulin 100 units in 100-mL 0.9% NaCl solution.

  **a.** Estimated flow rate in mL/ hr? _____
  **b.** Ordered flow rate in mL/ hr:

    DA equation:

  **c.** Evaluation: _____

2 Ordered: Insulin lispro, Humalog IV at 4 units/ hr, for a patient with a glucose level of 325 mg/ dL. Available: 50 units Humalog insulin in 100 mL 0.9% NaCl solution.

  **a.** Estimated flow rate in mL/ hr? _____
  **b.** Ordered flow rate in mL/ hr:

    DA equation:

  **c.** Evaluation: _____

3 Ordered: Humulin R insulin IV at 6 units/ hr, for a patient with a glucose level of 400 mg/ dL. Draw a plasma glucose test stat to verify the capillary monitor level and recheck in 1 hour. Available: 50 units Humulin R insulin in 100 mL 0.9% NaCl solution.

  **a.** Estimated flow rate in mL/ hr? _____
  **b.** Ordered flow rate in mL/ hr:

    DA equation:

  **c.** Evaluation: _____

4 Ordered: to wean the patient (refer to example in problem 3) and reduce the flow rate by 50% because the blood glucose level has dropped to 185 mg/ dL.

  **a.** Estimated flow rate in mL/ hr? _____
  **b.** Ordered flow rate in mL/ hr:

    DA equation:

  **c.** Evaluation: _____

5 Ordered: Iletin II R insulin IV at 2 units/ hr. Infusing: IV of D5W 100 mL with 50 units Iletin II R insulin added flowing at 2 mL/ hr.

   **a.** Estimated flow rate ordered: _____

   **b.** Ordered flow rate in mL/ hr:

   DA equation:

   **c.** Evaluation: _____

   **d.** What nursing actions, if any, should be taken? _____

---

**RAPID PRACTICE 11-10** Insulin Differences

**Estimated completion time: 10-15 minutes**   Answers on page **588**

**Directions:** *Answer the questions pertaining to the differences among the insulin solutions available.*

1 **a.** Which are the only types of insulin that may be given intravenously?

   _____

   **b.** Are they clear or cloudy in the bottle? _____

2 Which two types of insulin within the same brand are most frequently given in mixed combination: short-, intermediate-, or long-acting?

   _____

3 **a.** What are the two concentrations of insulin supplied? _____

   **b.** Of the two, which one is more commonly used? _____

4 Are there intermediate- or long-acting forms of Humalog or Novolog?

   _____

5 **a.** When short- and intermediate-acting insulin are combined, which of the two is usually given in the larger dose? _____

   **b.** Why do you think this is so? _____

---

# Insulin Administration Devices

New products on the market are developed to make insulin administration more convenient, easier, and less painful.

- Finer needles are being developed to reduce the discomfort of injections (Figure 11-18).

## Prefilled Pens

Prefilled insulin pens contain regular insulin, intermediate-acting insulin, and mixtures of the two for ease of use by patients who have difficulty manipulating syringe equipment. The dose can be dialed easily. Pens are less noticeable than are syringes for injection in public places (Figure 11-19).

BD Ultra-Fine™ 33 Lancet (magnified)

Figure **11-18.** BD Ultra-Fine™ 33 Lancet. (From Becton, Dickinson and Company, Franklin Lakes, NJ.)

Figure **11-19. A,** Humulin® 70/ 30 and Humulin® N insulin pens. **B,** NovoPen® Junior. **C,** NovoLog® FlexPen. **D,** NovoLog® Mix 70/ 30 FlexPen®. (**A** copyright Eli Lilly and Company. All rights reserved. Used with permission. **B** to **D** from Novo Nordisk Inc., Princeton, NJ.)

Figure **11-20.** InnoLet®. (From Novo Nordisk Inc., Princeton, NJ.)

The InnoLet is a hand-held device used with either the NovoFine® 30G or NovoFine® 31G needles to administer subcutaneous insulin. Prefilled with 300 units available in two types of insulin, the large dial permits easy visualization of the number of units to administer. A window provides an estimate of how much insulin remains. This device eliminates the need to prepare an individual syringe for administration (Figure 11-20).

<table>
<tr><td>**Clinical Relevance**</td><td>Teaching patients about diabetes is a challenge. Consider all the content in this chapter, which is limited to medication administration only. The diabetic patient has a great deal more to learn about the disease than just medication administration. The patient most often is not a healthcare professional. Usually it is helpful to plan the teaching around the reason for hospitalization: is this a newly diagnosed patient, or did illness, travel, or noncompliance with the medication regimen cause the hospitalization in a person who has had diabetes for a long time? What is the patient's assessment of the reason for hospitalization?</td></tr>
</table>

**✳ Communication**

"What brought you to the hospital?" "Has this happened before?" "What has been the most difficult part of this disease for you?" "What parts of the diet are difficult?" Be prepared to listen to the patient's answers to these questions. Then, assess the teaching needs and formulate a prioritized practical teaching plan that takes into account what the patient already knows and urgently needs to know.

Figure **11-21.** Paradigm Link® blood glucose monitor and Paradigm® 515 insulin pump. (From Medtronic Inc., Minneapolis, MN.)

## Insulin Pumps

Insulin pumps are devices worn by patients who are unresponsive to intermittent subcutaneous injections and need more frequent administration to maintain control of glucose levels (Figure 11-21). Two types are available: implantable and portable. A programmed, continuous, subcutaneously injected basal (flat, low, continuous) dose of fast-acting insulin is delivered through a subcutaneous access site throughout the day and night. The basal dose does not cover mealtime needs or other elevations. Added boluses are administered on the pump to cover meals and glucose elevations. Only *short-acting* insulins are used in insulin pumps. Frequent blood glucose monitoring is recommended for these patients to normalize their glucose levels.

## CHAPTER 11 MULTIPLE-CHOICE REVIEW

**Estimated completion time: 30 minutes    Answers on page 588**

**Directions:** *Select the best answer for the following questions.*

1 Which insulin must never be mixed with any other? _____
 1. Humulin N
 2. Humalog
 3. Novolin R
 4. glargine (Lantus)

2 Which route is most commonly prescribed for administering insulin?
 _____
 1. Intradermal
 2. Subcutaneous
 3. Intramuscular
 4. Intravenous

3 Which types of insulin should be clear? _____
 1. Regular, insulin glargine, and insulin detemir
 2. Humulin N
 3. All insulin preparations
 4. Novolin N

4 At which level of blood glucose may a patient be likely to experience symptoms of hypoglycemia? _____
 1. >400 mg/dL
 2. 100-200 mg/dL
 3. 100 mg/dL
 4. <70 mg/dL

5 How may a nurse's action be *most likely* to cause a hypoglycemic episode for a patient? _____
 1. Administer too low a dose of insulin for a patient of a particular weight.
 2. Give a dextrose-containing beverage to a patient.
 3. Administer a dose of regular or fast-acting insulin that is not followed by a meal.
 4. Set up an insulin pump for a patient with the prescribed basal dose.

6 What does a prepared insulin mix such as Humulin N 70/30 contain?
 _____
 1. Lower doses than if each insulin was administered separately
 2. 70% fast-acting insulin and 30% intermediate-acting insulin
 3. 100% Humulin N
 4. 70% intermediate-acting insulin and 30% fast-acting insulin

7 Which insulin schedule requires a bedtime snack? _____
1. Regular insulin in the morning and before lunch
2. Short-acting insulin before lunch
3. Intermediate-, long-acting, and any evening insulins
4. Insulin lispro before lunch

8 Which explanation reflects the most likely serious and unwelcome result of reversing the dosage for an order for 6 units of Regular Insulin and 30 units of NPH? _____
1. Early onset of hypoglycemic episode
2. Late onset of hypoglycemic episode
3. Early onset of hyperglycemic episode
4. Late onset of hyperglycemic episode

9 What expectation is reasonable for nurses to have about most prescribed doses of fast-acting insulin? _____
1. They are usually high doses.
2. They are usually low doses.
3. They are always combined with intermediate-acting insulins.
4. They contain additives to extend their action.

10 Which phrase best describes diabetes mellitus? _____
1. A metabolic disorder of the alpha cells formed in the islet cells of Langerhans
2. A neuroendocrine disorder that affects the pituitary gland characterized by thirst, high urine output, and frequent hypoglycemic episodes
3. An endocrine disorder that affects carbohydrate, protein, and fat metabolism, characterized by hyperglycemia
4. A multisystem disorder characterized by excessive glucagon production and lack of ADH

## CHAPTER 11 FINAL PRACTICE

**Estimated completion time: 1-1½ hours**    Answers on page **589**

**Directions:** *Answer the following questions using DA equations to verify doses and flow rates. Use a calculator for long division and multiplication. Label answers.*

1 a. What is the most common concentration of insulin preparations? _____
   b. When preparing an insulin mix, which insulin must be protected and withdrawn first from the vial? _____
   c. Why? _____

2 Ordered: Novolin N 30 units subcut AM and PM, 30 minutes before meals. Select the appropriate syringe. Draw an arrow touching the calibration for the correct dose.

**3** Ordered:

Humulin R 10 units }
Humulin N 44 units } Subcut 30 minutes before breakfast and dinner.

**a.** Which insulin will you withdraw first? _____

**b.** Mark the syringe to the total dose. Place an arrow touching the calibration for the amount of intermediate-acting insulin.

4 Ordered:

Novolin R 6 units
Novolin N 20 units } Subcut 30 minutes before breakfast and dinner.

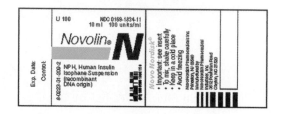

a. Which insulin will you withdraw first? _____

b. Mark the syringe to the total dose. Place an arrow touching the calibration for the amount of intermediate-acting insulin.

5 Ordered: insulin lispro 6 units tid 10 minutes before meals.

a. Is this a rapid-, intermediate-, or long-acting insulin? _____

b. Place an arrow touching the calibration for the amount of the insulin.

Problems 6-9 refer to the patient in problem 6.

**6** Ordered: Humulin Regular insulin IV infusion in 0.9% NaCl to start at rate of 5 units/ hr, for a patient with a blood level glucose >400 mg/ dL. Available: Humulin Regular 100 units/ 100 mL of 0.9% NaCl solution. Obtain BGM test results every hour. Discontinue any other insulin orders.

**a.** How many units/ mL are contained in the available solution? _____

**b.** Estimate the flow rate with mental arithmetic and verify with a DA equation.

DA equation:

**c.** Evaluation: _____

**d.** Should the infusion be administered on a electronic infusion pump?

_____

**7** The patient referred to in problem 6 has a blood glucose level of 325 mg/ dL.

**a.** Using the sliding scale below, what flow rate in milliliters per hour will be administered?

| Blood Glucose Level (mg/ dL) | Infusion Rate (units/ hr) |
|---|---|
| 151-200 | 1 |
| 201-250 | 2 |
| 251-300 | 3 |
| 301-400 | 4 |
| >400 | 5 |

**b.** Use a DA equation to back up mental arithmetic flow rate estimate:

**c.** Evaluation: _____

**8** The physician also orders an IV of D5W at 100 mL/ hr to avoid hypoglycemia while on insulin infusion. This IV solution has a small amount of glucose in it.

**a.** How many grams of glucose are contained in a 1000-mL container of D5W? (Refer to "Hyperalimentation: Total Parental Nutrition," in Chapter 10.)

DA equation:

**b.** Evaluation: _____

**9** The next blood glucose level obtained for the patient is 210 mg/ dL. The order calls for decreasing the flow rate by 50%. Refer to problem 7 flow rate sliding scale.

**a.** Estimate the rate the nurse will set on the pump and verify with a DA equation. _____

DA equation:

**b.** Evaluation: _____

**10 a.** What are the three major types of exogenous insulin available in terms of onset of insulin activity in the body?

_____

**b.** What type of nutrient will the nurse promptly administer if the patient is conscious, is symptomatic, and can swallow and the blood glucose level falls below 70 mg/ dL? _____

_____

## Suggestions for Further Reading

www.bd.com
www.diabetes.niddk.nik.gov/dm
www.diabetes.org
www.diabetes.org/diabetes-statistics/native-americans.jsp
www.hospira.com
www.ismp.org
www.jcaho.org
www.joslin.org
www.lillydiabetes.com
www.medtronic.com
www.mydna.com/health/diabetes/
www.novonordisk-us.com

 Additional practice problems can be found in the Advanced Calculations section on the enclosed companion CD.

Chapter 12 focuses on anticoagulants, which are also delivered in units. Many of the principles learned in this chapter can be applied to Chapter 12.

*"Our greatest weakness lies in giving up. The most certain way to succeed is to try just one more time."*

—THOMAS EDISON

# 12

# ANTICOAGULANT AGENTS

## Objectives

- Differentiate oral and parenteral anticoagulant agents and related tests.
- Calculate doses for oral and parenteral anticoagulant agents.
- Evaluate and titrate anticoagulant doses based upon relevant laboratory tests.
- Identify antidotes for anticoagulant therapy.
- Identify critical patient safety issues related to anticoagulant therapy.

## Essential Prior Knowledge

Mastery of Chapters 1-11

## Equipment

- None needed

## Estimated Time To Complete Chapter

- 1-2 hours

## Introduction

Safe administration of anticoagulants, like that of insulin, requires comprehension of the underlying theory of the action of the medications, the antidotes, related pathophysiologic conditions, and relevant clinical assessments, including interpretation of laboratory test results. The dose calculations are relatively simple but, because of variations in patients' dose response, the dose must be carefully titrated based on results of frequent patient-based laboratory testing. The goal is to extend clotting time sufficiently to prevent adverse clotting event. Normal clotting time poses a risk of thromboembolic events for a variety of conditions.

Anticoagulants are now prescribed for many conditions, for example:

- Prolonged immobility
- Pre-, intra-, and postoperative lower extremity orthopedic surgery
- Potential, intra-, and post-cardiac events, such as arrhythmias, myocardial infarcts, and cardiac surgery
- Intra- and post-pelvic surgery
- History of thromboembolic conditions, such as deep vein thromboses, pulmonary emboli, and stroke
- Maintenance of patency of IV lines

Nurses are expected to evaluate and administer oral, subcutaneous, and IV anticoagulants. These medications may be encountered in the hospital, clinic, office, and home settings.

Students need to consult pharmacology, pathophysiology, and medical surgical nursing texts, as well as clinical skills texts, for complete understanding of anticoagulant therapy. Clinical mentors are required for supervised experience and practice of the skills required for safe anticoagulation therapy.

**413**

## ESSENTIAL Vocabulary

| | |
|---|---|
| **Embolus** | Blood clot that travels from its original location, usually a pelvic or leg vein. May block circulation in another vessel, such as a pulmonary artery. |
| **Thrombus** | Blood clot that forms in a blood vessel, usually a vein. |
| **Petechiae** | Pinpoint bruises seen on skin and mucous membranes, indicative of a bleeding disorder. **Mnemonic:** PPP (Petechiae PinPoint) |
| **Thromboembolic Disorders** **Deep Vein Thrombus (DVT)** | Blood clot usually located in the deeper veins of leg or pelvis. |
| **Pulmonary Embolus (PE)** | Blood clot (often a DVT) that has traveled through the circulation and blocked an artery of the lung. |
| **Thrombocytopenia** | Decreased platelet count. Contraindication for heparin therapy. (See "Coagulation Tests, Platelet Count," p. 415.) |

**Q:** *Ask Yourself*

**1** What is the difference between DVT and PE?

**A:** *My Answer*

_____

## Medications

| | |
|---|---|
| **Anticoagulants** | Drugs that interfere with specific clotting factors, thus prolonging the coagulation time. They are used for patients with potential or current heart, lung, and vessel disease. They do *not* dissolve established clots, nor do they "thin" blood, although they are commonly referred to as blood thinners. |
| **Oral Anticoagulants: Warfarin Sodium (Coumadin)** | Frequently prescribed outpatient oral anticoagulant that inhibits vitamin K–dependent clotting factors. Tests to monitor coagulation with warfarin are the international normalized ratio (INR) test and prothrombin time (PT). |
| **Parenteral Anticoagulants** **Heparin Sodium** **Heparin Calcium** | Heparin sodium or calcium acts on multiple coagulation factors. From bovine intestinal source, heparin is given by IV or subcutaneous route. Activated partial thromboplastin time (PTT) test results must be monitored closely q4-6h until levels are stabilized, after dose adjustments, and then daily. Not suitable for home use. Interact with many drugs. Drug interactions can be fatal. |
| **Clotting Factors** | Proteins and enzymes in the blood that are essential for coagulation. Tests are performed to identify specific factor deficiencies as well as to monitor anticoagulant therapy. |
| **Heparin Flush Solutions (Heplock Flush)** | Low-dose heparin (10-100 units/ mL) used to maintain patency of indwelling IV devices. Up to 500 units/ mL may be ordered for central lines. |
| **Low-Molecular-Weight Heparin (LMWH)** **Dalteparin (Fragmin)** **Enoxaparin (Lovenox)** **IV Ardeparin (Normaflo)** | Altered (fractionated) heparin with lower risk of thrombocytopenia than unfractionated heparins, thus lower risk of bleeding. Dose based on patient's *weight*. It is given by subcutaneous or IV route. Does *not* need to be monitored frequently, as with unfractionated heparin, which requires frequent monitoring with the activated partial thromboplastin time test. Can be administered at home with selected patients. Used for prevention of thromboemboli for high-risk patients, including orthopedic surgical patients. |

CHAPTER 12

| Heparinoid (Danaparoid Sodium) | Heparin-like drug that does not contain heparin (*-oid* means "like") used for postoperative DVT prophylaxis. |
| --- | --- |
| Protamine Sulfate | Antidote for heparin and heparinoid drugs. |
| Thrombolytic Agents Streptokinase Alteplase Recombinant Tissue Plasminogen Activator (tPA) | Drugs that "lyse," or dissolve, clots if given within a specified amount of time. Used for patients with acute stroke or pulmonary embolism. |
| Vitamin K | Antidote for warfarin products. |

**1**    What are some of the differences between heparin and warfarin products?

Q:*Ask Yourself*

A:*My Answer*

## COAGULATION Tests

| Control Values | Laboratory derived "average normal values" for specific test results. May vary from laboratory to laboratory, depending on agents used for testing. Determined daily by laboratory tests for prothrombin time, partial thromboplastin time, and activated partial thromboplastin time tests to ensure efficacy of agents used for each batch of tests for accurate measurement. |
| --- | --- |
| International Normalized Ratio (INR) | Standardized formula-derived laboratory value *preferred* for monitoring *warfarin* therapy. Normal blood has an INR of 1. Therapeutic target range for blood of anti-coagulated patients is 2.0-3.0 INR value, derived from patient-specific prothrombin time value. |
| Prothrombin Time (PT, or Pro Time) | Formerly used for monitoring warfarin therapy, it now may be used as adjunct to INR. It is not as reliable as INR. Normal control values in *uncoagulated* patients vary from laboratory to laboratory by from 11 to 15 seconds. |
| Activated Partial Thromboplastin Time (aPTT) | *Shortened* form of the PT test with activators added, *preferred* for monitoring *heparin* therapy, *not to be confused with PT test for warfarin or the longer partial thromboplastin time (PTT) test. "Normal" control aPTT time is about 30-40 seconds (about $\frac{1}{2}$ minute), depending on test agents used. |
| Platelet Count | Actual count of number of thrombocytes in blood (normal adult value, 150,000-400,000/ mcL). Less than 50,000/ mcL poses risk of bleeding from minor trauma and surgery. Less than *20,000/ mcL* poses *great risk* of spontaneous hemorrhage. |
| Other Tests that May Be Ordered for Patients Receiving Anticoagulant Therapy or Those with Coagulation Disorders | Bleeding time Hematocrit (Hct) Hemoglobin (Hgb) Stool test for occult blood Urine test for blood Liver function tests (LFTs) Renal function tests Whole blood clotting time (WBCT) Activated coagulation time (ACT) Specific clotting factor assays D-dimer test |

Q: *Ask Yourself*

A: *My Answer*

1 What is the preferred test for patients receiving heparin products, as opposed to the test for those receiving warfarin products?

2 What is the main risk for patients who have thrombocytopenia?

---

**FAQ** | *What is the difference between a normal* (control) *value for a PT or an aPTT and a therapeutic level?*

**ANSWER:** The normal control value is the coagulation time in seconds for a specific test, such as the aPTT, for a person who is *not* receiving anticoagulants. It varies from test to test and laboratory to laboratory, depending on the agents used for the test.

When patients receive anticoagulants, they receive a *"therapeutic amount"* of drug that will *extend* their coagulation time to reduce their risk of having a thromboembolic event. Anticoagulant doses are individualized for each patient, or "patient-specific," based on the patient's test results.

The therapeutic level is based on the laboratory daily control value. It is the desired *target* coagulation range in seconds that prevents clot formation in patients who are at risk. It is *longer than* the normal control finding for an aPTT coagulation test, which is 30-40 seconds for a person who is *not* receiving heparin.

The therapeutic level for an aPTT test is within *1.5 to 2.5 times the control value in seconds* (45-100 seconds), a narrow therapeutic range that will prolong clot formation but not be excessive enough to cause bleeding.

To evaluate a patient-specific coagulation test result:
- Obtain the therapeutic target range by multiplying the control value by the desired factors for the range.
- Compare the patient's test result to see if it falls within the range.

---

**EXAMPLES**

1/1/06, Control value for aPTT tests: 30 seconds

Therapeutic target range: 1.5 to 2.5 times the control value (45 to 100 seconds)

aPTT results for Patient X, a patient receiving heparin: 130 seconds

Decision: Hold the anticoagulant. It is not within the desired therapeutic range. Notify the prescriber promptly. Obtain orders. Document. Monitor the patient for bleeding events.

Analysis: Patient's aPTT coagulation time has been *extended* too long with recent doses of anticoagulants. Patient is at risk for bleeding. Antidote may be prescribed.

Note that if the value was *below* the therapeutic range, the patient would be at risk for a thromboembolic event.

---

Q: *Ask Yourself*

A: *My Answer*

1 If a *control value* for a coagulation test is 12 seconds and the *therapeutic range* is 1.5 to 2.5 times the control value, would the patient's test result be within therapeutic range if it was *24 seconds?* (Use simple arithmetic with or without a calculator.)

---

**RAPID PRACTICE 12-1** Vocabulary Review: Anticoagulants and Tests

**Estimated completion time: 5-10 minutes** **Answers on page 590**

**Directions:** *Study the introduction and the vocabulary list. Select the correct response.*

**Test Tip:** Quickly place a single line through the incorrect responses to narrow your choices.

1 Anticoagulants are used for the following purposes: _____

   **1.** To dissolve well-established clots in high-risk patients

   **2.** To decrease coagulation time

   **3.** To treat hemorrhage

   **4.** To prevent thrombi and emboli formation

2 An oral anticoagulant that is ordered for outpatient use is _____

   **1.** Warfarin sodium (Coumadin, Sofarin, Warfilone)

   **2.** Enoxaparin (Lovenox)

   **3.** Streptokinase and alteplase

   **4.** Danaparoid sodium

3 The standardized relevant laboratory test for monitoring therapeutic levels of warfarin is called _____

   **1.** INR                **3.** Vitamin K level

   **2.** PTT                **4.** aPTT

4 The most commonly used laboratory test to monitor therapeutic levels of heparin is _____

   **1.** aPTT             **3.** INR

   **2.** PT               **4.** Vitamin K level

5 The main danger of *excessive* anticoagulant therapy is _____

   **1.** DVT formation         **3.** Hemorrhage

   **2.** PE               **4.** Increased platelet count

---

## RAPID PRACTICE 12-2 Anticoagulant Agents and Antidotes

**Estimated completion time: 5-10 minutes**    Answers on page **591**

**Directions:** *Identify the correct agent, term, purpose, or antidote for anticoagulant therapy.*

1 The drug antidote for warfarin excess is _____

   **1.** Blood transfusion        **3.** Vitamin K (phytonadione)

   **2.** Iron                **4.** Protamine sulfate

2 The drug antidote for heparin excess is _____

   **1.** Blood transfusion        **3.** Vitamin K (phytonadione)

   **2.** Iron                **4.** Protamine sulfate

3 Intravenous heparin flush solutions are used for which purpose? _____

   **1.** Occult blood in stool and hematuria    **3.** Petechiae and ecchymoses

   **2.** Epistaxis                     **4.** Patency of IV access devices

4 The difference between a control value and a therapeutic value for a specific anticoagulant test is _____

   **1.** The control value is the extended blood coagulation time in seconds needed to prevent clots, whereas the therapeutic desired value is the normal coagulation time in seconds for a patient not receiving anticoagulants.

   **2.** The control value is the level that the prescriber orders for the patient to control his or her blood coagulation. The therapeutic coagulation levels or range is less time in seconds than the control value.

   **3.** The control value is the laboratory-derived normal coagulation time in seconds for a particular test for a patient who is not receiving anticoagulants. The therapeutic value is the desired extended time in seconds for the patient receiving a specific anticoagulant.

   **4.** The control value and the therapeutic time in seconds for coagulation are the same for all patients receiving a specific anticoagulant.

**5** Drugs that dissolve clots are classified as _____

  **1.** Anticoagulants              **3.** Thrombolytic enzyme agents

  **2.** Hormones                   **4.** Salicylates

---

**FAQ** | *What is the relationship between the PT value and the INR value?*

**ANSWER:** The INR standardized test value introduced by the World Health Organization in 1983 is used by most prescribers to adjust or titrate warfarin doses. The patient's therapeutic INR range is determined daily by the individual laboratory based in part on the PT value. The INR is not a separate test. It is a formula-derived value:

$$INR = \frac{Patient's\ PT\ Value}{Mean\ Normal\ PT\ Value^*} \Big\} ISI$$

The INR value is used to evaluate the patient's response to treatment. Some prescribers also require the PT value to be reported with the INR.

*ISI: International Sensitivity Index, a value assigned to the thromboplastin reagent by the manufacturer of the specific laboratory test material.

---

**FAQ** | *How can I remember the differences between heparin therapy and warfarin therapy?*

**ANSWER:** Write out a brief outline of the differences. Be able to reproduce this critical information. Following is one suggested format that emphasizes the differences.

---

## Comparison of Anticoagulant Products

|  | Warfarin | Heparin (unfractionated) | Low molecular weight heparin (LMWH) |
|---|---|---|---|
| **Name** | Coumadin | Heparin | dalteparin (Fragmin) enoxaparin (Lovenox) ardeparin (Normaflow) |
| **Route** | Oral | Subcutaneous or IV | Subcutaneous or IV |
| **Tests** | INR usual test; also PT | Frequently aPTT | aPTT infrequently needed |
| **Action** | Interferes with extrinsic (tissue injury site) vitamin K–dependent clotting mechanisms | Interferes with intrinsic (within vessel) clotting mechanisms | Interferes with intrinsic and extrinsic clotting mechanisms Less chance for bleeding than unfractionated heparin |
| **Drug antidote** | Vitamin K | Protamine sulfate | Protamine sulfate |

➤ Heparin and LMWH doses are *not* interchangeable.

➤ Do not confuse PT with PTT.

➤ Plasma, plasma expanders, and blood also may be needed to counteract loss of blood from overdoses of anticoagulants.

➤ Examine the drug labels as you work through the chapter.

**RAPID PRACTICE 12-3** Interpreting INR and PT Results for Patients Receiving Warfarin Therapy

**Estimated completion time: 20 minutes**    Answers on page **591**

**Directions:** *Study the Essential Vocabulary, Coagulation Tests, and explanations on pp. 414-415. Examine the test results supplied in the problems. Provide the requested answers.*

1  A patient, Mr. X, was discharged post–myocardial infarction on Coumadin 5 mg PO bedtime daily. The patient has been requested to return to the office twice a week for INR test follow-up to ensure that the Coumadin dose is within therapeutic range. The medication is prescribed at bedtime so that, if the following morning laboratory test result requires dose adjustment, it can be made the same evening.

   A prescription was given for warfarin 5 mg #60 pills. "Take 5 mg at bedtime as directed." The tablets are scored so that, if the dose needs to be reduced, the patient can take 2.5 mg if prescribed without purchasing another prescription.

   > **COUMADIN®    5 mg**
   > (Warfarin Sodium Tablets, USP)
   > Crystalline
   > **DuPont Pharma**
   > Wilmington, Delaware 19880
   > LOT KA009A
   > EXP

   The normal therapeutic range of INR for Mr. X on anticoagulant therapy is 2 to 3. For the first laboratory test in the office, the INR value was 2.6. What is the expected decision for Mr. X? (Circle one.)

   **a.** Continue on 5-mg/ day dose and return to office in 3 days for next INR.
   **b.** Hold the Coumadin. Come in for vitamin K (phytonadione) injection.
   **c.** Increase the Coumadin dose to 7.5 mg/ day.
   **d.** Order an aPTT test.

2  Mr. X, named in problem 1, has a PT test ordered in addition to the INR. PT was reported at 25 seconds. The laboratory control PT value was 11.5 seconds.

   ➤ The therapeutic PT time for an anticoagulated patient such as Mr. X is 2 to 2.5 times the laboratory control value.

   What is the desired PT range for Mr. X in seconds? _____

3  What is the nurse's evaluation of Mr. X's PT time (25 seconds)? (Circle one.)

   **a.** 25 seconds is within the desired range for extended coagulation for Mr. X.
   **b.** Mr. X needs a higher dose of anticoagulant and is at risk for thrombus or embolus formation.
   **c.** Mr. X is receiving too much anticoagulant.
   **d.** Mr. X's PT value should be 11.5 seconds.

4  A few weeks later, Mr. X's INR result is 7, and he is complaining of bleeding when he brushes his teeth as well as dark-colored urine and stools, which test positive for presence of blood. The PT value is 49 seconds. The therapeutic INR value is 2 to 3 for Mr. X. The control PT is 12 seconds.

   **a.** What is the nurse's evaluation of the laboratory results? (Circle one.)
     **1.** Mr. X is in danger of forming thrombi or emboli.
     **2.** Mr. X is in danger of bleeding from excessive anticoagulation.
     **3.** Mr. X's results are within normal limits for anticoagulation.

The physician orders vitamin K 2 mg subcut stat.

**b.** How many mL of vitamin K will the nurse prepare for injection after the dilution? Use mental arithmetic, and verify with a DA equation. _____

DA equation:

Evaluation: _____

Mr. X is instructed to hold the Coumadin dosage until results of his next INR test.

**5** Three days later, Mr. X's INR is 3. The physician lowers the Coumadin dose to 2.5 mg/ day. Mr. X's tablets are scored. He is instructed to buy a pill cutter at a local pharmacy and to keep a record of when he takes his nightly Coumadin dose. His next few laboratory tests will be scheduled weekly.

**COUMADIN®**    **5 mg**
(Warfarin Sodium Tablets, USP)
Crystalline
**DuPont Pharma**
Wilmington, Delaware 19880
LOT KA009A
EXP

**a.** How many pills will Mr. X take daily? _____
**b.** Which of the following Coumadin doses would be safest for Mr. X to have prescribed for his next prescription, assuming that his INR remains stable?
_____

Coumadin® is available in a wide range of dosages
(crystalline warfarin sodium)

1   2   $2\frac{1}{2}$   4   5   $7\frac{1}{2}$   10

to more easily meet your patient's therapeutic needs

| **Clinical Relevance** | Assess patients for the variety of doses they may have on hand at home and the precautions they take to avoid taking the wrong dose. It is not unusual to have doses adjusted. Keeping track of changing doses of the same medication can be challenging for anyone. |

**✳ Communication**

"Mr. X, how do you keep track of your anticoagulant medications when you take them at home?"

➤ Noncompliance with anticoagulant therapy can be fatal. Forgetting to take a medication or doubling up is not a rare occurrence, even in the most alert patient population. Remember that there is a difference between what is taught and what is learned. Communication for teaching need not be formal. For example, the patient will have little interest in learning the chain of physiologic clotting mechanisms from a flow chart.

1   Take a minute to browse your most comprehensive current pharmacology text for drug interactions with Coumadin. Besides aspirin, other nonsteroidal anti-inflammatory drugs, and antibiotics, what other medications do you recognize on the list? What effect do they have on the anticoagulant?

*Q:Ask Yourself*

*A:My Answer*

2   Does the length of the list illustrate the need to check the medications each patient is currently receiving? (While you are in that section of the text, browse the side effects also.)

---

Teaching of outpatients receiving anticoagulants is critical. One example of a preventable tragedy was a patient who suffered lacerations in a relatively minor automobile accident and who died from loss of blood. The patient did not carry a wallet card with information about the medication (warfarin) and the dose, nor did the patient wear an identification bracelet. Another example is illustrated by the case of a patient on anticoagulants who became seasick on a cruise and had several episodes of hematemesis. He stayed in bed and sent his wife to the cruise ship front desk for oral pills for seasickness for 2 days but could not keep them down. Eventually, he sought care from the ship's physician. Units of blood had to be delivered by helicopter to save the patient's life.

**Clinical Relevance**

➤ A responsible family member must have all the priority information about the anticoagulant dose, timing, testing, and follow-up visits. Patients need to be reminded to carry a list of their medicines and doses on their person.

**Clinical Relevance**

# Injectable Anticoagulants

The prototypical parenteral anticoagulant is heparin sodium, which must be administered IV in the hospital because of its short half-life and the need for frequent titration to laboratory results. Subcutaneous heparin is also only administered by nurses. Derived from pork and bovine intestinal mucosa, it interacts with many drugs. The nurse must check the medications the patient is receiving against the lengthy drug interaction list for heparin.

If ordered IV, heparin should be administered on an infusion pump with an IV line dedicated for heparin administration only. Check institutional policies. If this is not feasible, a saline flush must be administered before and after using an existing line.

Take a moment to examine some examples of the varied doses of heparin available. It helps to have a general understanding of the purpose of the range of doses because the selection of the correct concentration is a critical nursing decision.

➤ As with most liquid injectables for adults, drug amounts in mL are usually rounded to the nearest tenth of a mL.

# Low-Dose Heparin Concentrations used to Maintain Patency of Intravenous Devices (Flushes)

Flushes of very low-dose heparin are administered to maintain the patency of venous access sites. They are *not* given to anticoagulate a patient (Figure 12-1).

➤ The flush solution—saline or heparin—is selected according to agency protocol. Saline solution may be preferred as a flush for certain venous access devices.

The prescriber does not write the volume in milliliters of the flush to be used. The volume of the flush depends on the fluid capacity of the indwelling device and

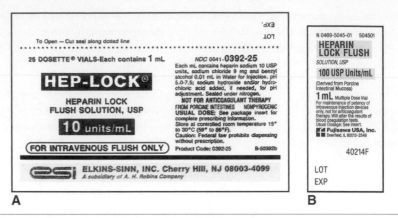

Figure 12-1. **A,** Hep-Lock 10 units/ mL. **B,** Heparin Lock Flush 100 units/ mL.

institutional policy. The longer the catheter, the more volume will be needed to "flush" the line.

➤ Consult agency guidelines and equipment literature for precise concentrations and volumes for each type of flush.

➤ Know the difference when you see these acronyms:

SASH, acronym for heparin flush: Saline, Administer (drug), Saline, Heparin
SAS, acronym for saline flush: Saline, Administer (drug), Saline

**1** As I check my pharmacology reference for heparin drug interactions, why do I realize it would be critical to flush IV lines with saline solution *before* and *after* administering heparin?

_____

**2** Which drug listed is one I have most frequently seen or heard about?

_____

**3** Why would it be preferable to use a separate IV line and imperative to use an infusion pump for heparin infusions?

_____

# Heparin Concentrations used for Subcutaneous Administration and Bolus Intravenous Doses

Like many other drugs, heparin is supplied in several concentrations. Three examples are shown in Figure 12-2.

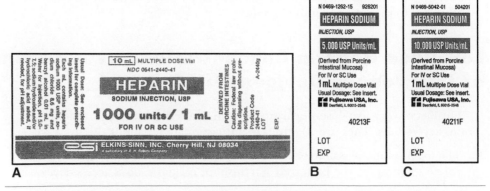

Figure 12-2. **A,** Heparin 1000 units/ mL. **B,** Heparin 5000 units/ mL. **C,** Heparin 10,000 units/ mL.

➤ Heparin has been identified as a high-risk drug by the Institute for Safe Medication Practices (ISMP). It is critical to select the correct ordered concentration of a powerful drug such as heparin.

1 What is the difference in the heparin product concentrations shown in Figure 12-2 and in Figure 12-3 on p. 422?

Q:*Ask Yourself*

A:*My Answer*

➤ A dose of 5000 units/ 1 mL is 5 times more concentrated than 1000 units/ mL. A dose of 10,000 units/ 1 mL is 10 times more concentrated than 1000 units/ mL.

➤ The more concentrated the dose, the greater the anticoagulant effect and the greater the risk of bleeding.

➤ Adding or subtracting a zero from an order or misreading a *U* as a zero must be avoided.

• Many at-risk patients receive a standard dose of 5000 units of heparin subcutaneously q12h for DVT prevention. This dose does not require aPTT monitoring. Platelet counts may be ordered every few days.

➤ Injection sites are rotated. Refer to "Sites for Insulin Injection" in Chapter 11 (p. 390).

➤ Heparin injections are not aspirated before administration.

➤ Avoid massaging the site.

• Needle angle depends on patient size.

   ➤ A bolus of low-dose heparin, 5000 units, may be given as a loading dose (fast startup) and/or as a test for reactions such as allergies before an IV infusion.

➤ Heparin is never given via the IM route.

➤ When a label such as a heparin label states the concentration as 1:1000 or 1:10,000, it is interpreted as g/ mL. Thus, 1:1000 means 1 g/ 1000 mL, which is 10 times stronger than a solution of 1 g/ 10,000 mL.

➤ Check agency policies for rounding heparin doses. They may vary from the *nearest* 50 to 100 units.

## Heparin Concentrations used for Intravenous Infusions

The general guidelines for continuous heparin infusions are *20,000 to 40,000* units every 24 hours, depending on the patient's condition and test results.

Although in some settings, nurses may prepare and mix IV heparin solutions, the trend is to use premixed preparations to ensure the patient's safety.

There are also premixed preparations of heparin of 12,500 units/ 250 mL NS and 25,000 to 40,000 units in 250 or 500 mL NS in vials and ampules. Heparin is also available premixed in Ad-Vantage vials to accompany Ad-Vantage IV solution containers. Refer to Chapter 9 for a review of Ad-Vantage IV systems.

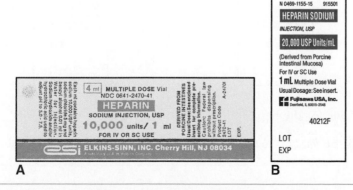

Figure 12-3. **A,** Heparin 10,000 units/ mL. **B,** Heparin 20,000 units/ mL.

## RAPID PRACTICE 12-4 Heparin Preparations

**Estimated completion time: 10 minutes**   Answers on page **591**

**Directions:** *Examine the preceding information about heparin and the labels on the opposite page, and review the vocabulary to answer the following questions.*

**1** The volume for the heparin flush solutions shown on the labels is _____

**2** Which is the *lowest* concentration of flush solution provided on the labels above? _____

**3** The purpose of a flush solution is _____

**4** The key difference between SASH and SAS is _____

_____

**5** Which is more concentrated: 1000 units/ mL or 10,000 units/ mL? _____

**6** Which is more concentrated: a 1:1000 solution or a 1:10,000 solution? _____

**7** Which is more concentrated: 5,000 units/ mL or 10,000 units/ mL? _____

**8** If a *U* for *units* was misread as a zero, the kind of adverse consequence to the patient receiving the heparin dose could be _____

**9** The maximum dose of heparin units over a 24-hour period is about (can be exceeded, depending on patient's condition) _____

**10** Heparin solutions must be isolated from other IV medications a patient is receiving because _____

**1** What is the general difference among heparin solution doses used for flush versus prophylaxis versus therapeutic administration? (Answer in brief phrases.)

_____

**2** Which heparin solution shown on p. 424 has the *highest* concentration?

_____

*Ask Yourself*

*My Answer*

# Calculating Heparin Flow Rates in Milliliters per Hour (mL/ hr) and Units per Hour Using DA-Style Equations

Calculations are the same as for any other DA-style equation.

---

**EXAMPLES**

The following example illustrates the calculation of the flow rate in mL/ hr when the number of units per hour is known.

Ordered: heparin 500 units/ hr.

Available: heparin 20,000 units in 500 mL D5W. Desired answer units: mL/ hr to nearest mL.

Undesired factors in answer: units.
- Set up the equation.
- Check to see that only desired factors remain: mL/ hr.
- Simplify the equation: reduce 500/ 20,000 by canceling zeros.
- Cancel zeros in the remaining 500/ 200, and then calculate.

$$\frac{mL}{hr} = \frac{500 \text{ mL}}{20{,}000 \text{ units}} \times \frac{500 \text{ units}}{1 \text{ hr}} = \frac{25}{2} = 12.5, \text{ or } 13 \text{ mL/ hr}$$

Evaluation: The equation is balanced. Only mL/ hr remains.

➤ The nurse always needs to know that the units per hour flowing match the prescriber's order, whether the nurse or someone else set up the infusion. This can be determined very easily from the flow rate using DA style equation.

The following example illustrates the calculation of the flow rate in units per hour when the number of mL/ hr is known:

Desired answer units: units per hour to the nearest 100 units.

Existing infusion: heparin flowing at 20 mL/ hr in 500 mL D5W infusion labeled *20,000 units heparin*.

- Set up the equation.
- Check to see that only the desired factors, units per hour, remain after cancellation and that the undesired factors (mL) are canceled.
- Simplify the equation: reduce and cancel zeros.

$$\frac{\text{units}}{\text{hr}} = \frac{\overset{40}{\cancel{20,000}} \text{ units}}{\underset{1}{\cancel{500 \text{ mL}}}} \times \frac{20 \cancel{\text{ mL}}}{1 \text{ hr}} = 800 \text{ units/ hr}$$

Evaluation: Equation is balanced. Only units/ hr remain.

➤ Do *not* confuse *units* per hour with *mL/ hr* in an order or in calculations.

➤ Contrast the mL/ hr flow rate with the number of heparin units per hour. Units per hour is a relatively large amount. The mL/ hr flow rate is relatively small.

## RAPID PRACTICE 12-5 Titrating Heparin Doses to aPTT Values

**Estimated completion time: 20-30 minutes**  Answers on page **591**

**Directions:** *Read the following case history information for the patient on heparin therapy. Calculate the doses and provide the requested nursing evaluations. Round all doses to the nearest 100 units. Label all work. Use a calculator for long division and multiplication.*

Mr. Y has been hospitalized with arterial fibrillation, a condition that predisposes him to thromboembolus formation. The physician has ordered a complete blood screening for clotting and bleeding times, including a baseline platelet count and aPTT. Mr. Y's baseline aPTT is 30 seconds.* He is not receiving anticoagulants yet. The platelet count is: 250,000/ mm³.

Because both of Mr. Y's values are within the normal range, the physician institutes heparin therapy to extend coagulation time.

Initial order for Mr. Y: heparin 5000-unit bolus loading test dose IV slowly. Pharmacology references state to infuse the first 1000 units over 1 minute, then give the rest of the IV loading dose before starting a continuous infusion. Follow with continuous infusion at 1000 units/ hr. Obtain an aPTT in 4 hours.

➤ Some patients have reactions to heparin, including allergies to the pork or bovine components. Read labels carefully. Refer to Figure 12-10.

Thus, the slow bolus test dose is ordered.

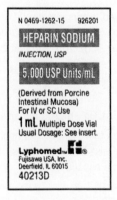

N 0469-1262-15    926201

**HEPARIN SODIUM**

*INJECTION, USP*

**5,000 USP Units/mL**

(Derived from Porcine Intestinal Mucosa)
For IV or SC Use

**1 mL** Multiple Dose Vial
Usual Dosage: See insert.

**Lyphomed**™ ®
Fujisawa USA, Inc.
Deerfield, IL 60015
40213D

---

*Think of a *half-minute* as a rough, approximate normal aPTT. The normal range is about 20 to 35 seconds. Use the precise range supplied by the individual laboratory for heparin administration.

**1** Why is thrombocytopenia, as measured by a platelet count under 100,000, a contraindication to the institution of heparin therapy? Refer to Essential Vocabulary if necessary. (Give a brief answer.)

_____

**2** The physician leaves the following order: Start infusion at 1000 units/ hr. Available: 25,000 units/ 250 mL of NS. Heparin infusions are administered on infusion pumps.

**a.** The nurse will set the flow rate at how many mL/ hr?

DA equation:

**b.** Evaluation: _____

Prescriber orders IV heparin for Mr. Y, whose weight is 80 kg. Titrate (adjust) heparin q4h to maintain aPTT. Up to 44 seconds, increase infusion by 1 unit/ kg/ hr. 45 to 75 seconds: no adjustment. 76 to 80 seconds: decrease infusion by 1 unit/ kg/ hr. aPTT greater than 80 seconds: hold infusion. Call physician for orders.

**3** Mr. Y's next aPTT is 50 seconds. Control is 30 seconds. Desired aPTT for patient receiving heparin anticoagulant therapy is 1.5 to 2.5 times control.

**a.** Desired therapeutic range in seconds for Mr. Y: _____
**b.** Is Mr. Y's current result within the aPTT therapeutic range? (Yes/No) _____
**c.** Does an adjustment need to be made in IV heparin units/ hr and IV flow rate based upon the aPTT result and the titration schedule? (Brief phrases)

_____
_____

DA equation if applicable:

**d.** Evaluation: _____

**4** Mr. Y's next aPTT is 76 seconds. Control is 30 seconds. Desired aPTT for patient receiving anticoagulant therapy is 1.5 to 2.5 times control.

**a.** What is the desired therapeutic aPTT range in seconds for Mr. Y?

_____
**b.** Is it within the desired therapeutic range? _____
**c.** Will an adjustment in units/ hr be needed based on the aPTT result and the titration schedule ordered in problem 2? (Answer briefly.)

_____
_____

**d.** If so, how many units/ hr should Mr. Y receive? Round answer to nearest 100 units/ hr.

DA equation:

**e.** Will there be an adjustment needed in Mr. Y's IV flow rate? _____
**f.** If so, how many mL/ hr should he receive?

DA equation:

5 The orders for a new patient read: Heparin infusion: 1600 units/ hr. The nurse on the oncoming shift sees that the existing flow rate is 32 mL /hr.

    a. How many units/ hr to the nearest 100 units is the patient receiving based on the existing concentration of heparin 12,500 units/ 250 mL of NS?

    _____

    DA equation:

    b. Evaluation: (Is the flow rate correct or incorrect for the order?)

    _____

    c. Is this amount within the usual recommended 24-hour range of 20,000 to 40,000 units/ hr for IV heparin infusions? (Yes/No) _____

## RAPID PRACTICE 12-6  Heparin and Heparinoid Preparations

**Estimated completion time: 20 minutes**   Answers on page **592**

**Directions:** *Read each patient's history. Calculate the doses using a DA equation and a calculator for long division and multiplication.*

1 Mr. M is receiving heparin continuous infusion of 12 units/ kg/ hr. Available: premixed heparin 25,000 units in 500 mL. Mr. M's weight is 90 kg.

    a. How many units per hour of heparin should Mr. M receive to the nearest 100 units? _____

    b. What rate will the nurse set on the infusion pump to the nearest mL?

    DA equation:

    c. Evaluation: _____

2 Mr. M.'s aPTT exceeds 90 seconds. The control aPTT is 35 seconds. The physician orders laboratory tests, including a platelet count, and protamine sulfate 1 mg IV for every 100 units of half the *hourly heparin dose administered in the past hour.*

    a. Is Mr. M. at risk of thrombi or bleeding? (Circle one.)

    b. Number of units of heparin administered in the past hour rounded to the nearest 100 units per hr: _____

    c. Half the amount of units of heparin administered in the past hour (to the nearest 100 units): _____

    d. Number of milligrams of protamine sulfate to be administered based on the order: _____

    DA equation:

    e. Evaluation: _____

**3** A current drug reference states to administer the protamine sulfate IV ordered in problem 2 *slowly over 1 to 3 minutes.* ➤ Too-rapid administration can result in anaphylaxis, severe hypotension, hypertension, bradycardia, and dyspnea.

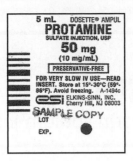

**a.** How many mL (to the nearest tenth) of protamine sulfate IV will be administered to Mr. M (problem 2)? _____

DA equation:

**b.** Evaluation: _____

**4** Mrs. J is scheduled for a hip replacement. She is placed on prophylactic anticoagulation with a LMWH agent, dalteparin (Fragmin):

2500 international units subcut 2 hours before surgery
2500 international units subcut 8 hours after surgery
5000 international units subcut daily for 14 days postoperatively in the hospital and at home

Periodic complete blood count, platelet count, and stool test for occult blood were ordered.

How many mL will Mrs. J need to receive preoperatively (to the nearest tenth of a mL)?

**a.** Estimated dose:
**b.** DA verification:

**c.** Evaluation _____

**5** Fragmin 80 international units/ kg is ordered prophylactically q12h subcut for Mrs. V, a patient with unstable angina. Mrs. V weighs 110 lb.

10 x 0.2 mL single dose syringes, preassembled with needle guards
NDC 0013-2426-91

## Fragmin®

### dalteparin sodium injection

## 5000 IU (anti-Xa) per 0.2 mL

## For subcutaneous injection

**2,500 IU Single-dose prefilled syringe**

What is Mrs. V's weight in kg?

**a.** Estimate: _____

DA equation:

**b.** Evaluation: _____

**c.** How many units will the nurse prepare for Mrs. V.?

DA equation:

**d.** Evaluation: _____

**e.** How many mL will the nurse prepare to the nearest hundredth of a mL?

**f.** Estimate: _____

DA equation:

**g.** Evaluation: _____

➤ Do *not* interchange units with milligrams for dose. Check the order and label, and compare units ordered to units supplied.

## CHAPTER 12 MULTIPLE-CHOICE REVIEW

**Estimated completion time: 20-30 minutes**   Answers on page **593**

**Directions:** *Select the correct answer.*

1 Which of the following medications require(s) INR testing? _____
   **1.** Streptokinase
   **2.** Heparinoids
   **3.** Heparin sodium or calcium
   **4.** Warfarin products

2 Which medication is given orally? _____
   **1.** Warfarin products
   **2.** Heparinoids
   **3.** Heparin sodium
   **4.** Heparin calcium

3 Which bests describes the "control value" for aPTT and PT testing? _____
   **1.** It reflects the patient's current laboratory value before treatment.
   **2.** It is a measure of therapeutic response to anticoagulation.
   **3.** It reflects the current laboratory norm based on the batch of materials used for testing that day.
   **4.** It is the general range of norms for all patients receiving anticoagulants.

4 The general recommended flow rate for initial continuous heparin infusions for adults, which can vary widely depending on the patient's condition and test results, is _____
   **1.** 1000 to 1700 units/ hr
   **2.** 5 units/ hr
   **3.** 5000 units/ hr
   **4.** 25,000 units/ hr

5 The main reason unwanted amounts of medicine need to be discarded from prefilled syringes before administering the prescribed volume to the patient is
_____
   **1.** Remainders are to be discarded from all prefilled syringes.
   **2.** The nurse might inadvertently administer more than the ordered amount.
   **3.** There is risk of undermedication and a potential thromboembolic event.
   **4.** It is usually hospital policy.

6 Which of the following statements is true about the relationship between international units and milligrams? _____
   **1.** Milligrams are a measure of weight, and international units are a standardized amount that produces a particular biologic effect.
   **2.** Milligrams and corresponding units can be determined by the nurse using a standard formula for all drugs.
   **3.** The effect of 1 mg is equal to the effect of 1 international unit of the same product.
   **4.** Milligrams, milliliters, and international units can be used interchangeably.

7 When may a physician have to consider aspirin only for anticoagulation for a patient needing anticoagulation therapy? _____
   **1.** The patient is at high risk for DVT.
   **2.** The patient is at very high risk for developing clots.
   **3.** The patient is noncompliant with medication and test regimens.
   **4.** The patient is elderly and lives with children.

8 The preferred test for monitoring heparin therapy is _____
   **1.** PT
   **2.** aPTT
   **3.** PTT
   **4.** INR

9 Which of the following dose concentrations are commonly used for heparin flushes? _____

   **1.** 10 to 25,000 units/ 250 mL     **3.** 5000 to 10,000 units/ mL
   **2.** 10 to 100 units/ mL         **4.** 1000 to 5000 units/ mL

10 Which antidote should be on hand for patients receiving heparin therapy?
_____

   **1.** Activated charcoal        **3.** Potassium chloride
   **2.** Vitamin K             **4.** Protamine sulfate

## CHAPTER 12 FINAL PRACTICE

**Estimated completion time: 1-2 hours**   Answers on page **593**

**Directions:** *Answer the anticoagulant-related questions. Use a calculator for long division and multiplication. Evaluate your equations. Label all answers.*

1 Ordered: Coumadin (warfarin sodium) 5 mg at bedtime for an elderly patient for discharge post–myocardial infarction. INR values are ordered twice weekly for the first month. The target therapeutic INR is 2 to 3 for this patient. The laboratory reports the patient's INR result at 5.

   **a.** What will the physician probably do regarding the dosage of Coumadin— rise it or lower it? (Circle one.)
   **b.** If the patient has several different strengths of Coumadin at home because of dosage adjustments, what sort of advice would be advisable to give the patient regarding drug storage?

   _____

   _____

2 Ordered: heparin infusion of 2000 units/ hr based on patient's weight. A heparin infusion of 25,000 units in 250 mL is being administered at 20 mL/ hr.

   **a.** How many *units per hour,* to nearest 100 units, are being infused?

     DA equation:

   **b.** Evaluation: _____

3 Ordered: heparin 18 units/ kg/ hr in a continuous infusion. Available: heparin 25,000 units in 500 mL D5W. Patient's weight: 70 kg

   **a.** How many units/ hr are ordered:

     DA equation:

   **b.** Evaluation: _____
   **c.** The nurse will set the flow rate at how many mL/ hr: _____

     DA equation:

   **d.** Evaluation: _____

CHAPTER 12

**4** Ordered: Heparin infusion of 1500 units/ hr. Available: Heparin 25,000 units/ 500 mL NS. The IV is infusing at 20 mL/ hr when the nurse arrives on the shift.

   **a.** Is the existing flow rate correct? If not, what should it be?

   DA equation:

   **b.** Evaluation: _____

**5** Ordered: Lovenox 30 mg subcut daily at bedtime: It is supplied in a prefilled syringe.

LOVENOX®
(enoxaparin
sodium) Injection
**40 mg/0.4 mL**
Syringe
RHÔNE-POULENC RORER
PHARMACEUTICALS INC.
COLLEGEVILLE, PA 19426
Made in France    L-5560A
LOT 506572A    EXP

   **a.** What type of drug is Lovenox: heparin, LMWH, warfarin, or thrombolytic derivative? _____

   **b.** How many mL will the nurse prepare?

   DA equation:

   **c.** Evaluation: _____

**6** Ordered: continuous heparin infusion to maintain the aPTT between 60 and 70 seconds, for a patient with atrial fibrillation. After the initial slow bolus loading dose of 5000 units IV, draw a stat aPTT and begin the infusion at 1000 units/ hr. Obtain the aPTT q6h. Patient weight is 70 kg. The following sliding scale is given to titrate the heparin infusion:

| aPTT | Action |
|---|---|
| 30-45 seconds | Increase the drip by 3 units/ kg/ hr. |
| 46-70 seconds | No change. |
| 71-85 seconds | Reduce the drip by 2 units/ kg/ hr. |
| Over 85 seconds | Hold the infusion for 1 hr. Call the physician for orders. |

Available: 20,000 units of heparin in 500 mL D5W. The first aPTT drawn is 40 seconds.

   **a.** Current flow rate in mL/ hr at 1000 units/ hr should be set at:

   DA equation:

   **b.** Evaluation: _____

   **c.** Nurse's evaluation of the aPTT. (Give a brief answer.)

   _____

   **d.** Adjusted number of units/ hr if applicable:

   DA equation:

   **e.** Evaluation: _____

    **f.** Adjusted number of mL/ hr if applicable: _____

    DA equation:

    **g.** Evaluation: _____

7 The patient described in problem 6 has another aPTT drawn 6 hours later. The result is 65 seconds.

    **a.** Adjustment in mL/ hr if applicable. _____

    DA equation:

    **b.** Evaluation: _____

8 A nurse checks an infusion of heparin 25,000 units/ 500 mL Ringer's solution. It is flowing at 40 mL/ hr.

    **a.** How many units of heparin per hour are being delivered?

    DA equation:

    **b.** Evaluation: _____
    **c.** Is this order within the recommended 24-hour dose for heparin infusions? _____

9 The order for the infusion in problem 8 is for 1200 units/ hr.

    **a.** For how many mL/ hr will the nurse set the infusion?

    DA equation:

    **b.** What adverse effect will the nurse monitor for, in addition to obtaining another aPTT? _____

10 **a.** What does "extended coagulation time" mean to you? _____
    **b.** Why should a heparin infusion be administered on an infusion pump? _____

## Suggestions for Further Reading

http://clotcare.com/clotcare/search.aspx?by=med
www.aafp.org/afp/990201ap/635.html
www.ahrq.gov/downloads/pub/advances/vol3/Harder.doc
www.cdc.gov.mmwr/preview
www.ismp.org
www.ncbi.nim.nih.gov
www.nlm.nih.gov/medlineplus/druginfo/uspdi/202280.html

 Additional practice problems can be found in the Advanced Calculations section on the enclosed companion CD.

Chapter 13 focuses on pediatric dose calculations. These determinations are often multi-step calculations of fractional doses of medications using the familiar techniques of dimensional analysis.

# PART VI
## MEDICATIONS FOR INFANTS AND CHILDREN

CHAPTER 13  PEDIATRIC MEDICATION CALCULATIONS

*"Children have neither past nor future; they enjoy the present, which very few of us do."*

—JEAN DE LA BRUYERE

# PEDIATRIC MEDICATION CALCULATIONS

## Objectives

- Distinguish the milligram (mg), microgram (mcg), gram (g), and square meter (m2) units of measurement.
- Evaluate orders for minimum and maximum pediatric SDR doses.
- Calculate pediatric weight-based doses for oral and parenteral routes.
- Calculate pediatric doses based on body surface area.
- Calculate flow rates for IV volume-control devices.
- State measures to prevent medication errors for pediatric patients.

## Essential Prior Knowledge

Chapters 1-12

## Equipment

- A calculator is useful for converting pounds to kilograms and calculating SDR.

## Estimated Time To Complete Chapter

- 2-2½ hours

## Introduction

To have therapeutic value and to avoid injury, medication doses must be highly individualized for pediatric populations. The requirements for body fluid and electrolyte balance in infants and children, as well as immature renal and liver function, dictate a need for great care with fluid and medication administration. The necessary departures from average adult unit doses have resulted in medication errors for a vulnerable population.

Medications for children may be referred to as *"fractional doses"* if they consist of a partial dose of the amount supplied. Doses for children are usually based on *weight*—micrograms, milligrams, or grams per kilogram of body weight—or on *surface area:* micrograms or milligrams per square meter of body surface area. Therapeutic doses for children are included in most current medication references. The trend is for the pharmacy to supply more pediatric-specific pre-prepared medications to reduce the chance of calculation error.

Occasionally, young patients receive a higher-than-usual adult dose because of the severity of illness, the threat to life, or the lack of response to lower doses and other medications. The particular emphases for safe medication administration with pediatric populations, beyond the selection of appropriate equipment and sites for the medications, are:

1  Verifying that the order is within the SDR for the target population
2  Distinguishing microgram, milligram, and square meter units of measurement

3  Calculating accurate fractional doses and fluid needs for all routes
4  Identifying the correct patient when the patient cannot speak
5  Assessing side effects and complications in nonverbal patients

The nurse has extra responsibilities to protect the safety of the pediatric patient.

➤ Pediatric patients cannot protect themselves from medication errors. Many cannot identify themselves and are not in a position to question medications and medication orders or to verbalize physical complaints. In addition to using printed identification bracelets, bar codes, and other methods, the nurse should have a family member verify the identity of a pediatric patient.

The preceding chapters provide a considerable foundation for quickly mastering the calculations in this chapter.

> ▲ **Cultural Note**
>
> Cultural awareness of naming practices is important in avoiding misidentification of a patient who is to receive medications and treatments. When identifying a pediatric patient, keep in mind that naming practices of parents and children vary widely among cultures. Family members may have different last names, based on particular paternal and maternal naming practices.

## ESSENTIAL Vocabulary

| | |
|---|---|
| **Body Surface Area (BSA)** | Area covered by the skin measured in square meters. Used for accurate dosing of powerful drugs and for at-risk populations. |
| **Square Meter (m²)** | Metric unit of area measurement. Powerful medications, particularly anti-cancer medications, may be based on square meters of BSA. |
| **Milligrams per Kilogram (mg/ kg)** | Drug amount in milligrams based on kilograms of body weight. The most common unit of measurement for prescribed doses of medications for pediatric and frail patients and for powerful drugs. |
| **Nomogram** | Graphic representation of numerical relationships. A BSA nomogram is used to estimate square meters of body surface area. |
| **Safe Dose Range (SDR)** | Minimum-to-maximum therapeutic dose range for a target population: adult, child, infant, neonate, or elderly. |

## RAPID PRACTICE 13-1  Vocabulary Review

**Estimated completion time: 5 minutes**   Answers on page **595**

**Directions:** *Read the vocabulary and introductory material to provide the answers to the questions.*

1  Medication dose that is less than the usual adult dose:

_____

2  Abbreviation for the minimum-to-maximum therapeutic dose range cited by manufacturers:

_____

3  The most common measurement used for determining the dose for pediatric patients:

_____

4  Units of measurement that may be used to calculate doses for pediatric populations:

_____

5  Which metric unit is used to measure BSA?

_____

# Comparing Adult and Pediatric Medication Doses and Schedules

➤ Examine the selected examples in Table 13-1, and note the differences in dosing and units of measurement for adults and children.

There may be many more subclassifications of drug dose based on precise age groups of neonates, infants, and children and on various conditions for which one drug may be prescribed.

**Q** *Ask Yourself*

**A** *My Answer*

**1** Which of the recommended SDRs for amoxicillin is weight-based: the adult or the child?

_____

➤ Taking 2 or 3 minutes to verify a safe dose order with a current pediatric drug reference and/or pharmacy may prevent a tragic error.

| TABLE 13-1 | IV Dose Comparison by Age Group for Selected Drugs |
|---|---|
| **Name of Drug** | **Dose Comparison** |
| **Potassium chloride (KCl)*** | SDR, **Adult,** Individualized: IV 20-60 mEq q24h |
| | 200 mEq/ 24 hr for hypokalemia is usually not exceeded. 40 mEq dilution per Liter preferred |
| | SDR, **Child,** Individualized: IV 1-4 mEq/ kg of body weight / 24 hr |
| | OR |
| | 10 mEq/ hr, whichever is <u>less</u>, not to exceed 40 mEq/ 24 hr. Must be at least 40 mEq dilution per Liter. |
| | Monitor serum potassium levels. |
| | Contact prescriber if patient is fluid-restricted. |
| | Monitor ECG for symptoms of hypo- and hyperkalemia. |
| | Pediatrics: KCl must be infused on electronic infusion pump. Obtain written order for *each* infusion. |
| **Morphine sulfate** | |
| Pain relief | **Adult,** IV: 2.5-15 mg q4h |
| Postoperative analgesia | **Child,** IV: 0.01-0.04 mg/ kg/ hr |
| | **Neonate,** IV: 0.015-0.02 mg/ kg/ hr[†] |
| Severe chronic cancer pain | **Child,** IV: 0.025-2.6 mg/ kg/ hr |
| **Prazosin HCl** | **Adult,** PO: 1 mg at bedtime to start |
| | **Child,** PO: 5 mcg/ kg q6h to start |
| **Amoxicillin** | **Adult,** PO: 250-500 mg q8h |
| | **Child,** PO: 25-50 mg/ kg/ d (max 60-80 mg/ kg/ d divided q8h) |
| **Clindamycin** | **Child,** IM/IV: 25-40 mg/ kg/ d divided q6-8h |
| | **Neonate,** IM/IV, ≤7 d: 10-15 mg/kg/d divided q8-12h |
| | **Neonate,** IM/IV, >7 d: 10-20 mg / kg/ d divided q6-12h |

*Potassium chloride has been identified as a high-risk medication, one with higher than average potential for causing injury if an error occurs. Doses are highly individualized, based on purpose (e.g., maintenance or replacement), current serum K levels, weight, and renal function.

[†]A neonate refers to an infant in the first 4 weeks of life. Consult drug references for child age-related dose guidelines. They vary.

## RAPID PRACTICE 13-2 Medication Dosing Differences for Children and Adults

**Estimated completion time: 10-15 minutes**   **Answers on page 595**

**Directions:** *Examine Table 13-1 to answer the questions pertaining to SDR guidelines.*

1 What is the difference in the drug *unit of measurement* for adults and children for the antihypertensive drug prazosin? (How many mcg are there in a mg?)

_____

2 What is the difference in the initial *frequency schedules* for the antihypertensive drug prazosin for adults and children?

_____

3 What is the difference in the *maximum* doses of morphine sulfate for a child with postoperative pain and a child with severe chronic cancer pain?

_____

4 What is the difference in the doses of clindamycin for neonates ≤7 days of age and neonates >7 days of age?

_____

5 What action must be taken if a patient is fluid restricted and potassium is ordered?

_____

# Calculating Kilograms to Nearest Tenth from Pounds and Ounces

A patient's body weight in kilograms is usually calculated to the *nearest tenth* for determining pediatric doses.

➤ It is important to note that ounces must be converted to tenths of a pound *before* kilograms are calculated. 5 lb 4 oz is *not* equal to 5.4 lb.

---

**EXAMPLES**

1 Convert 5 lb 4 oz to pounds. Conversion formula: 16 oz = 1 lb.

$$lb = \frac{1 \text{ lb}}{16 \text{ oz}} \times 4 \text{ oz} = 0.25 \text{ lb, rounded to } 0.3 \text{ lb}$$

2 Add the lb: 5 + 0.3 = 5.3 Total lb
3 Convert 5.3 lb to kilograms. Conversion formula: 2.2 lb = 1 kg.

$$kg = \frac{1 \text{ kg}}{2.2 \text{ lb}} \times 5.3 \text{ lb} = 2.4 \text{ kg}$$

Evaluation: Dividing 5.3 by 2 gives a rough estimate of 2.5 kg. Experienced nurses use a calculator to divide ounces by 16 to obtain pounds and add that result to the number of pounds in the given weight (4 oz ÷ 16 = 0.25, or 0.3 lb; 5 lb + 0.3 lb = 5.3 lb total). Next, using the conversion formula 2.2 lb = 1 kg, the total number of pounds, 5.3 lb, is divided by 2.2 to obtain 2.4 kg.

---

➤ The nurse must know how to set up a DA equation to calculate doses in case a functioning calculator is not available.

## RAPID PRACTICE 13-3 Converting Pounds to Kilograms Review

**Estimated completion time: 20-25 minutes**    Answers on page **596**

**Directions:** *Estimate the weight in kg. Calculate the weight in kg to the nearest tenth of a kilogram using DA-style equations. Verify the result with a calculator. Remember to change ounces to pounds if necessary.*

1  12 lb 3 oz
   **a.** Estimated kg wt: _____
   **b.** Actual wt in kg:

   DA equation:

   **c.** Evaluation: _____

2  20 lb 6 oz
   **a.** Estimated kg wt: _____
   **b.** Actual wt in kg:

   DA equation:

   **c.** Evaluation: _____

3  4 lb 8 oz
   **a.** Estimated kg wt: _____
   **b.** Actual wt in kg:

   DA equation:

   **c.** Evaluation: _____

4  25 lb 9 oz
   **a.** Estimated kg wt: _____
   **b.** Actual wt in kg:

   DA equation:

   **c.** Evaluation: _____

5  18 lb 12 oz
   **a.** Estimated kg wt: _____
   **b.** Actual wt in kg:

   DA equation:

   **c.** Evaluation: _____

Consult TJC recommendations for Pediatric Patient Medication at
www.jointcommission.org/Sentine1Events/Sentine1EventAlert/sea_35.htm

# Sequence for Calculating Safe Dose Range

➤ Review the logic and example of the multi-step process for evaluating an order for safe dose. A calculator is helpful.

STEPS

1 Obtain the total body weight in the desired terms.
2 Calculate the SDR.
3 Compare and evaluate the order with the SDR. Contact the prescriber if the order is not within the SDR.
4 If the order is safe, estimate, calculate, and evaluate the dose.

---

EXAMPLES

Ordered: Drug Y 60 mg/ day

Patient's wt: 26 lb 6oz

SDR: 5-10 mg/ kg/ day in a single dose

Supplied: Drug Y 100 mg/ 5 mL

Conversion formulas: 16 oz = 1 lb and 2.2 lb = 1 kg

Kilogram estimate: 26 lb ÷ 2 = 13 kg.

(1) Total lb = $\dfrac{1\ lb}{16\ oz} \times 6\ oz = 0.375$, rounded to 0.4 lb, 26 lb + 0.4 lb = 26.4 total lb

SDR for this child:

$$mg = \frac{5\ mg}{kg} \times \frac{1\ \cancel{kg}}{2.2\ \cancel{lb}} \times 26.4\ \cancel{lb} = 60\ mg/\ day\ \text{low safe dose}$$

$$mg = \frac{10\ mg}{kg} \times \frac{1\ \cancel{kg}}{2.2\ \cancel{lb}} \times 26.4\ \cancel{lb} = 120\ mg/\ day\ \text{high safe dose}$$

(2) SDR = 60-120mg/ day.

(Ordered: 60 mg/ day.)

(3) Evaluation: It can be seen at a glance that the dose ordered is within the SDR both for the total amount and the schedule. Therefore, give the medication.

Estimate: Will be giving less than unit dose of 100 mg/ 5 mL supplied.

(4) $$mL = \frac{\overset{1}{\cancel{5}}\ mL}{\underset{\underset{1}{20}}{\cancel{100}}\ mg} \times \overset{3}{\cancel{60}}\ mg = 3\ mL$$

Evaluation: The equation is balanced. This is a reasonable dose because the order was for slightly more than one-half the number of mg supplied in 5 mL.

---

• Note that once the *total number of pounds* is determined, it is entered in the SDR equations with the conversion formula to kilograms.
• For purposes of comparison, it is helpful to put the amount ordered directly *below* the SDR for the patient in order to visualize that the order is within the SDR.
• Experienced nurses use a calculator to obtain the SDR and kg wt.
• You need to be able to set up a DA equation to recall data entry order.

1 What are the four main steps in the sequence for evaluating and calculating the recommended safe dose? (State your answer using 1 to 3 key words for each step.)

Q: *Ask Yourself*

A: *My Answer*

**Estimated completion time: 25 minutes** Answers on page **597**

**Directions:** *Obtain total lb and change to kg if needed. Calculate the SDR. Compare the ordered dose with the SDR in same units of measurement (compare mcg to mcg, mg to mg, and g to g using metric conversion formulas). Evaluate the order for safe dose. Use a calculator for long division and multiplication.*

1  Ordered: Drug Y 500 mcg/ hr IV. SDR for children: 10-20 mcg/ kg/ hr. Patient's weight: 66 lb.

   **a.** Estimated kg wt: _____ Actual kg wt: _____
   **b.** SDR for this child: _____

   DA equation:

   **c.** Evaluation: *Safe to give or Hold and clarify promptly with prescriber? (Circle one.)*

2  Ordered: Drug Y 5 mg IV q8h. SDR for children: 200-500 mcg/ kg/ day in 3 divided doses. Patient's weight: 12 lb.

   **a.** Estimated kg wt: _____ Actual kg wt: _____
   **b.** SDR for this child: _____

   DA equation:

   **c.** Evaluation: *Safe to give or Hold and clarify promptly with prescriber. (Circle one.)*

3  Ordered: Drug Y 250 mg PO 4 times daily. SDR for children: 1-1.5 g per day in 4 divided doses. Use mental arithmetic to convert mg and g.

   **a.** SDR for children: _____
   **b.** Evaluation of order: _____
   **c.** Evaluation: *Safe to give or Hold and clarify promptly with prescriber? (Circle one.)*

4  Ordered: Drug Y 2 mg PO q6h. SDR for children: 500-800 mcg/ kg/ day in 4-6 divided doses. Patient's weight: 22 lb.

   **a.** Estimated kg wt: _____ Actual kg wt: _____
   **b.** SDR for this child: _____

   DA equation:

   **c.** Evaluation: *Safe to give or Hold and clarify promptly with prescriber? (Circle one.)*

5  Ordered: Drug Y 35 mg IM stat

   SDR for children: 1-3 mg/ kg q4-6h

   Patient wt: 20 lb 4 oz

   **a.** Estimated kg wt: _____ Actual kg wt: _____
   **b.** SDR for this child: _____

   DA equation:

   **c.** Evaluation: *Safe to give or Hold and clarify promptly with prescriber? (Circle one.)*

# Body Surface Area (BSA)

The weight-based medication orders for mg/kg and mcg/kg are the most frequently encountered units of measurement found in medication orders for children. Occasionally, the nurse will encounter an order based on body surface area (BSA) in square meters ($m^2$) of skin. BSA-based dosing is considered superior to weight-based dosing for powerful medications.

Most medications ordered in square meters of BSA are calculated by the pharmacist or prescriber and frequently are antineoplastic drugs administered by a nurse who has chemotherapy certification. Square meters of BSA may also be used for the SDR of drugs other than anticancer agents, particularly for infants, children, and geriatric patients. In addition, BSA may be used for calculating fluid and ventilation requirements.

➤ The nurse is expected to be able to define BSA, identify square meters, and, *most important*, distinguish among $m^2$ and mg and mcg metric measurements when reading orders, medication records, and current drug references and when calculating SDR.

The BSA is derived from formulas based on weight and height. There are two BSA formulas, one for the metric system and one for the English system.

**Metric Formula**                 **English Formula**

$$\sqrt{\frac{\text{weight (kg)} \times \text{height (cm)}}{3600}} = \text{BSA (m}^2)$$   $$\sqrt{\frac{\text{weight (lb)} \times \text{height (in)}}{3131}} = \text{BSA (m}^2)$$

1  A meter is just a little larger than a yard (1 meter = 1.09 yard). If you estimated your BSA in square yards, would you expect the amount to be very small?

Q: *Ask Yourself*

A: *My Answer*

2  What is my BSA? Use your weight and a calculator to apply one of the BSA formulas. Multiply the numerators, divide by the denominator, and then enter the square root sign. Does the term *square meters* provide a clue as to size of the result?

## Reading Body Surface Area in Square Meters on a Nomogram

The BSA nomogram is an *estimation* of BSA and is faster to use than the formulas. Figure 13-1 is an example of a nomogram of a BSA-derived medication dose.

## Calculating Milligrams per Square Meter (mg/m²)

In calculating the mg/$m^2$ of BSA, the sequence is the same as that used in mcg- and mg-based SDR calculations.

➤ The calculation of milligrams per square meter is performed using a DA-style equation or simple multiplication, just as it is for calculating milligrams per kilogram (e.g., 2 mg/$m^2$ means "2 milligrams of medicine for each square meter of body surface area").

Figure 13-1. Modified West Nomogram for Body Surface Area Estimation. The red line denoted by arrow *A* in the highlighted column, "Children of Normal Weight for Height," illustrates a BSA of 0.7 m² for a child weighing 7 lb. Calculations for children who are *not* at normal height for weight, as determined by standard pediatric growth charts, will have a different BSA for their weight. The outside columns are used to plot height and weight. The BSA is read at the intersection as indicated by the red arrow over line B on the column titled "SA" by connecting the two plotted measurements with a straight line *(B)*. There are additional nomograms for adults. (Nomogram modified with data from Berhrman RE, Kleigman R, Jenson HB: Nelson textbook of pediatrics, ed. 17, Philadelphia, 2004, Saunders.)

---

**EXAMPLES**

Examine the following example.

Ordered: Drug Y 4 mg qid

Patient's BSA: 0.8 m². SDR: 20 mg/ m² daily in 4 divided doses.

$$\frac{mg}{day} = \frac{20\ mg}{m^2} \times 0.8\ m^2 = 16\ mg/\ day \div 4 = 4\ mg/\ dose$$

SDR= 16 mg total per day divided in 4 doses

Order: 16 mg total per day, 4 mg per dose

Evaluation: The total dose and the frequency schedule are in accordance with the SDR. Give 4 mg.

---

➤ Pay close attention to the placement of decimal points. Square meters of BSA are *very small amounts.* A missing decimal point would result in a tenfold dose error.

➤ Pediatric doses are calculated to the *nearest hundredth* of a mL. Check agency policies.

> **FAQ** | *Where will the staff nurse find the BSA of the patient?*
>
> **ANSWER:** The pharmacy usually provides the BSA and the dose on a MAR or a separate chemotherapy medication sheet. The nurse uses the pharmacy-provided BSA calculation to check the SDR obtained from a current pharmacology reference or drug package insert. If the BSA is not available and a nomogram for the appropriate age group is not available, the pharmacy can be contacted.

## RAPID PRACTICE 13-5    Evaluating Pediatric SDR

**Estimated completion time: 15-20 minutes**    Answers on page **598**

**Directions:** *Evaluate the following orders. For BSA in square meters, read the nomogram in Figure 13-1 and calculate the safe dose. Set up a DA equation, and verify your answer with a calculator. State reason for giving or withholding the medication.*

1  Ordered: An IV infusion of heparin 225 units/ hr for a baby of normal weight for height weighing 10 lb.

   SDR: 20,000 units/ $m^2$ q24h continues IV infusion
   **a.** BSA for this child: _____
   **b.** SDR for this patient: _____

   DA equation:

   **c.** Evaluation: *Safe to give* or *Hold and clarify promptly with prescriber?* (Circle one and state reason.) _____

2  Ordered: vincristine 1 mg IV once a week, for a child with Hodgkin's disease of normal weight for height weighing 30 lb. SDR: 1.5-2 mg/ $m^2$/ week.

   **a.** BSA for this child: _____
   **b.** SDR for this patient: _____

   DA equation:

   **c.** Evaluation: *Safe to give* or *Hold and clarify promptly with prescriber?* (Circle one and state reason.) _____

3  Ordered: methotrexate 15 mg PO, for a child with leukemia of normal weight for height weighing 70 lb. SDR: 3.3 mg/ $m^2$/ day.

   **a.** BSA for this child: _____
   **b.** SDR for this patient: _____

   DA equation:

   **c.** Evaluation: *Safe to give* or *Hold and clarify promptly with prescriber?* (Circle one and state reason.) _____

4  Ordered: gentamicin 125 mg every 8 hours IV, for a child with severe infection weighing 50 kg. SDR: 2-2.5 mg/ kg q8h.

   **a.** BSA for this child: _____ (Is it needed? Why or why not?) _____
   **b.** SDR for this patient: _____

DA equation:

**c.** Evaluation: *Safe to give* or *Hold and clarify promptly with prescriber?* (Circle one and state reason.) _____

**5** Ordered: dopamine 20 mcg/ min IV, for an infant with respiratory distress syndrome weighing 5 kg. SDR: starting dose 1-5 mcg/ kg/ min.
   **a.** BSA for this child: _____ (Is it needed? Why or why not?)_____
   **b.** SDR for this patient: _____

   DA equation:

**c.** Evaluation: *Safe to give* or *Hold and clarify promptly with prescriber?* (Circle one and state reason.) _____

➤ There may be a good reason for a very high dose order, such as severity of illness or nonresponsiveness to a lower dose. The nurse must clarify and document the response from the prescriber, as in the following example:

"4/25/05, 1800: High dose of Drug Y, 5mg/ hr IV for 22-kg child, verified with prescriber per TC. John Smith, R.N. "

# Equipment for Medication Administration to Pediatric Patients and Patients Unable to Chew Tablets and Pills

In addition to dose modifications, the equipment used to deliver medication to a child may be different from that used for the average adult. Droppers, bottle nipples, measuring teaspoons, special oral syringes, and regular syringes *with the needle removed,* with or without a short tubing extension, may be used.

| **Clinical Relevance** | The medications may be administered with pleasant-tasting, nonessential foods (never milk) to disguise an unfamiliar or unwelcome taste. A pill-crushing device or mortar and pestle may be needed to grind and mix non–enteric-coated pills, if permitted (Figure 13-2). Water, applesauce, or sherbet may be used to mix the medication or formula to follow the medication, depending on diet orders, swallowing ability, and age. Popsicles may be permitted immediately after a medicine to offset the taste. Some children prefer to drink from a 1-oz medicine cup. |
|---|---|

If a nipple is used to deliver medication, rinse the nipple with water first so that the medicine will flow rather than stick to the nipple. Follow the medicine with water or formula *within the fluid limitations* permitted for the patient (Figure 13-3).

When family members are present, they can be very helpful by holding the child and/or giving the oral medication and something more pleasant-tasting to follow.

Remember that medications can be measured accurately with a syringe and transferred to another device.

➤ Take extra measures to assess swallowing ability before attempting to give any medications by mouth to at-risk populations. This may include checking the gag reflex with a tongue blade.
➤ The presence of a gag reflex alone is not enough to assume swallowing ability. Follow up with a test of swallowing some sips of water. Do not assume that a baby can always drink from a bottle. Infants and children can have swallowing problems, just as adults can.

**Figure 13-2. A,** Using a mortar and pestle to grind pills. **B,** Using a pill-crushing device. Pills may also be left in a blister package for crushing. (From Elkin MK, Perry AG, Potter PA: Nursing interventions and clinical skills, ed. 3, St. Louis, 2004, Mosby.)

**Figure 13-3.** Using a nipple to deliver medication. (From Clayton BD, Stock YN: Basic pharmacology for nurses, ed. 13, St. Louis, 2004, Mosby.)

Giving medications to pediatric patients can be a challenge. Some nurses have the intuitive skills necessary to obtaining cooperation, and others acquire skills through experience. It helps the pediatric nursing student to shadow an experienced pediatric nurse. The records and report should provide clues as to the child's behaviors and preferences. Clinical experience in pediatric units is often limited, and there may not be enough time to have several successes.

**Clinical Relevance**

**RAPID PRACTICE 13-6** Pediatric Oral Medications

**Estimated completion time: 30-60 minutes** Answers on page **598**

**Directions:** *Determine the patient's weight in kg to the nearest tenth if needed. Calculate SDR, and evaluate the order for appropriate dose and schedule. Use a calculator for long division and multiplication. If the order is safe to administer, calculate liquid doses to nearest tenth and doses less than 1 mL to nearest hundredth of a mL. If the drug is to be held, state the reason but do not calculate the dose.*

1 Ordered: Keflex (cephalexin for oral suspension) 150 mg PO qid for a child with a mild upper respiratory infection.

Read the label to obtain the SDR.

Patient's weight: 36 lb

**a.** SDR for this child: _____

DA equation:

**b.** Evaluation: *Safe to give* or *Hold and clarify promptly with prescriber?* (Circle one and state reason.) _____

**c.** Total number of mg in container: _____

**d.** Dilution directions (use brief phrases):

_____

**e.** Amount to be administered if safe dose: _____

2 Ordered: leucovorin 20 mg PO 6 hr after administration of the antineoplastic methotrexate today to prevent toxicity.

SDR: 10 mg/ m²

Patient's weight: 70 lb (31.8 kg). BSA: 1.10 m²*

---

*Trailing zeros (e.g., 1.10 m²) are not permitted (per JCAHO) in patient medication-related documents. They are encountered in printed laboratory, drug, and scientific references and are appropriate for BSA nomograms.

**a.** SDR for this child: _____

DA equation:



**b.** Evaluation: *Safe to give* or *Hold and clarify promptly with prescriber?* (Circle one and state reason.) _____
**c.** Amount to be administered if safe dose: _____

DA equation:



**d.** Evaluation: _____

1   What amount would have been administered if the nurse was unfamiliar with square meters and used the weight in kilograms or pounds instead of square meters in problem 2 to calculate the dose?

_____

3   Ordered: Biaxin (clarithromycin oral suspension) 150 mg PO bid, for a child with otitis media.

SDR for this child: 15 mg/ kg/ day in 2 divided doses

Patient's weight: 44 lb

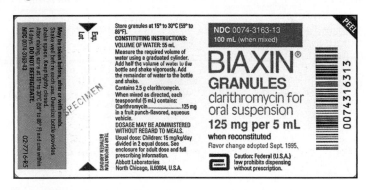

**a.** SDR for this child: _____

DA equation:



**b.** Evaluation: *Safe to give* or *Hold and clarify promptly with prescriber?* (Circle one and state reason.) _____
**c.** Dilution directions: _____
**d.** Amount to be administered if safe dose: _____

**4** Ordered: Lanoxin (digoxin) elixir 0.1 mg PO bid maintenance dose, for a 4-year-old child with congestive heart failure who has already received a loading dose

SDR for children >2 years: loading dose 0.02-0.04 mg/ kg divided q8h over 24 hr; maintenance dose 0.006-0.012 mg/ kg in divided doses q12h

Patient's weight: 20 kg

**a.** SDR for this child: _____

DA equation:

**b.** Evaluation: *Safe to give* or *Hold and clarify promptly with prescriber* (Circle one and state reason.) _____

**c.** Amount to be administered if safe dose:

Estimated dose: _____

DA equation:

**d.** How many mcg/ mL are provided in the medication container? _____

**5** Ordered: Epivir solution (lamivudine), an antiviral agent, 30 mg PO bid for a baby with HIV infection

SDR for children <50 kg: 2 mg/ kg/ day in divided doses q8h with zidovudine

Patient's weight: 20 lb

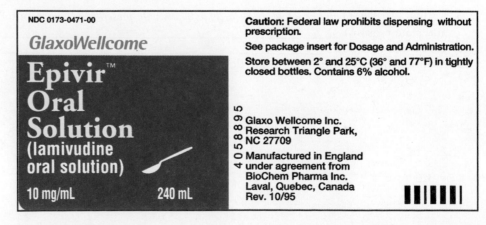

**a.** SDR for this child: _____

DA equation:




**b.** Evaluation: *Safe to give* or *Hold and clarify promptly with prescriber?* (Circle one.)
**c.** Amount to be administered if safe dose: _____

# Injection Sites for Pediatric Patients

Check agency policies regarding injection sites. With all injections, the potential site must be fully visible and carefully assessed.

The vastus lateralis muscle is preferred for injections for babies <7 months of age (Figure 13-4).

The ventrogluteal muscle is preferred for children >7 months of age and for adults (Figure 13-5).

**Figure 13-4.** Vastus lateralis intramuscular injection site. (In Lilley LL, Harrington S, Snyder JS: Pharmacology and the nursing process, ed. 4, St. Louis, 2005, Mosby. From Rick Brady, Riva, MD.)

**Figure 13-5.** Ventrogluteal intramuscular injection site. (In Lilley LL, Harrington S, Snyder JS: Pharmacology and the nursing process, ed. 4, St. Louis, 2005, Mosby. From Rick Brady, Riva, MD.)

Figure **13-6.** Dorsogluteal intramuscular injection site. (In Lilley LL, Harrington S, Snyder JS: Pharmacology and the nursing process, ed. 4, St. Louis, 2005, Mosby. From Rick Brady, Riva, MD.)

Figure **13-7.** Deltoid intramuscular injection site. (In Lilley LL, Harrington S, Snyder JS: Pharmacology and the nursing process, ed. 4, St. Louis, 2005, Mosby. From Rick Brady, Riva, MD.)

➤ Site rotation and site documentation are required.
➤ The dorsogluteal site is not a preferred site. There is a danger of damaging the sciatic nerve and striking blood vessels in an underdeveloped gluteal muscle (Figure 13-6). Children who have not walked for a year and underweight or frail persons are at especially high risk for injury. Check your agency policy.

The deltoid site may be used for small-volume medications in older children with well-developed deltoid muscles (Figure 13-7).

# Injection Volumes for Pediatric Populations

Injection volumes must be adjusted downward, depending on the size and condition of the area to be injected.

➤ 0.5 mL is the maximum for subcutaneous injections in infants and small children.
➤ 1 mL is the maximum for IM injections in children *<2 years*. Assess the potential sites for older children before making a decision to increase the volume per site.

As with adults, subcutaneous and IM medications in children must be administered with the correct size and angle of needle for the area being injected. A 45-degree angle may be needed for IM injections for underweight patients.

The syringe is selected based on the volume of the medication. A 1-mL syringe may be used for medication doses of <1 mL. This syringe permits administration to the *nearest hundredth* of a milliliter.

Supervised practice and reference to current clinical skills textbooks are needed to develop these injection skills.

## RAPID PRACTICE 13-7  Subcutaneous and Intramuscular Injections for Children

**Estimated completion time: 25-30 minutes**   Answers on page **599**

**Directions:** *Evaluate the following orders. If the dose is safe to administer, calculate the dose. Evaluate all your equations. Indicate the nearest measurable dose with an arrow on the syringe provided. Use a calculator for long division and multiplication.*

**1** Ordered: atropine sulfate 0.2 mg subcut on call to the operating room, as prophylaxis for excess secretions and salivation during anesthesia.

SDR for children: 0.01 mg/ kg subcut

Patient's weight: 22.9 kg

| | |
|---|---|
| NDC 0641-**2210-43**<br>**10 X 20 mL** Multiple Dose Vials<br>**ATROPINE**<br>SULFATE INJECTION, USP<br>**400 mcg/mL**<br>(0.4 mg/mL.)<br>FOR SC, IM OR IV USE | Each mL contains atropine sulfate 400 mcg (0.4 mg), sodium chloride 9 mg and benzyl alcohol 0.015 mL in Water for Injection. pH 3.0-6.5; sulfuric acid added, if needed, for pH adjustment.<br>**POISON**<br>USUAL DOSE: See package insert.<br>Store at controlled room temperature 15°-30°C (59°-86°F).<br>Caution: Federal law prohibits dispensing without prescription.<br>Product Code<br>2210-43                    B-32210 |

ELKINS-SINN, INC. Cherry Hill, NJ 08003-4099
*A subsidiary of A. H. Robins Company*

**a.** SDR for this child: _____

DA equation:

**b.** Evaluation: *Safe to give* or *Hold and clarify promptly with prescriber?* (Circle one and state reason.) _____

**c.** Amount to be administered if safe to give:

DA equation:

**d.** Evaluation: _____

Draw an arrow pointing to the dose on the syringe.

**2** Ordered: AquaMEPHYTON (phytonadione) 4 mg IM once a week prophylactically for hypothrombinemia, for a child on prolonged TPN therapy who has
not walked in several months.

SDR for children: 2-5 mg once weekly IM

Patient's weight: 30 lb

**a.** SDR for this child: _____

DA equation:

**b.** Evaluation: *Safe to give* or *Hold and clarify promptly with prescriber?* (Circle one
and state reason.) _____
**c.** Amount to be administered if safe to give:

DA equation:

**d.** Evaluation: _____

Draw an arrow pointing to the dose on the syringe.

**3** Ordered: Humalog insulin 3 units subcut 4 times daily ac and at bedtime, for a
newly diagnosed 10-year-old child with diabetes type 1.

SDR for children: initial 2-4 units subcut 4 times daily ac and at bedtime (SDR
for adults: initial 5-10 units ac and at bedtime)

**a.** SDR for this child: _____
**b.** Evaluation: *Safe to give* or *Hold and clarify promptly with prescriber?* (Circle one
and state reason.) _____

**c.** Draw an arrow pointing to the dose on the syringe that would be easier to read for this dose.

**d.** Would a bedtime snack be needed? If so, why? _____

➤ Remember that you may encounter *SC* and *HS* as abbreviations for "subcutaneous" and "bedtime." Do not use them when writing on MARs. They can be misinterpreted.

**4** Ordered: adrenaline HCl 1:1000 (epinephrine injection) 0.1 mg subcut stat, a bronchodilator for asthma.

SDR for children: IM or SC 0.01-0.03 mg/ kg q5min if needed

Patient's weight: 66 lb.

**a.** SDR for this child: _____

DA equation:


**b.** Evaluation: *Safe to give* or *Hold and clarify promptly with prescriber?* (Circle one and state reason.) _____

**c.** Which solution would you select if you had a choice? Why? _____
_____

**d.** Amount to be administered if safe to give:

DA equation:

**e.** Evaluation: _____

5 Ordered: codeine 10 mg IM, an analgesic for a child with pain

SDR for children: IM 0.5 mg/ kg q4-6h (IV codeine not used for children)

Patient's weight: 45 lb.

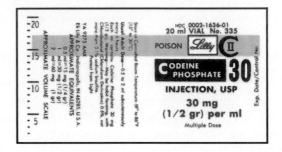

**a.** SDR for this child (kg to nearest tenth; mg to nearest whole number):

DA equation:

**b.** Evaluation: *Safe to give* or *Hold and clarify promptly with prescriber?* (Circle one
and state reason.) _____

**c.** Amount to be administered if safe to give to nearest hundredth of a mL:

DA equation:

**d.** Evaluation: _____
**e.** Which unit of measurement on the label is an apothecary unit? _____

# Fluid Requirements for Pediatric Patients

Volume needs vary and need to be adjusted for the weight and age of the
child. Infants have a larger percentage of fluid volume as a percentage of body
weight than do older children and adults. They also have a greater BSA in relation
to body mass, which causes them to lose more water through the skin than do
older children and adults. They lose a higher percentage of fluids from the lungs
because of their more rapid respirations and excrete more urine because it is less
concentrated.

➤ Overhydration and dehydration can present a grave risk to pediatric patients.
There are several formulas for calculating fluid requirements. They are adjusted for maintenance and replacement as well as for conditions requiring
*fluid restrictions.* Some formulas are based on caloric metabolism and others
on BSA. Keep these concepts and the data in Table 13-2, which follows, in
mind when administering any kind of fluids and oral or parenteral medications to pediatric patients.

| TABLE 13-2 | Fluid Requirements of Healthy Children and Adults | | | | |
|---|---|---|---|---|---|
| | | | | **AVERAGE FLUID INTAKE REQUIREMENT** | |
| **Weight** | **Normal fluid volume need** | **Sample weight (kg)** | **Daily** | **Hourly** | |
| Neonate | 90 mL/ kg/ 24 hr | 3 kg | 270 mL | 11 mL | |
| Up to 10 kg | 120 mL/ kg/ 24 hr after age 7 days | 8 kg | 960 mL | 40 mL | |
| 11-20 kg | 1000 mL + 50 mL/ kg over 10 kg | 15 kg | 1,250 mL | 52 mL | |
| Over 20 kg | 1500 mL + 20 mL/ kg over 20 kg | 25 kg | 1600 mL | 67 mL | |
| Average adult | 2-3 liters/ day | 68 kg | 2-3 mL | 125 mL | |

Table 13-2 illustrates the average fluid requirements of *healthy* adults, babies, and children of various weights.

1   What would be the normal 24-hr fluid intake requirement for a baby weighing 6 kg (13.2 lb) compared with a 150-lb adult?

**Q** *Ask Yourself*

**A** *My Answer*

➤ A child with cardiac, respiratory, or renal dysfunction may have severe fluid restrictions imposed. Such restrictions would affect the amount of fluid to be administered with medications as well as IV solution flow rates.

➤ If a pediatric patient is receiving fluids from other sources, such as bottles and cups, the IV volume must be adjusted downward accordingly. This is also the case with adults.

**Clinical Relevance**

# Intravenous Injections for Infants and Children

➤ Infusion volumes for infants and children are much *smaller* and infusion rates *slower* than for average adults. Use of a volumetric infusion pump for IV fluids and medications is preferred for pediatric patients. Check agency policies.

## Using a Volume-Control Device

The use of a volume-control device protects patients from accidental fluid and drug overload if the flow rate is programmed correctly (Figure 13-8, p. 458). Volume-control devices may be used for two purposes:

1   They protect from possible fluid overload from the main IV line. This is achieved by opening the clamp from the main IV line to fill the chamber with 1 or 2 hours worth of IV fluid, according to agency policy.

2   The medication may be added to the solution from the main IV bag or to a separate solution placed in the volume-control device. This would be an alternative to attaching a piggyback medicated solution to a port on a primary IV line.

### Using Volume-Control Chambers to Protect Patients from Fluid and Drug Overload

Ordered: Drug Y in a continuous IV infusion at 1.5 mg/ kg/ hr

Available: 100 mg in 100 mL NS

Patient's weight: 8 kg

SDR: maximum 6 mg/ kg/ hr

**EXAMPLES**

*Continued*

Agency policy: 1 hour's worth of fluid volume is maximum amount permitted in volume control chamber.

$$\frac{mg}{hr} = \frac{1.5\ mg}{1\ \cancel{kg}} \times \frac{8\ \cancel{kg}}{hr} = 12\ mg/hr$$

To calculate the volume in mL/ hr needed to deliver 12 mg/ hr,

$$\frac{mL}{hr} = \frac{\overset{1}{\cancel{100}}\ mL}{\underset{1}{\cancel{100}}\ \cancel{mg}} \times \frac{12\ \cancel{mg}}{1\ hr} = 12\ mL/hr$$

The nurse opens the clamp on the main IV line, puts 1 hour's worth of medicated fluid (12 mL) in the volume-control device, and shuts the clamp to the main IV line (Figure 13-8). An alarm will be set off to alert staff to a need for chamber refill.

➤ Agency flush procedures must be followed.

**Q: Ask Yourself**

**A: My Answer**

1  An IV infusion contains 100 mg of drug in 250 mL of solution. What is the maximum amount of fluid and medicine that can flow into the patient very rapidly if the main IV line malfunctions (assuming there is no volume-control device in place)?

**Using a Volume-Control Device to Administer Intravenous Medication** The medication dose may be added with a syringe through the port to the chamber after the IV diluent is placed in the volume-control device (Figure 13-9).

➤ If a *different medication* than that shown on the label of the main IV fluid is added to a volume-control device, a medication label must be attached to the volume-control device.

Figure **13-8.** Volume-control device. (From Perry AG, Potter PA: Clinical nursing skills and techniques, ed. 5, St. Louis, 2004, Mosby.)

Figure 13-9. Adding medication to a volume-control device. (From Perry AG, Potter PA: Clinical nursing skills and techniques, ed. 6, St. Louis, 2006, Mosby.)

For example, with a main IV solution of potassium in D5W and an ordered antibiotic of amikacin to be infused over 30 minutes, a label such as the following would be attached to the volume-control device:

> MEDICATION ADDED
>
> 1/01/06, 1800, amikacin sulfate 200 mg/ 50 mL D5W.
> Flow rate: 100 mL/ hr.
>
> John Smith, R.N.

This label will alert the staff that a *flush* and possible flow rate change will be necessary after the medication infusion is completed.

## Flushing a Volume-Control Device

The volume-control device and tubing must be cleared of medication residue with a "flush" *before* and *after* the medication has been infused. If the flush solution is different from the main IV solution, a new label must be placed on the volume-control device to alert the staff that a flush is taking place. The label alerts the staff to wait before adding another medication to the system.

> FLUSH
>
> 1/01/06, 1830, 15 mL D5W infusing
>
> John Smith, R.N.

Check agency policies for types and amounts of flushes. A flush may be indicated before and after a medication is administered and may consist of 5-10 mL or more of solution. It should be of an amount sufficient to clear the volume-control device and the rest of the IV line to the venous entry site.

## Calculating the Medicated Fluid Amount
## for a Volume-Control Device

- Calculate the *total amount of fluid* for the dose and diluent (e.g., 5 mL antibiotic to be diluted to 30 mL with NS) as stated in the drug insert or pediatric drug reference.
- Shut the clamp to the main IV line. Flush line according to agency policy. Place the diluent *minus* the amount of medicine in the calibrated chamber of the volume-control device (e.g., 30 mL − 5 mL medicine = 25 mL NS).
- Add the medicine and gently mix the medicine and diluent in the calibrated chamber.
- Administer the medicine at the ordered flow rate. Label the volume-control device.
- Flush the volume-control device with the needed amount and type of flush solution. Label the volume-control device for the flush. Reset the flow rate as needed.

➤ If an infusion pump is not available, a microdrip pediatric administration set with a DF of 60 is used with a volume-control device. Recall that the hourly drop/ min flow rate for a microdrip set is equal to the number of mL/ hr ordered (Figure 13-10).

**Figure 13-10. A,** Electronic infusion pump with volume-control device. **B,** Gravity infusion with volume-control device and microdrip tubing. (From Brown M, Mulholland JL: Drug calculations: process and problems for clinical practice, ed. 7, St. Louis, 2004, Mosby.)

## RAPID PRACTICE 13-8 Volume-Control Device Flow Rates

**Estimated completion time: 10 minutes**   Answers on page **601**

**Directions:** *Examine the example in problem 1. Calculate the amount of medicine and flush to be administered. Refer to "Intravenous Piggyback Solutions," in Chapter 9 (p. 304), for review if necessary.*

1 Ordered: 2 mL medicine to be diluted to 25 mL D5W in a volume-control device on a volumetric pump and infused over 30 minutes.

   **a.** Amount of diluent to place in volume-control device:
   25 mL − 2 mL = 23 mL diluent
   **b.** Amount of medicine to place in volume-control device: 2 mL medicine
   **c.** IV flow rate to set on the pump: 50 mL/ hr

   DA equation:

   $$\frac{mL}{hr} = \frac{25\ mL}{\underset{1}{\cancel{30\ min}}} \times \frac{\overset{2}{\cancel{60\ min}}}{1\ hr} = 50\ mL/\ hr$$

   **d.** Evaluation: The equation is balanced. An IV flow rate of 50 mL over 60 minutes will deliver 25 mL in 30 minutes.

   Follow the medication with a 5- to 10-mL flush. Check agency policy for content and volume of flush.

2 Ordered: 10 mL medicine to be diluted to 20 mL NS in a volume-control device on a volumetric infusion pump and infused over 30 minutes.

   **a.** Amount of diluent to place in volume-control device: _____
   **b.** Amount of medicine to place in volume-control device: _____
   **c.** IV flow rate to set on pump: _____

   DA equation:




   **d.** Evaluation: _____

   Follow the medication with a 5- to 10-mL flush. Check agency policy.

3 Ordered: 25 mL of medicine to be diluted to 50 mL in NS in a volume-control device attached to a gravity infusion device with a pediatric microdrip tubing set to be administered over 1 hour. (Refer to Chapter 9 for a review of flow rate calculations for microdrip sets).

   **a.** Amount of diluent to place in volume-control device: _____
   **b.** Amount of medicine to place in volume-control device: _____
   **c.** Flow rate to set on microdrip pediatric set: _____ drops/ min

   Follow the medication with a 5- to 10-mL flush. Check agency policy.

4 Ordered: 15 mL of medication to be diluted to 30 mL in D5W on a volumetric infusion pump to be administered over 20 minutes.

   **a.** Amount of diluent to place in volume-control device: _____
   **b.** Amount of medicine to place in volume-control device: _____
   **c.** Flow rate to set on microdrip pediatric set: _____ drops/ min

   DA equation:




   **d.** Evaluation: _____

   Follow the medication with a 5- to 10-mL flush. Check agency policy.

5 Ordered: 3 mL of medication to be diluted to 15 mL in NS in a volume-control device on gravity infusion with microdrip tubing to be administered over 30 minutes.

   **a.** Amount of medicine to place in volume-control device: _____

   **b.** Flow rate to set on microdrip pediatric set: _____ drops/ min

   DA equation:

   **c.** Evaluation: _____

   Follow the medication with a 5- to 10-mL flush. Check agency policy.

## Syringe Pump Infusers

A syringe pump system may be used to deliver *small-volume intermittent* infusions, which can also protect the patient from fluid and drug overload if the flow rate is programmed correctly. Syringe pump infusers can now be programmed for flow rates and alarms (Figure 13-11).

Figure **13-11.** Freedom 60 syringe infusion pump system. (From Repro-Med Systems, Inc., Chester, NY.)

## Calculating Medicated Intravenous Infusion Rates Review

| **EXAMPLES** | If the ordered dose is within the SDR, the nurse calculates the flow rate in mL/ hr to the nearest whole mL. |
| --- | --- |
| | Ordered: Drug Y continuous infusion at 30 mcg/ hr |
| | Patient's weight: 66 lb, or 30 kg |
| | SDR for children: 20-35 mcg/ kg/ 24 hr in IV infusion |
| | Available: 2 mg ampule in 250 mL. |

SDR for this patient:  20 mcg × 30 kg = 600 mcg low safe dose q 24 h

(Use calculator)      35 mcg × 30 kg = 1050 mcg high safe dose q 24 h

Ordered dose:        30 mcg × 24 hr = 720 mcg/ hr

(Use calculator)

Evaluation: The ordered daily dose is within the SDR and safe to give.

$$\text{mL/ hr flow rate: } \frac{mL}{hr} = \frac{\overset{\overset{1}{\cancel{125}}}{\cancel{250}} \, mL}{\underset{1}{\cancel{2} \, mg}} \times \frac{1 \, \cancel{mg}}{\underset{8}{\cancel{1000 \, mcg}}} \times \frac{30 \, \cancel{mcg}}{1 \, hr} = 3.75, \text{ or } 4 \, mL/ hr$$

Administer at 4 mL per hour.

# Comparing Safe Dose Range and Order

➤ Remember to compare the SDR and the ordered dose in the *same* units of measurement and for the same time frame: mg to mg, mcg to mcg, and hours to hours. Do not confuse the SDR and the order when performing the comparisons. When an underdose or overdose has been ordered, contact the prescriber.

## RAPID PRACTICE 13-9  Intravenous Medication Calculations

**Estimated completion time: 30 minutes to 1 hour**    Answers on page **601**

**Directions:** *Examine the example shown above. Solve the IV problems using DA equations and a calculator for long division and multiplication.*

1 Ordered: Trisenox (arsenic trioxide) IV infusion for a child with leukemia to flow at 5 mcg/ min daily.

Available: Trisenox 10 mg/ 250 mL NS

**a.** How many mcg/ hr are ordered? _____

**b.** How many total mcg are in the available infusion? _____

**c.** How many mcg/ mL are in the total available solution?

DA equation:

**d.** Evaluation: _____

**e.** What flow rate, to the nearest mL/ hr, should be set?

DA equation:

**f.** Evaluation: _____

2 Use the information from problem 1. The agency has a policy that a volume-control device must be used. Agency policy states that a maximum of 2 hours' worth of volume can be placed in the device.

   **a.** How many mL will be placed in the volume-control device? _____

   **b.** The prescriber ordered that the dose be increased by 3 mcg/ min. What will the new flow rate be?

   DA equation:

   **c.** Evaluation: _____

3 Ordered: furosemide, a diuretic, 25 mg IV q12h, for an infant with edema

   SDR: 0.5-2 mg/ kg/ dose q6-12h

   Patient's weight: 9 kg

   **a.** SDR for this infant: _____

   **b.** Evaluation: *Safe to give* or *Hold and clarify promptly with prescriber?* (Circle one and state reason.) _____

   **c.** Dose in mL to be administered if the order is safe to give:

   DA equation:

   **d.** Evaluation: _____

4 Ordered: KCl IV infusion 0.1 mEq/ kg/ hr in 100 mL D5W, ordered for a child with hypokalemia

   Available from pharmacy: KCl 10 mEq/ 100 mL D5W

   SDR for children: up to 3 mEq/ kg/ 24 hr, not to exceed 40 mEq/ 24 hr

   Patient's weight: 8 kg

   Directions in reference: Must dilute in compatible solution. 40 mEq/ L concentration is preferred, although can be diluted in 100 mL or more for replacement therapy for patient on fluid restrictions with a prescriber's order. Must be administered on infusion pump. Monitor electrocardiogram. Obtain order for subsequent infusion. Infuse using volume-control device with no more than 1 hour's worth of ordered fluid amount. Check potassium level every 2 hours.

a. SDR for this infant: _____

b. Amount ordered for 24 hours: _____

c. Evaluation: *Safe to give* or *Hold and clarify promptly with prescriber?* (Circle one and state reason.)_____

d. Hourly flow rate:

   DA equation:

e. Evaluation: _____

5 Ordered: phenobarbital sodium 50 mg IV stat, for preoperative sedation of a child. SDR for children: 1-3 mg/ kg/ 24 hr 60-90 minutes before procedure. Patient's weight: 14 lb 8 oz.

a. Patient's weight in kg to nearest tenth: _____

b. SDR for this child: _____

   DA equation:

c. Evaluation: *Safe to give* or *Hold and clarify promptly with prescriber?* (Circle one and state reason.) _____

d. Dose to be administered if the order is safe to give:

   DA equation:

e. Evaluation: _____

## CHAPTER 13 MULTIPLE-CHOICE REVIEW

**Estimated completion time: 30-60 minutes**    Answers on page **602**

**Directions:** *Select the best answer. Use a calculator for long division and multiplication. Calculate kg to the nearest tenth. Calculate medications to nearest hundredth of a milliliter if less than 1 mL or to the nearest tenth if more than 1 mL.*

1 The nurse should avoid mixing medicines for an infant or toddler in which product: ____

   **1.** Applesauce                    **3.** Water

   **2.** Sherbet                       **4.** Milk

2 Which statement about body fluid volume in infants is true? ____

   **1.** Infants have a smaller amount of total body water as a percentage of body weight than do adults and therefore receive less fluid per kg than do adults.

   **2.** Infants and adults have approximately the same amount of total body water as a percentage of body weight.

   **3.** Infants have a greater fluid volume as a percentage of body weight than do adults and are subject to grave injury from dehydration.

   **4.** Infants are immune from body fluid deficits because of reduced intake needs.

3 The first suggested step for safe dose calculations for unfamiliar medications after reading the medication order and relevant laboratory tests is _____

   **1.** Call the prescriber.

   **2.** Calculate the SDR.

   **3.** Calculate the dose.

   **4.** Visit the parents and explain what you plan to do.

4 Two devices used in pediatric settings to help prevent drug or fluid volume overload for IV orders are _____

   **1.** Add-Vantage systems and premixed medications

   **2.** Gravity infusion sets and macrodrip tubing

   **3.** Syringe pumps and volume-control burette chambers

   **4.** PCA pumps and syringe pumps

5 If an electronic pump is not available to deliver a continuous infusion to a pediatric patient, which infusion device would be the best choice? _____

   **1.** Gravity infusion device with microdrip tubing and a volume-control device

   **2.** Gravity infusion device with macrodrip tubing DF 10

   **3.** Direct injection with a syringe administered very slowly

   **4.** PCA pump

6 An IV solution of 100 mL containing 10 mg of a drug is to be infused at 20 mcg/ min. The mL/ hr flow rate should be set at ____

   **1.** 12         **3.** 100

   **2.** 20         **4.** 120

7 An IV solution of 250 mL with 250 mg of drug is to be infused at 8 mL/ hr. The number of mg/ hr to be delivered is _____

   **1.** 1         **3.** 10

   **2.** 8         **4.** 20

8 Ordered: 0.05 mg of a drug for a child. Available: 0.5 mg/ 10 mL. How many mL will you administer? ____

   **1.** 15         **3.** 5

   **2.** 10         **4.** 1

9 A continuous IV of D5W at 15 mL/ hr is ordered for a toddler. In the absence of an electronic infusion device, what is the correct action by the nurse? _____

   **1.** Infuse the IV solution using a gravity device, macrodrip DF 15, at 4 mL/ hr.

   **2.** Infuse the IV solution using a gravity device, microdrip DF 60, at 15 drops/ min.

   **3.** Infuse the IV solution using a gravity device, DF 10, at 3 mL/ hr.

   **4.** Wait for an electronic infusion device to become available.

**10** Ordered: phenobarbital sodium 80 mg IM for a 40-kg child who needs sedation. SDR: 6 mg/ kg/ day in 3 divided doses.

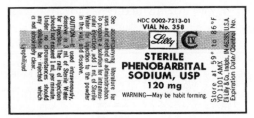

Which amount would you prepare?

**1.** 0.66 mL

**2.** 0.67 mL

**3.** 0.8 mL

**4.** Hold drug and contact prescriber.

## CHAPTER 13 FINAL PRACTICE

**Estimated completion time: 1-2 hours**   Answers on page **602**

**Directions:** *Use a calculator for long division and multiplication. Label all answers.*

**1** Ordered: diphenhydramine HCl (Benadryl Children's Liquid) 12.5 mg, for a 10-year-old child who has developed hives from an antibiotic. He is on a regular diet.

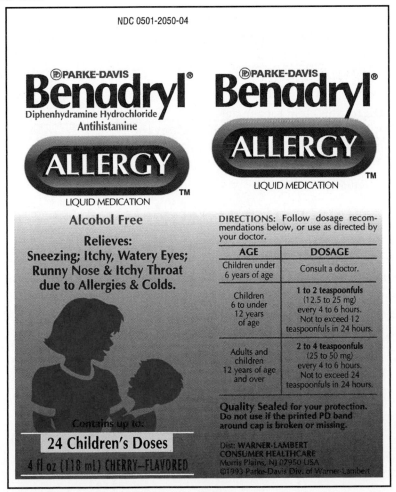

**a.** How many mL will you administer? _____

**b.** What might you offer to follow the dose if the child does not like the taste of the medicine? _____

**2** Ordered: Duricef (cefadroxil) oral suspension 600 mg daily PO, for a 7-year-old child with tonsillitis.

SDR: 30 mg/ kg/ day or in 2 divided doses for 10 days

Patient's weight: 20 kg.

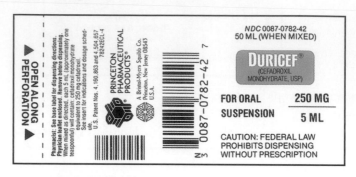

**a.** SDR for this child: _____

**b.** Evaluation: *Safe to give* or *Hold and clarify promptly with prescriber?* (Circle one and state reason.) _____

**c.** Calculate the dose if safe.

DA equation:

**d.** Evaluation: _____

**3** Ordered: cytarabine, an antineoplastic drug, 0.1 g/ day IV to be infused in NS over 4 hours.

SDR: 100 mg/ m$^2$/ day

Patient's weight: 31 lb. BSA: 0.6 m$^2$.

**a.** SDR for this child for the day: _____

**b.** Evaluation: *Safe to give* or *Hold and clarify promptly with prescriber?* (Circle one and state reason.) _____

**c.** Calculate the dose if safe.

DA equation:

**d.** Evaluation: _____

**4** Ordered: Mycostatin (nystatin) oral syrup 250,000 units for a 4-month-old infant with thrush (oral candidiasis).

SDR for children and infants >3 months: 250,000-500,000 units/ day

Directions: Place half the dose in either side of the mouth.

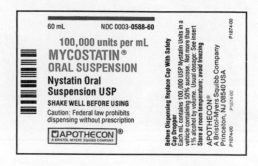

**a.** If order is safe, how many mL will you prepare? _____

DA equation:

**b.** Evaluation: _____

**c.** What device among those on p. 446 might be appropriate to administer this order to an infant of this age? _____

**d.** Which directions on the label must the nurse follow before pouring the medicine? _____

5  Ordered: Infants' Tylenol (acetaminophen) 1 mL PO for a 2½-year-old child. Patient's weight: 12 kg.

**Label A**                                           **Label B**

**Directions:**
1. Shake well before using.
2. Find right dose on chart below. If possible, use weight to dose; otherwise use age.
3. Only use enclosed measuring cup.
4. If needed, repeat dose every 4 hours.
5. Do not use more than 5 times a day.

| WEIGHT (lb) | AGE (yr) | DOSE (tsp) |
|---|---|---|
| Under 24 | Under 2 | Consult Physician |
| 24–35 | 2–3 | 1 |
| 36–47 | 4–5 | 1 ½ |
| 48–59 | 6–8 | 2 |
| 60–71 | 9–10 | 2 ½ |
| 72–95 | 11 | 3 |

**Attention:**
Specially designed for use with enclosed measuring cup. Use only enclosed measuring cup to dose this product. Do not use any other dosing device.

**Inactive Ingredients:** Butylparaben, Cellulose, Citric Acid, Corn Syrup, Flavors, Glycerin, Propylene Glycol, Purified Water, Sodium Benzoate, Sorbitol, Xanthan Gum and FD&C Red #40.

● Tylenol® products are the first choice of Pediatricians.

● Children's Tylenol® Liquids are not the same concentration as Infants' Tylenol® Drops. For accurate dosing, follow the dosing instructions on this label.

● Use only enclosed measuring cup to dose.
● Items like kitchen teaspoons may not be accurate.
● Never use spoons, droppers or cups that come with other medicines.

Store at room temperature.
See bottom panel of carton for expiration date and lot number.

**McNEIL**
McNEIL CONSUMER PRODUCTS CO.
DIVISION OF McNEIL-PPC, INC.
FORT WASHINGTON, PA 19034 USA    U.S. Patent No. 5,272,137  © McN-PPC, Inc.'97

GREAT CHERRY TASTE!
**CHILDREN'S TYLENOL®**
Fever Reducer-Pain Reliever  acetaminophen
**SUSPENSION LIQUID**
See New Label
**FOR AGES 2-11**
RICH CHERRY FLAVOR
Alcohol Free
Aspirin Free
Ibuprofen Free
Read Instructions Carefully
4 fl oz (120 mL)
80 mg per 1/2 teaspoon
(160 mg per 5 mL)

ASPIRIN FREE
ALCOHOL FREE
IBUPROFEN FREE

**Directions:**
1. Shake well before using.
2. Find right dose on chart below. If possible, use weight to dose; otherwise, use age.
3. Only use enclosed dropper; fill to prescribed level and dispense liquid slowly into child's mouth toward inner cheek.
4. Replace dropper tightly to maintain child resistance.
5. If needed, repeat dose every 4 hours.
6. Do not use more than 5 times a day.

| WEIGHT (lb) | AGE (yr) | DOSE |
|---|---|---|
| Under 24 | Under 2 | Consult Doctor |
| 24-35 | 2-3 | 2 Dropperfuls (2 x 0.8 mL) |

**Attention:**
This product has been specifically designed for use only with enclosed dropper. Do not use any other dosing device with this product.

● Tylenol® products are the first choice of Pediatricians.
● Infants' Tylenol® Drops are more concentrated than Children's Tylenol® Liquids. For accurate dosing, follow the dosing instructions on this label.
● Only use enclosed dropper to dose.
● Never use spoons, droppers or cups that come with other medicines.

Infants'
**TYLENOL®**
Acetaminophen
**CONCENTRATED DROPS**
Fever Reducer - Pain Reliever
Pediatricians' First Choice
NEW !
SAFE-TY-LOCK™ Bottle
Unique Safety Barrier
Stage 1 One  TYLENOL INFANTS
Grape Flavor
1/2 FL OZ (15 mL) 80 mg per 0.8 mL

**a.** Which label would you select?_____ With which device would you administer the medication? _____

**b.** What is the concentration, in mg/ mL, of Children's Tylenol susp? With which device would you administer the medication?

_____

**c.** What is the concentration in mg/ mL, of Infants' Tylenol Concentrated Drops? _____

**d.** Which is more concentrated, Infants' or Children's Tylenol preparation?

_____

These products have been confused by nurses as well as consumers. The labels are very clearly marked. However, the uninformed think that the concentrated drops are interchangeable with the children's suspension and are safe to give to children in the dose prescribed for the suspension. The infant drops are much more concentrated in order to achieve a very low volume of medication for infants. This has caused fatal errors.

Parents have also overdosed their children at home by giving too much of the over-the-counter product either by using household utensils or by giving it more often than the label states. Keep this in mind when teaching parents.

➤ Aspirin (acetylsalicylic acid) is not given to infants, children, and teenagers under *19 years* of age who have fever due to flu or viral symptoms. Aspirin has been associated with Reye's syndrome in those age groups.

*Q: Ask Yourself*

*A: My Answer*

1 What is the difference in unit dose between the concentrated drops and children's suspension acetaminophen?

_____

2 Would it be safer always to clarify orders that specify only mL and do not state the total dose desired, such as 80 or 160 mg?

_____

6 Ordered: codeine 20 mg IM stat, for analgesia.

SDR for children: 0.5 mg/ kg q4-6h

Patient's weight: 88 lb

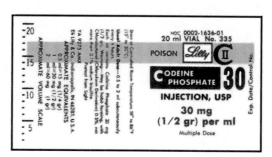

**a.** SDR for this child: _____

DA equation:

**b.** Evaluation: *Safe to give* or *Hold and clarify promptly with prescriber?* (Circle one.)
**c.** If safe, will you give more or less than the unit dose on hand?

DA equation:

**d.** What is the nearest measurable dose you will prepare for the available syringe?

DA equation:

**e.** Evaluation: _____

Draw a vertical line through the calibrated line on the syringe to indicate the nearest measurable dose.

**7** Ordered: KCl 10 mEq/ hr as a continuous infusion, for a child with hypokalemia. Check potassium levels every 4 hours.

Available: 40 mEq KCl in 250 mL D5W

SDR for children: 0.5 to 1 mEq/ kg/ 24 hr

Patient's weight: 42 lb.

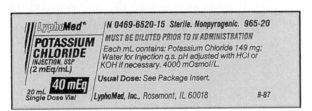

**a.** Weight in kg to the nearest tenth: _____
**b.** SDR for this child: _____
**c.** Ordered dose for this child: _____
**d.** Evaluation: *Safe to give* or *Hold and clarify promptly with prescriber?* (Circle one and state reason.) _____
**e.** If safe, what should the flow rate on the infusion pump be?

_____

DA equation:

**f.** Evaluation: _____

8  Ordered: atropine sulfate 0.5 mg IV, for a 5 year-old-child with brad-yarrhythmia. SDR for child with bradyarrhythmia: 0.01-0.03 mg/ kg to achieve pulse rate >60 beats per minute. Maximum dose for child: 500 mcg. Patient's weight: 44 lb.

| | |
|---|---|
| EXP  LOT  *NDC 0641-2210-43* 10 X 20 mL Multiple Dose Vials **ATROPINE** SULFATE INJECTION, USP **400 mcg/mL** (0.4 mg/mL) **FOR SC, IM OR IV USE** | Each mL contains atropine sulfate 400 mcg (0.4 mg), sodium chloride 9 mg and benzyl alcohol 0.015 mL in Water for Injection. pH 3.0–6.5; sulfuric acid added, if needed, for pH adjustment. **POISON** USUAL DOSE: See package insert. Store at controlled room temperature 15°–30° C (59°–86° F). Caution: Federal law prohibits dispensing without prescription. Product Code 2210-43                              B-32210 |

*esi*   ELKINS-SINN, INC. Cherry Hill, NJ 08003-4099
A subsidiary of A. H. Robins Company

a. Weight in kg to the nearest tenth: _____
b. SDR for this child: _____

   DA equation:

c. Ordered dose for this child in mcg: _____
d. Evaluation: *Safe to give* or *Hold and clarify promptly with prescriber?* (Circle one and give reason.) _____
e. If safe, will you give more or less than the unit dose on hand? _____
f. How many mL will you give?

   DA equation:

g. Evaluation: _____

9  Ordered: Vancocin (vancomycin hydrochloride) 1500 mg IVPB infusion bid for a 12-year-old child with a staphylococcus infection.

   SDR IV for children: 40 mg/ kg/ day divided q6-12 hr not to exceed 2 g/ day.

   Patient's weight: 77 lbs

| |
|---|
| FOR INTRAVENOUS USE  IMPORTANT—Read literature for precautions and directions before use. Usual Adult Dose—2 g daily. Dilute with 10 mL of Sterile Water for Injection. After Dilution—Refrigerate. Prior to Reconstitution Store at 59° to 86°F. MUST BE FURTHER DILUTED BEFORE USE—SEE LITERATURE  Lyophilized  YD 2651 AMX  Mfd. by Eli Lilly Industries, Inc. Carolina, Puerto Rico 00630, a subsidiary of Eli Lilly & Co., Indianapolis, IN U.S.A.    NDC 0002-1444-01 **VIAL No. 657** R *Lilly* **VANCOCIN®HCl** sterile vancomycin hydrochloride, usp **INTRAVENOUS** Equiv. to **500 mg** Vancomycin |

a. Estimated pt wt in kg: _____   Actual wt in kg: _____
b. SDR: _____

   DA equation:

c. Evaluation: _____

**10** Ordered: digoxin 0.5 mg IV, for child with congestive heart failure

SDR: 0.015-0.35 mg/ kg. Patient's weight 24 lb 6 oz

Directions: Administer IV over *5 minutes*. Safe to give undiluted. If needed, dilute each mL of drug in 4 mL SW (to permit small amounts of drug to be infused over time). Use a calculator to determine SDR.

> **LANOXIN®**     **2mL**
> **(digoxin) Injection**
> 500 µg (0.5 mg) in 2 mL
> (250 µg [0.25 mg] per mL)
> Store at 15° to 25°C (59° to 77°F).
> PROTECT FROM LIGHT.
> Glaxo Wellcome Inc.
> Research Triangle Park, NC 27709
> Rev. 1/96
>
> **542308**
>
> **LOT**
> **EXP**

**a.** Weight in kg to the nearest tenth: _____

**b.** SDR for this child to the nearest tenth mg: _____

DA equation:

**c.** Ordered dose for this child: _____

**d.** Evaluation: *Safe to give* or *Hold and clarify promptly with prescriber?* (Circle one and state reason.) _____

**e.** If safe, will you give more or less than the unit dose on hand? _____

**f.** How many mL of digoxin will you prepare before dilution? _____

## Suggestions for Further Reading

➤ To access many Internet references on rates and types of medication errors in pediatrics, type "children's medication errors" in your favorite search engine.

Gahart B, Nazareno A: 2005 Intravenous medications, ed. 21, St. Louis, 2005, Mosby
www.childrenshospital.org
www.fda.gov/fdac/default.htm
www.fda.gov/fdac/features/2003/303_meds.html
www.ismp.org/pr/pediatricpharmacy guidelines
www.jointcommission.org/Sentine1Events/Sentine1EventAlert/sea_35.htm
www.jcaho.org
www.medlineplus.gov
www.pedseducation.org/online
www.wo-pub2.med.cornell.edu

 Additional practice problems can be found in the Pediatric Calculations section on the enclosed companion CD.

# MULTIPLE-CHOICE FINAL REVIEW

**Directions:** *Select the correct response for the following questions. Estimate a reasonable answer whenever you can; use a calculator for weights and safe dose ranges, and use DA for verification of doses. Evaluate your answer. Do not "guess" the answer. Put a checkmark to the right of questions that need review. After completion of the rest of the test, review any checkmarked question(s).*

1 The metric equivalent of 1500 mg is:

**1.** 0.015 g

**2.** 0.15 g

**3.** 1.5 g

**4.** 15 g

2 The metric equivalent of 0.75 g is:

**1.** 0.75 mg

**2.** 7.5 mg

**3.** 75 mg

**4.** 750 mg

3 The metric equivalent of 5000 mcg is:

**1.** 0.5 g

**2.** 5 mg

**3.** 50 mg

**4.** 500 mg

4 A patient weighs 150 lb. How many kilograms does the patient weigh (to the nearest tenth)?

**1.** 330 kg

**2.** 150 kg

**3.** 75.5 kg

**4.** 68.2 kg

Did your estimate support the answer?

5 Tetracycline 0.5 g orally (PO) four times daily is ordered for a patient with an infection. Tetracycline 250 mg/capsule is available. How many capsules will you prepare?

**1.** ½ capsule

**2.** 1 capsule

**3.** 2 capsules

**4.** 4 capsules

Did your estimate support the answer?

6 Digoxin 0.0625 mg PO daily is ordered for a patient with heart failure.

How many tablets will you prepare?

**1.** 4 tablets

**2.** 2 tablets

**3.** 1 tablet

**4.** 0.5 tablet

Did your estimate support the answer?

**7** Ordered: amoxicillin capsules. 0.5 g PO four times daily for 7 days.

How many capsules will you prepare?

**1.** ½ capsule          **3.** 2 capsules
**2.** 1 capsule          **4.** 4 capsules

Did your estimate support the answer?

**8** Ordered: cefaclor suspension 200 mg PO q6h for a patient with an infection.

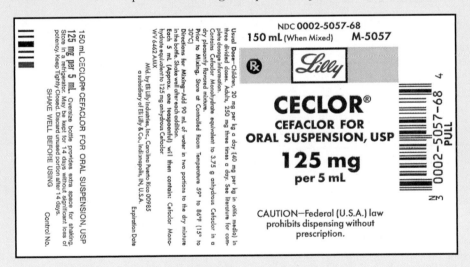

How many milliliters will you prepare?

**1.** 15 mL          **3.** 8 mL
**2.** 12 mL          **4.** 4 mL

Did your estimate support the answer?

9 Ordered: fluphenazine hydrochloride 3 mg intramuscularly (IM) three times a day (t.i.d.) for a patient with schizophrenia.

How many milliliters will you prepare, to the nearest measurable dose, on the syringe provided?

**1.** 0.75 mL                    **3.** 1.2 mL

**2.** 1 mL                       **4.** 1.5 mL

Did your estimate support the answer?

10 Ordered: Solu-Cortef 150 mg IM stat for a patient with a severe allergic reaction.

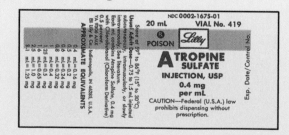

How many milliliters will you prepare?

**1.** 0.8 mL                     **3.** 1.8 mL

**2.** 1.2 mL                     **4.** 2.5 mL

Did your estimate support the answer?

11 Ordered: atropine sulfate 0.3 mg.

How many milliliters will you prepare, to the nearest tenth of a milliliter?

**1.** 0.3 mL                     **3.** 0.8 mL

**2.** 0.4 mL                     **4.** 1.3 mL

Did your estimate support the answer?

12 Ordered: intravenous (IV) infusion of D5LR q8h. Available: 1-liter bag of D5LR. At how many milliliters per hour will the flow rate be set?

**1.** 125 mL                     **3.** 175 mL

**2.** 150 mL                     **4.** 200 mL

**13** What would be an average expected D5W or LR IV maintenance flow rate range of unmedicated isotonic solution for an adult patient in good health who will be on nothing-by-mouth (NPO) status for 1 or 2 days?

**1.** 200-250 mL/hour
**2.** 75-125 mL/hour
**3.** 25-50 mL/hour
**4.** 10-25 mL/hour

**14** Ordered: 1000 mL D5W at 50 mL/hour. Available: macrodrip administration set with a drop factor of 15. What flow rate will you set?

**1.** 50 mL/hour
**2.** 50 drops/minute
**3.** 12.5 drops/minute
**4.** 13 drops/minute

**15** Ordered: 250 mL D5W at 30 mL/hour. Available: microdrip pediatric administration set. What flow rate will you set?

**1.** 30 mL/hour
**2.** 30 drops/minute
**3.** 60 mL/hour
**4.** 60 drops/minute

Did your estimate support your answer?

**16** Ordered: 500 mL N/S at 100 mL/hour. Available: macrodrip administration set with a drop factor of 20. What flow rate will you set?

**1.** 166 mL/hour
**2.** 166 drops/minute
**3.** 33 mL/hour
**4.** 33 drops/minute

**17** What is the fastest reasonable rate of drops per minute that can be counted when using a pediatric administration set according to the text?

**1.** 30 drops/minute
**2.** 60 drops/minute
**3.** 90 drops/minute
**4.** 100 drops/minute

**18** Ordered: a transfusion of 250 mL of packed red cells for a patient with anemia. What solution must be used to prime the IV line Y tubing before and after the blood is administered?

**1.** NS
**2.** D5W
**3.** L/R
**4.** D10W

**19** Ordered: a transfusion for a patient. Agency policy calls for 2 mL/minute flow rate for the first 30 minutes while the patient is observed for possible adverse reactions. What flow rate in milliliters per hour will you set on an infusion pump for the first 30 minutes?

**1.** 30 mL/hour
**2.** 60 mL/hour
**3.** 90 mL/hour
**4.** 120 mL/hour

Did your estimate support your answer?

**20** Ordered: a blood transfusion for a patient. Available: IV gravity device and tubing administration sets with drop factors of 10, 15, 20, and 60. Which set has the largest diameter, permitting the largest drop, and is used to administer blood?

**1.** DF 10
**2.** DF 15
**3.** DF 20
**4.** DF 60

Did your estimate support your answer?

**21** Ordered: an IVPB of 40 mL to be infused over 30 minutes on an infusion pump. What will be the flow rate in milliliters per hour?

**1.** 30 mL/hour
**2.** 75 mL/hour
**3.** 80 mL/hour
**4.** 90 mL/hour

Did your estimate support your answer?

**22** Ordered: an IVPB of 20 mL to be infused over 20 minutes on an infusion pump. What will be the flow rate in milliliters per hour?

1. 20 mL/hour
2. 40 mL/hour
3. 60 mL/hour
4. 80 mL/hour

Did your estimate support your answer?

**23** Ordered: an IVPB of 30 mL to be infused over 30 minutes on a gravity device with microdrip tubing. What will be the flow rate?

1. 30 mL/hour
2. 60 mL/hour
3. 30 drops/minute
4. 60 drops/minute

Did your estimate support your answer?

**24** How many grams of carbohydrate are there in an IV of 500 mL of D5NS?

1. 25 g
2. 50 g
3. 75 g
4. 100 g

**25** How many kilocalories of carbohydrate are there in an IV of 1000 mL D5W?

1. 1000 kcal
2. 500 kcal
3. 200 kcal
4. 50 kcal

**26** Ordered: heparin 800 units/hr IV. Available: 25,000 units of heparin in 500 mL of NS. How many milliliters per hour will deliver 800 units/hr?

1. 4 mL/hour
2. 8 mL/hour
3. 12 mL/hour
4. 16 mL/hour

**27** Infusing: heparin IV at 10 mL/hour. Available: 25,000 units of Heparin in 250 mL of NS. How many units per hour are infusing?

1. 25 units/hour
2. 100 units/hour
3. 250 units/hour
4. 1000 units/hour

**28** Ordered: IV of Nipride (nitroprusside sodium) at 0.5 mcg/kg/min to maintain a patient's blood pressure. Available: Nipride 50 mg in 500 mL D5W. Patient weight: 70 kg.

What flow rate in milliliters per hr should be set on the IV infusion pump?

1. 12 mL/hour
2. 21 mL/hour
3. 42 mL/hour
4. 70 mL/hour

**29** Which is the most appropriate action for the nurse to take for insulin mix orders?

1. Check the labels of the two insulins to be sure they are compatible.
2. Call the prescriber before preparing the insulin mix.
3. Administer dextrose before administering the insulin mix.
4. Be prepared to administer glucagon after administering the insulin mix.

**30** Ordered: insulin glargine (Lantus) 15 units subcut at bedtime. The patient's current blood glucose (BG) is 55. The patient complains of shakiness and nervousness. What decision will the nurse make?

1. Give the patient a diet cola and administer the insulin because it is long acting.
2. Prepare and administer the insulin because it does not have a peak.
3. Hold the insulin, follow agency and prescriber protocols, and contact the prescriber promptly because the patient is hyperglycemic.
4. Hold the insulin, follow agency and prescriber protocols for hypoglycemic episodes, and contact the prescriber promptly.

**31** Which type(s) of insulin can be administered via the IV route?

1. NPH and Lente
2. Insulin glargine
3. Regular insulins and insulin lispro (Humalog)
4. Insulin zinc suspensions and Humulin U

**32** The insulin bottle label states U 100. Identify the correct meaning of U 100 on the label.

**1.** It refers to the total contents. There are 100 units in the bottle.
**2.** It refers to the concentration. There are 100 units/mL.
**3.** It refers to the recommended adult dose: 100 units.
**4.** It refers to the number of units per 100 mL.

**33** Ordered: carbamazepine susp 50 mg PO four times daily for a 10-year-old child who is experiencing seizures. SDR for the 24-hr period for a child less than 12 years old: 10 to 20 mg/kg/day in three or four divided doses. The child weighs 44 lb. The SDR is:

**1.** 100 -200 mg/day
**2.** 200-400 mg/day
**3.** 500-1000 mg/ day
**4.** 998-1936 mg/day

**34** Select the statement that best describes the difference between $m^2$ and mg:

**1.** mg is a metric measurement of weight, and $m^2$ refers to micrograms
**2.** mg is a metric measurement of volume, and $m^2$ refers to lean body mass
**3.** mg is a metric measurement of weight, and $m^2$ refers to square meters of body surface area (BSA)
**4.** mg is a metric measurement of weight, and $m^2$ refers to square milligrams of weight

**35** Ordered: prednisone maintenance dose: 30 mg/$m^2$ PO twice a week for a child with leukemia. The child's BSA is 0.5 $m^2$. How many milligrams will you administer?

**1.** 150 mg
**2.** 30 mg
**3.** 15 mg
**4.** 2.5 mg

# COMPREHENSIVE FINAL PRACTICE

**Directions:** *Estimate and calculate doses using DA style equations where requested. Evaluate your answer in terms of the estimate and the equation result. If you cannot estimate the dose, estimate whether it will be more or less of unit dose supplied. Use a calculator for long division and multiplication. Label all answers.*

**1** Ordered: benztropine mesylate 1 mg PO daily for a patient with Parkinson's disease.

How many tablets will you administer?

**a.** Estimated dose:

DA equation:

**b.** Evaluation:

**2** Ordered: alprazolam 0.5 mg PO at bedtime for a patient with high anxiety.

How many tablets will you administer?

**a.** Estimated dose:

DA equation:

**b.** Evaluation:

**3** Ordered: digoxin 250 mcg PO daily for an adult with heart failure.

How many tablets will you administer?

**a.** Estimated dose:

DA equation:

**b.** Evaluation:

**c.** Which is the generic name of this medication? _____

**4** Ordered: ciprofloxacin hydrochloride 1.5 g PO for a patient with a severe infection.

How many tablets will you administer?

**a.** Estimated dose:

DA equation:

**b.** Evaluation:

**c.** Which is the generic name of this medication? _____

**5** Ordered: dexamethasone 0.5 mg PO stat for a patient with acute allergy attack.

How many tablets will you administer?

**a.** Estimated dose:

DA equation:

**b.** Evaluation:

**6** Ordered diltiazem sustained-release tablets 0.12 g PO daily at bedtime for a patient with hypertension.

**Label A**                                                **Label B**

 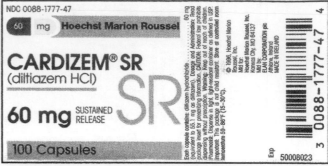

Which medication will you administer? _____

How many tablets will you administer?

**a.** Estimated dose:

  DA equation:

**b.** Evaluation:

**7** Ordered: 20% potassium chloride liquid 20 mEq PO daily for a patient taking a diuretic.

How many mL will you administer?

**a.** Estimated dose:

DA equation:

**b.** Evaluation:

Shade in the medicine cup to the nearest 5 mL. Mark the syringe at the additional amount to be added.

8 Ordered: codeine 45 mg PO q4-6h prn pain.

**a.** What is the metric unit dose available? _____

**b.** What is the apothecary system equivalent unit dose noted on the label?

_____

**c.** How many tablets will you administer?

**d.** Estimated dose:

DA equation:

**e.** Evaluation:

**9** Ordered: metformin 1.5 g PO daily with breakfast for a diabetic patient.

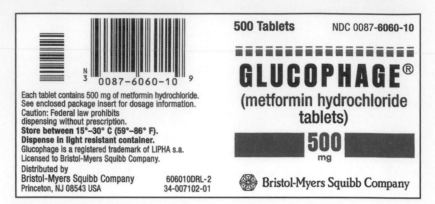

How many tablets will you administer?

**a.** Estimated dose:

DA equation:

**b.** Evaluation:

**10** Ordered: levothyroxine 0.1 mg PO daily in AM for a patient who is hypothyroid.

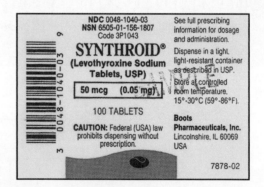

How many tablets will you administer?

**a.** Estimated dose:

DA equation:

**b.** Evaluation:

**c.** What is the equivalent of the dose ordered in micrograms? _____

**11** Ordered: morphine sulfate 10 mg IM stat for a patient in pain.

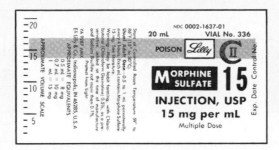

How many mL will you administer?

**a.** Estimated dose:

DA equation:

**b.** Evaluation:

Mark the syringe to the nearest measurable amount.

**12** Ordered: furosemide 30 mg IM stat for a patient with urinary retention.

How many mL will you administer?

**a.** Estimated dose:

DA equation:

**b.** Evaluation:

Mark the syringe to the nearest measurable amount.

**13** Ordered: digoxin 0.3 mg IM on admission for a patient in heart failure.

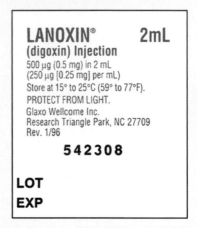

LANOXIN®     2mL
(digoxin) Injection
500 μg (0.5 mg) in 2 mL
(250 μg [0.25 mg] per mL)
Store at 15° to 25°C (59° to 77°F).
PROTECT FROM LIGHT.
Glaxo Wellcome Inc.
Research Triangle Park, NC 27709
Rev. 1/96

**542308**

LOT
EXP

How many mL will you administer?

**a.** Estimated dose:

DA equation:

**b.** Evaluation:

Mark the syringe to the nearest measurable amount.

**14** Ordered: hydromorphone HCl 2 mg
        prochlorperazine 2.5 mg  } IM stat for a patient in pain.

How many mL of hydromorphone will you prepare?

**a.** Estimate: hydromorphone dose: _____

DA equation:


**b.** Evaluation:


**c.** How many mL of prochlorperazine will you prepare?

**d.** Estimated prochlorperazine dose: _____

DA equation:


**e.** Evaluation:


**f.** What is the total dose in mL to be administered?

Shade in the syringe with the total dose to the nearest measurable amount:

**15** Ordered: Penicillin G Procaine susp 400,000 units IM stat for a patient with a skin infection.

How many mL will you administer (to the nearest tenth of a mL)?

**a.** Estimated dose:

DA equation:

**b.** Evaluation:

**16** Ordered: ticarcillin disodium 600 mg IM q6h daily for a patient with a respiratory infection.

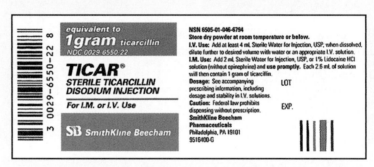

How many mL will you administer (to the nearest tenth of a mL)?

**a.** What is the concentration of the solution after reconstitution for IM injection? _____

**b.** Estimated dose:

DA equation:

**c.** Evaluation:

**17** Ordered: Novolin Regular Insulin for a diabetic patient on a sliding scale tid 30 minutes ac and at bedtime. Current BGM is 190.

Using the sliding scale that follows, how many units of insulin will be administered? _____

| Sliding Scale BG mg/ dL | Insulin dose (Novolin) |
| --- | --- |
| 70 – 180 | 0 Units |
| 181 – 200 | 2 Units |
| 201 – 250 | 4 Units |
| 251 – 300 | 6 Units |
| Over 300 | Call physician |

**a.** Mark the syringe to the nearest measurable dose:

**b.** Is this a fast, intermediate, or long acting insulin? _____
**c.** Will insulin raise or lower the blood glucose level? _____

**18** Ordered: Humulin R 6 Units
           Humulin N 20 Units } subcut 30 minutes ac breakfast daily.

From which bottle should the insulin be withdrawn first? _____

Mark total dose on the insulin syringe provided. Place an arrow pointing to the calibration which reflects the intermediate acting insulin dose.

19 Ordered: Insulin glargine 24 units subcut daily at bedtime.

Mark in total dose on the insulin syringe provided.

**a.** Is this insulin a fast, intermediate or long acting insulin? _____

**b.** Which is the advantage of the 50 unit 0.5 mL syringe as opposed to the 100 unit 1 mL syringe? _____

20 Ordered: Heparin IV infusion 1000 Units per hour.
Available: Heparin 20,000 Units in 500 mL D5/W.

How many mL per hour will you infuse?

DA equation:

**a.** Evaluation:

**b.** Which lab test must be monitored for patients receiving heparin therapy?
_____

**21** Infusing: Heparin at 30 mL per hour in an IV of D5W 250 mL containing Heparin 10,000 Units.

How many units per hour are infusing?

DA equation:

**a.** Evaluation:

**b.** What is the major potential adverse effect of heparin overdose?
_____

**22** Infusing: Regular Insulin at 7 mL per hour IV.
Available: Humulin Regular insulin 100 units in 100 mL of NS.

How many units per hour are infusing?

**a.** Estimated units per hour:

DA equation:

**b.** Evaluation:

**c.** What is the major potential adverse effect of an insulin overdose?
_____

**23** Ordered: IV KCl to infuse at 10 mEq/ hour for a patient with hypokalemia.
Available: 500 mL NS with 40 mEq of KCl added premixed by pharmacy.

➤ "Recheck serum K levels when 40 mEq of KCl have been infused."

What flow rate will you set on the infusion pump? _____

DA equation:

**a.** Evaluation:

**b.** The IV was started at 1300 hours. At what time would the nurse need to order and recheck a serum K level? _____

**24** Ordered: IV antibiotic to be piggybacked on a primary line: 50 mL to infuse over 30 minutes.

How many mL per hour will you set the infusion pump?

**a.** Estimated flow rate:

DA equation:

**b.** Evaluation:

**25** Ordered: IV antibiotic 100 mg q6h times 3 days. Available from pharmacy: IV antibiotic solution in 30 mL of D5W to be piggybacked to a primary line. Directions: *"Infuse over 20 minutes."*

How many mL per hour will you set the infusion pump?

**a.** Estimated flow rate:

DA equation:

**b.** Evaluation:

**26** Ordered: IV antibiotic 250 mg q4h for 48 hrs. Available from pharmacy: IV antibiotic solution in 20 mL to be piggybacked on a primary line: Directions: *"Infuse over 60 minutes."*

Which kind of infusion administration set would you select for this order if an infusion pump was not available? _____

**a.** What flow rate will you set? _____
**b.** Estimated flow rate:

DA equation:

**c.** Evaluation:

**27** Ordered: IV D5W of 500 mL every 4 hours. Available: A gravity device. Drop factor on the tubing: 15.

What flow rate will you set? _____

DA equation:

**a.** Evaluation:

**28** IV is infusing at 10 ml/ hr in a pediatric patient. Ordered: IV medication of 100 mg diluted to a total volume of 20 mL in NS to be administered over 30 minutes. Agency policy states that a volume control device must be used for all medicated IV's for pediatric patients.

Available: Medication 100 mg/ 2 mL.

How many mL will be placed in the volume control device?
_____

**a.** What flow rate will be set on the infusion pump for the medication administration? _____

DA equation:

**b.** What procedure must be followed (according to agency policy) before and after a medication is infused on a primary line? _____

**29** Ordered: Hyperalimentation (TPN) continuous infusion in a central line at 60 mL per hour for a patient who has a gastrointestinal disorder. Among the contents ordered:
15% dextrose solution
4.25% amino acids

How many grams of dextrose are contained in a liter of the TPN solution?

DA equation:

**a.** Evaluation:

**b.** How many approximate carbohydrate kilocalories will the dextrose provide per liter of TPN solution?

DA equation:

**c.** Evaluation:

**d.** How many grams of amino acids are contained in a liter of TPN solution?

DA equation:

**e.** Evaluation:

**f.** How many approximate* protein kilocalories will the amino acids provide per liter of TPN solution?

DA equation:

**g.** Evaluation:

30 The prescriber also orders a lipid solution for the patient mentioned in problem # 29: 200 mL of 20% fat emulsion to be added to the total volume once a day.

How many grams of lipid are contained in the liter?

DA equation:

**a.** Evaluation:

**b.** How many kilocalories will each lipid solution provide?

DA equation:

**c.** Evaluation:

31 Ordered: Start Pitocin IV at 2 milliunits/ minute.

Available: Pitocin 5 units in 500 mL of D5W.
Conversion formulas: 1000 milliunits = 1 unit; 60 minutes = 1 hour
At how many mL per hour will the flow rate be set?

DA equation:

**a.** Evaluation:

---

*A calculation of 4 calories per g of CHO, 4 calories per g of amino acids, and 9 calories per gram of fat yield an approximate amount of calories.

**32** Ordered: Dobutamine HCl 3 mcg/ kg/ minute. Patient weight: 154 lb.

Available: Dobutamine 250 mg in 500 mL.

Estimated wt in kg: _____

**a.** Actual wt in kg: _____

DA equation:


**b.** Evaluation:


**c.** Dose ordered in mcg/ min: _____

**d.** Dose ordered in mg/ min: _____

**e.** At how many mL per hour will the flow rate be set?

DA equation:


**f.** Evaluation:


**33** Ordered: diazepam 10 mg direct IV before endoscopy procedure.

Directions: Injection undiluted at a rate of 5 mg/ minute.

Total mL to be injected: _____

**a.** Estimated dose: _____

DA equation:


**b.** Evaluation:


**c.** Using a 3-mL syringe, how many mL per minute will you inject?

_____

DA equation:

**d.** Evaluation:


**e.** Over how many total minutes will you inject? _____
seconds? _____

**f.** How many seconds per calibration will you inject? _____

**34** Ordered: phenytoin oral suspension 175 mg PO daily in the AM for a child with seizures.

N 0071-2214-20     *Shake Well*

**Dilantin-125**®
(Phenytoin Oral Suspension, USP)

**125 mg per 5 mL potency**

**Important—**Another strength available; verify unspecified prescriptions.

**Caution—**Federal law prohibits dispensing without prescription.

**8 fl oz (237 mL)**

**PARKE-DAVIS**
Div of Warner-Lambert Co/Morris Plains, NJ 07950 USA

6505-00-890-1110

**Shake well before using.**

Each 5 mL contains phenytoin, 125 mg with a maximum alcohol content not greater than 0.6 percent.

**Usual Dose—**Adults, 1 teaspoonful three times daily; Children, see package insert.

See package insert for complete prescribing information.

**Store below 30° C (86° F). Protect from freezing.**

Keep this and all drugs out of the reach of children.

Exp date and lot

2214G013

SDR child: 250 mg/ $m^2$/ day as single dose or divided in 2 doses.

Child's BSA: 0.7 $m^2$

What is the safe dose for this child? _____

    DA equation:


**a.** Evaluation:


**b.** If safe dose ordered, how many mL will you administer?

    DA equation:


**c.** Evaluation:

Shade in medicine cup to nearest measurable dose. Mark the syringe at the additional amount to be added.

**35** Ordered: cefaclor oral susp. 0.8 g PO bid for a child with otitis media weighing 44 lb.

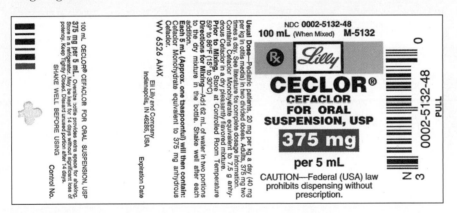

What is the child's wt in kg? _____

**a.** Estimated:

DA equation:

**b.** Actual:

DA equation:

**c.** Evaluation:

**d.** SDR (refer to label) for this patient:

DA equation:

**e.** Evaluation:

**f.** How many mL of water are needed to reconstitute this medication?
**g.** If a safe dose ordered, how many mL will you prepare to nearest tenth of a mL?

DA equation:

**h.** Evaluation:

Shade in medicine cup to nearest measurable dose. Mark the syringe at the additional amount to be added.

## Essential Math Self-Assessment

1 greater than

2 less than

3 greater than or equal to

4 less than or equal to

5 $\geq$

6 $\dfrac{300}{1}$

7 425.

8 434

9 $\dfrac{256}{256}$

10 V

11 10

12 90

13 1, 2, 4, 8, 16

14 1, 2, 5, 10

15 15, 30, 45

16 $10 \times 10 \times 10 = 1000$

17 $5^2 = 25$

18 $\sqrt{36} = 6$

19 10

20 8

21 $\dfrac{2}{5}$

22 $\dfrac{2}{3}\dfrac{\text{Numerator}}{\text{Denominator}}$

23 $\dfrac{1}{10}; \dfrac{1}{6}$

24 $5\frac{1}{6}$

25 $\dfrac{36}{5}$

26 8; 30

27 5

28 $\dfrac{4}{5}\dfrac{1}{25}$

29 $\frac{17}{12} = 1\frac{5}{12}; \frac{11}{18}$

30 $\dfrac{17}{24}; \dfrac{3}{8}$

31 $\frac{1}{2}; \frac{19}{5} = 3\frac{4}{5}$

32 $\frac{9}{2} = 4\frac{1}{2}; 16$

33 $\dfrac{10\ \text{Diapers}}{1\ \text{pkg}}; \dfrac{\$2}{1\ \text{gallon}}\dfrac{\$30}{1\ \text{hour}}$

34 0.25; 0.83

35 $\frac{461}{1000}; 5\frac{9}{100}$

36 0.5; 0.1

37 1.34

38 0.235

39 0.23

40 0.1

41 $\dfrac{3}{10}; \dfrac{16}{100} = \dfrac{4}{25}; \dfrac{125}{1000} = \dfrac{1}{8}$

42 0.416

43 4

44 10%; 32%; 3.2%

45 1600 (Find 10%, then take $\frac{1}{2}$ or multiply $\$32,000 \times 0.05$.)

46 75

47 60

48 "Times" - a multiplication sign ($5 \times 6 \times 3$)

49 baseline (1.2)

50 $\dfrac{1}{2} \times \dfrac{1}{6} = \dfrac{1}{12}$

# Chapter 1

## Rapid Practice 1-1

| | | | |
|---|---|---|---|
| 1 | 3 | 4 | 2 |
| 2 | 1 | 5 | 3 |
| 3 | 4 | | |

## Rapid Practice 1-2

| | | | |
|---|---|---|---|
| 1 | $<$ | 4 | $>$ |
| 2 | $\leq$ | 5 | $\sqrt{\phantom{x}}$ |
| 3 | $\geq$ | | |

## Rapid Practice 1-3

| | | | |
|---|---|---|---|
| 1 | 4 | 4 | 1 |
| 2 | 3 | 5 | 4 |
| 3 | 1 | | |

## Rapid Practice 1-4

1 $\dfrac{100}{1}$

2 100.0

3 192.02

4 Avoid errors: The decimal may be misread as the number one "1".

5 $\dfrac{100}{100}$

## Rapid Practice 1-5

| | | | |
|---|---|---|---|
| 1 | 15 | 6 | 41 |
| 2 | 14 | 7 | 59 |
| 3 | 22 | 8 | 300 |
| 4 | 8 | 9 | 400 |
| 5 | 4 | 10 | 3000 |

## Rapid Practice 1-6

1 X

2 XV

3 XXX

4 IL

5 LX

6 LXIV

7 XIV

8 MCMIII

9 MM

10 XLIV

## Rapid Practice 1-7

1 $10 \times 4 = 40$

2 2, 3, 4, 6

3 2, 4

4 12

5 5, 10, 15, . . .

## Rapid Practice 1-8

1 5

2 0.5

3 2000

4 50

5 $\frac{1}{2}$

## Rapid Practice 1-9

1 2

2 4

3 4

4 1

5 2

## Rapid Practice 1-10

1 12

2 $7^2 = 7 \times 7 = 49$

3 Divisor $= \frac{1}{2}$

4 100

5 15

## Rapid Practice 1-11

1 $10 \times 10$

2 $2 \times 2 \times 2 \times 2 \times 2$

3 $10^8$

4 10

5 4

## Rapid Practice 1-12

| | | | | |
|---|---|---|---|---|
| 1 | 2 | | 4 | 3 |
| 2 | 3 | | 5 | 3 |
| 3 | 2 | | | |

## Rapid Practice 1-13

| Number | | ÷ 10 | ÷ 100 | ÷ 1000 | Number | | × 10 | × 100 | × 1000 |
|---|---|---|---|---|---|---|---|---|---|
| 1 | 50 | 5 | 0.5 | 0.05 | 6 | 0.125 | 1.25 | 12.5 | 125 |
| 2 | 125 | 12.5 | 1.25 | 0.125 | 7 | 0.5 | 5 | 50 | 500 |
| 3 | 10 | 1 | 0.1 | 0.01 | 8 | 0.25 | 2.5 | 25 | 250 |
| 4 | 250 | 25 | 2.5 | 0.25 | 9 | 0.005 | 0.05 | 0.5 | 5 |
| 5 | 1000 | 100 | 10 | 1 | 10 | 0.1 | 1 | 10 | 100 |

## Rapid Practice 1-14

1 $\frac{5}{10}$

2 $\frac{3}{1000}$

3 $\frac{25}{100}$

4 $1\frac{56}{100}$

5 $2\frac{345}{10,000}$

## Rapid Practice 1-15

| | | | | |
|---|---|---|---|---|
| 1 | 0.25 | | 6 | 0.15 |
| 2 | 0.2 | | 7 | 0.6 |
| 3 | 0.25 | | 8 | 0.1 |
| 4 | 0.4 | | 9 | 0.04 |
| 5 | 0.05 | | 10 | 0.005 |

## Rapid Practice 1-16

| | | | | |
|---|---|---|---|---|
| 1 | 0.3 | | 6 | 0.006 |
| 2 | 1.32 | | 7 | 0.05 |
| 3 | 0.01 | | 8 | 0.5 |
| 4 | 0.6 | | 9 | 1.06 |
| 5 | 0.5 | | 10 | 0.5 |

## Rapid Practice 1-17

1 $\frac{8}{10}$

2 $\frac{35}{100}$

3 $\frac{5}{1000}$

4 $1\frac{25}{100}$

5 $3\frac{5}{10}$

6 $\frac{25}{100}$

7 $\frac{15}{1000}$

8 $\frac{9}{10}$

9 $2\frac{8}{100}$

10 $\frac{4}{10,000}$

## Rapid Practice 1-18

1 **a.** 0.3
  **b.** 1.3
  **c.** 0.8
  **d.** 1.9
  **e.** 0.1

2 **a.** 0.69
  **b.** 3.75
  **c.** 0.89
  **d.** 2.38
  **e.** 0.05

3 **a.** 2
  **b.** 11
  **c.** 1
  **d.** 2
  **e.** 3

## Rapid Practice 1-19

1 0.8

2 0.0642

3 0.15

4 9.0

5 0.000014

## Rapid Practice 1-20

1 $4\overline{)10}$

2 $3.05\overline{)20.32}$ → $305\overline{)2032.}$

3 $0.25\overline{)100.00}$ → $25\overline{)10000.}$

4 $1.2\overline{)5.06}$ → $12\overline{)50.6}$

5 $0.025\overline{)0.100}$ → $25\overline{)100.}$

6 $0.1\overline{)0.5}$ → $1\overline{)5.}$

7 $9\overline{)12.035}$ → No change

8 $2.6\overline{)4.003}$ → $26\overline{)40.03}$

9 $0.04\overline{)2.10}$ → $4\overline{)210.}$

10 $0.125\overline{)2.500}$ → $125\overline{)2500.}$

## Rapid Practice 1-21

1 $5 \overline{)20.5}$ → $4.1$

2 $5 \overline{)205.}$ → $41.$

3 $2 \overline{)3.0}$ → $1.5$

4 $4 \overline{)1.00}$ → $0.25$

5 $250 \overline{)200.}$ → $0.8$

## Rapid Practice 1-22

1 2          4 2

2 4          5 2

3 4

## Rapid Practice 1-23

1 3          4 3

2 4          5 1

3 2

## Rapid Practice 1-24

1 18          4 50

2 30          5 200

3 12

## Rapid Practice 1-25

1 $\dfrac{2}{6}$          4 $\dfrac{6}{8}$

2 $\dfrac{12}{15}$          5 $\dfrac{9}{24}$

3 $\dfrac{4}{8}$

## Rapid Practice 1-26

| Greater Fraction | LCD | Equivalent Fractions Result |
|---|---|---|
| 2 $\frac{1}{8}$ | 24 | $\frac{3}{24} > \frac{2}{24}$ |
| 3 $\frac{1}{100}$ | 200 | $\frac{2}{200} > \frac{1}{200}$ |
| 4 $\frac{5}{6}$ | 30 | $\frac{24}{30} < \frac{25}{30}$ |
| 5 $\frac{4}{50}$ | 250 | $\frac{1}{250} < \frac{20}{250}$ |

## Rapid Practice 1-27

1  2    $\frac{1}{2} + \frac{1}{2} = \frac{2}{2} = 1$

2  4    $\frac{2}{4} + \frac{1}{4} = \frac{3}{4}$

3  24    $\frac{12}{24} + \frac{8}{24} = \frac{20}{24} = \frac{5}{6}$

4  40    $\frac{30}{40} + \frac{24}{40} = \frac{54}{40} = 1\frac{7}{20}$

5  12    $\frac{8}{12} + \frac{3}{12} = \frac{11}{12}$

## Rapid Practice 1-28

| LCD | Answer |
|---|---|
| 1  2 | $1\frac{1}{2} - \frac{1}{2} = 1$ |
| 2  10 | $\frac{6}{10} - \frac{5}{10} = \frac{1}{10}$ |
| 3  12 | $\frac{14}{12} - \frac{9}{12} = \frac{5}{12}$ |
| 4  8 | $9\frac{10}{8} - 4\frac{5}{8} = 5\frac{5}{8}$ |
| 5  20 | $3\frac{21}{20} - 3\frac{7}{20} = \frac{14}{20} = \frac{7}{10}$ |

## Rapid Practice 1-29

1  $\frac{1}{27}$

2  $\frac{3}{8}$

3  $\frac{2}{30} = \frac{1}{15}$

4  $\frac{1}{25,000}$

5  $\frac{27}{50}$

## Rapid Practice 1-30

1  $\dfrac{3}{8}$     $\left(\dfrac{1}{\underset{1}{\cancel{2}}} \times \dfrac{\overset{3}{\cancel{6}}}{8} = \dfrac{3}{8}\right)$

4  $\dfrac{2}{3}$     $\left(\dfrac{\overset{1}{\cancel{4}}}{\underset{1}{\cancel{5}}} \times \dfrac{\overset{2}{\cancel{10}}}{\underset{3}{\cancel{12}}} = \dfrac{2}{3}\right)$

2  $1$     $\left(\dfrac{\overset{1}{\cancel{2}}}{\underset{1}{\cancel{3}}} \times \dfrac{\overset{1}{\cancel{3}}}{\underset{1}{\cancel{2}}} = 1\right)$

5  $\dfrac{2}{5}$     $\left(\dfrac{\overset{2}{\cancel{100}}}{\underset{1}{\cancel{200}}} \times \dfrac{\overset{1}{\cancel{200}}}{\underset{5}{\cancel{250}}} = \dfrac{2}{5}\right)$

3  $\dfrac{1}{2}$     $\left(\dfrac{3}{\cancel{5}} \times \dfrac{\overset{1}{\cancel{5}}}{6} = \dfrac{3}{6} = \dfrac{1}{2}\right)$

## Rapid Practice 1-31

1  $\dfrac{5}{16}$     $\left(\dfrac{1}{4} \times \dfrac{5}{4} = \dfrac{5}{16}\right)$

4  $\dfrac{13}{15}$     $\left(\dfrac{1}{5} \times \dfrac{13}{3} = \dfrac{13}{15}\right)$

2  $\dfrac{38}{9} = 4\dfrac{2}{9}$     $\left(\dfrac{19}{\underset{3}{\cancel{6}}} \times \dfrac{\overset{2}{\cancel{4}}}{3} = \dfrac{38}{9} = 4\dfrac{2}{9}\right)$

5  $\dfrac{17}{48}$     $\left(\dfrac{1}{6} \times \dfrac{17}{8} = \dfrac{17}{48}\right)$

3  $\dfrac{5}{4} = 1\dfrac{1}{4}$     $\left(\dfrac{5}{2} \times \dfrac{1}{2} = \dfrac{5}{4} = 1\dfrac{1}{4}\right)$

## Rapid Practice 1-32

1  $3$     $\left(\dfrac{1}{\underset{1}{\cancel{2}}} \times \dfrac{\overset{3}{\cancel{6}}}{1} = \dfrac{3}{1} = 3\right)$

4  $5$     $\left(\dfrac{5}{\underset{1}{\cancel{4}}} \times \dfrac{\overset{1}{\cancel{4}}}{1} = 5\right)$

2  $2\dfrac{2}{3}$     $\left(\dfrac{1}{3} \times \dfrac{8}{1} = \dfrac{8}{3} = 2\dfrac{2}{3}\right)$

5  $5$     $\left(\dfrac{5}{\underset{1}{\cancel{2}}} \times \dfrac{\overset{1}{\cancel{2}}}{1} = 5\right)$

3  $1\dfrac{3}{5}$     $\left(\dfrac{2}{5} \times \dfrac{4}{1} = \dfrac{8}{5} = 1\dfrac{3}{5}\right)$

## Rapid Practice 1-33

1  25%

6  $\dfrac{1}{10}$

2  75%

7  $\dfrac{3}{20}$

3  16.7%

8  $\dfrac{1}{2}$

4  33.3%

9  $\dfrac{1}{8}$

5  83.3%

10  $\dfrac{1}{4}$

## Rapid Practice 1-34

| | | | |
|---|---|---|---|
| 2 | 0.35 | 7 | 5% |
| 3 | 0.75 | 8 | 12.5% |
| 4 | 0.055 | 9 | 5.25% |
| 5 | 2 | 10 | 50% |
| 6 | 10% | | |

## Rapid Practice 1-35

| | Fraction | Decimal | Percentage |
|---|---|---|---|
| 1 | $\frac{2}{10}$ | 0.2 | 20% |
| 2 | $1\frac{5}{10}$ | 1.5 | 150% |
| 3 | $\frac{75}{100}$ | 0.75 | 75% |
| 4 | $\frac{1}{5}$ | 0.2 | 20% |
| 5 | $\frac{6}{10}$ | 0.6 | 60% |

## Rapid Practice 1-36

2 $960 \div 4 = 240$ mL per cup

3 $300 \div 12 = 25$ miles per gallon

4 $6000 \div 6 = 1000$ megabytes per gigabyte

5 $320 \div 80 = 4$ calories per gram of carbohydrate

## Chapter 1 Multiple-Choice Review

1 4
**Comment:** Do not handwrite this symbol in medical records. It may be misinterpreted.

2 2

3 4

4 4

5 1

6 2

| | | | |
|---|---|---|---|
| 7 | 3 | 14 | 3 |
| 8 | 2 | 15 | 3 |
| 9 | 2 | 16 | 2 |
| 10 | 3 | 17 | 3 |
| 11 | 2 | 18 | 4 |
| 12 | 1 | 19 | 4 |
| 13 | 3 | 20 | 1 |

## Chapter 1 Final Practice

1 For children *"less than"* two

2 $\sqrt{9}$

3 greater than or equal to

4 $\dfrac{85}{1}$

5 $85.0 = 85$

6 $500.00 = 500$

7 $\dfrac{500}{500}$

8 15

9 XVI

10 $8 + 7 = 15$

11 $8 \times 7 = 56$

12 1, 2, 3, 4, 6, 12

13 2, 5, 10

14 12

15 10, 15, 20, . . .

16 $\dfrac{1}{2}$

17 $10 \times 10 \times 10 \times 10 \ (= 10{,}000)$

18 $12^2 = 12 \times 12 = 144$

19 $\sqrt{100} = 10$

20 10

21 8

22 $\dfrac{3}{4}$

23 Numerator = 7; Denominator = 8

24 $\dfrac{1}{100}$ (the denominator is a power of 10)

25 One hundred fourteen thousandths

26 0.42

27 1.259 (1.25.9)

28 8030 (8.030.)

29 0.9

30 0.01

31 50

32 $\dfrac{5}{10} = \dfrac{1}{2}$

33 $\dfrac{25}{1000} = \dfrac{1}{40}$

34 0.05

35 0.232

36 3.39

37 $\dfrac{1}{8}$

38 $\dfrac{1}{15}$

39 $\dfrac{1}{100} = 1\%$

40 $6\frac{1}{4}$

41 $\dfrac{7}{6}$

42 12

43 $\dfrac{2}{3} = \dfrac{4}{6} = \dfrac{6}{9} = \dfrac{8}{12} \ldots$

44 greater than

45 $\dfrac{5}{6}$

46 4

47 $\dfrac{15}{60} = \dfrac{1}{4}$

48 $\dfrac{12}{24} + \dfrac{4}{24} + \dfrac{3}{24} = \dfrac{19}{24}$

**49**  $\dfrac{8}{40} - \dfrac{5}{40} = \dfrac{3}{40}$

**50**  $\dfrac{5}{4} \times \dfrac{17}{7} = \dfrac{85}{28} = 3\frac{1}{28}$

**51**  $\dfrac{2}{\overset{1}{3}} \times \dfrac{\overset{2}{6}}{1} = 4$

**52**  **a.** 0.6    **b.** 60%

**53**  **a.** 1%    **b.** $\dfrac{1}{100}$

**54**  $\dfrac{\$75}{50} = \$1.50$ per syringe

**55**  $10 \times 8 = 80$

# Chapter 2

## Rapid Practice 2-1

**1**  **a.** Desired answer
   **b.** Conversion formulas
   **c.** Original factors

**2**  Quantity is a number, unit is dimension.

**3**  A conversion formula is a ratio that expresses equivalent amounts for two entities.

**4**  3 is the numerator

**5**  8 is the denominator

## Rapid Practice 2-2

**1**  $\dfrac{12 \text{ eggs}}{1 \text{ Dozen}}$

**2**  $\dfrac{1 \text{ km}}{0.6 \text{ miles}}$

**3**  $\dfrac{4 \text{ qts}}{1 \text{ gallon}}$

**4**  $\dfrac{60 \text{ seconds}}{1 \text{ minute}}$

**5**  $\dfrac{1000 \text{ mg}}{1 \text{ gram}}$

## Rapid Practice 2-3

| Desired Answer Units | Conversion Formula | Original Factors to Convert |
|---|---|---|
| 2 quarts | $\dfrac{1 \text{ quart}}{4 \text{ cups}}$ | 8 cups |
| 3 yards | $\dfrac{1 \text{ yard}}{1 \text{ meter}}$ | 50 meters |
| 4 dozen | $\dfrac{12 \text{ dozen}}{1 \text{ gross}}$ | 2 gross |
| 5 Eurodollars | $\dfrac{1 \text{ Eurodollar}}{\$1.20}$ | $500 |

**Comment:** Note that original numbers and units to be converted do not have a denominator and are placed in the numerator position with an implied denominator of 1.

## Rapid Practice 2-4

1 **a.** Yes
  **b.** N/A
  **c.** Larger

2 **a.** No
  **b.** $\dfrac{1 \text{ kg}}{2.2 \text{ lb}}$
  **c.** Smaller

3 **a.** No
  **b.** $\dfrac{1 \text{ L}}{1000 \text{ mL}}$
  **c.** Smaller

4 **a.** Yes
  **b.** N/A
  **c.** Larger

5 **a.** Yes
  **b.** N/Λ
  **c.** Larger

## Rapid Practice 2-5

2 hours $= \dfrac{1 \text{ hour}}{20 \text{ dollars}} \times 500 \text{ dollars} = 25$ hours

3 megabytes $= \dfrac{1000 \text{ megabytes}}{1 \text{ gigabyte}} \times 4 \text{ gigabytes} = 4000$ megabytes

4 gallons $= \dfrac{1 \text{ gallon}}{4 \text{ liters}} \times 40 \text{ liters} = 10$ gallons

5 LPNs $= \dfrac{2 \text{ LPNs}}{5 \text{ CNAs}} \times 40 \text{ CNAs} = 16$ LPNs

## Rapid Practice 2-6

1 A cups $= \dfrac{2 \text{ cups}}{1 \text{ pint}} \times \dfrac{2 \text{ pints}}{1 \text{ quart}} \times 5 \text{ quarts} = 20$ cups

**2** B inches $= \dfrac{12 \text{ inches}}{1 \text{ foot}} \times \dfrac{3 \text{ feet}}{1 \text{ yard}} \times 20 \text{ yards} = 720 \text{ inches}$

**3** B mm $= \dfrac{10 \text{ mm}}{1 \text{ cm}} \times \dfrac{2.5 \text{ cm}}{1 \text{ inch}} \times 10 \text{ inches} = 250 \text{ mm}$

**4** B weeks $= \dfrac{4 \text{ weeks}}{1 \text{ month}} \times \dfrac{12 \text{ months}}{1 \text{ year}} \times 4 \text{ years} = 192 \text{ weeks}$

**5** B grams $= \dfrac{1 \text{ gram}}{1000 \text{ mg}} \times \dfrac{1 \text{ mg}}{1000 \text{ mcg}} \times 4000 \text{ mcg} = \dfrac{4000}{1{,}000{,}000} = 0.004 \text{ grams}$

## Rapid Practice 2-7

**1** lbs $= \dfrac{2.2 \text{ lbs}}{1 \text{ kg}} \times 80 \text{ kg} = 176 \text{ lbs}$

**2** pints $= \dfrac{2 \text{ pints}}{1 \text{ qt}} \times \dfrac{4 \text{ qts}}{1 \text{ gallon}} \times 5 \text{ gallon} = 40 \text{ pints}$

**3** inches $= \dfrac{1 \text{ inch}}{2.5 \text{ cm}} \times \dfrac{1 \text{ cm}}{10 \text{ mm}} \times 25 \text{ mm} = 1 \text{ inch}$

**4** hours $= \dfrac{1 \text{ hr}}{60 \text{ min}} \times \dfrac{1 \text{ min}}{60 \text{ sec}} \times 7200 \text{ sec} = 2 \text{ hours}$

**5** grams $= \dfrac{1 \text{ gram}}{1000 \text{ mg}} \times \dfrac{1 \text{ mg}}{1000 \text{ mcg}} \times 25{,}000 \text{ mcg} = 0.025 \text{ grams}$

## Chapter 2 Multiple-Choice Review

**1** 3        **6** 1

**2** 1        **7** 3

**3** 2        **8** 3

**4** 2        **9** 1

**5** 3        **10** 4

## Chapter 2 Final Practice

**1** **a.** Desired answer units
**b.** Conversion formula(s)
**c.** Original factors to convert

**2** Eggs $= \dfrac{12 \text{ eggs}}{1 \text{ dozen}} \times 10 \text{ dozen} = 120 \text{ eggs}$

**3** Km $= \dfrac{1 \text{ km}}{0.6 \text{ miles}} \times 50 \text{ miles} = 83.3 \text{ km}$

**4** lbs $= \dfrac{2.2 \text{ lbs}}{1 \text{ Kg}} \times 60 \text{ Kg} = 132 \text{ lbs}$

**5** Inches $= \dfrac{12 \text{ Inches}}{1 \text{ foot}} \times \dfrac{3 \text{ feet}}{1 \text{ yard}} = 50 \text{ yards} = 1800 \text{ inches}$

**6** $mm = \dfrac{10\ mm}{1\ \text{cm}} \times \dfrac{2.5\ \text{cm}}{1\ \text{inch}} \times 1\ \text{inch} = 25\ mm$ (millimeters)

**Comment:** 2.5 cm is an approximate equivalent. There are 2.54 cm in an inch.

**7** $meters = \dfrac{1\ meter}{1.09\ \text{yards}} \times 30\ \text{yards} = 27.5\ meters$

**8** $DVDs = \dfrac{1\ DVD}{8\ \text{Dollars}} \times 100\ \text{Dollars} = 12.5\ DVD\text{'s}$ (12 DVD's with \$4 remaining)

**9** $Rx = \dfrac{1\ Rx}{50\ \text{Dollars}} \times 2000\ \text{Dollars} = 40\ Rx$

**10** $Nurses = \dfrac{1\ nurse}{12\ \text{beds}} \times 480\ \text{beds} = 40\ nurses$

**11** $Liters = \dfrac{1\ liter}{1\ \text{qt}} \times \dfrac{4\ \text{qt}}{1\ \text{gallon}} \times 8\ \text{gallons} = 32\ liters\ (L)$

**12** $Inches = \dfrac{12\ inches}{1\ \text{foot}} \times \dfrac{3\ \text{feet}}{1\ \text{yard}} \times 100\ \text{yards} = 360\ inches$

**13** $Tablespoons = \dfrac{3\ tbs}{1\ \text{oz}} \times \dfrac{8\ \text{oz}}{1\ \text{cup}} \times 1\ \text{cup} = 24\ tbs$ (tablespoons)

**14** $Cups = \dfrac{2\ cups}{1\ \text{pt}} \times \dfrac{2\ \text{pt}}{1\ \text{qt}} \times 2\ \text{qt} = 8\ cups$

**15** $Seconds = \dfrac{60\ seconds}{1\ \text{minute}} \times \dfrac{60\ \text{minutes}}{1\ \text{hr}} \times 2\ \text{hrs} = 7200\ seconds$

**16** $mL = \dfrac{5\ mL}{1\ \text{tsp}} \times \dfrac{3\ \text{tsp}}{1\ \text{tbs}} \times 3\ \text{tbs} = 45\ mL$ (milliliters)

**17** $NA = \dfrac{2\ NA}{1\ \text{RN}} \times \dfrac{1\ \text{RN}}{\underset{1}{\cancel{10\ \text{beds}}}} \times \overset{30}{\cancel{300\ \text{beds}}} = 60\ NA$

**18** $Inches = \dfrac{2.5\ inches}{1\ \text{cm}} \times \dfrac{100\ \text{cm}}{1\ \text{meter}} \times 1\ \text{meter} = 250\ inches$

**19** $cm = \dfrac{2.5\ cm}{1\ \text{inch}} \times \dfrac{12\ \text{inches}}{1\ \text{ft}} \times 1\ \text{ft} = 30\ cm$ (centimeters)

**20** $mcg = \dfrac{1000\ mcg}{1\ \text{mg}} \times \dfrac{1000\ \text{mg}}{1\ \text{gram}} \times 2\ \text{grams} = 2{,}000{,}000\ mcg$ (micrograms)

# Chapter 3

## Rapid Practice 3-1

**1** grain

**2** gram, liter, meter

**3** To avoid confusion with the number 1

4 Inconsistent capacities of household measures

5 modern metric system

## Rapid Practice 3-2

| | | | | | |
|---|---|---|---|---|---|
| 1 | milli- | m | 6 | liter | L |
| 2 | centi- | c | 7 | meter | m |
| 3 | micro- | mc | 8 | gram | g |
| 4 | deci- | d | 9 | meter | |
| 5 | kilo- | k | 10 | milli- | |

## Rapid Practice 3-3

1 L

2 k

3 80 milligrams per deciliter

4 mcg

5 g = gram; L = liter; m = meter

## Rapid Practice 3-4

1 4

2 2

3 1

4 2

5 3

## Rapid Practice 3-5

1 mg

2 mcg

3 mm

4 mL

5 kg

## Rapid Practice 3-6

1 L = liter

2 m = meter

3 L = liter

4 g = gram

5 g = gram

## Rapid Practice 3-7

1 4

2 1

3 3

4 1

5 1

## Rapid Practice 3-8

1  150 mg = 0.15 g          3.5 g = 3500 mg

2  500 mg = 0.5 g          0.25 g = 250 mg

3  2000 mg = 2 g           0.6 g = 600 mg

4  250 mg = 0.25 g         0.125 g = 125 mg

5  100 mg = 0.1 g          0.04 g = 40 mg

6  1500 mg = 1.5 g         2 g = 2000 mg

7  375 mg = 0.375 g        0.3 g= 300 mg

8  60 mg = 0.06 g          0.75 g = 750 mg

9  175 mg = 0.175 g        5 g = 5000 mg

10  400 mg = 0.4 g         0.006 g = 6 mg

## Rapid Practice 3-9

1  $mg = \dfrac{1000\ mg}{1\ \cancel{g}} \times 1.5\ \cancel{g} = 1500\ mg$

2  $mg = \dfrac{1000\ mg}{1\ \cancel{g}} \times 0.15\ \cancel{g} = 150\ mg$

3  $mg = \dfrac{1000\ mg}{1\ \cancel{g}} \times 4\ \cancel{g} = 4000\ mg$

4  $g = \dfrac{1\ g}{\underset{2}{\cancel{1000\ mg}}} \times \overset{1}{\cancel{500\ mg}} = 0.5\ g$       **Comment:** Reduce large numbers to make the calculations easier.

5  $g = \dfrac{1\ g}{1000\ \cancel{mg}} \times 60\ \cancel{mg} = 0.06\ g$

## Rapid Practice 3-10

1  3          4  1

2  2          5  4

3  1

## Rapid Practice 3-11

|    | mg      | mcg      | mcg and mg |
|----|---------|----------|------------|
| 1  | 5 mg    | 2000 mcg | 1000 mcg   |
| 2  | 0.3 mg  | 500 mcg  | 0.5 g      |
| 3  | 1.5 mg  | 1800 mcg | 200 mcg    |
| 4  | 20 mg   | 150 mcg  | 0.01 g     |
| 5  | 2.5 mg  | 600 mcg  | 30,000 mcg |

## Rapid Practice 3-12

| | | | |
|---|---|---|---|
| 1 | centimeter | 6 | L |
| 2 | milliliter | 7 | m |
| 3 | milligram | 8 | kg |
| 4 | millimeter | 9 | km |
| 5 | microgram | 10 | cL |

## Rapid Practice 3-13

| | | | |
|---|---|---|---|
| 1 | 1000 mg | 6 | 1000 mL |
| 2 | 1000 g | 7 | 2500 mg |
| 3 | 10 mm | 8 | 0.5 g |
| 4 | 1000 mcg | 9 | 2.5 g |
| 5 | 1,000,000 mcg | 10 | 50,000 mg |

## Rapid Practice 3-14

| | | | |
|---|---|---|---|
| 1 | 15 grains | 4 | 15 mL |
| 2 | 10 mL | 5 | 30 mL |
| 3 | 15 mL | | |

## Chapter 3 Multiple-Choice Quiz

| | | | |
|---|---|---|---|
| 1 | 1 | 6 | 2 |
| 2 | 2 | 7 | 4 |
| 3 | 3 | 8 | 1 |
| 4 | 3 | 9 | 2 |
| 5 | 1 | 10 | 3 |

## Chapter 3 Final Practice

1. **a.** meter = m
   **b.** liter = L
   **c.** gram = g
   **d.** kilo-1000 = k
   **e.** milli- $\dfrac{1}{1000}$ = m
   **f.** centi- $\dfrac{1}{100}$ = c
   **g.** micro- $\dfrac{1}{1,000,000}$ = mc

**2** $mg = \dfrac{1000\ mg}{1\ \cancel{g}} \times 0.15\ \cancel{g} = 150\ mg$

**Comment:** The first numerator, mg, matches the described answer units, mg. Only mg remains in the answer.

**3** $g = \dfrac{1\ g}{1000\ \cancel{mg}} \times 400\ \cancel{mg} = 0.4\ g$

**4** $mL = \dfrac{1000\ ml}{1\ \cancel{L}} \times 0.25\ \cancel{L} = 250\ mL$

**5** $mg = \dfrac{1\ mg}{1000\ \cancel{mcg}} \times 150\ \cancel{mcg} = 0.15\ mg$

**6** $g = \dfrac{1000\ g}{1\ \cancel{kg}} \times 1.5\ \cancel{kg} = 1500\ g$

**7** $mg = \dfrac{1000\ mg}{1\ \cancel{g}} \times 0.1\ \cancel{g} = 100\ mg$

**8** $cm = \dfrac{\overset{1}{\cancel{100}}\ cm}{1\ \cancel{m}} \times \dfrac{1\ \cancel{m}}{\underset{10}{\cancel{1000}\ mm}} \times 15\ \cancel{mm} = \dfrac{15}{10} = 1.5\ cm$

**Comment:** Notice the diagonal direction of the cancelled units.

**9** $mcg = \dfrac{1000\ mcg}{1\ \cancel{mg}} \times 0.2\ \cancel{mg} = 200\ mcg$

**10** $g = \dfrac{1\ gram}{1000\ \cancel{mg}} \times \dfrac{1\ \cancel{mg}}{1000\ \cancel{mcg}} \times 256{,}000\ \cancel{mcg} = 0.256\ g$

**11** $mL = \dfrac{5\ mL}{1\ \cancel{tsp}} \times 3\ \cancel{tsp} = 15\ mL$

**12** $mL = \dfrac{15\ mL}{1\ \cancel{tbs}} \times 2\ \cancel{tbs} = 30\ mL$

**13** $mL = \dfrac{30\ mL}{1\ \cancel{oz}} \times 1.5\ \cancel{oz} = 45\ mL$

**14** $tsp = \dfrac{3\ tsp}{1\ \cancel{tbs}} \times 1\ \cancel{tbs} = 3\ tsp$

**15** $tbs = \dfrac{2\ tbs}{1\ \cancel{oz}} \times 2\ \cancel{oz} = 4\ tbs$

**16** $1000\ \cancel{g}$

**17** $2.2\ \cancel{lbs}$

**18** $mL = \dfrac{1000\ mL}{1\ \cancel{L}} \times 0.5\ \cancel{L} = 500\ mL$

**19 a.** 84 mg per mL
**b.** 1 mEq per mL

**20 a.** 149 mg per mL
**b.** 2 mEq per mL

# Chapter 4

## Rapid Practice 4-1

1. 1
2. 3
3. 2

4. 2
5. 2

## Rapid Practice 4-2

1. cap
2. DS
3. XR
4. supp
5. tab

6. LA
7. XL
8. ENT.
9. CD
10. UNG

## Rapid Practice 4-3

1. scored tablet
2. cap
3. enteric-coated tablet; capsules

4. compound
5. XR; XL; SR; CD; LA

## Rapid Practice 4-4

1. susp.
2. mixt.
3. sol.

4. elix.
5. aq.

## Rapid Practice 4-5

1. bucc
2. SL
3. NG
4. left ear
5. GT

6. top
7. PO
8. MDI
9. vag
10. NPO

## Rapid Practice 4-6

1 after meals

2 twice a day

3 as needed

4 without

5 immediately (and only one dose)

6 every 4 hours

7 nothing by mouth

8 before meals

9 with (as "with meals")

10 give as desired (pertaining to fluids or activity)

11 c̄

12 prn

13 D/C (e.g., specific medication [D/C aspirin] or treatment [D/C catheter])

14 ent

15 ac

16 each, every

17 tid

18 q2h

19 s̄

20 q12h

## Rapid Practice 4-7

1 T = tricycle; B = bicycle
   (3 wheels)    (2 wheels)

2 PRN

3 q4h = 6 times a day

4 **a.** Give "Tears No More" 2 (two) drops in each eye as needed for itching or burning
   **b.** Give Mylanta antacid 1 (one) ounce three times a day before meals
   **c.** Pharmacy

5 4; 6

## Rapid Practice 4-8

1  susp

2  elix

3  sol

4  fld

5  fld ext

6  prn

7  NPO

8  IM

9  stat

10  top

11  cheek (to be dissolved, not swallowed)

12  as desired (for fluids, activity)

13  metered dose inhaler

14  two times daily

15  intradermal

16  as needed; when necessary

17  nothing by mouth

18  intravenous push

19  Give medication when X-ray calls for the patient.

20  every 6 hours

## Rapid Practice 4-9

1  sublingual

2  solution

3  intramuscular

4  double strength

5  every hour

6  elixir

7  every six hours

8  nasogastic tube

9  every four hours

10  nothing by mouth

11  oral, by mouth

12  gastrostomy tube

13  before meals

14  cheek

15  after meals

16  as needed, when necessary

17  two times daily

18  every eight hours

19  three times daily

20  immediately (for only one dose)

## Rapid Practice 4-10

1  **a.** Sinemet
   **b.** 2 (it is a compound drug)
   **c.** Carbidopa 10 mg, Levodopa 100 mg

2  **a.** lorazepam
   **b.** 100 tab
   **c.** 0.5 mg

3  **a.** multiple dose vial
   **b.** 400 mcg/ mL
   **c.** 0.4 mg/ mL

4  **a.** Potassium Chloride
   **b.** 40 mEq/ 15 mL
   **c.** One pint

5  **a.** Biaxin
   **b.** clarithromycin
   **c.** 0.25 g

6  **a.** Lopressor
   **b.** metoprolol tartrate
   **c.** 50 mg per tablet

7 **a.** Elixir
**b.** 20 mg/ 5 mL
**c.** 14%

8 **a.** gemfibrozil
**b.** 0.6 g
**c.** multidose

9 **a.** benztropine mesylate
**b.** 500 mcg/ tablet
**c.** 100

10 **a.** 800 mcg/ mL
**b.** 0.8 mg/ mL
**c.** IV

## Rapid Practice 4-11

2 **a.** capsules
**b.** 250 mg/ capsule
**c.** 0.5 g
**d.** 1000 mg = 1 gram
**e.** 1.5 g or 1500 mg (q8h = 3 times in 24 hrs)
**f.** 0.5 g = 0.500. = 500 mg

3 **a.** mL
**b.** 125 mg/ 5 mL
**c.** 0.25 g
**d.** 1000 mg = 1 g
**e.** 1 g (0.25 g × 4 doses) = 1 gram per day
**f.** 0.250 g = 250 mg

4 **a.** mL
**b.** 15 mg/ mL
**c.** intramuscular
**d.** immediately
**e.** intramuscular, subcutaneous, intravenous

5 **a.** loracarbef
**b.** Suspension
**c.** 200 mg/ 5 mL—label B (0.2 g = 200 mg)
**d.** 0.2 g
**e.** 1000 mg = 1 gram

## Rapid Practice 4-12

1 with $= \bar{c}$; without $= \bar{s}$

2 the prescriber

3 medication errors due to misinterpretation, forgetting, not hearing, etc.

4 Prepare and mix medications together; deliver immediately by intramuscular route.

5 They may look like other numbers such as 1 and 0.

## Rapid Practice 4-13

| | | | |
|---|---|---|---|
| 1 | 3 | 4 | 1 |
| 2 | 3 | 5 | 4 |
| 3 | 2 | | |

## Rapid Practice 4-14

1  PENICILLIN; ASA (aspirin)

2  1800

3  Humalog

4  Lasix. Document the clarification. Report to nurse supervisor.

5  2400

6  NKDA–No

7  Losartan (Cozaar). Blood pressure assessment needed.

8  Acetaminophen

9  **a.** both eyes
   **b.** consult prescriber, document

10  every 4 hours

## Rapid Practice 4-15

| | | | |
|---|---|---|---|
| 1 | d | 4 | b |
| 2 | a | 5 | c |
| 3 | e | | |

## Chapter 4 Multiple-Choice Review

| | | | |
|---|---|---|---|
| 1 | 1 | 11 | 2 |
| 2 | 2 | 12 | 2 |
| 3 | 3 | 13 | 2 |
| 4 | 4 | 14 | 2 |
| 5 | 2 | 15 | 1 |
| 6 | 1 | 16 | 2 |
| 7 | 3 | 17 | 2 |
| 8 | 2 | 18 | 3 |
| 9 | 4 | 19 | 1 |
| 10 | 2 | 20 | 1 |

1  immediately

2  every hour

3  as needed

4  intravenously

5  nothing by mouth

6  by mouth

7  total parenteral nutrition

8  nasogastric

9  intravenously

10  subcutaneously

11  nasogastric

12  by mouth

13  every 2 hours

14  every night at bedtime

15  intramuscularly every 4 hours as needed

16  suppositories

17  by mouth. Distinguish total drug from total volume.

18  elixirs and suspensions two times daily

19  without

20  sublingually

21  right patient

22  right drug

23  right dose

24  right time

25  right route

26  right documentation

27  right to refuse

28  2 capsules

$$\text{capsules} = \frac{1 \text{ capsule}}{\cancel{50 \text{ mg}}_{1}} \times \frac{\cancel{1000 \text{ mg}}^{20}}{1 \cancel{g}} \times 0.1 \cancel{g} = 2 \text{ capsules}$$

29  **a.** the ordered dose; the unit dose concentration
    **b.** one or more conversion formulas

30 **a.** ERY-TAB
**b.** $0.5 \text{ g} \times 2 = 1 \text{ g}$ per day or 1000 mg per day
**c.** 250 mg per tablet
**d.** 2 tablets per dose

$$\text{tab} = \frac{1 \text{ tab}}{\underset{1}{\cancel{250 \text{ mg}}}} \times \frac{\overset{4}{\cancel{1000 \text{ mg}}}}{1 \cancel{\text{ g}}} \times 0.5 \cancel{\text{ g}} = 2 \text{ tabs}$$

# Chapter 5

## Rapid Practice 5-1

1 True      4 False

2 True      5 True

3 True

## Rapid Practice 5-2

1 2 tablets      6 2 tablets

2 1.5 tablets      7 0.5 tablet

3 2 capsules      8 2 capsules

4 0.5 tablet      9 2.5 tablets

5 2 tablets      10 0.5 tablet

## Rapid Practice 5-3

2 **a.** 1000 mg = 1 gram
**b.** 2 tablets ($250 = 2 \times 125$)
**c.** 2 tablets
$$\text{tablet} = \frac{1 \text{ tablet}}{\cancel{125 \text{ mg}}} \times \overset{2}{\cancel{250 \text{ mg}}} = 2 \text{ tablets}$$
**d.** Equation is balanced. Answer = estimate.

3 **a.** No conversion formula needed
**b.** 2 tablets ($0.1 = 2 \times 0.5$)
**c.** 2 tablets

$$\text{tablet} = \frac{1 \text{ tablet}}{\underset{1}{\cancel{0.05 \text{ g}}}} \times \overset{2}{\cancel{0.1 \text{ g}}} = 2 \text{ tablets}$$

**d.** Equation is balanced. Answer = estimate.

**4 a.** No conversion formula needed

**b.** $1\frac{1}{2}$ tablets $(75 = 1\frac{1}{2} \times 50)$

**c.** 1.5 tablets

$$\text{tablet} = \frac{1 \text{ tablet}}{\underset{2}{\cancel{50 \text{ mcg}}}} \times \overset{3}{\cancel{75 \text{ mcg}}} = 1.5 \text{ tablets}$$

**d.** Equation is balanced. Answer = estimate.

**5 a.** No conversion formula needed

**b.** 2 tablets $(20 = 2 \times 10)$

**c.** 2 tablets

$$\text{tab} = \frac{1 \text{ tab}}{\underset{1}{\cancel{10 \text{ mEq}}}} \times \overset{2}{\cancel{20 \text{ mEq}}} = 2 \text{ tabs}$$

**d.** Equation is balanced. Answer = estimate.

**6 a.** 1000 mg = 1 gram

**b.** 0.2 g = 200 mg; 2 capsules $(200 = 2 \times 100)$

**c.** 2 capsules

$$\text{capsule} = \frac{1 \text{ capsule}}{\underset{1}{\cancel{100 \text{ mg}}}} \times \frac{\overset{10}{\cancel{1000 \text{ mg}}}}{1 \text{ g}} \times 0.2 \text{ g} = 2 \text{ capsules}$$

**d.** Equation is balanced. Answer = estimate.

**7 a.** 1000 mg = 1 g

**b.** 250 mg = 0.25 g; 1 capsule

**c.** 1 capsule

$$\text{capsule} = \frac{1 \text{ capsule}}{0.25 \text{ g}} \times \frac{1 \text{ g}}{\underset{4}{\cancel{1000 \text{ mg}}}} \times \overset{1}{\cancel{250 \text{ mg}}} = \frac{1}{1} = 1 \text{ capsule}$$

**d.** Equation is balanced. Answer = estimate.

**8 a.** 1000 mg = 1 g

**b.** $0.25 = 2 \times 0.125$; 2 capsules

**c.** 2 capsules

$$\text{capsule} = \frac{1 \text{ capsule}}{\underset{1}{\cancel{125 \text{ mg}}}} \times \frac{\overset{8}{\cancel{1000 \text{ mg}}}}{1 \text{ g}} \times 0.25 \text{ g} = 2 \text{ capsules}$$

**d.** Equation is balanced. Answer = estimate.

**9 a.** 1000 mcg = 1 mg

**b.** 0.175 mg = 175 mcg

**c.** 0.5 tablet

$$\text{tab} = \frac{1 \text{ tab}}{350 \cancel{\text{ mcg}}} \times \frac{1000 \cancel{\text{ mcg}}}{1 \cancel{\text{ mg}}} \times 0.175 \cancel{\text{ mg}} = \frac{175}{350} = 0.5 \text{ tab}$$

**d.** Equation is balanced. Answer = estimate.

**10 a.** 1000 mcg = 1 mg

**b.** 0.1 mg = 100 mcg

**c.** 2 tablets (100 = 50 × 2)

$$\text{tab} = \frac{1 \text{ tablet}}{\underset{1}{\cancel{50 \text{ mcg}}}} \times \frac{\overset{20}{\cancel{1000 \text{ mcg}}}}{1 \cancel{\text{ mg}}} \times 0.1 \cancel{\text{ mg}} = 2 \text{ tablets}$$

**d.** Equation is balanced. Answer = estimate.

## Rapid Practice 5-4

**2** 100 mg          100,000 mcg

**3** 8 mg          0.008 g

**4** 25 mg          0.025 g

**5** 300 mg          0.3 g

## Rapid Practice 5-5

| No. | Decimal Place | Direction | Answer |
| --- | --- | --- | --- |
| 2 | 3 | L | 0.2 mg |
| 3 | 3 | R | 500 mcg |
| 4 | 6 | L | 0.015 g |
| 5 | 6 | R | 4000 mcg |
| 6 | 3 | L | 2.2 g |
| 7 | 3 | L | 0.35 mg |
| 8 | 6 | L | 0.005 g |
| 9 | 3 | R | 50 mg |
| 10 | 3 | L | 0.05 g |

## Rapid Practice 5-6

**1 a.** 30 mg = 2 × 15 mg

**b.** 2 tablets

$$\text{tab} = \frac{1 \text{ tab}}{\cancel{15 \text{ mg}}} \times \cancel{30 \text{ mg}} = 2 \text{ tablets}$$

**c.** Equation is balanced. Estimate = answer.

**2 a.** 1 mg = 2 × 0.5 mg

**b.** 2 tablets

$$\text{tab} = \frac{1 \text{ tab}}{\cancel{0.5 \text{ mg}}} \times \cancel{1 \text{ mg}} = 2 \text{ tablets}$$

**c.** Equation is balanced. Estimate = answer.

**3 a.** $0.25 \text{ g} = 250 \text{ mg}$

**b.** 1 tablet

$$\text{tab} = \frac{1 \text{ tab}}{\underset{1}{\cancel{250 \text{ mg}}}} \times \frac{\overset{4}{\cancel{1000 \text{ mg}}}}{1 \cancel{\text{g}}} \times 0.25 \cancel{\text{g}} = 1 \text{ tablet}$$

**c.** Equation is balanced. Estimate = answer.

**4 a.** $0.1 \text{ g} = 100 \text{ mg}; 50 \times 2 = 100$

**b.** 2 tablets

$$\text{tab} = \frac{1 \text{ tab}}{\underset{1}{\cancel{50 \text{ mg}}}} \times \frac{\overset{20}{\cancel{1000 \text{ mg}}}}{1 \cancel{\text{g}}} \times 0.1 \cancel{\text{g}} = 2 \text{ tablets}$$

**c.** Equation is balanced. Estimate = answer.

**5 a.** $0.5 \text{ mg} \times 2 = 1 \text{ mg}$

**b.** 2 tablets

$$\text{tab} = \frac{1 \text{ tab}}{\cancel{0.5 \text{ mg}}} \times \overset{2}{\cancel{1 \text{ mg}}} = 2 \text{ tablets}$$

**c.** Equation is balanced. Estimate = answer.

## Rapid Practice 5-7

**1 a.** $0.25 \times 2 \text{ tablets} = 0.5$

$$\text{tab} = \frac{1 \text{ tab}}{\underset{1}{\cancel{0.25 \text{ mg}}}} \times \overset{2}{\cancel{0.5 \text{ mg}}} = 2 \text{ tablets}$$

**b.** Equation is balanced. Answer = estimate.

**2 a.** $0.5 \text{ g} = 500 \text{ mg}; 500 \times 2 = 1000 \text{ mg}; 2 \text{ tablets}$

$$\text{tab} = \frac{1 \text{ tablet}}{0.5 \cancel{\text{g}}} \times \frac{1 \cancel{\text{g}}}{1000 \cancel{\text{mg}}} \times 1000 \cancel{\text{mg}} = \frac{1}{0.5} = 2 \text{ tablets}$$

**b.** Equation is balanced. Answer = estimate.

**3 a.** $0.1 \text{ mg} = 100 \text{ mcg}; 1 \text{ tablet}$

$$\text{tab} = \frac{1 \text{ tab}}{0.1 \cancel{\text{mg}}} \times \frac{1 \cancel{\text{mg}}}{\underset{10}{\cancel{1000 \text{ mcg}}}} \times \overset{1}{\cancel{100 \text{ mcg}}} = 1 \text{ tablet}$$

**b.** Equation is balanced. Answer = estimate.

**4 a.** $100 \text{ mg} = 0.1 \text{ g}; 1 \text{ tablet}$

$$\text{cap} = \frac{1 \text{ cap}}{\underset{1}{\cancel{100 \text{ mg}}}} \times \frac{\overset{10}{\cancel{1000 \text{ mg}}}}{1 \cancel{\text{g}}} \times 0.1 \cancel{\text{g}} = 1 \text{ capsule}$$

**b.** Equation is balanced. Answer = estimate.

**5 a.** $0.12 \text{ g} = 120 \text{ mg}; 1 \text{ tablet}$

$$\text{tab} = \frac{1 \text{ tab}}{120 \cancel{\text{mg}}} \times \frac{1000 \cancel{\text{mg}}}{1 \cancel{\text{g}}} \times 0.12 \cancel{\text{g}} = \frac{\cancel{120}}{\cancel{120}} = 1 \text{ tablet}$$

**b.** Equation is balanced. Answer = estimate.

## Rapid Practice 5-8

2  5000 mcg = 5 mg     more     2 mL

3  0.1 g = 100 mg     less     0.3 mL

4  0.5 g = 500 mg     more     1.5 mL

5  0.1 g = 100 mg     more     2 mL

## Rapid Practice 5-9

1  **a.** Give over 2× the dose per 5 mL supplied (more than 10 mL)

$$mL = \frac{5\ mL}{\underset{2}{\cancel{10\ mg}}} \times \overset{5}{\cancel{25\ mg}} = \frac{25}{2} = 12.5\ mL$$

   **b.** Equation is balanced. Estimate supports answer.

2  **a.** Give more than dose per 5 mL supplied but less than 2×

$$mL = \frac{5\ mL}{\cancel{5\ mg}} \times 8\ \cancel{mg} = 8\ mL$$

   **b.** Equation is balanced. Estimate supports answer.

3  **a.** Give slightly more than 5 mL (15 mg is more than 12.5 mg)

$$mL = \frac{5\ mL}{12.5\ \cancel{mg}} \times 15\ \cancel{mg} = \frac{75}{12.5} = 6\ mL$$

   **b.** Equation is balanced. Estimate supports answer.

4  **a.** Give half the dose per mL supplied (50 is 2 × 25).

$$mL = \frac{1\ mL}{\underset{2}{\cancel{50\ mcg}}} \times \overset{1}{\cancel{25\ mcg}} = \frac{1}{2} = 0.5\ mL$$

   **b.** Equation is balanced. Estimate supports answer.

5  **a.** Give about $1\frac{1}{2} \times 5$ mL.

$$mL = \frac{5\ mL}{\underset{2}{\cancel{4\ mg}}} \times \overset{3}{\cancel{6\ mg}} = \frac{15}{2} = 7.5\ mL$$

   **b.** Equation is balanced. Estimate supports answer.

## Rapid Practice 5-10

| | Amt to prepare | Place in cup | Place in Syringe | Syringe size |
|---|---|---|---|---|
| 1 | 6.5 mL | 5 | 1.5 | 3 |
| 2 | 14 mL | 10 | 4 | 5 |
| 3 | 9 mL | 5 | 4 | 5 |
| 4 | 17 mL | 15 | 2 | 3 |
| 5 | 27.4 mL | 25 | 2.4 | 3 |

528  •  A<small>NSWER</small> K<small>EYS</small>

## Rapid Practice 5-11

**1 a.** Give $1\frac{1}{2}$ times the available unit dose of 1 mL or 1.5 mL

$$mL = \frac{1\ mL}{\underset{2}{50\ mg}} \times \overset{3}{\cancel{75\ mg}} = 1.5\ mL$$

**b.** Equation is balanced. Estimate = answer.

**2 a.** Give $4 \times 5$ mL.

$$\frac{\cancel{5}\ mL}{\cancel{5\ mg}} \times 20\ \cancel{mg} = 20\ mL$$

**b.** Equation is balanced. Answer = estimate.

**3 a.** Give slightly more than $2 \times 2$ mL.

$$\frac{2\ mL}{\underset{3}{15\ mg}} \times \overset{7}{\cancel{35\ mg}} = \frac{14}{3} = 4.7\ mL$$

**b.** Equation is balanced. Answer = estimate.

**4 a.** Give more than 8 mL but less than 16 mL.

$$mL = \frac{8\ mL}{\underset{3}{75\ mg}} \times \overset{5}{\cancel{125\ mg}} = \frac{40}{3} = 13.3\ mL$$

**b.** Equation is balanced. Estimate supports answer.

**5 a.** Give slightly less than 20 mL.

$$mL = \frac{10\ mL}{\underset{5}{25\ mg}} \times \overset{9}{\cancel{45\ mg}} = \frac{90}{5} = 18\ mL$$

**b.** Equation is balanced. Estimate supports answer.

## Rapid Practice 5-12

**1 a.** Give slightly more than 5 mL.

$$mL = \frac{5\ mL}{\underset{4}{20\ mg}} \times \overset{5}{\cancel{25\ mg}} = \frac{25}{4} = 6.25 \rightarrow 6.3\ mL$$

**b.** Equation is balanced. Estimate supports answer.

**2 a.** Give less than 15 mL, more than 7.5 mL.

$$mL = \frac{15\ mL}{\underset{8}{40\ mEq}} \times \overset{5}{\cancel{25\ mEq}} = \frac{75}{8} = 9.37 \rightarrow 9.4\ mL$$

**b.** Equation is balanced. Estimate supports answer.

**3 a.** Give more than 1 mL but less than 2 mL.

$$mL = \frac{1\ mL}{\underset{3}{30\ mg}} \times \overset{5}{\cancel{50\ mg}} = \frac{5}{3} = 1.7\ mL$$

**b.** Equation is balanced. Answer approximates estimate

**4 a.** Give about $2\frac{1}{2} \times 5$ mL.

$$mL = \frac{5\ mL}{\underset{2}{10\ mg}} \times \overset{5}{\cancel{25\ mg}} = \frac{25}{2} = 12.5\ mL$$

**b.** Equation is balanced. Estimate = answer.

**5 a.** 0.6 g = 600 mg; give 2 × 5 mL.

$$\frac{5 \text{ mL}}{\underset{3}{\cancel{300 \text{ mg}}}} \times \frac{\overset{10}{\cancel{1000 \text{ mg}}}}{1 \text{ g}} = 0.16 \text{ g} = \frac{30}{3} = 10 \text{ mL}$$

**b.** Equation is balanced. Answer = estimate.

## Rapid Practice 5-13

| SDR | Patient's weight (lb) | Estimated weight (kg) to the nearest whole number | Actual weight (kg) to the nearest tenth | Total SDR to nearest tenth |
|---|---|---|---|---|
| 2 100-200 mcg/ kg/ day (100 mcg = 0.1 mg) | 40 | 20 | 18.2 | 0.1 mg × 18.2 kg = 1.82 → 1.8 mg/ day<br>0.2 mg × 18.2 kg = 3.64 → 3.6 mg/ day<br>SDR = 1.8-3.6 mg/ day |
| 3 0.2-0.5 g/ kg/ day | 44 | 22 | 20 | 0.2 × 20 = 4 g/ day<br>0.5 × 20 = 10 g/ day<br>SDR = 4-10 g/ day |
| 4 0.25-1.5 mg/ kg/ day | 150 | 75 | 68.2 | 0.25 × 68.2 = 17.1 mg/ day<br>1.5 × 68.2 = 102.3 mg/ day<br>SDR = 17.1-102.3 mg/ day |
| 5 2-5 mcg/ kg/ day | 180 | 90 | 81.8 | 2 × 81.8 = 163.8 mcg/ day<br>5 × 81.8 = 409 mcg/ day<br>SDR = 163.8-409 mcg/ day |
| 6 0.1-0.2 g/ kg/ day | 95 | 48 | 43.2 | 0.1 × 43.2 = 4.3 g/ day<br>0.2 × 43.2 = 8.6 g/ day<br>SDR = 4.3-8.6 g/ day |
| 7 5-10 mcg/ kg/ day | 88 | 44 | 40 | 5 × 40 = 200 mcg/ day<br>10 × 40 = 400 mcg/ day<br>SDR = 200-400 mcg/ day |
| 8 10-20 mg/ kg/ day in 3 divided doses | 200 | 100 | 90.9 | 10 × 90.9 = 909 mg/ day<br>20 × 90.9 = 1818 mg/ day<br>SDR = 909-1818 mg/ day |
| 9 1-5 mcg/ kg/ day | 30 | 15 | 13.6 | 1 × 13.6 mcg/ day<br>5 × 13.6 = 68 mcg/ day<br>SDR = 13.6-68 mcg/ day |
| 10 0.05-0.1 g/ day in 4 divided doses | 150 | 75 | 68.2 | 0.05 × 68.2 = 3.4 g/ day<br>0.1 × 68.2 = 6.8 g/ day<br>SDR = 3.4-6.8 g/ day |

2 **a.** Estimated weight in kg = 80 kg; actual weight in kg = 72.7 kg
   **b.** SDR low, $1 \times 72.7 = 72.7$ mg/ day; SDR high, $2 \times 72.7 = 145.4$ mg/ day
   **c.** 50 mg $\times$ 6 = 300 mg
   **d.** No. The ordered dose exceeds the high safe dose.
   **e.** Hold medication and clarify promptly with prescriber.

3 **a.** Estimated weight in kg = 60 kg; actual weight in kg = 54.5 kg
   **b.** SDR low, $2 \times 54.5 = 109$ mg/ day; SDR high, $4 \times 54.5 = 218$ mg/ day
   **c.** 50 mg $\times$ 4 = 200 mg
   **d.** Yes
   **e.** Order within SDR and safe to give.

4 **a.** Estimated weight in kg = 50 kg; actual weight in kg = 45.5 kg
   **b.** SDR low, $10 \times 45.5 = 455$ mg/ day; SDR high, $20 \times 45.5 = 910$ mg/ day
   **c.** 250 mg $\times$ 3 = 750 mg (0.25 g = 250 mg)
   **d.** Yes
   **e.** Order within SDR and safe to give.

5 **a.** Estimated weight in kg = 30 kg; actual weight in kg = 27.3 kg
   **b.** SDR low, $5 \times 27.3 = 136.5$ mg/ day; SDR high, $10 \times 27.3 = 273$ mg/ day
   **c.** 25 mg $\times$ 2 = 50 mg
   **d.** No. The ordered dose is significantly less than the low safe dose.
   **e.** Hold medication and clarify promptly with prescriber.

## Rapid Practice 5-15

2 **a.** 300 mg/ 5 mL
   **b.** 1000 mg = 1 g; 0.6 g = 600 mg
   **c.** Yes
   **d.** Safe to give
   **e.** Give two times the unit dose volume of 5 mL.
   **f.** 10 mL

$$mL = \frac{5 \text{ mL}}{300 \text{ mg}} \times \frac{1000 \text{ mg}}{1 \text{ g}} \times 0.6 \text{ g} = \frac{30}{3} = 10 \text{ mL}$$

   **g.** Equation is balanced. Estimate supports answer.

3 **a.** No conversions needed
   **b.** Yes
   **c.** Safe to give
   **d.** Give two times dose per volume supplied: 10 mL

**e.** 10 mL

$$mL = \frac{5\ mL}{1\ \cancel{mg}} \times 2\ \cancel{mg} = 10\ mL$$

**f.** Equation is balanced. Estimate supports answer.

4 **a.** No conversions needed
   **b.** Yes
   **c.** Safe to give
   **d.** Give slightly more than 15 mL
   **e.** 16.9 mL

$$\frac{15\ mL}{\underset{8}{\cancel{40\ mEq}}} \times \overset{9}{\cancel{45\ mEq}} = \frac{135}{8} = 16.9\ mL$$

**f.** Equation is balanced. Estimate supports answer.

5  Estimated weight in kg: 22 kg; actual weight in kg: 20 kg

   **a.** No conversions needed
   **b.** No
   **c.** Hold. 120 mg ordered for one dose is overdose. Contact prescriber promptly. Document.
   **d.** N/A
   **e.** N/A
   **f.** N/A

## Chapter 5 Multiple-Choice Review

| | | | |
|---|---|---|---|
| 1 | 2 | 6 | 3 |
| 2 | 1 | 7 | 4 |
| 3 | 2 | 8 | 3 |
| 4 | 4 | 9 | 4 |
| 5 | 1 | 10 | 3 |

## Chapter 5 Final Practice

1  **a.** SDR 325-625 mg q4h up to 12 tablets per day or 2-3 tablets (325-975 mg)
   q6h up to 12 tablets in 24 hr.
   Order: 0.65 g (625 mg) 6 times a day (12 tablets)
   **b.** Safe to give
   **c.** 2; less
   **d.** Will give 2 tabs (325 mg mEq $\times$ 2 = 650 mg)

   $$\text{tab} = \frac{1 \text{ tab}}{325 \text{ mg}} \times \frac{1000 \text{ mg}}{1 \text{ g}} \times 0.65 \text{ g} = 2 \text{ tablets}$$

   **e.** Equation is balanced. Answer = estimate.

2  **a.** SDR: 325-650 mg q4-6h up to 4 g (4000 mg) daily.
   Order: 0.65 g (650 mg 4$\times$ daily = 2600 mg [2.6 g] daily)
   **b.** Safe to give
   **c.** 2 $\times$ 10.15 mL (2 $\times$ 325 mg)
   **d.** 20.3 mL

   $$\text{mL} = \frac{10.15 \text{ mL}}{325 \text{ mg}} \times \frac{1000 \text{ mg}}{1 \text{ g}} \times 0.65 \text{ g} = \frac{6597.5}{325} = 20.3 \text{ mL}$$

   **e.** Equation is balanced. Answer = estimate.

**3 a.** SDR 60 mg daily.

Order: 0.06 g (60 mg) × 2 = 120 mg ordered daily

**b.** Unsafe. Order exceeds SDR. Hold medication. Call prescriber promptly.

**c.** N/A

**d.** N/A

**e.** N/A

**4 a.** SDR: 20-40 mEq/ day.

Order: 30 mEq/ day.

**b.** Safe to give

**c.** Give less than dose per volume supplied of 15 mL

**d.** 11.3 mL

$$mL = \frac{15\ mL}{\cancel{40\ mEq}_{4}} \times \cancel{30\ mEq}^{3} = \frac{45}{4} = 11.25 \rightarrow 11.3\ mL$$

**e.** Equation is balanced. Estimate supports answer.

**5 a.** SDR: 10-50 mg 3-4 times per day.

Order: 50 mg (0.05 g) 3× per day.

**b.** Safe to give

**c.** Give more than 1 mL, less than 2 mL

**d.** 1.7 mL

$$mL = \frac{1\ mL}{30\ \cancel{mg}} \times \frac{1000\ \cancel{mg}}{1\ \cancel{g}} \times 0.05\ \cancel{g} = \frac{50}{30} = 1.66 \rightarrow 1.7\ mL$$

**e.** Equation is balanced. Estimate supports answer.

**6 a.** SDR 100-300 mg/ day in divided doses or at bedtime.
Order: 0.09 g (90 mg) $\times$ 2 doses = 180 mg/ day.

**b.** Safe to give

**c.** 3 tablets (0.09 g ordered = 90 mg); 30 mg $\times$ 3 = 3 tablets (90 mg).

**d.** 3 tablets

$$\text{tab} = \frac{1 \text{ tab}}{30 \text{ mg}} \times \frac{1000 \text{ mg}}{1 \text{ g}} \times 0.09 \text{ g} = \frac{90}{30} = 3 \text{ tabs}$$

**e.** Equation is balanced. Estimate = answer.
**Comment:** Recheck orders for doses exceeding 1 or 2 tablets. In this case the patient diagnosis and the current drug literature support the administration of 90 mg.

**7 a.** SDR: 200 mg bid to start.
Order: 0.2 g (200 mg) bid.

**b.** Safe to give

**c.** 2 tablets = 100 mg $\times$ 2 = 200 mg = 2 tablets

**d.** 2 tablets

$$\text{tab} = \frac{1 \text{ tab}}{100 \text{ mg}} \times 1000 \text{ mg} \times 0.2 \text{ g} = 2 \text{ tabs}$$

**e.** Equation is balanced. Estimate = answer.

**8 a.** SDR maintenance: 75-125 mcg daily.
Order: 0.1 mg = 100 mcg daily.

**b.** Safe to give

**c.** 2 tablets (0.05 $\times$ 2 = 0.1)

**d.** 2 tablets

$$\text{tab} = \frac{1 \text{ tab}}{\underset{1}{0.05 \text{ mg}}} \times \overset{2}{0.1 \text{ mg}} = 2 \text{ tabs}$$

**e.** Equation is balanced. Estimate = answer.

**9 a.** SDR: 5 mg $\times$ 22.7 kg (50 lb) = 113.5 mg total daily dose.
Order: 75 mg $\times$ 2 = 150 mg/ day.

**b.** Order is unsafe. 150 mg exceeds SDR. Withhold medication. Contact prescriber promptly. Document.

**c.** N/A

**d.** N/A

**e.** N/A

**10 a.** SDR: 125-250 mg q6-8h.
Order: 0.25 g (250 mg) q8h.

**b.** Safe to give

**c.** 1 tablet (0.25 g = 250 mg)

**d.** 1 tablet

$$\text{tab} = \frac{1 \text{ tab}}{\underset{1}{250 \text{ mg}}} \times \overset{4}{1000 \text{ mg}} \times 0.25 \text{ g} = 1 \text{ tab}$$

**e.** Equation is balanced. Estimate = answer.

# Chapter 6

## Rapid Practice 6-1

1 calibrations

2 intradermal; 1 mL

3 parenteral

4 gauge

5 smaller

1  20 mL

2  5

3  1 mL

4

5

6  10 mL

7  5

8  0.2 mL

9

10

1  5 mL

2  5

3  0.2 mL

4

5

**Note:** There are 5-mL syringes with 10 calibrations per mL.

6  1 mL

7  10

8  0.01 mL

9

10

**Comment:** Pay special attention to the decimal place when preparing small doses.

# Rapid Practice 6-4

**1** 3 mL

**2** 0.1 mL

**3**

**4**

**5**

# Rapid Practice 6-5

| | Ordered Dose | Syringe Size (in mL) | | Ordered Dose | Syringe Size (in mL) |
|---|---|---|---|---|---|
| 1 | 2.8 mL | 3 | 6 | 9.6 mL | 10 |
| 2 | 3.2 mL | 5 | 7 | 12.6 mL | 20 |
| 3 | 6.4 mL | 10 | 8 | 0.6 mL | 1 |
| 4 | 0.08 mL | 1 | 9 | 1.5 mL | 3 |
| 5 | 1.7 mL | 3 | 10 | 0.1 mL | 1 |

In some clinical situations a larger syringe may be selected.

# Rapid Practice 6-6

**1** The volume of medication to be administered

**2** No. They must be placed in biohazard or sharps container.

**3** 1 mL

**4** 5 mL; 3.2 mL

**5** 10 mL; 5.8 mL

1  a. 5 mL
   b. 5
   c. 0.2 mL
   d. 3.6 mL

2  a. 1 mL
   b. 10
   c. 0.01 mL
   d. 0.45 mL

3  a. 3 mL
   b. 10
   c. 0.1 mL
   d. 1.3 mL

4  a. 10 mL
   b. 5
   c. 0.2 mL
   d. 5.8 mL

5  a. 20 mL
   b. 1
   c. 1 mL
   d. 18 mL

## Rapid Practice 6-8

1

2

3

4

5

## Rapid Practice 6-9

1

2

3

4

5

## Rapid Practice 6-10

**1**

**2**

**3**

**4**

**5**

## Rapid Practice 6-11

**1** **a.** 5 mL
**b.** 3
**c.** 0.2 mL
**d.**

**2  a.** 1 mL
**b.**

**c.** 0.01 mL
**d.**

**3  a.** 20 mL
**b.**

**c.** 1 mL
**d.**

**4  a.** 10 mL
**b.**

**c.** 0.2 mL
**d.**

**5 a.** 3 mL
   **b.**

   **c.** 0.1 mL
   **d.**

## Chapter 6 Multiple-Choice Review

| | | | |
|---|---|---|---|
| 1 | 1 | 6 | 3 |
| 2 | 2 | 7 | 1 |
| 3 | 2 | 8 | 1 |
| 4 | 1 | 9 | 1 |
| 5 | 1 | 10 | 3 |

## Chapter 6 Final Practice

**1 a.** more
   **b.** give twice unit dose

$$mL = \frac{mL}{\overset{}{\underset{1}{100\ mg}}} \times \overset{2}{\cancel{200\ mg}} = 2\ mL$$

   **c.** Equation is balanced; estimate supports answer.

**2 a.** less
   **b.** give half of unit dose.

$$mL = \frac{mL}{\overset{}{\underset{2}{30\ mg}}} \times \overset{1}{\cancel{15\ mg}} = 0.5\ mL$$

**c.** Equation is balanced; estimate supports answer.

**3  a.** more
  **b.** 6.4 mL

$$mL = \frac{mL}{50\ \text{mg}} \times 320\ \text{mg} = 6.4\ mL$$

  **c.** Equation is balanced; estimate supports answer.

**4  a.** more than 1 mL, less than 2 mL
  **b.** 1.1 mL

$$mL = \frac{mL}{75\ \text{mg}} \times 80\ \text{mg} = 1.066\ \text{rounded to}\ 1.1\ mL$$

  **c.** Equation is balanced. Estimate supports answer

**5  a.** more; order is five times unit dose concentration
  **b.** 5 mL

$$mL = \frac{mL}{\underset{1}{10\ \text{mg}}} \times \overset{5}{50\ \text{mg}} = 5\ mL$$

  **c.** Equation is balanced; Estimate supports answer.

**6** **a.** less than 1 mL
   **b.** 0.8 mL

$$mL = \frac{mL}{\underset{5}{\cancel{50\ mg}}} \times \overset{4}{\cancel{40\ mg}} = 0.8\ mL$$

   **c.** Equation is balanced; estimate supports answer.

**7** **a.** slightly more than 1 mL
   **b.** 1.2 mL

$$mL = \frac{mL}{\underset{5}{\cancel{100\ mg}}} \times \overset{6}{\cancel{120\ mg}} = 1.2\ mL$$

   **c.** Equation is balanced; estimate supports answer.

**8** **a.** less
   **b.** 0.15 mL

$$mL = \frac{mL}{100\ \cancel{mg}} \times 15\ \cancel{mg} = 0.15\ mL$$

   **c.** Equation is balanced; estimate supports answer.

**9** **a.** Total mL volume of the order
   **b.** After calculating dose

**10** **a.** Never recap used needles. Use sharps container promptly for used needles and syringes.
   **b.** Hepatitis B and C and AIDS

# Chapter 7

## Rapid Practice 7-1

**1** 2

**2** 4

**3** 2

**4** 1

**5** 2

## Rapid Practice 7-2

**1 a.** Oral suspension when reconstituted from powder
 **b.** Water
 **c.** 140 mL
 **d.** Slowly add and shake vigorously.
 **e.** 200 mg/ 5 mL
 **f.** Multidose
 **g.** 200 mL
 **h.** 40 unit doses
 **i.** Room temperature
 **j.** Refrigerator
 **k.** After 10 days

**2 a.** Oral suspension when reconstituted from powder
 **b.** Water
 **c.** 78 mL
 **d.** Tap until all powder flows freely. Add $\frac{1}{3}$ of 78 mL (24 mL). After shaking vigorously, add remaining $\frac{2}{3}$ (52 mL) and shake vigorously.
 **e.** 125 mg/ 5 mL
 **f.** 250-500 mg every 8 hrs
 **g.** 20-40 mg/ kg/ day in divided doses every 8 hours, depending on age, weight, or infection severity.
 **h.** Multidose
 **i.** Discard suspension after 14 days

**3 a.** oral suspension when reconstituted from powder
 **b.** 39 mL of water
 **c.** 50 mL
 **d.** 200 mg/ 5 mL
 **e.** Refrigeration preferable but not required.
 **f.** Shake well before using.
 **g.** Discard suspension after 14 days.

**4 a.** 1-g vial (IM) 3-mL diluent; 1-g vial (IV) 10 mL diluent
 **b.** (IM) 300 mg/ mL; (IV) 95 mg/ mL

**5 a.** Duricef
 **b.** cefadroxil monohydrate
 **c.** oral suspension when reconstituted from powder
 **d.** 500 mg/ 5 mL
 **e.** 359-PR-246
 **f.** 10/15/06

**1** **a.** 45 mL of water

  **b.** more (0.3 g = 300 mg, which is more than 250 mg)

  **c.** 6 mL

$$mL = \frac{5 \text{ mL}}{\underset{1}{\cancel{250 \text{ mg}}}} \times \frac{\overset{4}{\cancel{1000 \text{ mg}}}}{1 \text{ g}} \times 0.3 \text{ g} = 6 \text{ mL}$$

  **d.** Equation is balanced. Estimate supports answer.

**2** **a.** Add 60 mL water followed by 30 mL of water for a total of 90 mL.

  **b.** Estimate will give more than 2 times unit dose of 5 mL (0.25 g = 250 mg).

  **c.** 10 mL

$$mL: \frac{5 \text{ mL}}{\underset{1}{\cancel{125 \text{ mg}}}} \times \frac{\overset{8}{\cancel{1000 \text{ mg}}}}{1 \text{ g}} \times 0.25 \text{ g} = 10 \text{ mL}$$

  **d.** Equation is balanced. Estimate supports answer

**3  a.** More than 5 mL (0.2 g = 200 mg)

  **b.** 8 mL

$$mL = \frac{5 \text{ mL}}{\underset{1}{\cancel{125 \text{ mg}}}} \times \frac{\overset{8}{\cancel{1000 \text{ mg}}}}{1 \text{ g}} \times 0.2 \text{ g} = 8 \text{ mL}$$

  **c.** Equation in balanced. Estimate supports answer

**4  a.** 24 mL distilled or Purified Water

  **b.** More than 1 mL or 3 times more (10 × 3 = 30)

  **c.** 3 mL

$$mL = \frac{1 \text{ mL}}{\underset{1}{\cancel{10 \text{ mg}}}} \times \overset{3}{\cancel{30 \text{ mg}}} - 3 \text{ mL}$$

  **d.** Equation is balanced. Estimate supports answer

**5  a.** 63 mL of water in 2 portions

  **b.** Less than 5 mL

  **c.** 3 mL

$$mL = \frac{5 \text{ mL}}{\underset{5}{\cancel{125 \text{ mg}}}} \times \cancel{75 \text{ mg}} \overset{3}{=} \frac{15}{5} = 3 \text{ mL}$$

  **d.** Equation is balanced. Estimate supports answer

**Comment:** The medicine cup is inappropriate for measurement of this dose.     **ANSWER KEYS** • **549**

## Rapid Practice 7-4

2 **a.** 4 mL (0.1 g = 100 mg)
 **b.** 100 mg/ mL
 **c.** 1 mL (100 mg = 0.1 g)

3 **a.** 2 mL (0.25 g = 250 mg)
 **b.** 250 mg/ mL
 **c.** 1 mL (250 mg = 0.25 g)

4 **a.** 2 mL (0.3 g = 300 mg)
 **b.** 250 mg/ mL
 **c.** 1.2 mL (300 mg is more than 250 mg)

$$1 \text{ mL} = \frac{1 \text{ mL}}{\underset{1}{\cancel{250 \text{ mg}}}} \times \frac{\overset{4}{\cancel{1000 \text{ mg}}}}{1 \text{ g}} \times 0.3 \cancel{\text{ g}} = 4 \times 0.3 = 1.2 \text{ mL}$$

 **d.** Equation is balanced. Estimate supports answer.

5 **a.** 12 mL
 **b.** 50 mg/ mL
 **c.** 10 mL

$$1 \text{ mL} = \frac{1 \text{ mL}}{\underset{1}{\cancel{50 \text{ mg}}}} \times \frac{\overset{20}{\cancel{1000 \text{ mg}}}}{1 \text{ g}} \times 0.5 \cancel{\text{ g}} = 10 \text{ mL}$$

 **d.** Equation is balanced. Estimate supports answer.

## Rapid Practice 7-5

2 **a.** Sterile water
 **b.** 2.7 mL
 **c.** 250 mg/ 1.5 mL
 **d.** 200 mg is less than 250 mg; estimated dose less than 1.5 mL.
 **e.** 1.2 mL

$$\text{mL} = \frac{1.5 \text{ mL}}{\underset{5}{\cancel{250 \text{ mg}}}} \times \overset{4}{\cancel{200 \text{ mg}}} = 1.2 \text{ mL}$$

 **f.** Equation is balanced. Estimate supports answer.

3 **a.** Sterile water for injection
 **b.** 2.5 mL
 **c.** 330 mg/ mL
 **d.** more than 1 mL (0.4 g = 400 mg; 330 mg/ mL unit dose available)

**e.** 1.2 mL

$$mL = \frac{1\ mL}{330\ \cancel{mg}} \times \frac{1000\ \cancel{mg}}{1\ \cancel{g}} \times 0.4\ \cancel{g} = \frac{400}{330} = 1.2\ mL$$

**f.** Equation is balanced. Estimate supports answer.

**4 a.** Sterile water or bacteriostatic water
**b.** 2 mL
**c.** 500 mg/ 1.2 mL
**d.** equal (0.5g = 500 mg)
**e.** more than 1 mL
**f.** 1.2 mL

$$mL = \frac{1.2\ mL}{\cancel{500\ mg}_{1}} \times \overset{2}{\cancel{1000\ mg}} \times 0.5\ \cancel{g} = 1.2\ mL$$

**g.** Equation is balanced. Estimate supports answer.
**h.** Discard after 12 hours at room temperature, 10 days if refrigerated.

**5 a.** 5 g; 5000 mg in vial
**b.** 1 g/ 2.5 mL
**c.** less than 2.5 mL
**d.** 2 mL

$$mL = \frac{2.5\ mL}{1\ \cancel{g}} \times 0.8\ \cancel{g} = 2\ mL$$

**e.** Equation is balanced. Estimate supports answer.
**f.** After reconstitution, discard unused portion after 24 hours if stored at room temperature or after 72 hours if refrigerated.

## Rapid Practice 7-6

| | Fractional Strength | Ratio | Percent | Amount Active Ingredient | Amount Diluent Inactive Ingredient |
|---|---|---|---|---|---|
| 2 | $\frac{3}{5}$ | 3:2 | 60% | 36 mL | 24 mL |
| 3 | $\frac{3}{4}$ | 3:1 | 75% | 750 mL | 250 mL |
| 4 | $\frac{1}{5}$ | 1:4 | 20% | 48 mL | 192 mL |
| 5 | $\frac{1}{10}$ | 1:9 | 10% | 5 mL | 45 mL |

## Chapter 7 Multiple-Choice Review

1 3        6 1

2 4        7 2

3 1        8 1

4 2        9 2

5 1        10 2

## Chapter 7 Final Practice

1 **a.** slightly more than 10 mL
  **b.** 12 mL

$$mL = \frac{5 \text{ mL}}{\underset{1}{\cancel{125 \text{ mg}}}} \times \frac{\overset{8}{\cancel{1000 \text{ mg}}}}{1 \text{ g}} \times 0.3 \text{ g} = 12 \text{ mL}$$

  **c.** Equation is balanced. Estimate supports answer.

2 **a.** less than 5 mL (0.2 g = 200 mg)
  **b.** 4 mL

$$mL = \frac{5 \text{ mL}}{\underset{1}{\cancel{250 \text{ mg}}}} \times \frac{\overset{4}{\cancel{1000 \text{ mg}}}}{1 \text{ g}} \times 0.2 \text{ g} = 4 \text{ mL}$$

**c.** Equation is balanced. Estimate supports answer.

**Comment:** Medicine cup is not appropriate for an amount less than 5 mL.

**3 a.** more than 5 mL

**b.** 6.3 mL

$$mL = \frac{5\ mL}{\cancel{200\ mg}_{1}} \times \frac{\overset{5}{\cancel{1000\ mg}}}{1\ g} \times 0.25\ \cancel{g} = 6.25\ mL,\ rounded\ to\ 6.3\ mL$$

**c.** Equation is balanced. Estimate supports answer.

**4 a.** slightly more than 5 mL

**b.** 5.3 mL

$$mL = \frac{5\ mL}{187\ \cancel{mg}} \times \frac{1000\ \cancel{mg}}{1\ \cancel{g}} \times 0.2\ \cancel{g} = 5.34,\ rounded\ to\ 5.3\ mL$$

**c.** Equation is balanced. Estimate supports answer.

**5  a.** slightly more than 5 mL
   **b.** 6 mL

$$\text{mL} = \frac{5 \text{ mL}}{\underset{1}{\cancel{125 \text{ mg}}}} \times \frac{\overset{8}{\cancel{1000 \text{ mg}}}}{1 \text{ g}} \times 0.15 \cancel{\text{ g}} = 6 \text{ mL}$$

   **c.** Equation is balanced. Estimate supports answer.

**6  a.** 1:3
   **b.** $\frac{1}{4}$
   **c.** mL = 200 mL × 0.25 = 50 mL (or 200 mL × $\frac{1}{4}$ = 50 mL Ensure)
   **d.** 200 mL − 50 mL = 150 mL water

**7  a.** 33%
   **b.** 1:2
   **c.** mL = 30 mL × 0.33 = 10 mL (or 30 × $\frac{1}{3}$ = 10 mL formula)
   **d.** 30 mL − 10 mL = 20 mL diluent of SW

**8  a.** 50%
   **b.** $\frac{1}{2}$
   **c.** mL = 30 mL × 0.5 = 15 mL (or 30 × $\frac{1}{2}$ = 15 mL formula)
   **d.** 30 mL − 15 mL = 15 mL diluent of SW

**9  a.** Less (1% × $\frac{1}{100}$) (0.9% = $\frac{0.9}{100}$)
   **b.** 0.9 g solute
   **c.** 9 g

$$\text{g} = \frac{0.9 \text{ g}}{\underset{1}{\cancel{100 \text{ mL}}}} \times \overset{10}{\cancel{1000 \text{ mL}}} = 9 \text{ g solute}$$

**10  a.** 1:1
   **b.** 25 mL
   **c.** 25 mL (25 + 25 = 50 mL)

# Chapter 8

## Rapid Practice 8-1

1  1

2  2

3  3

4  4

5  3

## Rapid Practice 8-2

1 **a.** 250 mg/ mL
  **b.** 0.45 g = 450 mg. Give almost 2 mL.
  **c.** 1.8 mL

$$mL = \frac{1 \text{ mL}}{\underset{1}{250 \text{ mg}}} \times \frac{\overset{4}{\cancel{1000 \text{ mg}}}}{1 \text{ g}} \times 0.45 \text{ g} = 1.8 \text{ mL}$$

  **d.** Equation is balanced. Estimate supports answer.

2 **a.** 2 mg/ 2 mL
  **b.** between 1 and 2 mL (1500 mcg = 1.5 mg)
  **c.** 1.5 mL

$$mL = \frac{\cancel{2} \text{ mL}}{\underset{2}{\cancel{2} \text{ mg}}} \times \frac{1 \text{ mg}}{\cancel{1000 \text{ mcg}}} \times \overset{3}{\cancel{1500 \text{ mcg}}} = \frac{3}{2} = 1.5 \text{ mL}$$

  **d.** Equation is balanced. Estimate supports answer.

3 **a.** 15 mg/ mL
  **b.** give slightly more than 0.5 mL
  **c.** 0.6 mL

$$mL = \frac{1 \text{ mL}}{\underset{5}{15 \text{ mg}}} \times \overset{3}{\cancel{9 \text{ mg}}} = \frac{3}{5} = 0.6 \text{ mL}$$

  **d.** Equation is balanced. Estimate supports answer.

**4**  **a.** 4 mg/ mL

   **b.** give one half or 0.5 mL

   **c.** 0.5 mL

$$mL = \frac{1\ mL}{\underset{2}{\cancel{4\ mg}}} \times \overset{1}{\cancel{2\ mg}} = \frac{1}{2} = 0.5\ mL$$

   **d.** Equation is balanced. Estimate supports answer.

**5**  **a.** 0.5 mg/ 2 mL

   **b.** 0.125 mg is $\frac{1}{4}$ of 0.5 mg. Give $\frac{1}{4}$ of 2 mL or 0.5 mL.

   **c.** 0.5 mL

$$mL = \frac{\overset{4}{\cancel{2\ mL}}}{\underset{1}{\cancel{0.5\ mg}}} \times 0.125\ \cancel{mg} = 0.5\ mL$$

   **d.** Equation is balanced. Estimate supports answer.

## Rapid Practice 8-3

**1**  **a.** give less than 1 mL (0.02 g = 20 mg)

   **b.** 0.7 mL

$$mL = \frac{1\ mL}{30\ \cancel{mg}} \times \frac{100\cancel{0\ mg}}{1\ \cancel{g}} \times 0.02\ \cancel{g} = \frac{2}{3} = \begin{matrix}0.66\ \text{rounded to} \\ 0.7\ mL\end{matrix}$$

   **c.** Equation is balanced. Estimate supports answer.

**2**  **a.** give less than 4 mL

   **b.** 3.5 mL

$$mL = \frac{\overset{1}{\cancel{4\ mL}}}{\underset{10}{\cancel{40\ mg}}} \times 38\ \cancel{mg} = \frac{38}{10} = 3.8\ mL$$

**c.** Equation is balanced. Estimate supports answer.

**d.** 0.2 mL

**3 a.** give more than 2 mL
**b.** 2.4 mL

$$mL = \frac{2\ mL}{\underset{1}{250\ mg}} \times \overset{4}{\cancel{1000\ mg}} \times 0.3\ \cancel{g} = 2.4\ mL$$

**c.** Equation is balanced. Estimate supports answer.

**4 a.** give less than 1 mL
**b.** 0.75 mL

$$mL = \frac{1\ mL}{0.4\ \cancel{mg}} \times 0.3\ \cancel{mg} = 0.75\ mL$$

**c.** Equation is balanced. Estimate supports answer.

**5**

**2  a.** give less than 1 mL

   **b.** 0.4 mL

$$mL = \frac{1\ mL}{4\ \cancel{mg}} \times 1.5\ \cancel{mg} = 0.37 \text{ rounded to } 0.4\ mL \text{ Dilaudid}$$

   **c.** Equation is balanced. Estimate supports answer.

   **d.** 1 mL

   **e.** 1 mL

$$\frac{mg}{mL} = \frac{1\ mL}{\cancel{0.4\ mg}} \times \cancel{0.4\ mg} = 1\ mL \text{ Atropine}$$

   **f.** Equation is balanced. Estimate supports answer.

   **g.**    0.4 Dilaudid

   $$\underline{+\ 1.0\ \text{Atropine}}$$

   1.4 mL Total Volume

**3  a.** prepare slightly less than 1 mL

   **b.** 0.8 mL

$$mL = \frac{1\ mL}{\underset{5}{\cancel{10\ mg}}} \times \overset{4}{\cancel{8\ mg}} = 0.8\ mL \text{ Morphine}$$

   **c.** Equation is balanced. Estimate supports DA equation.

   **d.** Prepare more than 1 mL.

   **e.** 1.5 mL

$$mL = \frac{1\ mL}{\underset{2}{\cancel{0.4\ mg}}} \times \overset{3}{\cancel{0.6\ mg}} = 1.5\ mL \text{ Atropine}$$

   **f.** Equation is balanced. Estimate supports DA equation.

   **g.**    0.8 mL Morphine

   $$\underline{+\ 1.5\ mL\ \text{Atropine}}$$

   2.3 mL Total Volume

**4  a.** less than 1 mL.

   **b.** $mL = \dfrac{1\ mL}{4\ \cancel{mg}} \times 3\ \cancel{mg} = 0.75\ mL$ rounded to 0.8 mL Dilaudid

   **c.** Equation is balanced. Estimate supports answer.

   **d.** Prepare more than 1 mL.

**e.** mL = $\dfrac{1 \text{ mL}}{5 \text{ mg}}$ × 8 ~~mg~~ = 1.6 mL Compazine

**f.** Equation is balanced. Estimate supports answer.

**g.**   0.8 mL Dilaudid

  + 1.6 mL Compazine

  ───────────────

  2.4 mL Total Volume

**5 a.** prepare more than 1 mL.

**b.** 1.5 mL

  mL = $\dfrac{\text{mL}}{10 \text{ mg}}$ × 15 ~~mg~~ = 1.5 mL Morphine

**c.** Equation is balanced. Estimate supports answer.

**d.** less than 1 mL.

**e.** 0.7 mL

  mL = $\dfrac{1 \text{ mL}}{\underset{10}{\cancel{50 \text{ mg}}}}$ × $\overset{7}{\cancel{35 \text{ mg}}}$ = 0.7 mL Vistaril

**f.** Equation is balanced. Estimate supports answer.

**g.**   1.5 mL Morphine

  + 0.7 mL Vistaril

  ───────────────

  2.2 mL Total Volume

## Chapter 8 Multiple-Choice Review

**1**  4 (1 mL Dilaudid + 0.7 mL Vistaril)    **6**  2

**2**  2                                      **7**  3

**3**  3                                      **8**  4

**4**  1                                      **9**  1

**5**  3                                      **10**  4

1 **a.** less than 1 mL

   **b.** 0.8 mL

   $$mL = \frac{1\ mL}{4\ \cancel{mg}} \times 3\ \cancel{mg} = 0.75\ mL\ Dilaudid \rightarrow 0.8\ mL$$

   **c.** less than 1 mL

   **d.** 0.8 mL

   $$mL = \frac{1\ mL}{\cancel{50\ mg}\ _5} \times \cancel{40\ mg}^{\ 4} = 0.8\ mL$$

   **e.** Total combined volume = 0.8 mL Dilaudid

   $$\underline{+\ 0.8\ mL\ Vistaril}$$
   $$1.6\ mL$$

2 **a.** less than 1 mL

   **b.** 0.7 mL

   $$mL = \frac{1\ mL}{\cancel{50\ mg}\ _{10}} \times \cancel{35\ mg}^{\ 7} = 0.7\ mL$$

   **c.** 2 mL
   **d.** 2 mL

   $$mL = \frac{1\ mL}{\cancel{5\ mg}\ _1} \times \cancel{10\ mg}^{\ 2} = 2\ mL$$

   **e.** Total combined volume = 0.7 mL Meperidine

   $$\underline{+\ 2.0\ mL\ Compazine}$$
   $$2.7\ mL$$

3 **a.** Slightly less than 1 mL
   **b.** 0.8 mL

   $$mL = \frac{1\ mL}{\cancel{15\ mg}\ _5} \times \cancel{12\ mg}^{\ 4} = \frac{4}{5} = 0.8\ mL$$

   Equation is balanced. Estimate supports answer.

   **c.** $\frac{3}{4}$ of 2 mL or 1.5 mL

   **d.** 1.5 mL

$$mL = \frac{2\text{ mL}}{0.4\text{ mg}} \times 0.3\text{ mg} = \frac{0.6}{0.4} = 1.5\text{ mL}$$

**e.** $1.5 + 0.8 = 2.3$ mL total

**4 a.** less than 1 mL

**b.** 0.3 mL

$$mL = \frac{1\text{ mL}}{\underset{3}{\cancel{30\text{ mg}}}} \times \overset{1}{\cancel{10\text{ mg}}} = 0.33 \to 0.3\text{ mL}$$

Equation is balanced. Estimate supports answer.

**5 a.** 2 grams

**b.** 6.6 mL

**c.** 250 mg/ mL

**d.** more than 1.5 mL

**e.** 1.6 mL

$$mL = \frac{1\text{ mL}}{\underset{1}{\cancel{250\text{ mg}}}} \times \frac{\overset{4}{\cancel{1000\text{ mg}}}}{1\text{ g}} \times 0.4\text{ g} = 1.6\text{ mL}$$

**6 a.** 1 gram

**b.** 3.5 mL

**c.** 250 mg/ mL

**d.** more than 0.5 mL

**e.** 0.8 mL

$$mL = \frac{1\text{ mL}}{\underset{1}{\cancel{250\text{ mg}}}} \times \frac{\overset{4}{\cancel{1000\text{ mg}}}}{1\text{ g}} \times 0.2\text{ g} = 0.8\text{ mL}$$

**7** **a.** 120 mg

   **b.** 1 mL SW for injection

   **c.** 120 mg/ mL

   **d.** Slightly less than 1 mL

   **e.** 0.8 mL

   $$mL = \frac{1\ mL}{120\ \cancel{mg}} \times \frac{1000\ \cancel{mg}}{1\ \cancel{g}} \times 0.1\ \cancel{g} = \frac{10}{12} = \frac{5}{6} = 0.83\ mL \text{ rounded to } 0.8\ mL \text{ for this syringe}$$

   Equation is balanced. Estimate supports answer.

**8** **a.** 1,000,000 units

   **b.** 4.6 mL

   **c.** 200,000 units/ mL unit dose concentration

   **d.** 2 mL

   **e.** 2 mL

   $$mL = \frac{1\ mL}{\frac{200{,}000\ units}{1}} \times \overset{2}{\cancel{400{,}000\ units}} = 2\ mL$$

**9** **a.** less than 1 mL

   **b.** 400 mg/ mL

   **c.** $\frac{3}{4}$ of a mL

   **d.** 0.8 mL

   $$mL = \frac{1\ mL}{\underset{4}{\cancel{400\ mg}}} \times \overset{3}{\cancel{300\ mg}} = 0.75\ mL \rightarrow 0.8\ mL$$

   Answer supports estimate.

**10 a.** 0.4 mg/ mL = 400 mcg/ mL
**b.** 0.5 mL (0.2 mg = 200 mcg)
**c.** 0.5 mL

$$mL = \frac{1 \ mL}{\underset{2}{0.4 \ mg}} \times \overset{1}{0.2 \ mg} = 0.5 \ mL$$

Answer supports estimate.

# Chapter 9

## Rapid Practice 9-1

1 A continuous IV does not have a stop date or time. Intermittent IVs are delivered at intervals; they do not continue indefinitely.

2 A primary line is the main IV line. A secondary line connects to ports on the primary tubing line for additional medications and solutions to be added.

3 **a.** DF refers to the number of drops per mL delivered through IV tubing, on gravity infusion equipment.
**b.** A microdrip (pediatric) set delivers the smallest drops (60 drops per mL).

4 Nonvolumetric EID are gravity dependent. Volumetric pumps are not gravity dependent. They deliver fluids under positive pressure.

5 mL per hr

## Rapid Practice 9-2

1 3                              4 1

2 2                              5 3

3 2

## Rapid Practice 9-3

| Order | Abbreviation(s) for solution | Flow Rate (mL/ hr) | Time to infuse (hr and min if applicable) |
|---|---|---|---|
| 1 Infuse 500 mL normal saline over 6 hr | NS | 83 | 6 hr |
| 2 1000 mL 5% dextrose in water @ 125 mL/ hr | D5W 5DW | 125 | 8 hr |
| 3 1 L lactated Ringer's q10h | LRS RLS | 100 | 10 hr |
| 4 250 mL half-strength normal saline q4h | 0.45% NaCl Sol $\frac{1}{2}$ NS $\frac{1}{2}$ strength NS | 63 | 4 hr |
| 5 500 mL 5% dextrose in lactated Ringer's @ 40 mL per hr | D5 L/R D5 R/L | 40 | 12 hr, 30 min |

## Rapid Practice 9-4

2 **a.** 83 mL/ hr (1000 ÷ 12)

   **b.** 28 drops/ min

$$\frac{drops}{minute} = \frac{\overset{1}{\cancel{20}} \ drops}{1 \ \cancel{mL}} \times \frac{1000 \ \cancel{mL}}{12 \ \cancel{hr}} \times \frac{1 \ \cancel{hr}}{\underset{3}{\cancel{60}} \ min} = \frac{1000}{36} = 27.7 \rightarrow 28 \ drops/ \ min$$

   **c.** Equation is balanced. Only drops/ min remain. Min had to be entered in a conversion formula in the denominator to match the desired answer.

   **Comment:** Remember that a slash means "per" and is a dividing line.

3 **a.** 75 mL/ hr

   **b.** 13 drops/ min

$$\frac{drops}{min} = \frac{\overset{1}{\cancel{10}} \ drops}{1 \ \cancel{mL}} \times \frac{75 \ \cancel{mL}}{1 \ \cancel{hr}} \times \frac{1 \ \cancel{hr}}{\underset{6}{\cancel{60}} \ min} = \frac{75}{6} = 12.5 \rightarrow 13 \ drops/ \ min$$

   **c.** Equation is balanced. Only drops/ min remain.

4 **a.** 83 mL/ hr

$$\frac{mL}{hr} = \frac{500 \ mL}{6 \ hr} = 83.3 \rightarrow 83 \ mL \ per \ hr$$

   **b.** 28 drops/ min

$$\frac{drops}{minute} = \frac{\overset{1}{\cancel{20}} \ drops}{1 \ \cancel{mL}} \times \frac{500 \ \cancel{mL}}{6 \ \cancel{hr}} \times \frac{1 \ \cancel{hr}}{\underset{3}{\cancel{60}} \ min} = \frac{500}{18} = 27.7 \rightarrow 28 \ drops/ \ min$$

   **c.** Equation is balanced. Only drops/ min remain.

   **Comment:** $\frac{83 \ mL}{1 \ hr}$ could have been substituted for $\frac{500 \ mL}{6 \ hr}$ in the equation.

**5 a.** 10 hours; $100 \div 10 = 10$ hr duration

**b.** 10 drops/ min

$$\frac{\text{drops}}{\text{minute}} = \frac{\cancel{60}\,\text{drops}}{1\,\cancel{\text{mL}}} \times \frac{10\,\cancel{\text{mL}}}{1\,\cancel{\text{hr}}} \times \frac{1\,\cancel{\text{hr}}}{\cancel{60}\,\text{min}} = 10 \text{ drops per minute}$$

**c.** Equation is balanced. Only drops/ min remain.

**Comment:** Note that the 60 DF and 60 min cancel each other so that mL/ hr (10) = drops/ min (10).

## Rapid Practice 9-5

**1** 75 mL/ hr

$$\frac{\text{mL}}{\text{hr}} = \frac{600\,\text{mL}}{8\,\text{hr}} = 75 \text{ mL/ hr}$$

**2 a.** 25 mL/ hr will equal 25 drops/ min because the DF is 60.

**b.** 25 drops/ min

$$\frac{\text{drops}}{\text{min}} = \frac{\cancel{60}\,\text{drops}}{1\,\cancel{\text{mL}}} \times \frac{25\,\cancel{\text{mL}}}{1\,\cancel{\text{hr}}} \times \frac{1\,\cancel{\text{hr}}}{\cancel{60}\,\text{min}} = 25 \text{ drops/ min}$$

**c.** Equation is balanced. Estimate equals answer.

**3 a.** 13 drops/ min

$$\frac{\text{drops}}{\text{min}} = \frac{\overset{1}{\cancel{10}}\,\text{drops}}{1\,\cancel{\text{mL}}} \times \frac{80\,\cancel{\text{mL}}}{1\,\cancel{\text{hr}}} \times \frac{1\,\cancel{\text{hr}}}{\underset{6}{\cancel{60}}\,\text{min}} = \frac{80}{6} = 13 \text{ drops/ min}$$

**b.** Equation is balanced. Only $\dfrac{\text{drops}}{\text{minute}}$ remain.

**c.** Yes. The flow rate can be converted.

**4 a.** 6 drops/ min

$$\frac{\text{drops}}{\text{min}} = \frac{\overset{1}{\cancel{15}}\,\text{drops}}{1\,\cancel{\text{mL}}} \times \frac{25\,\cancel{\text{mL}}}{1\,\cancel{\text{hr}}} \times \frac{1\,\cancel{\text{hr}}}{\underset{4}{\cancel{60}}\,\text{min}} = \frac{25}{4} = 6.25 \to 6 \text{ drops/ min}$$

**b.** Equation is balanced. Only drops/ min remain.

**c.** Yes. 6 drops per minute can be counted.

**Comment:** It is a very slow rate. The site may coagulate. It would be better to change to smaller tubing such as DF60. Then the flow rate would be 25 drops/ min.

**5 a.** 33 drops/ min

$$\frac{\text{drops}}{\text{min}} = \frac{\overset{1}{\cancel{20}}\,\text{drop}}{1\,\cancel{\text{mL}}} \times \frac{100\,\cancel{\text{mL}}}{1\,\cancel{\text{hr}}} \times \frac{1\,\cancel{\text{hr}}}{\underset{3}{\cancel{60}}\,\text{min}} = \frac{100}{3} = 33.3 \to 33 \text{ drops/ min.}$$

**b.** Equation is balanced. Only drops/ min remain.

**c.** Yes. 20 drops per minute can be counted.

## Rapid Practice 9-6

**1 a.** 10 drops/ min because DF is 60.

**b.** Microdrip

**c.** A needle-like projection delivers the small drops for the microdrip (pediatric) tubing.

**2 a.** 17 drops/ min

$$\frac{\text{drops}}{\text{min}} = \frac{\overset{1}{\cancel{10}}\ \text{drops}}{1\ \cancel{\text{mL}}} \times \frac{100\ \cancel{\text{mL}}}{1\ \cancel{\text{hr}}} \times \frac{1\ \cancel{\text{hr}}}{\underset{6}{\cancel{60}}\ \text{min}} = \frac{100}{6} = 16.6 \rightarrow 17\ \text{drops/ min}$$

**b.** Equation is balanced. Only drops/ min remain. Note that 1 hr = 60 min is often the last entry in DF equations.

**3 a.** 31 drops/ min

$$\frac{\text{drops}}{\text{minute}} = \frac{\overset{1}{\cancel{15}}\ \text{drops}}{1\ \cancel{\text{mL}}} \times \frac{125\ \cancel{\text{mL}}}{1\ \cancel{\text{hr}}} \times \frac{1\ \cancel{\text{hr}}}{\underset{4}{\cancel{60}}\ \text{min}} = \frac{125}{4} = 31\ \text{drops/ min}$$

**b.** Equation is balanced. Only drops/ min remain.

**4 a.** 25 drops/ min

$$\frac{\text{drops}}{\text{min}} = \frac{\overset{1}{\cancel{20}}\ \text{drops}}{1\ \cancel{\text{mL}}} \times \frac{75\ \cancel{\text{mL}}}{1\ \cancel{\text{hr}}} \times \frac{1\ \cancel{\text{hr}}}{\underset{3}{\cancel{60}}\ \text{min}} = \frac{75}{3} = 25\ \text{drops/ min}$$

**b.** Equation is balanced. Only drops/ min remain.

**5 a.** 20 drops/ min

$$\frac{\text{drops}}{\text{minute}} = \frac{\overset{1}{\cancel{10}}\ \text{drops}}{1\ \cancel{\text{mL}}} \times \frac{120\ \cancel{\text{mL}}}{1\ \cancel{\text{hr}}} \times \frac{1\ \cancel{\text{hr}}}{\underset{6}{\cancel{60}}\ \text{min}} = \frac{120}{6} = 20\ \text{drops/ min}$$

**b.** Equation is balanced. Only drops/ min remain.

## Rapid Practice 9-7

**1 a.** 21 drops/ min

$$\frac{\text{drops}}{\text{minute}} = \frac{\overset{1}{\cancel{10}}\ \text{drops}}{1\ \cancel{\text{mL}}} \times \frac{125\ \cancel{\text{mL}}}{1\ \cancel{\text{hr}}} \times \frac{1\ \cancel{\text{hr}}}{\underset{6}{\cancel{60}}\ \text{min}} = 20.8 \rightarrow 21\ \text{drops/ min}$$

**b.** Equation is balanced. Only drops/ min remain.

**2 a.** 13 drops/ min

$$\frac{\text{drops}}{\text{minute}} = \frac{\overset{1}{\cancel{15}}\ \text{drops}}{1\ \cancel{\text{mL}}} \times \frac{50\ \cancel{\text{mL}}}{1\ \cancel{\text{hr}}} \times \frac{1\ \cancel{\text{hr}}}{\underset{4}{\cancel{60}}\ \text{min}} = 12.5 \rightarrow 13\ \text{drops/ min}$$

**b.** Equation is balanced. Only drops/ min remain.

**3 a.** 17 drops/ min

$$\frac{\text{drops}}{\text{minute}} = \frac{\overset{1}{\cancel{20}}\ \text{drops}}{1\ \cancel{\text{mL}}} \times \frac{50\ \cancel{\text{mL}}}{1\ \cancel{\text{hr}}} \times \frac{1\ \cancel{\text{hr}}}{\underset{3}{\cancel{60}}\ \text{min}} = \frac{50}{3} = 16.6 \rightarrow 17\ \text{drops/ min}$$

**b.** Equation is balanced. Only drops/ min remain.

**4 a.** 13 drops/ min

$$\frac{\text{drops}}{\text{minute}} = \frac{\overset{1}{\cancel{10}}\ \text{drops}}{1\ \cancel{\text{mL}}} \times \frac{75\ \cancel{\text{mL}}}{1\ \cancel{\text{hr}}} \times \frac{1\ \cancel{\text{hr}}}{\underset{6}{\cancel{60}}\ \text{min}} = \frac{75}{6} = 12.5 \rightarrow 13\ \text{drops/ min}$$

**b.** Equation is balanced. Only drops/ min remain.

**5 a.** 40 drops/ min

$$\frac{drops}{min} = \frac{\cancel{60}\ drops}{1\ \cancel{mL}} \times \frac{40\ \cancel{mL}}{1\ \cancel{hr}} \times \frac{1\ \cancel{hr}}{\cancel{60}\ min} = 40\ drops/\ min$$

**b.** Estimate = answer. Equation is balanced.

## Rapid Practice 9-8

**2 a.** 160 mL/ hr (80 × 2)

$$\frac{mL}{hr} = \frac{80\ mL}{\underset{1}{\cancel{30\ min}}} \times \frac{\overset{2}{\cancel{60\ min}}}{1\ hr} = 160\ mL/\ hr$$

**b.** Equation is balanced. Estimate = answer.

**3 a.** 3 × 50 = 150 mL/ hr

$$\frac{mL}{hr} = \frac{50\ mL}{\underset{1}{\cancel{20\ min}}} \times \frac{\overset{3}{\cancel{60\ min}}}{1\ hr} = 150\ mL/\ hr$$

**b.** Equation is balanced. Estimate = answer.

**4 a.** 30 × 3 = 90 mL/ hr

$$\frac{mL}{hr} = \frac{30\ mL}{\underset{1}{\cancel{20\ min}}} \times \frac{\overset{3}{\cancel{60\ min}}}{1\ hr} = 90\ mL/\ hr$$

**b.** Equation is balanced. Estimate = answer.

**5 a.** 25 mL × 2 = 50 mL/ hr

$$\frac{mL}{hr} = \frac{25\ mL}{\underset{1}{\cancel{30\ min}}} \times \frac{\overset{2}{\cancel{60\ min}}}{1\ hr} = 50\ mL/\ hr$$

**b.** Equation is balanced. Estimate = answer.

## Rapid Practice 9-9

**1 a.** 150 mL per hr (50 × 3) (20 min periods)
**b.** 25 drops/ min

$$\frac{drops}{minute} = \frac{\overset{1}{\cancel{10}}\ drops}{1\ \cancel{mL}} \times \frac{50\ \cancel{mL}}{\underset{2}{\cancel{20}}\ min} = 25\ drops/\ min$$

**c.** Equation is balanced. Only drops/ min remain.

**2 a.** 100 × 2 (30 min periods) = 200 mL/ hr
**b.** 50 drops/ min

$$\frac{drops}{minute} = \frac{\overset{1}{\cancel{15}}\ drops}{1\ \cancel{mL}} \times \frac{100\ \cancel{mL}}{\underset{2}{\cancel{30}}\ min} = 50\ drops\ per\ min$$

**c.** Equation is balanced. Only drops/ min remain.

3 **a.** 75 mL/ hr
**b.** 25 drops/ min

$$\frac{\text{drops}}{\text{minute}} = \frac{\overset{1}{\cancel{20}}\text{ drops}}{1\ \cancel{\text{mL}}} \times \frac{75\ \cancel{\text{mL}}}{\underset{3}{\cancel{60}}\text{ min}} = \frac{75}{3} = 25\text{ drops/ min}$$

**c.** Equation is balanced. Only drops/ min remain.

4 **a.** 60 mL/ hr (30 min × 2) with microdrip mL/ hr = 60 drops/ min
**b.** 60 drops/ min

$$\frac{\text{drops}}{\text{minute}} = \frac{\overset{2}{\cancel{60}}\text{ drops}}{1\ \cancel{\text{mL}}} \times \frac{30\ \cancel{\text{mL}}}{\underset{1}{\cancel{30}}\text{ min}} = 60\text{ drops/ min}$$

**c.** Equation is balanced. Only drops/ min remain.

5 **a.** 150 mL/ hr (50 × 3) (three 20-min periods = 1 hr)
**b.** 25 drops/ min

$$\frac{\text{drops}}{\text{minute}} = \frac{\overset{1}{\cancel{10}}\text{ drops}}{1\ \cancel{\text{mL}}} \times \frac{50\ \cancel{\text{mL}}}{\underset{2}{\cancel{20}}\text{ min}} = 25\text{ drops/ min}$$

**c.** Equation is balanced. Only drops/ min remain.

## Rapid Practice 9-10

| Order | Estimated flow rate | DA |
|---|---|---|
| 2 30-mL anticancer medication to infuse in 20 min on EID | 90 mL/ hr (three 20-min volumes in 60 min/ 1 hr) | $\text{mL} = \dfrac{30\text{ mL}}{\underset{1}{\cancel{20\text{ min}}}} \times \dfrac{\overset{3}{\cancel{60\text{ min}}}}{1\text{ hr}} = 90\text{ mL/ hr}$ |
| 3 20-mL antibiotic solution to infuse in 30 min on Gravity Device DF60 | 40 ml/ hr (20 mL × 2) (2 × 30 min = 60 min) | $\dfrac{\text{drops}}{\text{min}} = \dfrac{\overset{2}{\cancel{60}}\text{ drops}}{1\ \cancel{\text{mL}}} \times \dfrac{20\ \cancel{\text{mL}}}{\underset{1}{\cancel{30}}\text{ min}} = 40\text{ drops/ min}$ $\left(\text{DF 60 }\dfrac{\text{drops}}{\text{min}} = \dfrac{\text{mL}}{\text{hr}}\right)$ |
| 4 60-mL antibiotic solution to infuse in 40 min on EID | 90 mL/ hr (half the rate of a 20-min order) (180 ÷ 2) | $\dfrac{\text{mL}}{\text{hr}} = \dfrac{60\text{ mL}}{\underset{2}{\cancel{40\text{ min}}}} \times \dfrac{\overset{3}{\cancel{60\text{ min}}}}{1\text{ hr}} = \dfrac{180}{2} = 90\text{ mL/ hr}$ |
| 5 25-mL antibiotic solution in 20 min on Gravity Infusion Device DF20 | 75 mL/ hr (3-20 min periods in 60 minutes) | $\dfrac{\text{drops}}{\text{min}} = \dfrac{\cancel{20}\text{ drops}}{1\ \cancel{\text{mL}}} \times \dfrac{25\ \cancel{\text{mL}}}{\cancel{20}\text{ min}} = 25\text{ drops/ min}$ |

## Rapid Practice 9-11

| Order | Equipment Available | Continuous or Intermittent | Flow Rate Equation (Label Answer) |
|---|---|---|---|
| 1 1000 mL D5W q10h | IV administration set DF 10 | Continuous | $\dfrac{drops}{min} = \dfrac{\cancel{10}\ drops}{1\ \cancel{mL}} \times \dfrac{1000\ \cancel{mL}}{\cancel{10}\ \cancel{hr}} \times \dfrac{1\ \cancel{hr}}{60\ min} = \dfrac{1000}{60}$ $= 17\ drops/\ min$ |
| 2 50 mL antibiotic solution to infuse over 20 minutes | Volumetric pump | Intermittent | $\dfrac{mL}{hr} = \dfrac{50\ mL}{\cancel{20\ min}_1} \times \dfrac{\cancel{60\ min}^3}{1\ hr} = 150\ mL/\ hr$ |
| 3 250 mL D5W over 4 hours | Electronic rate controller | Continuous | $\dfrac{mL}{hr} = \dfrac{250\ mL}{4\ hr} = 62.5 \to 63\ mL/\ hr$ |
| 4 500 mL NS q6h | IV administration set DF 15 | Continuous | $\dfrac{drops}{min} = \dfrac{\cancel{15}\ drops}{1\ \cancel{mL}} \times \dfrac{500\ \cancel{mL}}{\cancel{6}\ \cancel{hr}} \times \dfrac{1\ \cancel{hr}}{\cancel{60}\ min} = \dfrac{500}{24}$ $= 20.8 \to 21\ drops/\ min$ |
| 5 30 mL antibiotic solution to infuse over 30 minutes | Pediatric micro-drip administration set | Intermittent | $\dfrac{drops}{min} = \dfrac{60\ drops}{1\ \cancel{mL}} \times \dfrac{\cancel{30\ mL}}{\cancel{30}\ min} = 60\ drops/\ min$ |

## Rapid Practice 9-12

| Drop Count/ Time | Drops/ Min (Mental Calculation) | Administration Set DF | Flow Rate Equation |
|---|---|---|---|
| 8 drops/ 30 sec | 16 | 10 | $\dfrac{mL}{hr} = \dfrac{1\ mL}{\cancel{10}\ drops}_1 \times \dfrac{16\ \cancel{drops}}{1\ \cancel{min}} \times \dfrac{\cancel{60\ min}^6}{1\ hr} = 96\ mL/\ hr$ |
| 6 drops/ 15 sec | 24 | 60 | $\dfrac{mL}{hr} = \dfrac{1\ mL}{\cancel{60}\ drops} \times \dfrac{24\ \cancel{drops}}{1\ \cancel{min}} \times \dfrac{\cancel{60\ min}}{1\ hr} = 24\ mL/\ hr$ |
| 12 drops/ 30 sec | 24 | 15 | $\dfrac{mL}{hr} = \dfrac{1\ mL}{\cancel{15}\ drops}_1 \times \dfrac{24\ \cancel{drops}}{1\ \cancel{min}} \times \dfrac{\cancel{60\ min}^4}{1\ hr} = 96\ mL/\ hr$ |
| 15 drops/ 30 sec | 30 | 60 | $\dfrac{mL}{hr} = \dfrac{1\ mL}{\cancel{60}\ drops} \times \dfrac{30\ \cancel{drops}}{1\ \cancel{min}} \times \dfrac{\cancel{60\ min}}{1\ hr} = 30\ mL/\ hr$ |

## Rapid Practice 9-13

| | |
|---|---|
| **1** 2 | **4** 2 |
| **2** 4 | **5** 3 |
| **3** 3 | |

## Rapid Practice 9-14

**1 a.** macrodrip
   **b.** 150 mL/ hr
   **c.** 38 drops/ min

$$\frac{drops}{minute} = \frac{\overset{1}{\cancel{15}}\ drops}{1\ \cancel{mL}} \times \frac{150\ \cancel{mL}}{\underset{4}{\cancel{60}}\ min} = \frac{150}{4} = 37.5 \rightarrow 38\ drops/\ min$$

   **d.** Equation is balanced. Only drops/ min remain.
   **e.** 6 hr 42 min infusion duration time

$$hr = \frac{1\ hr}{\underset{3}{\cancel{150\ mL}}} \times \overset{20}{\cancel{1000\ mL}} = 6.66 \rightarrow 6.7\ hr$$

$$min = \frac{60\ min}{1\ \cancel{hr}} \times 0.7\ \cancel{hrs} = 42\ min$$

**2 a.** microdrip
   **b.** 50 drops/ min

$$\frac{drops}{minute} = \frac{\cancel{60}\ drops}{1\ \cancel{mL}} \times \frac{500\ \cancel{mL}}{10\ \cancel{hr}} \times \frac{1\ \cancel{hr}}{\cancel{60}\ min} = \frac{500}{10} = 50\ drops/\ min$$

   **c.** Equation is balanced. Only drops/ min remain.

**3 a.** macrodrip
   **b.** 21 drops/ min

$$\frac{drops}{minute} = \frac{\overset{1}{\cancel{10}}\ drops}{1\ \cancel{mL}} \times \frac{1000\ \cancel{mL}}{8\ \cancel{hr}} \times \frac{1\ \cancel{hr}}{\underset{6}{\cancel{60}}\ min} = \frac{1000}{48} = 20.8 \rightarrow 21\ drops/\ min$$

   **c.** Equation is balanced. Only drops/ min remain.

**4 a.** macrodrip
   **b.** 7 drops/ min

$$\frac{drops}{minute} = \frac{\overset{1}{\cancel{10}}\ drops}{1\ \cancel{mL}} \times \frac{40\ \cancel{mL}}{\underset{6}{\cancel{60}}\ min} = \frac{40}{6} = 6.6 \rightarrow 7\ drops/\ min$$

   **c.** Equation is balanced. Only drops/ min remain.

**5 a.** macrodrip
   **b.** 33 drops/ min

$$\frac{drops}{minute} = \frac{\overset{1}{\cancel{20}}\ drops}{1\ \cancel{mL}} \times \frac{100\ \cancel{mL}}{\underset{3}{\cancel{60}}\ min} = \frac{100}{3} = 33\ drops/\ min$$

   **c.** Equation is balanced. Only drops/ min remain.

# Rapid Practice 9-15

**1 a.** 21 drops/ min

$$\frac{\text{drops}}{\text{minute}} = \frac{\overset{1}{\cancel{15}}\text{ drops}}{1\text{ }\cancel{mL}} \times \frac{\overset{250}{\cancel{1000}\text{ }\cancel{mL}}}{12\text{ }\cancel{hr}} \times \frac{1\text{ }\cancel{hr}}{\underset{\underset{1}{4}}{\cancel{60}}\text{ min}} = \frac{250}{12} = 20.8 \rightarrow 21\text{ drops/ min}$$

**b.** Equation is balanced. Only drops/ min remain.

**2 a.** 125 mL/ hr

$$\frac{\text{mL}}{\text{hr}} = \frac{500}{4} = 125\text{ mL/ hr}$$

**b.** Equation is balanced. Only mL/ hr remain.

**3 a.** 125 mL/ hr

$$\frac{\text{mL}}{\text{hr}} = \frac{1000\text{ mL}}{8\text{ hr}} = 125\text{ mL/ hr}$$

**b. Comment:** mL/ hr can be dialed on a dial-a-flow device.

**4 a.** 14 drops/ min

$$\frac{\text{drops}}{\text{min}} = \frac{\overset{1}{\cancel{20}}\text{ drops}}{1\text{ }\cancel{mL}} \times \frac{250\text{ }\cancel{mL}}{6\text{ }\cancel{hr}} \times \frac{1\text{ }\cancel{hr}}{\underset{3}{\cancel{60}}\text{ min}} = \frac{250}{18} = 13.6 \rightarrow 14\text{ drops/ min}$$

**b.** Equation is balanced. Only mL/ hr remain.

**5 a.** 42 drops/ min

$$\frac{\text{drops}}{\text{min}} = \frac{\overset{1}{\cancel{60}}\text{ drops}}{1\text{ }\cancel{mL}} \times \frac{1000\text{ }\cancel{mL}}{24\text{ }\cancel{hr}} \times \frac{1\text{ }\cancel{hr}}{\underset{1}{\cancel{60}}\text{ min}} = \frac{1000}{24} = 41.6 \rightarrow 42\text{ drops/ min}$$

**b.** Equation is balanced. Only drops/ min remain.

**Comment:** With 60 DF and a continuous IV, mL/ hr = drops/ min.

# Rapid Practice 9-16

| IV Solution Volume and Ordered Duration | Estimated Flow Rate (ml/ hr) |
| --- | --- |
| **1** 25 mL to infuse in 30 min. | 50 (2 × 25) |
| **2** 50 mL to infuse in 20 min. | 150 (3 × 50) |
| **3** 60 mL to infuse in 60 min. | 60 (60 min = 1 hr) |
| **4** 100 mL to infuse in 60 min. | 100 (60 min = 1 hr) |
| **5** 75 mL to infuse in 40 min. | 112-113 (3 × 75 ÷ 2) |
|  | (The IV will flow half as fast as in 20 min.) |

$$\frac{\text{mL}}{\text{hr}} = \frac{75\text{ mL}}{\underset{2}{\cancel{40}\text{ min}}} \times \frac{\overset{3}{\cancel{60}\text{ min}}}{1\text{ hr}} = 112.5 \rightarrow 113\text{ mL/ hr}$$

Equation is balanced. Only mL/ hr remain.

## Rapid Practice 9-17

**1 a.** 100 grams

$$g = \frac{10 \text{ g}}{\underset{1}{\cancel{100 \text{ mL}}}} \times \overset{10}{\cancel{1000 \text{ mL}}} = 100 \text{ g Dextrose}$$

**b.** Equation is balanced. Only grams remain.

**2 a.** 75

$$g = \frac{5 \text{ g}}{\underset{1}{\cancel{100 \text{ mL}}}} \times \overset{15}{\cancel{1500 \text{ mL}}} = 75 \text{ g Dextrose}$$

**b.** Equation is balanced. Only grams remain.

**3 a.** 150 grams

$$g = \frac{5 \text{ g}}{\underset{1}{\cancel{100 \text{ mL}}}} \times \overset{30}{\cancel{3000 \text{ mL}}} = 150 \text{ g Dextrose}$$

**b.** Equation is balanced. Only grams remain.

**4 a.** 200 grams

$$g = \frac{10 \text{ g}}{\underset{1}{\cancel{100 \text{ mL}}}} \times \overset{20}{\cancel{2000 \text{ mL}}} = 200 \text{ g Dextrose}$$

**b.** Equation is balanced. Only grams remain.

**5 a.** 2.25 grams

$$g = \frac{0.45 \text{ g}}{\underset{1}{\cancel{100 \text{ mL}}}} \times \overset{5}{\cancel{500 \text{ mL}}} = 2.25 \text{ g NaCl}$$

**b.** Equation is balanced. Only grams remain. Remember that NS contains slightly less than 1% NaCl. Watch the decimal.

## Rapid Practice 9-18

**1 a.** 10
**b.** 3
**c.** 250 mL; 150 mL (50 mL × 3)
**d.** ahead
**e.** 7; 250
**f.** 36 mL/ hr (250 ÷ 7)

**2 a.** 10
**b.** 7
**c.** 900 mL; 700 mL (100 mL × 7 hr)
**d.** ahead
**e.** 3; 100
**f.** 33 mL/ hr (100 ÷ 3)

**3 a.** 5 (250 ÷ 50)
**b.** 2
**c.** 50 mL; 100 mL (50 mL × 2 hr)
**d.** behind
**e.** 3; 200
**f.** 67 mL/ hr (200 ÷ 3)

**4 a.** 4
**b.** 2
**c.** 400 mL; 250 mL
**d.** ahead
**e.** 2; 100
**f.** 50 mL/ hr (100 ÷ 2)

**5 a.** 10
**b.** 2
**c.** 50 mL; 50 mL
**d.** on time
**e.** 8; 200
**f.** Continue at 25 mL/ hr. No adjustment is needed.

## Chapter 9 Multiple-Choice Review

| | | | |
|---|---|---|---|
| **1** | 2 | **6** | 1 |
| **2** | 3 | **7** | 3 |
| **3** | 3 | **8** | 3 |
| **4** | 3 | **9** | 2 |
| **5** | 2 | **10** | 4 |

## Chapter 9 Final Practice

**1** Fluid maintenance, replacement of prior losses, and replacement of concurrent losses

**2** 0.9% NaCl, D5W, L/R (RLS)

**3** secondary

**4** The tubing delivers 10 drops/ mL.

**5 a.** 60
**b.** 60 drops/ min (60 mL/ hr)

**6 a.** 2.25

$$g = \frac{0.9 \text{ g}}{\underset{2}{100 \text{ mL}}} \times \overset{5}{\cancel{250 \text{ mL}}} = \frac{4.5}{2} = 2.25 \text{ g}$$

**b.** Equation is balanced.
**c.** 10 drops/ minute

$$\frac{\text{drops}}{\text{minute}} = \frac{\overset{1}{\cancel{10} \text{ drops}}}{1 \cancel{\text{ mL}}} \times \frac{250 \cancel{\text{ mL}}}{4 \cancel{\text{ hr}}} \times \frac{1 \cancel{\text{ hr}}}{\underset{6}{60} \text{ min}} = \frac{250}{24} = 10.4 \rightarrow 10 \text{ drops/ min}$$

**d.** Equation is balanced. Only drops/ min remain.

**7 a.** 5 hr
**b.** 225 mL

$$\frac{50 \text{ mL}}{1 \cancel{\text{ hr}}} \times 4.5 \cancel{\text{ hr}} = 225 \text{ mL}$$

**8 a.** 63 mL/hr

$$\frac{mL}{hr} = \frac{500\ mL}{8\ hr} = 62.5 \rightarrow 63\ mL/hr$$

**b.** 1200 + 7.5 hr = 1930 hr

**9** Ensure that the primary IV is flowing at its ordered rate.

**10** Cardiac arrest

**11** 120 mL/hr

$$\frac{mL}{hour} = \frac{2\ mL}{1\ \cancel{min}} \times \frac{60\ \cancel{min}}{1\ hr} = 120\ mL/hr$$

**12 a.**
$$\frac{drops}{minute} = \frac{\overset{1}{\cancel{10}}\ drops}{1\ \cancel{mL}} \times \frac{250\ \cancel{mL}}{2\ \cancel{hr}} \times \frac{1\ \cancel{hr}}{\underset{6}{60}\ min} = \frac{250}{6} = 41.6 \rightarrow 42\ drops/min$$

**b.** Equation is balanced. Only drops/min remain.

**Comment:** Equation can be simplified by substituting mL/hr for total mL/total hours.

**13 a.**
$$\frac{drops}{min} = \frac{\overset{1}{\cancel{15}}\ drops}{1\ \cancel{mL}} \times \frac{3000\ \cancel{mL}}{24\ \cancel{hr}} \times \frac{1\ \cancel{hr}}{\underset{4}{60}\ min} = 31.25 = 31\ drops/min$$

**b.** Equation is balanced. Only drops per min remain.

**14 a.**
$$\frac{drops}{min} = \frac{\overset{1}{\cancel{20}}\ drops}{1\ \cancel{mL}} \times \frac{500\ \cancel{mL}}{8\ \cancel{hr}} \times \frac{1\ \cancel{hr}}{\underset{3}{60}\ min} = 20.8 \rightarrow 21\ drops/min$$

**b.** Equation is balanced. Only drops/min remain.

**15 a.** 25 g Dextrose

$$g = \frac{50\ g}{\underset{2}{100\ mL}} \times \overset{1}{\cancel{50\ mL}} = 25\ g\ Dextrose$$

**b.** Equation is balanced. Only g remain.

**16 a.** Volume-control burette device
**b.** 1-2 hr worth of ordered fluid. Refer to agency policy.

**17 a.** 600 mL
**b.** 1800 hr
**c.** 6 hours
**d.** 116.6 → 117 mL/hr (700 ÷ 6)

**18** 100 mL/hr (50 × 2)

**19 a.** 60 drops/min (20 × 3)

$$\frac{mL}{hr} = \frac{\overset{3}{\cancel{60}}\ drops}{1\ \cancel{mL}} \times \frac{20\ \cancel{mL}}{\underset{1}{\cancel{20}}\ min} = 60\ drops/min$$

**b.** Equation is balanced. Only drops/min remain.

**20** Agency policies; reason for the delay (equipment/site patency/position); whether the solution is medicated; patient condition; amount of deficit; amount of time remaining in IV schedule

# Chapter 10

## Rapid Practice 10-1

1  2                                          4  1

2  3                                          5  4

3  3

## Rapid Practice 10-2

2  **a.** $120 \div 60 = 2$ mL/ min

$$\frac{mL}{min} = \frac{\overset{2}{\cancel{120}}\ mL}{1\ \cancel{hr}} \times \frac{1\ \cancel{hr}}{\underset{1}{\cancel{60}}\ min} = 2\ mL/\ min$$

**b.** Estimate = answer.

3  **a.** $4$ mg $\times 60 = 240$ mg/ hr

$$\frac{mg}{hr} = \frac{4\ mg}{1\ \cancel{min}} \times \frac{60\ \cancel{min}}{1hr} = 240\ mg/\ hr$$

**b.** Estimate = answer.

4  **a.** $60 \div 60 = 1$ mg/ min

$$\frac{mg}{min} = \frac{\overset{1}{\cancel{60}}\ mg}{1\ \cancel{hr}} \times \frac{1\ \cancel{hr}}{\underset{1}{\cancel{60}}\ min} = 1\ mg/\ min$$

**b.** Estimate = answer.

5  **a.** $20$ mg $\times 10$ kg $= 20$ mg/ min

$$\frac{mg}{min} = \frac{2\ mg}{1\ \cancel{kg}} \times \frac{10\ \cancel{kg}}{1\ min} = 20\ mg/\ min; 2\ mg \times 10\ kg = 20\ mg/\ min$$

**b.** Estimate = answer.

**c.** $20$ mg $\times 60$ min $= 1200$ mg/ hr

$$\frac{mg}{hour} = \frac{2\ mg}{1\ \cancel{kg}} \times \frac{10\ \cancel{kg}}{1\ \cancel{min}} \times \frac{60\ \cancel{min}}{1\ hr} = 1200\ mg/\ hour$$

**d.** Estimate = answer.

**Remember:** Units following "per" need to be in the divisor of equations, e.g., mL per hr ($\frac{mL}{hr}$) and mg per minute ($\frac{mg}{minute}$).

## Rapid Practice 10-3

1  **a.** $120$ mL/ hr

$$mL = \frac{\cancel{1000}\ mL}{\cancel{1000}\ mg} \times \frac{2\ \cancel{mg}}{1\ \cancel{min}} \times \frac{60\ \cancel{min}}{1\ hr} = 120\ mL/\ hr$$

**b.** Equation is balanced. Only mL/ hr remain. Note that mL must be entered in the first numerator, and hr must be entered in a denominator in the equation.

**2  a.** 120 mL/ hr

$$\frac{mL}{hr} = \frac{\overset{2}{\cancel{1000}}\ mL}{\underset{1}{\cancel{500}\ mg}} \times \frac{1\ \cancel{mg}}{1\ \cancel{min}} \times \frac{60\ \cancel{min}}{1\ hr} = 120\ mL/\ hr$$

**b.** Equation is balanced. Only mL/ hr remain.

**3  a.** 15 mL/ hr

$$\frac{mL}{hr} = \frac{\overset{1}{\cancel{250}}\ mL}{\underset{\underset{1}{2}}{\cancel{500}\ mg}} \times \frac{0.5\ \cancel{mg}}{1\ \cancel{min}} \times \frac{\overset{30}{\cancel{60}\ \cancel{min}}}{1\ hr} = 15\ mL/\ hr$$

**b.** Equation is balanced. Only mL/ hr remain.

**4  a.** 12 mL/ hr

$$\frac{mL}{hr} = \frac{\overset{1}{\cancel{100}}\ mL}{\underset{1}{\cancel{100}\ mg}} \times \frac{0.2\ \cancel{mg}}{1\ \cancel{min}} \times \frac{60\ \cancel{min}}{1\ hr} = 12\ mL/\ hr$$

**b.** Equation is balanced. Only mL/ hr remain.

**5  a.** 96 mL/ hr

$$\frac{mL}{hr} = \frac{\overset{4}{\cancel{1000}}\ mL}{\underset{1}{\cancel{250}\ mg}} \times \frac{0.4\ \cancel{mg}}{1\ \cancel{min}} \times \frac{60\ \cancel{min}}{1\ hr} = 96\ mL/\ hr$$

**Comment:** Experienced nurses convert 1 L to 1000 mL to shorten equations.

**b.** Equation is balanced. Only mL/ hr remain.

## Rapid Practice 10-4

**2  a.** 45 mL/ hr

$$\frac{mL}{hr} = \frac{\overset{1}{\cancel{100}}\ mL}{10\ \cancel{mg}} \times \frac{1\ \cancel{mg}}{\underset{\underset{1}{10}}{\cancel{1000}\ \cancel{mcg}}} \times \frac{75\ \cancel{mcg}}{1\ \cancel{min}} \times \frac{\overset{6}{\cancel{60}\ \cancel{min}}}{1\ hr} = \frac{450}{10} = 45\ mL/\ hr$$

**b.** Equation is balanced. Only mL/ hr remain.

**3  a.** 60 mL/ hr

$$\frac{mL}{hr} = \frac{\overset{1}{\cancel{200}}\ mL}{1\ \cancel{g}} \times \frac{1\ \cancel{g}}{\underset{5}{\cancel{1000}\ mg}} \times \frac{5\ \cancel{mg}}{1\ \cancel{min}} \times \frac{60\ \cancel{min}}{1\ hr} = \frac{300}{5} = 60\ mL/\ hr$$

**b.** Equation is balanced. Only mL/ hr remain.

**4  a.** 6 mL/ hr

$$\frac{mL}{hr} = \frac{\overset{1}{\cancel{250}}\ mL}{\underset{2}{\cancel{500}\ mg}} \times \frac{1\ \cancel{mg}}{\underset{5}{\cancel{1000}\ \cancel{mcg}}} \times \frac{\overset{1}{\cancel{200}\ \cancel{mcg}}}{1\ \cancel{min}} \times \frac{60\ \cancel{min}}{1\ hr} = \frac{60}{10} = 6\ mL/\ hr$$

**b.** Equation is balanced. Only mL/ hr remain.

**5 a.** 9 mL/ hr

$$\frac{mL}{hr} = \frac{\overset{1}{\cancel{200}}\ mL}{2\ \cancel{g}} \times \frac{1\ \cancel{g}}{\underset{5}{\cancel{1000}\ \cancel{mg}}} \times \frac{1.5\ \cancel{mg}}{1\ minute} \times \frac{60\ min}{1\ hr} = \frac{90}{10} = 9\ mL/\ hr$$

**b.** Equation is balanced. Only mL/ hr remain.

## Rapid Practice 10-5

**2 a.** 40 mg

$$mg = \frac{0.5\ mg}{1\ \cancel{kg}} \times 80\ \cancel{kg} = 40\ mg$$

**b.** None

**c.**
$$\frac{mL}{hr} = \frac{\overset{1}{\cancel{250}}\ mL}{\underset{2}{\cancel{500}\ \cancel{mg}}} \times \frac{40\ \cancel{mg}}{1\ hr} = \frac{40}{2} = 20\ mL/\ hr$$

**d.** Equation is balanced. Only mL/ hr remain.

**3 a.** 88 ÷ 2.2 = 40 kg

$$\frac{mcg}{min} = \frac{0.1\ mcg}{1\ \cancel{kg}} \times \frac{40\ \cancel{kg}}{1\ min} = 4\ mcg/\ min$$

$$kg = \frac{1\ kg}{2.2\ \cancel{lb}} \times 88\ \cancel{lb} = 40\ kg$$

**b.** 2 conversion formulas: min to hr, mcg to mg.

**c.**
$$\frac{mL}{hr} = \frac{\overset{1}{\cancel{250}}\ mL}{1\ \cancel{mg}} \times \frac{1\ \cancel{mg}}{\underset{4}{\cancel{1000}\ \cancel{mcg}}} \times \frac{4\ \cancel{mcg}}{1\ \cancel{min}} \times \frac{60\ \cancel{min}}{1\ hr} = 60\ mL/\ hr$$

**d.** Equation is balanced. Only mL/ hr remain.

**4 a.** 210 mcg

$$\frac{mcg}{min} = \frac{3\ mcg}{1\ kg} \times 70\ kg = 210\ mcg$$

**b.** 2 conversion formulas: mcg to mg, min to hr.

**c.**
$$\frac{mL}{hr} = \frac{\overset{1}{\cancel{500}}\ mL}{400\ \cancel{mg}} \times \frac{1\ \cancel{mg}}{\underset{2}{\cancel{1000}\ \cancel{mcg}}} \times \frac{210\ \cancel{mcg}}{1\ \cancel{min}} \times \frac{60\ \cancel{min}}{1\ hr} = \frac{60 \times 210}{400 \times 2} = 15.7 \rightarrow 16\ mL/\ hr$$

**d.** Equation is balanced. Only mL/ hr remain.

**5 a.** 2 mg/ min

**b.** 3 conversion formulas: g to mg, min to hr, L to mL (mental calculation).

**c.**
$$\frac{mL}{hr} = \frac{\overset{1}{\cancel{1000}}\ mL}{1\ \cancel{g}} \times \frac{1\ \cancel{g}}{\underset{1}{\cancel{1000}\ \cancel{mg}}} \times \frac{2\ \cancel{mg}}{1\ \cancel{min}} \times \frac{60\ \cancel{min}}{1\ hr} = 120\ mL/\ hr$$

**d.** Equation is balanced. Only mL/ hr remain.

1 a. 75 mL/ hr

$$\frac{mL}{hr} = \frac{\overset{5}{\cancel{250}} mL}{\underset{\underset{1}{4}}{\cancel{200}} mg} \times \frac{1 \cancel{mg}}{1 \cancel{min}} \times \frac{\overset{15}{\cancel{60\ min}}}{1\ hr} = 75\ mL/\ hr$$

b. Equation is balanced. Only mL/ hr remain.

2 a. 120 mL/ hr

$$\frac{mL}{hr} = \frac{2\ mL}{1 \cancel{min}} \times \frac{60 \cancel{min}}{1\ hr} = 120\ mL/\ hr$$

b. Equation is balanced. Only mL/ hr remain.
c. No, the microdrip flow rate (DF 60) in drops per minute = the mL/ hr rate. A rate greater than 60 drops per minute is too difficult to count.

3 a. 75 mL/ hr

$$\frac{mL}{hr} = \frac{\overset{1}{\cancel{250}} mL}{1 \cancel{g}} \times \frac{1 \cancel{g}}{\underset{\underset{1}{4}}{\cancel{1000}} mg} \times \frac{5 \cancel{mg}}{1 \cancel{min}} \times \frac{\overset{15}{\cancel{60\ min}}}{1\ hr} = 75\ mL/\ hr$$

b. Equation is balanced. Only mL/ hr remain.

4 a. 352 mcg

$$\frac{mcg}{min} = \frac{8\ mcg}{1 \cancel{kg}} \times \frac{44 \cancel{kg}}{1\ min} = 352\ mcg/\ min\ \text{initial dose}$$

b. 42 mL/ hr

$$\frac{mL}{hr} = \frac{\overset{1}{\cancel{1000}} mL}{\underset{125}{\cancel{500}} mg} \times \frac{1 \cancel{mg}}{\underset{1}{\cancel{1000}} mcg} \times \frac{\overset{88}{\cancel{352}} mcg}{1 \cancel{min}} \times \frac{60 \cancel{min}}{1\ hr} = \frac{88 \times 60}{125}$$

$$= 42.2 \rightarrow 42\ mL/\ hr$$
$$\text{initial flow rate}$$

c. Equation is balanced. Only mL/ hr remain.

5 a. 440 mcg

$$\frac{mcg}{min} = \frac{10\ mcg}{1 \cancel{kg}} \times \frac{44 \cancel{kg}}{1\ min} = 440\ mcg/\ min$$

b. 53 mL/ hr

$$\frac{mL}{hr} = \frac{\overset{1}{\cancel{1000}} mL}{500 \cancel{mg}} \times \frac{1 \cancel{mg}}{\underset{1}{\cancel{1000}} mcg} \times \frac{440 \cancel{mcg}}{1 \cancel{min}} \times \frac{60 \cancel{min}}{1\ hr} = \frac{440 \times 60}{500}$$

$$= 52.8 \rightarrow 53\ mL/\ hr$$

**Comment:** Experienced nurses mentally convert 1 L to 1000 mL.

c. Equation is balanced. Only mL/ hr remain.

**2** **a.** 0.25 mg/ mL

**b.** 125 mcg/ min

$$\frac{\text{mcg}}{\text{minute}} = \frac{\overset{1}{\cancel{1000}}\,\text{mcg}}{1\,\cancel{\text{mg}}} \times \frac{250\,\cancel{\text{mg}}}{\underset{1}{\cancel{1000\,\text{mL}}}} \times \frac{\overset{1}{\cancel{30\,\text{mL}}}}{1\,\cancel{\text{hr}}} \times \frac{1\,\cancel{\text{hr}}}{\underset{2}{60}\,\text{min}} = \frac{250}{2}$$

$$= 125\,\text{mcg/ min}$$

**c.** Equation is balanced. Only mg/ min remain.

**Comment:** The mcg to mg conversion formula had to be entered first because mcg were needed in the first numerator.

**3** **a.** 2 mg/ mL (500 mg/ 250 mL)

**b.** 83 mg/ min

$$\frac{\text{mg}}{\text{min}} = \frac{\overset{2}{\cancel{500}}\,\text{mg}}{\underset{1}{\cancel{250\,\text{mL}}}} \times \frac{\overset{5}{\cancel{25\,\text{mL}}}}{1\,\cancel{\text{hr}}} \times \frac{1\,\cancel{\text{hr}}}{\underset{12}{60}\,\text{min}} = 0.83\,\text{mg/ min}$$

**c.** Equation is balanced. Only mg/ min remain.

**4** **a.** 4 mg/ mL (1000 mg/ 250 mL)

**b.** 0.66 mg/ min

$$\frac{\text{mg}}{\text{minute}} = \frac{\overset{4}{\cancel{1000}}\,\text{mg}}{1\,\cancel{\text{g}}} \times \frac{1\,\cancel{\text{g}}}{\underset{1}{\cancel{250\,\text{mL}}}} \times \frac{\overset{1}{\cancel{10\,\text{mL}}}}{\cancel{\text{hr}}} \times \frac{1\,\cancel{\text{hr}}}{\underset{6}{60}\,\text{min}} = \frac{4}{6} = 0.66\,\text{mg/ min}$$

**c.** Equation is balanced. Only mg/ min remain.

**Comment:** The mg to g conversion formula had to be entered first because mg were needed in the first numerator.

**5** **a.** 1 mg/ mL (500 mg/ 500 mL)

**b.** 0.2 mg/ min

$$\frac{\text{mg}}{\text{min}} = \frac{\overset{1}{\cancel{500}}\,\text{mg}}{\underset{1}{\cancel{500\,\text{mL}}}} \times \frac{\overset{1}{\cancel{12\,\text{mL}}}}{1\,\cancel{\text{hr}}} \times \frac{1\,\cancel{\text{hr}}}{\underset{5}{60}\,\text{min}} = \frac{1}{5} = 0.2\,\text{mg/ min}$$

**c.** Equation is balanced. Only mg/ min remain.

## Rapid Practice 10-8

**1** **a.** 2 mL

$$\text{mL} = \frac{1\,\text{mL}}{\underset{1}{\cancel{0.4\,\text{mg}}}} \times \overset{2}{\cancel{0.8\,\text{mg}}} = 2\,\text{mL}$$

**b.** 5 mL

**c.** 1 minute

**d.** 5 mL/ min

**e.** 25 calibrations for 5 mL in a 10-mL syringe

**f.** 60 seconds (= 1 minute)

**g.** 2.4 seconds/ calibration

$$\frac{\text{seconds}}{\text{calibration}} = \frac{60}{25} = 2.4\,\text{seconds/ calibration}$$

**h.** Equation is balanced. Only seconds/ calibration remain.

**2 a.** 2 mL

$$mL = \frac{1\ mL}{\underset{1}{\cancel{5\ mg}}} \times \overset{2}{\cancel{10\ mg}} = 2\ mL\ (DA\ equation\ will\ go\ here)$$

**b.** N/A; 2 mL undiluted is total amount
**c.** 2 minutes
**d.** 1 mL/ min (5 mg/ min)
**e.** 20 calibrations for 2 mL on a 3-mL syringe
**f.** 120 seconds
**g.** 6 seconds/ calibration

$$\frac{sec}{calibration} = \frac{120}{20} = 6\ seconds/\ calibration$$

**h.** Equation is balanced. Only seconds/ calibration remain.

**3 a.** 0.8 mL

$$mL = \frac{1\ mL}{\underset{4}{\cancel{120\ mg}}} \times \overset{3}{\cancel{90\ mg}} \rightarrow 0.75\ rounded\ to\ 0.8\ mL$$

**b.** 3 mL
**c.** 3 minutes
**d.** 1 mL/ min
**e.** 30 calibrations on a 3-mL syringe
**f.** 180 seconds (3 minutes)
**g.** 12 seconds/ calibration

$$\frac{sec}{calibration} = \frac{180}{15} = 12\ seconds/\ calibration$$

**h.** Equation is balanced. Only seconds/ calibration remain.

**4 a.** 0.7 mL

$$mL = \frac{1\ mL}{\underset{3}{\cancel{75\ mg}}} \times \overset{2}{\cancel{50\ mg}} = 0.66\ rounded\ to\ 0.7\ mL$$

**b.** 5 mL
**c.** 5 minutes
**d.** 1 mL/ min
**e.** 25 calibrations
**f.** 300 (5 × 60) seconds
**g.** 12 seconds/ calibration

$$\frac{sec}{calibration} = \frac{300}{25} = 12\ seconds/\ calibration$$

**h.** Equation is balanced. Only seconds/ calibration remain.

**5 a.** 4 mL
**b.** N/A
**c.** 10 minutes (4 mg/ min)
**d.** 0.4 mL/ min
**e.** 20 calibrations in 5-mL syringe
**f.** 600 (10 × 60) seconds
**g.** 30 seconds/ calibration

$$\frac{sec}{calibration} = \frac{600}{20} = 30\ seconds/\ calibration$$

**h.** Equation is balanced. Only seconds/ calibration remain.

**1** 4

$$(2 \text{ mL} \times 60 \text{ min}/\text{hr})\left( \frac{2 \text{ mL}}{1 \text{ min}} \times \frac{60 \text{ min}}{1 \text{ hr}} = \frac{120 \text{ mL}}{\text{hr}} \right)$$

**2** 4

$$\frac{\text{mL}}{\text{hr}} = \frac{500 \text{ mL}}{\overset{}{\underset{4}{40 \text{ mEq}}}} \times \frac{\overset{1}{10 \text{ mEq}}}{1 \text{ hr}} - \frac{500}{4} = 125 \text{ mL}/\text{hr}$$

**3** 1

$$\frac{\text{mg}}{\text{mL}} = \frac{\overset{4}{1000} \text{ mg (1 g)}}{\underset{1}{250}} \ \ \text{mg} = 4 \text{ mg}/\text{mL}$$

**4** 4

$$\text{g} = \frac{25 \text{ g}}{\underset{1}{100 \text{ mL}}} \times \overset{10}{1000 \text{ mL}} = 250 \text{ g}$$

$$\text{kcal} = \frac{4 \text{ kcal}}{1 \text{ g}} \times 250 \text{ g} = 1000 \text{ kcal Dextrose}$$

**5** 2

$$\frac{\text{drops}}{\text{min}} = \frac{60 \text{ drops}}{1 \text{ mL}} \times \frac{\overset{1}{30 \text{ mL}}}{\underset{1}{30 \text{ min}}} = \frac{60 \text{ drops}}{\text{min}}$$

**6** 1

The diluted volume is used for the calculation: 5 mL in 5 minutes = 1 mL in 1 minute

**7** 4

**8** 2

$$\frac{500 \text{ mL remaining}}{3 \text{ hr remaining}} = 167 \text{ mL}/\text{hr}$$

**9** 3

1 mg for each mL is the most concentrated solution

**10** 2

$$\frac{\text{mg}}{\text{hr}} = \frac{\overset{1}{500} \text{ mg}}{\underset{2}{1000 \text{ mL}}} \times \frac{10 \text{ mL}}{1 \text{ hr}} = \frac{10}{2} = 5 \text{ mg}/\text{hr}$$

**1 a.** 3 mL

$$mL = \frac{4\ mL}{\underset{4}{40\ mg}} \times \overset{3}{\cancel{30\ mg}} = \frac{12}{4} = 3\ mL$$

**b.** 15 calibrations

**c.** 450 seconds

$$seconds = \frac{\overset{15}{\cancel{60}}\ sec}{1\ \cancel{min}} \times \frac{1\ \cancel{min}}{\underset{1}{4\ \cancel{mg}}} \times 30\ \cancel{mg} = 15 \times 30 = 450\ seconds$$

**d.** 30 seconds/ calibration

$$\frac{seconds}{calibration} = \frac{450\ seconds}{calibrations} = 30\ seconds/\ calibration$$

**2 a.** 11 mL/ hr

$$\frac{mg}{hr} = \frac{0.3\ mg}{1\ \cancel{kg}} \times 75\ \cancel{kg} = 22.5\ mg/\ hr\ ordered\ dose$$

$$\frac{mL}{hr} = \frac{\overset{1}{\cancel{250}}\ mL}{\underset{2}{\cancel{500}\ mg}} \times \frac{22.5\ \cancel{mg}}{1\ hr} = 11.25 \rightarrow 11\ mL/\ hr$$

Equations are balanced. Only mg/ hr and mL/ hr remain.

**b.** 15 mL/ hr

$$\frac{mg}{hr} = \frac{0.4\ mg}{1\ \cancel{kg}} \times 75\ \cancel{kg} = 30\ mg/\ hr\ ordered\ dose$$

$$\frac{mL}{hr} = \frac{\overset{1}{\cancel{250}}\ mL}{\underset{2}{\cancel{500}\ mg}} \times \frac{30\ \cancel{mg}}{1\ hr} = \frac{30}{2} = 15\ mL/\ hr$$

Equations are balanced. Only mg/ hr and mL/ hr remain.

**Comment:** See if you can set these problems up in one equation as shown on p. 341.

**3 a.** 0.2 mg/ mL

$$\frac{mg}{mL} = \frac{\overset{1}{\cancel{50}}\ mg}{\underset{5}{\cancel{250}\ mL}} = \frac{1}{5} = 0.2\ mg/\ mL\ concentration$$

Equation is balanced. Only mg/ mL remain.

**b.** 5 mL/ hr

$$\frac{mcg}{min} = \frac{0.3\ mcg}{1\ \cancel{kg}} \times \frac{60\ \cancel{kg}}{1\ min} = 18\ mcg/\ min\ ordered\ dose$$

$$\frac{mL}{hr} = \frac{\overset{\overset{1}{5}}{\cancel{250}}\ mL}{\underset{1}{\cancel{50}\ mg}} \times \frac{1\ \cancel{mg}}{\underset{200}{\cancel{1000}\ mcg}} \times \frac{18\ \cancel{mcg}}{1\ \cancel{min}} \times \frac{60\ \cancel{min}}{1\ hr} \times \frac{1080}{200} = 5.4$$

$$= 5\ mL/\ hr$$

Equations are balanced. Only mcg/ min and mL/ hr remain.

4 **a.** 0.5 mg/ mL

$$\frac{mg}{mL} = \frac{250 \text{ mg}}{500 \text{ mL}} = 0.5 \text{ mg/ mL}$$

**b.** 19 mL/ hr

$$\frac{mL}{hr} = \frac{\overset{1}{\cancel{500} \text{ mL}}}{250 \text{ } \cancel{mg}} \times \frac{1 \text{ } \cancel{mg}}{\underset{2}{1000 \text{ } \cancel{mcg}}} \times \frac{2.5 \text{ } \cancel{mcg}}{1 \text{ } \cancel{kg}} \times \frac{64 \text{ } \cancel{kg}}{1 \text{ } \cancel{min}} \times \frac{60 \text{ } \cancel{min}}{1 \text{ hr}} = 19.2$$

$$= \frac{19 \text{ mL}}{hr}$$

Equation is balanced. Only mL/ hr remain

5 125 mL/ hr

$$\frac{mL}{hr} = \frac{500 \text{ mL}}{\underset{4}{40 \text{ } \cancel{mEq}}} \times \frac{\overset{1}{\cancel{10 \text{ } mEq}}}{1 \text{ hr}} = 125 \text{ mL/ hr}$$

6 **a.** 15 mg/ hr

$$\frac{mg}{hr} = \frac{1 \text{ mg}}{1000 \text{ } \cancel{mcg}} \times \frac{3 \text{ } \cancel{mcg}}{1 \text{ } \cancel{kg}} \times \frac{82 \text{ } \cancel{kg}}{1 \text{ } \cancel{min}} \times \frac{60 \text{ } \cancel{min}}{1 \text{ hr}} = \frac{14760}{1000}$$

$$= 14.7 \text{ rounded to } 15 \text{ mg/ hr}$$

**b.** 19 mL/ hr

$$\frac{mL}{hr} = \frac{\overset{5}{\cancel{250} \text{ mL}}}{\underset{4}{\cancel{200} \text{ } \cancel{mg}}} \times \frac{15 \text{ } \cancel{mg}}{1 \text{ hr}} = \frac{75}{4} = 18.7 \text{ rounded to } 19 \text{ mL/ hr}$$

**Comment:** The nurse assesses the patient, contacts the prescriber, obtains an order to adjust the flow rate gradually to the ordered rate, and documents the incident.

7 **a.** 2.5 mL

$$mL = \frac{1 \text{ mL}}{0.4 \text{ } \cancel{mg}} \times 1 \text{ } \cancel{mg} = 2.5 \text{ mL}$$

**b.** 6 sec/ mL

$$\frac{seconds}{mL} = \frac{60 \text{ sec}}{10 \text{ mL}} = 6 \text{ sec/ mL}$$

**Comment:** Seconds per calibration are not needed for this large-volume injection.

8 **a.** 5 mL

$$mL = \frac{1 \text{ mL}}{0.4 \text{ } \cancel{mg}} \times 2 \text{ } \cancel{mg} = 5 \text{ mL}$$

**b.** 8 mL/ hr

$$\frac{mL}{hr} = \frac{500 \text{ mL}}{2 \text{ } \cancel{mg}} \times \frac{0.03 \text{ } \cancel{mg}}{1 \text{ hr}} = 7.5 \text{ mL rounded to } 8 \text{ mL/ hr}$$

**9 a.** 8 mL

$$mL = \frac{1 \text{ mL}}{\underset{1}{\cancel{500 \text{ mg}}}} \times \frac{\overset{2}{\cancel{1000 \text{ mg}}}}{1 \text{ g}} \times 4 \text{ g} = 8 \text{ mL}$$

**b.** 150 mL/ hr

$$\frac{mL}{hr} = \frac{2.5 \text{ mL}}{1 \cancel{\text{ min}}} \times \frac{60 \cancel{\text{ min}}}{1 \text{ hr}} = 150 \text{ mL/ hr}$$

**c.** 4 g = 4000 mg

$$\frac{mg}{min} = \frac{4\cancel{000} \text{ mg}}{25\cancel{0} \text{ mL}} \times \frac{2.5 \text{ mL}}{1 \text{ min}} = \frac{1000}{25} = 40 \text{ mg/ min}$$

**10 a.** 13.1 mL

$$mL = \frac{1 \text{ mL}}{\underset{8}{\cancel{80 \text{ mg}}}} \times \frac{15 \cancel{\text{ mg}}}{1 \cancel{\text{ kg}}} \times \overset{7}{\cancel{70 \text{ kg}}} = \frac{1050}{80} = 13.1 \text{ mL}$$

Equation is balanced. Only mL remain.

**b.** 63 mL/ hr

$$\frac{mL}{hr} = \frac{250 \text{ mL}}{4 \text{ hr}} = 62.5 \text{ rounded } 63 \text{ mL/ hr}$$

# Chapter 11

## Rapid Practice 11-1

**1** Stat BG—immediate, current level

FBS (fasting blood sugar)—level of blood sugar after fasting for at least 8 hours

2-hour postprandial—level 2 hours after a meal

fructosomine—average level over past 2 weeks

HbA1c (glycosylated hemoglobin)—average level over past 2 to 3 months

**2** SMBG

**3** 70-100 mg/ dL

**4** Insulin is a hormone lowers blood glucose levels by facilitating entry into muscle cells and other storage sites—insulin helps glucose get into cells

**5** Insulin shock—urgent *hypoglycemic* condition treated with glucose and other therapies

DKA—urgent *hyperglycemic* condition treated with insulin and other therapies.

## Rapid Practice 11-2

**1** Humalog (insulin lispro), Novolog (insulin aspart)

   **a. 1.** 100 units/ mL

      **2.** 1000 units (100 units × 10 mL), a multidose vial

   **b.** Dextrose

**2** Diet products do not contain dextrose

**3** Novolog (aspart), Humalog (lispro)

## Rapid Practice 11-3

1  Two injections per day, one AM and one PM.

2  No.

3  100 units/ mL

4  Cloudy

5  There is potential for overlapping duration. They are trying to avoid a hypo-glycemic episode during sleep

## Rapid Practice 11-4

1  Insulin glargine

2  Insulin glargine does not have a peak.

3  No. They contain additives.

4  100 units/ mL

5  No.

## Rapid Practice 11-5

1  16 units

2  22 units

3

4

5

## Rapid Practice 11-6

1

2 Give 12 units Humulin R subcut. Recheck BG in 1 hr.

3 Call physician immediately. Draw plasma BG.

4 To verify the accuracy of the fingerstick BG before instituting more aggressive treatment.

5 Hold insulin (0 units).

## Rapid Practice 11-7

2 **a.** intermediate
  **b.** suspension
  **c.** Yes. Some manufacturers recommend *gentle shaking*. Others recommend *rolling the vial*. Read the directions on the product.
  **d.** 6 to12 hr
  **e.** subcut
  **f.**

3 **a.** 30 minutes
  **b.** $2\frac{1}{2}$ to 5 hr
  **c.** 8 hr
  **d.**

4 **a.** 1000 units
  **b.** rapid
  **c.** 100 units/ mL

5 **a.** subcutaneous
  **b.**

## Rapid Practice 11-8

**2**

**3**

**4**

**5**

## Rapid Practice 11-9

**1 a.** 3 mL/ hr, because concentration is 1:1

   **b.** 3 mL/ hr

$$\frac{mL}{hr} = \frac{\overset{1}{\cancel{100}}\ mL}{\underset{1}{\cancel{100}\ units}} \times \frac{3\ \cancel{units}}{1\ hr} = 3\ mL/\ hr$$

   **c.** Equation is balanced. Estimate = answer.

   **Comment:** A "U" for units can be misread as a zero (0).

**2 a.** 8 mL/ hr, because concentration is 1 unit : 2 mL.

   **b.** 8 mL/ hr

$$\frac{mL}{hr} = \frac{\overset{2}{\cancel{100}}\ mL}{\underset{1}{\cancel{50}\ units}} \times \frac{4\ \cancel{units}}{1\ hr} = 8\ mL/\ hr$$

   **c.** Equation is balanced. Estimate = answer.

**3 a.** 12 mL/ hr, because concentration is 1:2.
**b.** 12 mL/ hr

$$\frac{mL}{hr} = \frac{\overset{2}{\cancel{100}}\ mL}{\underset{1}{\cancel{50}\ units}} \times \frac{6\ \cancel{units}}{1\ hr} = 12\ mL/\ hr$$

**c.** Evaluation: Equation is balanced. Estimate = answer.

**4 a.** 6 mL/ hr (half of original order)
**b.** 6 mL/ hr

$$\frac{mL}{hr} = \frac{\overset{2}{\cancel{100}}\ mL}{\underset{1}{\cancel{50}\ units}} \times \frac{3\ \cancel{units}}{hr} = 6\ mL/\ hr$$

**c.** 6 mL/ hr is 50% of original 12 mL ordered. Estimate supports answer.

**5 a.** 4 mL/ hr, because concentration is 1 unit : 2 mL.
**b.** 4 mL/ hr

$$\frac{mL}{hr} = \frac{\overset{2}{\cancel{100}}\ mL}{\underset{1}{\cancel{50}\ units}} \times \frac{2\ \cancel{units}}{1\ hr} = 4\ mL/\ hr\ ordered\ flow\ rate$$

**c.** Flow rate is incorrect. It is half the ordered rate.
**d.** Assess current BG level. Consult with prescriber for flow rate order changes. Document. Check agency policy about an incident report.

## Rapid Practice 11-10

**1 a.** Regular insulin and insulin lispro (Humalog)
**b.** clear

**2** short- and intermediate-acting

**3 a.** 100 units/ mL and 500 units/ m
**b.** U100 is the most commonly used.

**4** No.

**5 a.** The intermediate-acting insulin is usually the larger dose.
**b.** It is a modified product to cover a longer duration.

## Chapter 11 Multiple-Choice Review

**1** 4

**Comment:** If a short-acting insulin is needed, it can be given separately.

**2** 2

**3** 1

**4** 4

**5** 3

**6** 4

**7** 3

**Comment:** This helps prevent hypoglycemic episodes during sleep.

8  1

9  2

10  3

## Chapter 11 Final Practice

1  **a.** 100 units/ mL
   **b.** Regular insulin must be withdrawn first to protect it from contamination from an intermediate-acting insulin.
   **c.** Contamination would alter (lengthen) the action of the regular insulin.

2

   (The choice of syringe in the text is a 1-mL tuberculin syringe.)

3  **a.** Humulin R insulin
   **b.**

   The nurse must focus so as not to confuse the doses.

4  **a.** Novolin R
   **b.**

5  **a.** Insulin lispro is rapid acting.
   **b.**

**6 a.** 1 unit/ mL

$$\frac{\text{units}}{\text{mL}} = \frac{\overset{1}{\cancel{100}}\text{ units}}{\underset{1}{\cancel{100}}\text{ mL}} = 1 \text{ unit/ mL}$$

**b.** 5 mL/ hr of a 1:1 solution (for 5 units/ hr)

$$\frac{\text{mL}}{\text{hr}} = \frac{\overset{1}{\cancel{100}}\text{ mL}}{\underset{1}{\cancel{100}\text{ units}}} \times \frac{5\,\cancel{\text{units}}}{\text{hr}} = 5 \text{ mL/ hr}$$

**c.** Estimate = answer.

**d.** Yes. Insulin solutions for IV administration should be administered on an infusion pump.

**7 a.** 4 mL/ hr to deliver 4 units/ hr

**b.** $$\frac{\text{mL}}{\text{hr}} = \frac{\overset{1}{\cancel{100}}\text{ mL}}{\underset{1}{\cancel{100}\text{ units}}} \times \frac{4\,\cancel{\text{units}}}{1 \text{ hr}} = 4 \text{ mL per hr}$$

**c.** Estimate = Answer

**8 a.** 50 g

$$g = \frac{5 \text{ g}}{\underset{1}{\cancel{100}\text{ mL}}} \times \overset{10}{\cancel{1000 \text{ mL}}} = 50 \text{ g glucose}$$

**b.** Equation is balanced. Only grams remain.

**9 a.** $\frac{1}{2}$ of 4 mL/ hr = 2 mL/ hr

50% = 0.5 or $\frac{1}{2}$

$$\frac{\text{mL}}{\text{hr}} = \frac{\overset{2}{4}\text{ mL}}{\text{hr}} \times \frac{1}{\underset{1}{\cancel{2}}} = 2 \text{ mL/ hr}$$

**b.** Estimate = answer.

**10 a.** Short-, intermediate-, and long-acting.

**Comment:** *Endogenous insulin* refers to *insulin* produced by the individual's own beta cells. Exogenous and endogenous insulin can be differentiated by a C peptide assay test.

**b.** Dextrose, followed by a complex carbohydrate

# Chapter 12

## Rapid Practice 12-1

**1** 4

**2** 1

**3** 1

**4** 1

**5** 3

## Rapid Practice 12-2

1  3

2  4

3  4

4  3

5  3

## Rapid Practice 12-3

1  a

2  23-29 seconds ($2 \times 11.5$ sec and $2.5 \times 11.5$ sec)

3  a

4  **a.** 2
   **b.** 0.2 mL

$$mL = \frac{1\ mL}{10\ \cancel{mg}} \times 2\ \cancel{mg} = 0.2\ mL$$

   Equation is balanced. Only mL remain.

5  **a.** one half
   **b.** 2.5 mg

## Rapid Practice 12-4

1  1 mL

2  10 units/ mL

3  maintain patency of venous access devices

4  SASH includes heparin flush in addition to saline

5  10,000 units/ mL

6  1:1000

7  10,000 units/ mL

8  bleeding or hemorrhage

9  20,000 to 40,000 units

10  of possible adverse interactions

## Rapid Practice 12-5

1  Thrombocytopenia predisposes to bleeding. The addition of heparin would increase the risk.

2  **a.** 10 mL/ hr

$$\frac{mL}{hr} = \frac{\overset{1}{\cancel{250}}\ mL}{\underset{100}{\cancel{25,000\ units}}} \times 1000\ \cancel{units} = \frac{1000}{100} = 10\ mL/\ hr$$

   **b.** Equation is balanced. Only mL/ hr remains.

3 **a.** 45 to 75 seconds $(1.5 \times 30 = 45 \text{ seconds})(2.5 \times 30 = 75 \text{ seconds})$
  **b.** Yes
  **c.** No. Between 45 and 75, no adjustment is necessary.
  **d.** N/A
  **e.** N/A
  **f.** N/A

4 **a.** 45 to 75 seconds
  **b.** No
  **c.** Yes. The units/ hr need to be reduced by 1 unit/ kg/ hr.
  **d.** 80 units/ hr

$$\frac{\text{units}}{\text{hr}} = \frac{1 \text{ unit}}{1 \text{ kg}} \times \frac{80 \text{ kg}}{\text{hr}} = 80 \text{ units reduction per hour}$$

    1000 units $-$ 80 units $=$ 920 units rounded to 900 units/ hr
  **e.** Yes
  **f.** 9 mL/ hr

$$\frac{\text{mL}}{\text{hr}} = \frac{\overset{1}{\cancel{250}} \text{ mL}}{\underset{100}{\cancel{25,000 \text{ units}}}} \times 900 \,\cancel{\text{units}} = \frac{900}{100} = 9 \text{ mL/ hr}$$

5 **a.** 1600

$$\frac{\text{units}}{\text{hr}} = \frac{\overset{50}{\cancel{25,000}} \text{ units}}{\underset{1}{\cancel{500 \text{ mL}}}} \times \frac{32 \,\cancel{\text{mL}}}{\text{hr}} = 1600 \text{ units/ hr}$$

  **b.** Flow rate is correct.
  **c.** Yes $(1600 \times 24 = 38,400 \text{ units in 24 hr})$.

## Rapid Practice 12-6

1 **a.** 1100 units/ hr (1080 rounded to 1100)
  **b.** 22 mL/ hr

$$\frac{\text{mL}}{\text{hr}} = \frac{\overset{1}{\cancel{500}} \text{ mL}}{\underset{50}{\cancel{25,000 \text{ units}}}} \times 1100 \,\cancel{\text{units}} = 22 \text{ mL/ hr}$$

  **c.** Equation is balanced. Only mL/ hr remains.

2 **a.** bleeding
  **b.** 1100 units (1080 rounded to 1100)
  **c.** 550 units
  **d.** 5.5 mg

$$\text{mg} = \frac{1 \text{ mg}}{\underset{1}{\cancel{100 \text{ units}}}} \times \overset{5.5}{\cancel{550 \text{ units}}} = 5.5 \text{ mg protamine sulfate}$$

  **e.** Equation is balanced. Only mg remain.

3 **a.** 0.6 mL

$$\frac{1 \text{ mL}}{10 \text{ mg}} \times 5.5 \text{ mg} = 0.55 \text{ mL rounded to 0.6 mL}$$

  **b.** Equation is balanced. Only mL remain.

**4 a.** half of 0.2 mL = 0.1 mL

**b.** $mL = \dfrac{0.2\ mL}{\underset{2}{5000\ units}} \times \overset{1}{\cancel{2500\ units}} = \dfrac{0.2}{2} = 0.1\ mL$

**c.** Equation is balanced. Estimate supports answer.

**5 a.** 55 (110 ÷ 2)

$kg = \dfrac{1\ kg}{2.2\ \cancel{lb}} \times 110\ \cancel{lb} = \dfrac{110}{2.2} = 50\ kg$

**b.** Equation is balanced. Estimate supports answer.

**c.** 4000 units

$units = \dfrac{80\ units}{1\ \cancel{kg}} \times 50\ \cancel{kg} = 4000\ units$

**d.** Equation is balanced. Only units remain.

**e.** less than 1 mL

$mL = \dfrac{0.2\ mL}{\underset{5}{5000\ units}} \times \overset{4}{\cancel{4000\ units}} = \dfrac{0.8}{5} = 0.16\ mL$

**Comment:** Whether you give 0.16 or 0.2 mL depends on the calibration of the available syringe and agency and prescriber protocols.

**f.** Equation is balanced. Estimate supports answer.

## Chapter 12 Multiple-Choice Review

| | | | |
|---|---|---|---|
| **1** | 4 | **6** | 1 |
| **2** | 1 | **7** | 3 |
| **3** | 3 | **8** | 2 |
| **4** | 1 | **9** | 2 |
| **5** | 2 | **10** | 4 |

## Chapter 12 Comprehensive Final Practice

**1 a.** Lower it

**b.** Keep all the unused dosages (prescriptions) stored separately from the current dose strength.

**2 a.** 2000 units/ hr

$\dfrac{units}{hr} = \dfrac{\overset{100}{\cancel{25,000}}\ units}{\underset{1}{\cancel{250\ mL}}} \times \dfrac{20\ \cancel{mL}}{hr} = 2000\ units/\ hr$

**b.** The equation is balanced. The ordered units/ hr are being infused.

3  **a.** 1300 units/ hr

$$\frac{18 \text{ units}}{1 \text{ kg}} \times \frac{70 \text{ kg}}{1 \text{ hr}} = 1260 \text{ units/ hr rounded to } 1300 \text{ units/ hr}$$

   **b.** Equation is balanced. Only units/ hr remains.
   **c.** 26 mL/ hr

$$\frac{mL}{hr} = \frac{\overset{1}{\cancel{500}} \text{ mL}}{\underset{50}{\cancel{25,000 \text{ units}}}} \times 1300 \ \cancel{\text{units}} = 26 \text{ mL/ hr}$$

   **d.** Equation is balanced. Only mL/ hr remains.

4  **a.** IV rate is too slow and needs to be adjusted to 30 mL/ hr. Assess patient. Document. Check agency policy for IV rate adjustments.

$$\frac{mL}{hr} = \frac{\overset{1}{\cancel{500}} \text{ mL}}{\underset{\underset{1}{50}}{\cancel{25,000 \text{ units}}}} \times \frac{\overset{30}{\cancel{1500 \text{ units}}}}{1 \text{ hr}} = 30 \text{ mL/ hr}$$

   **b.** Equation is balanced. Only mL/ hr remain.

5  **a.** LMWH
   **b.** 0.3 mL

$$mL = \frac{0.4 \text{ mL}}{\underset{4}{\cancel{40 \text{ mg}}}} \times \overset{3}{\cancel{30 \text{ mg}}} = \frac{1.2}{4} = 0.3 \text{ mL}$$

   **c.** Equation is balanced. Only mL remain.

6  **a.** 25 mL/ hr

$$\frac{mL}{hr} = \frac{\overset{1}{\cancel{500}} \text{ mL}}{\underset{40}{\cancel{20,000 \text{ units}}}} \times \frac{1000 \ \cancel{\text{units}}}{hr} = \frac{1000}{40} = 25 \text{ mL/ hr}$$

   **b.** Equation is balanced. Only mL/ hr remains.
   **c.** The aPTT is too low at 40 seconds.
   **d.** 200 units increase/ hr

$$\frac{\text{units}}{hr} = \frac{3 \text{ units}}{1 \ \cancel{\text{kg}}} \times \frac{70 \ \cancel{\text{kg}}}{1 \text{ hr}} = 210 \text{ units/ hr increase needed}$$
$$\text{(rounded to 200 units increase/ hr)}$$

   **e.** Equation is balanced. Only units/ hr remains.
   **f.** 30 mL/ hr

$$\frac{mL}{hr} = \frac{\overset{1}{\cancel{500}} \text{ mL}}{\underset{\underset{1}{40}}{\cancel{20,000 \text{ units}}}} \times \frac{\overset{30}{\cancel{1200 \text{ units}}}}{hr} = 30 \text{ mL/ hr}$$

   **g.** Equation is balanced. Only mL/ hr remains. Flow rate needs to be increased to 30 mL/ hr.

7  **a.** No adjustment is needed.
   **b.** N/A

**8 a.** 2000 units/ hr

$$\text{units/ hr} = \frac{\overset{50}{\cancel{25{,}000}}\text{ units}}{\underset{1}{\cancel{500\text{ mL}}}} \times \frac{40\text{ }\cancel{\text{mL}}}{1\text{ hr}} = 2000\text{ units/ hr}$$

**b.** Equation is balanced. Only units/ hr remains.

**c.** No. 48,000 units for 24 hours (2000 units × 24) exceeds recommendations for up to 40,000 units/ 24 hr. Contact prescriber promptly about the order and document the response.

**9 a.** 24 mL/ hr

$$\frac{\text{mL}}{\text{hr}} = \frac{\overset{1}{\cancel{500}}\text{ mL}}{\underset{50}{\cancel{25{,}000}\text{ units}}} \times \frac{1200\text{ }\cancel{\text{units}}}{\text{hr}} = \frac{1200}{50} = 24\text{ mL/ hr}$$

**b.** Monitor for bleeding

**10 a.** "Delayed coagulation," "delayed clotted time," an effect of anticoagulants

**b.** It is a high-risk drug with potential for serious adverse effects of bleeding and hemorrhage. An infusion pump delivers a controlled rate.

# Chapter 13

## Rapid Practice 13-1

**1** Fractional

**2** SDR

**3** mg/ r kg

**4** mg/ kg; mcg/ kg; g/ kg, mg/ m$^2$; mcg/ m$^2$

**5** m$^2$

## Rapid Practice 13-2

**1** 1000 mcg = 1 mg

**2** Adult—once a day at bedtime; child—every 6 hours

**3** Child with postoperative pain: 0.04 mg/ kg/ hr; child with chronic cancer pain: 2.6 mg/ kg/ hr

**4** Neonate *less than* or equal to 7 days—10-15 mg/ kg/ day divided every 8-12 hours; neonate *over* 7 days of age—10-20 mg/ kg/ day divided every 6-12 hours.

**5** Contact prescriber.

1 **a.** 6 kg
 **b.** 5.5 kg

$$lb = \frac{1\ lb}{16\ \cancel{oz}} \times 3\ \cancel{oz} = \frac{3}{16} = 0.18 \text{ rounded to } 0.2\ lb$$

$$0.2\ lb + 12\ lb = 12.2\ lb$$

$$kg = \frac{1\ kg}{2.2\ \cancel{lb}} \times 12.2\ \cancel{lb} = 5.5\ kg$$

 **c.** Estimate supports answer. Equation is balanced.

2 **a.** $20 \div 2 = 10$ kg
 **b.** 9.3 kg

$$lb = \frac{1\ lb}{16\ \cancel{oz}} \times 6\ \cancel{oz} = 0.375 \text{ rounded to } 0.4\ lb$$

$$kg = \frac{1\ kg}{2.2\ \cancel{lb}} \times 20.4\ \cancel{lb} = 9.3\ kg$$

 **c.** Estimate supports answer. Equation is balanced.

3 **a.** $4 \div 2 = 2$ kg
 **b.** 2 kg

$$lb = \frac{1\ lb}{16\ \cancel{oz}} \times 8\ \cancel{oz} = 0.5\ lb$$

$$kg = \frac{1\ kg}{2.2\ \cancel{lb}} \times 4.5\ \cancel{lb} = 2.04 \text{ rounded to } 2\ kg$$

 **c.** Equation is balanced. Estimate supports answer.

4 **a.** $25 \div 2 = 12.5$ kg
 **b.** 11.6 kg

$$lb = \frac{1\ lb}{16\ \cancel{oz}} \times 9\ \cancel{oz} = \frac{9}{16} = 0.56\ lb \text{ rounded to } 0.6\ lb$$

$$kg = \frac{1\ kg}{2.2\ \cancel{lb}} \times 25.6\ \cancel{lb} = 11.63 \text{ rounded to } 11.6\ kg$$

 **c.** Equation is balanced. Estimate supports answer.

5 **a.** $18 \div 2 = 9$ kg
 **b.** 8.5 kg

$$lb = \frac{1\ lb}{16\ \cancel{oz}} \times 12\ \cancel{oz} = 0.75 \text{ rounded } 0.8\ lb$$

$$kg = \frac{1\ kg}{2.2\ \cancel{lb}} \times 18.8\ \cancel{lb} = 8.54 \text{ rounded to } 8.5\ kg$$

 **c.** Equation is balanced. Equation supports answer.

**1 a.** 66 lb = 30 kg; kg = $\dfrac{1 \text{ kg}}{2.2 \text{ lb}} \times 66 \text{ lb} = 30 \text{ kg}$

**b.** SDR: 300-600 mcg/ hr

mcg = $\dfrac{10 \text{ mcg}}{1 \text{ kg}} \times 30 \text{ kg} = 300 \text{ mcg/ hr low safe dose}$

mcg = $\dfrac{20 \text{ mcg}}{1 \text{ kg}} \times 30 \text{ kg} = 600 \text{ mcg/ hr high safe dose}$

**c.** Dose ordered 500 mcg/ hr is within SDR. Safe to give.

**2 a.** kg = $\dfrac{1 \text{ kg}}{2.2 \text{ lb}} \times 12 \text{ lb} = 5.45$ rounded to 5.5 kg

**Note:** kg are usually calculated to the nearest tenth.

**b.** SDR 1100-2750 mcg/ day

mcg = $\dfrac{200 \text{ mcg}}{1 \text{ kg}} \times 5.5 \text{ kg} = 1100 \text{ mcg/ day low safe dose}$

mcg = $\dfrac{500 \text{ mcg}}{1 \text{ kg}} \times 5.5 \text{ kg} = 2750 \text{ mcg/ day high safe dose}$

**c.** Hold and contact prescriber. Overdose.

**3 a.** SDR: 1-1.5 g in four divided doses
**b.** Ordered 250 mg × 4 = 1000 mg = 1 g/ day
**c.** Safe to give. Order is within SDR.

**4 a.** 22 ÷ 2 = 11 kg; 10 kg

kg = $\dfrac{1 \text{ kg}}{2.2 \text{ lb}} \times 22 \text{ lb} = 10 \text{ kg}$

**b.** SDR = 5000-8000 mcg per day in 4-6 divided doses

mcg = $\dfrac{500 \text{ mcg}}{1 \text{ kg}} \times 10 \text{ kg} = 5000 \text{ mcg low safe dose}$

mcg = $\dfrac{800 \text{ mcg}}{1 \text{ kg}} \times 10 \text{ kg} = 8000 \text{ mcg high safe dose}$

**c.** Safe to give (2 mg = 2000 mcg). Order is 2 mg four times a day (or 8000 mcg/ day).

**5 a.** 10 kg; 9.2 kg

lb = $\dfrac{1 \text{ lb}}{16 \text{ oz}} \times 4 \text{ oz} = 0.25$ rounded to 0.3 lb

kg = $\dfrac{1 \text{ kg}}{2.2 \text{ lb}} \times 20.3 \text{ lb} = \dfrac{20.3}{2.2} = 9.2 \text{ kg}$

**b.** SDR = 9.2-27.6 mg/ day.

SDR: mg = $\dfrac{3 \text{ mg}}{\text{kg}} \times 9.2 \text{ kg} = 27.6 \text{ mg/ day high safe dose}$

**c.** Hold and contact prescriber. Ordered dose exceeds SDR.

## Rapid Practice 13-5

**1 a.** $0.27 \text{ m}^2$

   **b.** units $= \dfrac{20{,}000 \text{ units}}{1 \, \cancel{\text{m}^2}} \times 0.27 \, \cancel{\text{m}^2} = 5400$ units every 24 hr

   **c.** Safe to give. The order is within in SDR ($5400 \div 24 = 225$ units/ hr).

**2 a.** $0.6 \text{ m}^2$

   **b.** 0.9-1.2 mg

     mg $= \dfrac{1.5 \text{ mg}}{1 \, \cancel{\text{m}^2}} \times 0.6 \, \cancel{\text{m}^2} = 0.9$ mg low safe dose once a week

     mg $= \dfrac{2 \text{ mg}}{1 \, \cancel{\text{m}^2}} \times 0.6 \, \cancel{\text{m}^2} = 1.2$ mg high safe dose once a week

   **c.** Safe to give. The order is within SDR.

**3 a.** $1.10 \text{ m}^2$

   **b.** mg $= \dfrac{3.3 \text{ mg}}{1 \, \cancel{\text{m}^2}} \times 1.10 \, \cancel{\text{m}^2} = 3.6$ mg safe daily dose

   **c.** Unsafe order. Overdose. Call prescriber promptly.

**4 a.** BSA is not needed. The SDR is not based on $\text{m}^2$ of BSA.

   **b.** 100-125 mg every 8 hr

     mg $= \dfrac{2 \text{ mg}}{1 \, \cancel{\text{kg}}} \times 50 \, \cancel{\text{kg}} = 100$ mg low safe dose q8h

     $\dfrac{2.5 \text{ mg}}{1 \, \cancel{\text{kg}}} \times 50 \, \cancel{\text{kg}} = 125$ mg high safe dose q8h

   **c.** Order is safe. It is within SDR.

**5 a.** B.S.A is not needed. The SDR is not based on $\text{m}^2$ of BSA.

   **b.** 5-25 mcg/ min

     mcg $= \dfrac{1 \text{ mcg}}{1 \, \cancel{\text{kg}}} \times 5 \, \cancel{\text{kg}} = 5$ mcg/ min low safe dose

     mcg $= \dfrac{5 \text{ mcg}}{\cancel{\text{kg}}} \times 5 \, \cancel{\text{kg}} = 25$ mcg/ min high safe dose

   **c.** Safe to give. The order is within SDR.

## Rapid Practice 13-6

**1 a.** 410-820 mg/ day.

     kg $= \dfrac{1 \text{ kg}}{2.2 \, \cancel{\text{lb}}} \times 36 \, \cancel{\text{lb}} = 16.36$ rounded to 16.4 kg

     mg $= \dfrac{25 \text{ mg}}{1 \, \cancel{\text{kg}}} \times 16.4 \, \cancel{\text{kg}} = 410$ mg low safe dose per day

     mg $= \dfrac{50 \text{ mg}}{1 \, \cancel{\text{kg}}} \times 16.4 \, \cancel{\text{kg}} = 820$ mg high safe dose per day

   **b.** Safe to give. Order is within SDR.

   **c.** mg $= \dfrac{125 \text{ mg}}{\underset{1}{\cancel{5 \text{ mL}}}} \times \overset{12}{\cancel{60 \text{ mL}}} = 1500$ mg

**d.** Add 36 mL in 2 portions; shake well after each addition.

**e.** 6 mL

$$\text{mL} = \dfrac{\overset{1}{\cancel{5}\ \text{mL}}}{\underset{1}{\cancel{\underset{25}{\cancel{125\ \text{mg}}}}}} \times \overset{6}{\cancel{150\ \text{mg}}} = 6\ \text{mL}$$

**2 a.** SDR $-\ \dfrac{10\ \text{mg}}{1\ \cancel{\text{m}^2}} \times 1.10\ \cancel{\text{m}^2} = 11\ \text{mg}$

**b.** Hold and clarify promptly. Ordered dose needs safe dose recommendation.

**c.** N/A

**d.** N/A

**3 a.** SDR = 15 mg/ kg/ day

44 lb ÷ 2.2 = 20 kg

$$\dfrac{\text{mg}}{\text{day}} = \dfrac{15\ \text{mg}}{1\ \cancel{\text{kg}}} \times \dfrac{20\ \cancel{\text{kg}}}{1\ \text{day}} = 300\ \text{mg/ day divided into two 150 mg doses}$$

**b.** Safe to give; within SDR.

**c.** Reconstitute with 55 mL of water in two portions. Shake after each addition.

**d.** 6 mL

$$\text{mL} - \dfrac{5\ \text{mL}}{\underset{5}{\cancel{125\ \text{mg}}}} \times \overset{6}{\cancel{150\ \text{mg}}} - \dfrac{30}{5} = 6\ \text{mL}$$

**4 a.** 0.12-0.24 mg/ day

$$\text{mg} = \dfrac{0.006\ \text{mg}}{1\ \cancel{\text{kg}}} \times 20\ \cancel{\text{kg}} = 0.12\ \text{mg low safe dose/ day}$$

$$\text{mg} = \dfrac{0.012\ \text{mg}}{1\ \cancel{\text{kg}}} \times 20\ \cancel{\text{kg}} = 0.24\ \text{mg high safe dose/ day}$$

**b.** Dose is safe; within safe dose range.

**c.** 2 mL (2 × 0.05 = 0.1 mg)

$$\text{mL} = \dfrac{1\ \text{mL}}{0.05\ \cancel{\text{mg}}} \times 0.1\ \cancel{\text{mg}} = \dfrac{0.1}{0.05} = 2\ \text{mL}$$

**d.** 50 mcg/ mL

**Note:** Microgram is abbreviated $\mu$g on the label. Use mcg in your written records.

**5 a.** 18.2 mg/ day

20 lb = 9.1 kg

$$\text{mg} = \dfrac{2\ \text{mg}}{1\ \cancel{\text{kg}}} \times 9.1\ \cancel{\text{kg}} = 18.2\ \text{mg/ day SDR}$$

**b.** Hold. Order exceeds amount: and frequency recommended.

**c.** N/A

## Rapid Practice 13-7

**1 a.** 0.2 mg

$$\text{mg} = \dfrac{0.01\ \text{mg}}{1\ \cancel{\text{kg}}} \times 22.9\ \cancel{\text{kg}} = 0.229\ \text{rounded to 0.2 mg}$$

**b.** Safe to give: within safe dose range.

**c.** 0.5 mL

$$mL = \frac{1\ mL}{0.1\ \cancel{mg}} \times 0.2\ \cancel{mg} = 0.5\ mL$$

**d.** Equation is balanced. Only mL remain.

**2 a.** SDR = 0.2 mg

$$kg = \frac{0.01\ mg}{1\ \cancel{kg}} \times 22.9\ \cancel{kg} = 0.22\ rounded\ to\ 0.2\ kg$$

**b.** Order is within SDR.

**c.** 0.5 mL

$$mL = \frac{mL}{0.4\ \cancel{mg}} \times 0.1\ \cancel{mg} = 0.5\ mL$$

**d.** Equations are balanced. Only kg and mL remain.

**3 a.** 2-4 units

**b.** Safe to give; within safe dose range.

**c.**

**d.** Yes. Bedtime snacks needed for long-acting, intermediate, and evening insulin administration to avoid hypoglycemic events during sleep.

**4 a.** 0.3-0.9 mg/ dose

$$kg = \frac{1\ kg}{2.2\ \cancel{lb}} \times 66\ \cancel{lb} = 30\ kg$$

$30 \times 0.01 = 0.3$ mg; $30 \times 0.03 = 0.9$ mg

**b.** Hold and clarify promptly with prescriber. Overdose ordered.

**c.** If the drug were safe to give, Adrenalin (upper label) 1:1000 is the correct concentration.

**d.** N/A

**e.** N/A

**5 a.** approximately 10 mg

$$kg = \frac{1\ kg}{2.2\ \cancel{lb}} \times 45\ \cancel{lb} = 20.4\ kg\ rounded\ to\ 20.5\ kg$$

$0.5 \times 20.5 = 10.25$ mg

**b.** Safe to give. At the maximum end of SDR, but within range.

**c.** 0.3 mL

$$mL = \frac{mL}{\overset{\displaystyle 30\ mg}{3}} \times \overset{1}{\cancel{10\ mg}} = 0.3\ mL$$

**d.** Equation is balanced. Only mL remain.

**e.** Grain (gr) is an apothecary unit of measurement.

## Rapid Practice 13-8

3 **a.** 20 − 10 = 10 mL

**b.** 10 mL

**c.** 40 mL/ hr

$$\frac{mL}{hr} = \frac{20\ mL}{\underset{1}{\cancel{30\ min}}} \times \frac{\overset{2}{\cancel{60\ min}}}{1\ hr} = 40\ mL/\ hr$$

**d.** Equation is balanced. Only mL/ hr remain.

3 **a.** 50 − 25 = 25 mL

**b.** 25 mL

**c.** 50 drops/ min (drops/ min = mL/ hr on a microdrip set)

4 **a.** 30 − 15 = 15 mL

**b.** 15 mL

**c.** 90 drops/ min

$$\frac{drops}{min} = \frac{\overset{3}{\cancel{60\ drops}}}{1\ \cancel{mL}} \times \frac{30\ \cancel{mL}}{\underset{1}{\cancel{20\ min}}} = 3 \times 30 = 90\ drops/\ min$$

**d.** Equation is balanced. Only drops/ min remains.

5 **a.** 3 mL

**b.** 30 drops/ min

$$\frac{drops}{min} = \frac{\overset{2}{\cancel{60\ drops}}}{1\ \cancel{mL}} \times \frac{15\ \cancel{mL}}{\underset{1}{\cancel{30\ min}}} = 30\ drops/\ min$$

**c.** Only drops/ min remain to be infused when the minutes are less than 1 hr; mL will not equal drops per minute.

## Rapid Practice 13-9

1 **a.** 5 mcg × 60 min = 300 mcg/ hr

**b.** 10 mg = 10,000 mcg (1000 mcg = 1 mg)

**c.** 40 mcg/ mL

$$\frac{mcg}{mL} = \frac{10,000\ mcg}{250\ mL} = 40\ mcg/\ mL$$

**d.** Equation is balanced. Only mcg/ mL remains.

**e.** 8 mL/ hr

$$\frac{mL}{hr} = \frac{\overset{1}{\cancel{250}}\ mL}{\underset{1}{\cancel{10\ mg}}} \times \frac{1\ \cancel{mg}}{\underset{4}{\cancel{1000\ mcg}}} \times \frac{5\ \cancel{mcg}}{1\ \cancel{min}} \times \frac{\overset{6}{\cancel{60\ min}}}{1\ hr} = \frac{15}{2} = 7.5\ \text{rounded to 8 mL/ hr}$$

**f.** Equation is balanced. Only mL/ hr remains.

**2 a.** 16 mL (8 mL × 2 hr)

**b.** 12 mL/ hr

$$\frac{mL}{hr} = \frac{\overset{1}{\cancel{250}} \, mL}{\underset{1}{\cancel{10} \, \cancel{mg}}} \times \frac{1 \, \cancel{mg}}{\underset{4}{\cancel{1000} \, \cancel{mcg}}} \times \frac{\overset{2}{\cancel{8} \, \cancel{mcg}}}{1 \, \cancel{min}} \times \frac{\overset{6}{\cancel{60} \, \cancel{min}}}{1 \, hr} = 12 \, mL/ \, hr$$

**c.** Equation is balanced. Only mL/ hr remain.

**Comment:** It should be estimated that the flow rate would be increased from 8 mL/ hr in problem #1, but not doubled.

**3 a.** SDR: 4.5-18 mg/ dose (0.5 × 9)(2 × 9)

**b.** Hold and contact prescriber immediately. Dose ordered is 7 mg above the SDR.

**c.** N/A

**d.** N/A

**4 a.** SDR:

$$\frac{3 \, mEq}{1 \, \cancel{kg}} \times 8 \, \cancel{kg} = 24 \, mEq \text{ q24h for this baby}$$

**b.** $mEq = \dfrac{0.1 \, mEq}{1 \, \cancel{kg}} \times 8 \, \cancel{kg} \times 24 \, hr = 19.2 \, mEq/ \, 24 \, hr$ ordered

**c.** Order is within SDR.

**d.** 8 mL/ hr

$$\frac{mL}{hr} = \frac{\overset{10}{\cancel{100}} \, mL}{\underset{1}{\cancel{10} \, \cancel{mEq}}} \times \frac{0.1 \, \cancel{mEq}}{1 \, \cancel{kg}} \times \frac{8 \, \cancel{kg}}{1 \, hr} = 8 \, mL/ \, hr$$

**e.** Equation is balanced. Only mL/ hr remains.

**5 a.** 6.6 kg $\left( \dfrac{1 \, kg}{2.2 \, \cancel{lb}} \times 14.5 \, \cancel{lb} = 6.6 \, kg \right)$

**Comment:** Remember to change oz (8) to lb (0.5) before solving equation.

**b.** SDR: 6.6-9.8 mg (1 × 6.6)(3 × 6.6)

**c.** Hold and clarify promptly with prescriber. Ordered dose exceeds SDR.

**d.** N/A

**e.** N/A

## Chapter 13 Multiple-Choice Review

| | |
|---|---|
| **1** 4 | **6** 1 |
| **2** 3 | **7** 2 |
| **3** 2 | **8** 4 |
| **4** 3 | **9** 2 |
| **5** 1 (Check agency polices.) | **10** 2 |

## Chapter 13 Final Practice

**1 a.** 5 mL (1 teaspoon)

**b.** popsicle

**2 a.** 20 × 30 = 600 mg/ day divided in 2 doses

**b.** Safe to give. It is within SDR.

**c.** $mL = \dfrac{\overset{1}{\cancel{5}} \text{ mL}}{\underset{\underset{1}{50}}{\cancel{250} \text{ mg}}} \times \overset{12}{\cancel{600} \text{ mg}} = 12 \text{ mL}$

**d.** Equation is balanced. Only mL remain.

**3 a.** $100 \times 0.6 = 60 \text{ mg/ day}$

**b.** Hold and clarify promptly with prescriber. Order is greater than SDR
**c.** N/A
**d.** N/A

**4 a.** 5 mL

$mL = \dfrac{1 \text{ mL}}{\underset{2}{\cancel{100,000} \text{ units}}} \times \overset{5}{\cancel{250,000} \text{ units}} = 2.5 \text{ mL total dose}$

**b.** Order is safe.
**c.** Needleless syringe or calibrated dropper
**d.** Place 1.25 mL on each side in the mouth of the child.

**5 a.** Label B, infant preparation; enclosed dropper
**b.** 32 mg/ mL (160 mg/ 5 mL); measuring cup
**c.** 80 mg/ 0.8 mL
**d.** The Infant preparation is much more concentrated. This reduces the volume of mL for the infant.

**6 a.** 20 mg every 4 to 6 hours
1 kg = 40 mg

$mg = \dfrac{0.5 \text{ mg}}{1 \text{ \cancel{kg}}} \times 40 \text{ \cancel{kg}} = 20 \text{ mg SDR per dose q4-6h}$

**b.** Safe to give; within SDR.
**c.** Will give less than 1 mL.
**d.** 0.66 mL

$mL = \dfrac{1 \text{ mL}}{\underset{3}{\cancel{30} \text{ mg}}} \times \overset{2}{\cancel{20} \text{ mg}} = 0.66 \text{ mL}$

**e.** Equation is balanced. Estimate supports answer.

**7 a.** $kg = \dfrac{1 \text{ kg}}{2.2 \text{ \cancel{lb}}} \times 42 \text{ \cancel{lb}} = 19.1 \text{ kg}$

**b.** 9.6-19.1 mEq/ hr

$mEq = \dfrac{0.5 \text{ mEq}}{1 \text{ \cancel{kg}}} \times 19.1 \text{ \cancel{kg}} = 9.55 \rightarrow 9.6 \text{ mEq/ hr low safe dose}$

$mEq = \dfrac{1 \text{ mEq}}{1 \text{ \cancel{kg}}} \times 19.1 \text{ \cancel{kg}} = 19.1 \text{ mEq/ hr high safe dose}$

**c.** 10 mEq/ hr
**d.** Safe to give; 10 mEq/ hr is within SDR.

**e.** 63 mL/ hr

$$\text{mL/ hr} = \frac{250 \text{ mL}}{40 \text{ mEq}} \times 10 \text{ mEq} = 62.5 \rightarrow 63 \text{ mL/ hr}$$

A volume control device would be used with 1 hour's worth of ordered mL/ hr at a time.

**f.** Equation is balanced. Only mL/ hr remain.

**8**  **a.** $\text{kg} = \dfrac{1 \text{ kg}}{2.2 \text{ lb}} \times 44 \text{ lb} = 20 \text{ kg}$

**b.** 0.2-0.6 mg (200-600 mcg)

**c.** 500 mcg

**d.** Safe to give; within SDR.

**e.** more than 1 mL

**f.** 1.3 mL

$$\text{mL} = \frac{\text{mL}}{\underset{4}{400 \text{ mcg}}} \times \overset{5}{500 \text{ mcg}} = 1.25 \text{ mL} \rightarrow 1.3 \text{ mL}$$

**g.** Equation is balanced. Only mL remain.

**9**  **a.** 33 kg (77 ÷ 2); 35 kg

**b.** SDR: $\dfrac{40 \text{ mg}}{1 \text{ kg}} \times 35 \text{ kg} = 1400 \text{ mg/ day}$

**c.** Hold medication and contact prescriber promptly. Order exceeds SDR for this child's weight. Order was 1500 mg bid or 3000 mg/ 24 hr.

**10**  **a.** 11.1 kg

24 lb 6 oz = 24.4 lb

6 oz ÷ 16 = 0.38 → 0.4 lb

$\text{kg} = \dfrac{1 \text{ kg}}{2.2 \text{ lb}} \times 24.4 \text{ lb} = 11.09 \rightarrow 11.1 \text{ kg}$

**b.** 0.2-3.9 mg

11.1 × 0.015 = 0.16 mg → 0.2 mg low safe dose

11.1 × 0.35 = 3.88 mg → 3.9 mg high safe dose

**c.** 0.5 mg

**d.** Safe to give. Ordered dose is within SDR.

**e.** The ordered mg, 0.5 mg, and the unit dose, 0.5 mg, are equal. You would give the unit dose.

**f.** 2 mL (0.5 mg = 500 mcg)

## Multiple-Choice Final Review

| | | | | |
|---|---|---|---|---|
| **1** | 3 | | **8** | 3 |
| **2** | 4 | | **9** | 3 |
| **3** | 2 | | **10** | 2 |
| **4** | 4 | | **11** | 3 |
| **5** | 3 | | **12** | 1 |
| **6** | 4 | | **13** | 2 |
| **7** | 3 | | **14** | 4 |

604 • ANSWER KEYS

| 15 | 2 | 26 | 4 |
|----|---|----|---|
| 16 | 4 | 27 | 4 |
| 17 | 2 | 28 | 2 |
| 18 | 1 | 29 | 1 |
| 19 | 4 | 30 | 4 |
| 20 | 1 | 31 | 3 |
| 21 | 3 | 32 | 2 |
| 22 | 3 | 33 | 2 |
| 23 | 4 | 34 | 3 |
| 24 | 1 | 35 | 3 |
| 25 | 3 |    |   |

# Comprehensive Final Review

**1 a.** 2 tabs ($0.5 \times 2 = 1$ mg)

$$\text{tab} = \frac{1 \text{ tab}}{0.5 \text{ mg}} \times 1 \text{ mg} = \frac{1}{0.5} = 2 \text{ tabs}$$

  **b.** Estimate supports answer.

**2 a.** 2 tabs ($0.25 \times 2 = 0.50$)

$$\text{tab} = \frac{1 \text{ tab}}{\underset{1}{0.25 \text{ mg}}} \times \overset{2}{0.5 \text{ mg}} = 2 \text{ tabs}$$

  **b.** Estimate supports answer.

**3 a.** 2 tabs ($0.125 \times 2 = 0.25$ mg $= 250$ mcg)

$$\text{tab} = \frac{1 \text{ tab}}{\underset{1}{125 \text{ mcg}}} \times \overset{2}{250 \text{ mcg}} = 2 \text{ tabs}$$

  **b.** Estimate supports answer.
  **c.** digoxin

**4 a.** 2 tabs

$$\text{tab} = \frac{1 \text{ tab}}{\underset{3}{750 \text{ mg}}} \times \frac{\overset{4}{1000 \text{ mg}}}{1 \text{ g}} \times 1.5 \text{ g} = \frac{6}{3} = 2 \text{ tabs}$$

  **b.** Estimate supports answer.
  **c.** ciprofloxacin hydrochloride

**5 a.** 2 tabs

$$\text{tab} = \frac{1 \text{ tab}}{\underset{1}{0.25 \text{ mg}}} \times \overset{2}{0.5 \text{ mg}} = 2 \text{ tab}$$

  **b.** Estimate supports answer.

**6** Label B, Cardizem SR

   **a.** 2 tabs

$$\text{tab} = \frac{1 \text{ tab}}{60 \text{ mg}} \times \frac{1000 \text{ mg}}{1 \text{ g}} \times 0.12 \text{ g} = \frac{120}{60} = 2 \text{ tabs}$$

   **b.** Equation is balanced. Answer = estimate.

**7** **a.** $\frac{1}{2}$ of 40 = 20; $\frac{1}{2}$ of 15 mL = 7.5 mL

$$\text{mL} = \frac{15 \text{ mL}}{\underset{2}{40 \text{ mEq}}} \times \overset{1}{20 \text{ mEq}} = \frac{15}{2} = 7.5 \text{ mL}$$

   **b.** Estimate supports answer.

**8** **a.** 15 mg/tab
   **b.** gr $\frac{1}{4}$/tab
   **c.** 45 ÷ 15 = 3 tabs

   **d.** $\text{tab} = \frac{1 \text{ tab}}{\underset{1}{15 \text{ mg}}} \times \overset{3}{45 \text{ mg}} = 3 \text{ tab}$

   **e.** Estimate supports answer.

**9** **a.** 1.5 g = 1500 mg ÷ 500 mg = 3 tabs

$$\text{tab} = \frac{1 \text{ tab}}{\underset{1}{500 \text{ mg}}} \times \frac{\overset{2}{1000 \text{ mg}}}{1 \text{ g}} \times 1.5 \text{ g} = 3 \text{ tabs}$$

   **b.** Estimate supports answer.

**10** **a.** 100 mcg ÷ 50 mcg = 2 tabs

$$\text{tab} = \frac{1 \text{ tab}}{\underset{1}{50 \text{ mcg}}} \times \frac{\overset{20}{1000 \text{ mcg}}}{1 \text{ mg}} \times 0.1 \text{ mg} = 20 \times 0.1 = 2 \text{ tab}$$

   **b.** Estimate supports answer.
   **c.** 0.1 mg = 100 mcg

**11 a.** Give less than 1 mL.

$$mL = \frac{1\ mL}{\underset{3}{\cancel{15\ mg}}} \times \overset{2}{\cancel{10\ mg}} = 0.67 \rightarrow 0.7\ mL$$

**b.** Estimate supports answer.

**12 a.** Give less than 4 mL, about one quarter less.

$$mL = \frac{4\ mL}{\underset{4}{\cancel{40\ mg}}} \times \overset{3}{\cancel{30\ mg}} = \frac{12}{4} = 3\ mL$$

**b.** Estimate supports answer.

**13 a.** Give less than 2 mL.

$$mL = \frac{2\ mL}{0.5\ \cancel{mg}} \times 0.3\ \cancel{mg} = \frac{0.6}{0.5} = 1.2\ mL$$

**b.** Estimate supports answer.

**14 a.** about 0.5 mL.

$$mL = \frac{1\ mL}{\underset{2}{\cancel{4\ mg}}} \times \overset{1}{\cancel{2\ mg}} = \frac{1}{2} = 0.5\ mL$$

**b.** Estimate supports answer
**c.** 0.5 mL
**d.** half of 5 mg (or 0.5 mL)

$$mL = \frac{1\ mL}{\underset{2}{\cancel{5\ mg}}} \times \overset{1}{\cancel{2.5\ mg}} = 0.5\ mL$$

**e.** Estimate supports answer.

**f.** $0.5 + 0.5 = 1$ mL

**15 a.** Will give slightly more than 1 mL

$$mL = \frac{1\ mL}{\underset{3}{300{,}000\ units}} \times \overset{4}{400{,}000\ units} = \frac{4}{3} = 1.3\ mL$$

**b.** Estimate supports answer.

**16 a.** Concentration after dilution is 1 g/ 2.6 mL.

**b.** Give less than 2.6 mL.

$$mL = \frac{2.6\ mL}{1\ g} \times \frac{1\ g}{\underset{5}{1000\ mg}} \times \overset{3}{600\ mg} = \frac{7.8}{5} = 1.56\ rounded\ to\ 1.6\ mL$$

**c.** Estimate supports answer.

**17** 2 units Novolin Regular insulin

**a.**

**b.** fast acting
**c.** lower

**18** Humulin R, the fast-acting clear insulin

**19**

**a.** long acting (up to 24 hours)
**b.** A 50-unit syringe permits easier visualization and more accurate measurement of insulin doses of 50 units or less.

**20** 2.5 mL/ hr

$$\frac{mL}{hr} = \frac{500 \text{ mL}}{\cancel{20,000}\text{ units}} \times \frac{\overset{1}{\cancel{1000}\text{ units}}}{1 \text{ hr}} = \frac{500}{20} = 2.5 \text{ mL/ hr}$$

**a.** Equation is balanced. Only mL/ hr remains.
**b.** The aPTT must be monitored.

**21** 1200 units/ hr

$$\frac{units}{hr} = \frac{\overset{40}{\cancel{10,000}}\text{ units}}{\underset{1}{\cancel{250}\text{ mL}}} \times \frac{30 \cancel{\text{ mL}}}{1 \text{ hr}} = 1200 \text{ units/ hr}$$

**a.** Equation is balanced. Only units/ hr remains.
**b.** hemorrhage

**22 a.** 7 units/ hr (100 units/ 100 mL is a 1:1 solution)

$$\frac{units}{hr} = \frac{\overset{1}{\cancel{100}}\text{ units}}{\underset{1}{\cancel{100}\text{ mL}}} \times \frac{7 \cancel{\text{ mL}}}{hr} = 7 \text{ units/ hr}$$

**b.** Equation is balanced. Only mL/ hr remains.
**c.** hypoglycemia

**23** 125 mL/ hr

$$\frac{mL}{hr} = \frac{\overset{125}{\cancel{500}}\text{ mL}}{\underset{\underset{1}{4}}{\cancel{40}\text{ mEq}}} \text{ KCl} \times \frac{\overset{1}{\cancel{10}\text{ mEq}}}{1 \text{ hr}} = 125 \text{ ml/ hr}$$

**a.** Equation is balanced. Only mL/ hr remains.
**b.** 1300 + 4 hr = 1700 hr. At 1700 the nurse needs to recheck serum K level.

$$hr = \frac{1 \text{ hr}}{10 \cancel{\text{ mEq}}} \times 40 \cancel{\text{ mEq}} = 4 \text{ hr}$$

**24 a.** 100 mL/ hr (30 min × 2 = 60 min; 50 × 2 = 100 mL/ hr)

$$\frac{mL}{hr} = \frac{50 \text{ mL}}{\underset{1}{\cancel{30}\text{ min}}} \times \frac{\overset{2}{\cancel{60}\text{ min}}}{1 \text{ hr}} = 100 \text{ mL/ hr}$$

**b.** Equation is balanced. Estimate supports answer.

**25 a.** 90 mL/ hr

$$\frac{mL}{hr} = \frac{30 \text{ mL}}{\underset{1}{\cancel{20}\text{ min}}} \times \frac{\overset{3}{\cancel{60}\text{ min}}}{1 \text{ hr}} = 90 \text{ mL/ hr}$$

**b.** Estimate supports answer.

**26** pediatric (microdrip) set

    **a.** 20 drops/ min with a DF60 set

    **b.** 20 drops/ min

$$\frac{\text{drops}}{\text{min}} = \frac{\overset{1}{\cancel{60}}\text{ drops}}{1\text{ }\cancel{mL}} \times \frac{20\text{ }\cancel{mL}}{\underset{1}{\cancel{60}}\text{ min}} = 20\text{ drops/ min}$$

    **c.** Estimate supports answer.

**27** 31 drops/ min

$$\frac{\text{drops}}{\text{min}} = \frac{\overset{1}{\cancel{15}}\text{ drops}}{1\text{ }\cancel{mL}} \times \frac{\overset{125}{\cancel{500}\text{ }\cancel{mL}}}{\underset{1}{\cancel{4}\text{ hr}}} \times \frac{1\text{ }\cancel{hr}}{\underset{4}{\cancel{60}}\text{ min}} = \frac{125}{4} = 31.25 \rightarrow 31\text{ drops/ min}$$

    **a.** Equation is balanced. Only drops/ min remains.

**28** 20 mL

    **a.** 40 mL/ hr

$$mL = \frac{20\text{ mL}}{\underset{1}{\cancel{30}\text{ min}}} \times \frac{\overset{2}{\cancel{60}\text{ min}}}{1\text{ hr}} = 40\text{ mL/ hr}$$

    **b.** The volume control device must be flushed with a compatible solution according to agency policies and manufacturer's recommendations.

**29** 150 g Dextrose

$$g = \frac{15\text{ g}}{\underset{1}{\cancel{100}\text{ mL}}} \times \overset{10}{\cancel{1000}\text{ mL}} = 150\text{ g of Dextrose}$$

    **a.** Equation is balanced. Only grams remain.

    **b.** 600 kcal CHO

$$kcal = \frac{4\text{ kcal}}{1\text{ }\cancel{g}} \times 150\text{ }\cancel{g} = 600\text{ kcal CHO}$$

    **c.** Equation is balanced. Only kcal remain.

    **d.** 42.5 g amino acids

$$g = \frac{4.25\text{ g}}{\underset{1}{\cancel{100}\text{ mL}}} \times \overset{10}{\cancel{1000}\text{ mL}} = 42.5\text{ g of amino acids}$$

    **e.** Equation is balanced. Only amino acids remain.

    **f.** $kcal = \dfrac{4\text{ kcal}}{1\text{ }\cancel{g}} \times 42.5\text{ }\cancel{g} = 170\text{ kcal amino acids}$

    **g.** Equation is balanced. Only kcal remain.

**30** 40 g lipids

$$g = \frac{20\text{ g}}{\underset{1}{\cancel{100}\text{ mL}}} \times \overset{2}{\cancel{200}\text{ mL}} = 40\text{ g lipids}$$

    **a.** Equation is balanced. Only grams remain.

**b.** 360 Kcal lipids

$$\text{Kcal} = \frac{9 \text{ Kcal}}{1 \text{ g}} \times 40 \text{ g} = 360 \text{ Kcal lipids}$$

**c.** Equation is balanced. Only Kcal remain.

**31** 12 mL/ hr

$$\frac{\text{mL}}{\text{hr}} = \frac{\overset{1}{\cancel{500}} \text{ mL}}{5 \text{ } \cancel{\text{units}}} \times \frac{1 \text{ } \cancel{\text{unit}}}{\underset{\underset{1}{2}}{1000 \text{ milliunits}}} \times \frac{\overset{1}{\cancel{2} \text{ } \cancel{\text{milliunits}}}}{1 \text{ } \cancel{\text{min}}} \times \frac{60 \text{ } \cancel{\text{min}}}{1 \text{ hr}} = 12 \text{ mL/ hr}$$

**a.** Equation is balanced. Only mL/ hr remains.

**32** 77 kg (154 lb ÷ 2)

**a.** 70 kg

$$\frac{1 \text{ kg}}{2.2 \text{ } \cancel{\text{lb}}} \times 154 \text{ } \cancel{\text{lb}} = 70 \text{ kg}$$

**b.** Only kg remain. Estimate supports answer.

**c.** $\dfrac{\text{mcg}}{\text{min}} = \dfrac{3 \text{ mcg}}{1 \text{ } \cancel{\text{kg}}} \times 70 \text{ } \cancel{\text{kg}} = 210 \text{ mcg/ min}$

**d.** $\dfrac{\text{mg}}{\text{min}} = 0.21 \text{ mg/ min } (210 \div 1000)$

**e.** $\dfrac{\text{mL}}{\text{hr}} = \dfrac{\overset{2}{\cancel{500}} \text{ mL}}{\underset{1}{\cancel{250} \text{ mg}}} \times \dfrac{1 \text{ } \cancel{\text{mg}}}{1000 \text{ } \cancel{\text{mcg}}} \times \dfrac{210 \text{ } \cancel{\text{mcg}}}{1 \text{ } \cancel{\text{min}}} \times \dfrac{60 \text{ } \cancel{\text{min}}}{1 \text{ hr}} = \dfrac{25200}{1000} = 25.2 \rightarrow 25 \text{ mL/ hr}$

**f.** Equation is balanced. Only mL/ hr remains.

**33 a.** 2 mL (5 mg × 2 = 10 mg)

$$\text{mL} = \frac{1 \text{ mL}}{\underset{1}{\cancel{5} \text{ mg}}} \times \overset{2}{\cancel{10} \text{ mg}} = 2 \text{ mL}$$

**b.** Equation is balanced. Only mL remain.

**c.** $\dfrac{\text{mL}}{\text{min}} = \dfrac{\overset{1}{\cancel{2}} \text{ mL}}{\underset{\underset{1}{2}}{\cancel{10} \text{ mg}}} \times \dfrac{\overset{1}{\cancel{5} \text{ mg}}}{1 \text{ min}} = 1 \text{ mL/ min}$

**d.** Equation is balanced. Only mL/ min remains.

**e.** Total minutes = 2 $\left( \dfrac{1 \text{ min}}{\underset{1}{\cancel{5} \text{ mg}}} \times \overset{2}{\cancel{10} \text{ mg}} = 2 \text{ min} \right)$

Total seconds = 120 $\left( \dfrac{60 \text{ sec}}{1 \text{ } \cancel{\text{min}}} \times 2 \text{ } \cancel{\text{min}} = 120 \text{ sec} \right)$

**f.** seconds/ calibration = $\dfrac{120 \text{ sec}}{20 \text{ calibrations}} = 6 \text{ sec/ calibration}$

**34** 175 mg/ day

$$mg = \frac{250 \text{ mg}}{1 \text{ m}^2} \times 0.7 \text{ m}^2 = 175 \text{ mg/ day safe dose}$$

**a.** Equation is balanced. Only mg remain.

**b.** 7 mL

$$mL = \frac{5 \text{ mL}}{\underset{5}{125 \text{ mg}}} \times \overset{7}{175 \text{ mg}} = \frac{35}{5} = 7 \text{ mL}$$

**c.** Equation is balanced. Only mL remain.

**35 a.** 44 lb ÷ 2 = 22 kg

**b.** 20 kg

$$kg = \frac{1 \text{ kg}}{\underset{1}{2.2 \text{ lb}}} \times \overset{20}{44 \text{ lb}} = 20 \text{ kg}$$

**c.** Estimate supports answer.

**d.** $\dfrac{mg}{day} = \dfrac{40 \text{ mg}}{1 \text{ kg}} \times \dfrac{20 \text{ kg}}{1 \text{ day}} = 800 \text{ mg/ day in 2 divided doses (400 mg/ dose)}$

**e.** The dose ordered is double the SDR for a child with otitis media. Hold and contact the prescriber promptly. Document the communication.

**f.** N/A

**g.** N/A

**h.** N/A

# INDEX

Page numbers followed by b indicate boxed material; f indicates figures; t, tables.

## A

**613**

## Metric Equivalents

| Weight | Volume |
|---|---|
| 1000 mcg (microgram) = 1 mg (milligram) | 1000 mL = 1 Liter |
| 1000 mg = 1 g (gram) | |
| 1000 g = 1 kg (kilogram) | |
| **lb to kg conversion** | |
| 2.2 lb = 1 kg | |

## Metric-Apothecary Conversion Clock

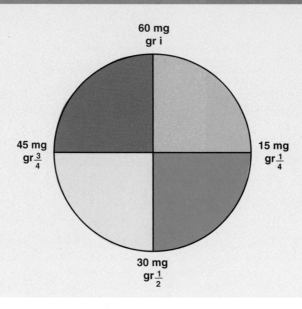

## Metric, Household, and Apothecary Liquid Equivalents*

| Metric | Household | Apothecary |
|---|---|---|
| 1 mL | | 15-16 minims* |
| 5 mL | 1 teaspoon (tsp) | 1 dram* |
| 15 mL | 1 tablespoon (tbs) | 4 drams* (oz ss) |
| | (½ ounce) (oz) | |
| 30 mL | 2 tablespoons (1 oz) | 8 drams (oz i) |
| 240 mL | 1 measuring cup (8 oz) | 8 oz (oz viii) |
| 500 mL | 1 pint (pt) (16 oz) | 1 pint (16 oz) |
| 1000 mL (1 liter ) | 1 quart (qt) (32 oz) | 1 quart (32 oz) |
| 4 liters | 1 gallon (gal) (4 quarts) | 1 gallon (4 quarts) |

Note: These equivalents are approximate.

*Minims and drams are no longer used in medication orders in the United States.